Compressed Video
over Networks

Signal Processing and Communications

Compressed Video
over Networks

edited by

Ming-Ting Sun
University of Washington
Seattle, Washington

Amy R. Reibman
AT&T Labs–Research
Red Bank, New Jersey

MARCEL DEKKER, INC.   NEW YORK · BASEL

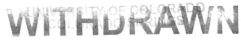
ISBN: 0-8247-9423-0

This book is printed on acid-free paper.

Headquarters
Marcel Dekker, Inc.
270 Madison Avenue, New York, NY 10016
tel. 212-696-9000; fax: 212-685-4540

Eastern Hemisphere Distribution
Marcel Dekker AG
Hutgasse 4, Postfach 812, CH-4001 Basel, Switzerland
tel: 41-61-261-8482; fax: 41-61-261-8896

World Wide Web
http://www.dekker.com
The publisher offers discounts on this book when ordered in bulk quantities. For more information, write to Special Sales/Professional Marketing at the headquarters address above.

Current printing (last digit):
10 9 8 7 6 5 4 3 2 1

PRINTED IN THE UNITED STATES OF AMERICA

Preface

Networked digital video applications are becoming more and more important in our everyday life. Videophone, video conferencing, video e-mail, video streaming, digital TV, high-definition TV (HDTV), video on demand (VoD), distance learning, remote collaboration, and surveillance are just some examples. In these applications, the digital video has to be compressed. Without compression, even a relatively low-quality digital color video with 352×288-pixel resolution, 15 frames/s, and 12 bits/pixel for videophone applications, will require about 18 Mbit/s. For digital TV, it will require more than 100 Mbit/s. With these high rates, it is not possible to have cost-effective video applications. In practical applications, digital video is compressed to lower bit rates down to a few tens of kilobits per second for videophone applications) so that it can be transported over wireless asynchronous transfer mode (ATM) networks, and networks based on, for example, public switched telephone network (PSTN), integrated service digital network (ISDN), asynchronous digital subscriber line (ADSL), cable and internet protocol (IP) service.

Compressed video, which uses the predictive coding algorithm and variable-length coding, is sensitive to network impairments, and transmission errors can cause error propagation. A single bit error can cause substantial degradation if no action is taken to stop or limit the extent of error propagation. Real-time two-way video communication applications are also sensitive to transport delay and delay variation. A packet of compressed video data arriving too late at the decoder will be useless if the decoding time of these data has passed. Since networks usually introduce various kinds of transmission impairment, providing high-quality, low-cost, ubiquitous compressed video applications is a tough technical challenge.

Compressed video signals are often transported over a heterogeneous network. Different networks have different characteristics. Some networks have constant bit rate while others have variable bit rate. Some networks are symmetrical (upstream bit rate is the same as the downstream bit rate) while others are asymmetrical. Some networks can guarantee quality of service while others cannot. Different networks can vary greatly in their different transmission performance in terms of bit rates, error rates, delay, and delay variation. All such factors impact the transport of the compressed video over the networks. To have an optimal end-to-end system, an overall understanding of the compressed video and the networks is essential.

This book is divided into four parts. Part 1 covers compressed video fundamentals and standards with focus on the aspects that are related to networking. Its two chapters focus on the H-series and MPEG video coding standards. Part 2 reviews the fundamentals of three different important networks: IP-based, wireless, and ATM networks, and focuses on aspects that impact the transport of compressed video. Part 3 focuses on issues and techniques related to the transport of compressed video over generic networks. Its chapters treat error concealment, layered coding, error resilience coding, variable bit rate coding, and the use of feedback of rate and loss information. These techniques are useful for achieving better end-to-end video quality. Part 4 covers the transport of compressed video over specific networks, including the Internet and wireless networks, and also presents some systems issues and standards.

We thank all the contributors to this book. It has been quite an enjoyable experience working with them. We also thank many reviewers for providing valuable comments and suggestions. We thank, as well, Mr. Jeongnam Youn for help during the development of this book. Finally, we thank Mr. B. J. Clark and Ms. Ann Pulido of Marcel Dekker, Inc. for their support in publishing this book.

Ming-Ting Sun
Amy R. Reibman

Contents

Contributors

Arthur W. Berger*   *Lucent Technologies, Holmdel, New Jersey*

Li Fung Chang   *AT&T Labs–Research, Red Bank, New Jersey*

Tsuhan Chen   *Department of Electrical and Computer Engineering, Carnegie Mellon University, Pittsburgh, Pennsylvania*

M. Reha Civanlar   *AT&T Labs–Research, Red Bank, New Jersey*

Guy Cote   *Department of Electrical Engineering, University of British Columbia, Vancouver, British Columbia, Canada*

N. G. Duffield   *AT&T Labs–Research, Florham Park, New Jersey*

Nikolaus Färber   *Telecommunications Laboratory, University of Erlangen–Nuremberg, Erlangen, Germany*

Mohammed Ghanbari   *Department of Electronic Systems Engineering, University of Essex, Colchester, England*

Bernd Girod   *Department of Electrical Engineering, Stanford University, Stanford, California*

Faouzi Kossentini   *Department of Electrical Engineering, University of British Columbia, Vancouver, British Columbia, Canada*

Sakae Okubo   *Waseda Research Center, Telecommunications Advancement Organization of Japan, Tokyo, Japan*

**Current affiliation:* Akamai Technologies, Cambridge, Massachusetts

Antonio Ortega   *Department of Electrical Engineering–Systems, University of Southern California, Los Angeles, California*

K. K. Ramakrishnan   *AT&T Labs–Research, Florham Park, New Jersey*

Henning Schulzrinne   *Department of Computer Science and Department of Electrical Engineering, Columbia University, New York, New York*

Thomas Sikora   *Department of Interactive Media–Human Factors, Heinrich-Hertz Institute for Communication Technology, Berlin, Germany*

Deepak Turaga   *Department of Electrical and Computer Engineering, Carnegie Mellon University, Pittsburgh, Pennsylvania*

Yao Wang   *Department of Electrical Engineering, Polytechnic University, Brooklyn, New York*

Stephan Wenger   *Technische Universitat Berlin, Berlin, Germany*

Qin-Fan Zhu   *Department of Engineering, Convergent Networks, Inc., Lowell, Massachusetts*

Part 1
Video

1
Fundamentals of Video Compression: H.263 as an Example

Deepak Turaga and Tsuhan Chen
Department of Electrical and Computer Engineering,
Carnegie Mellon University, Pittsburgh, Pennsylvania

1.1 INTRODUCTION

Standards define a common language that different parties can use, so that they can communicate with one another. Standards are thus a prerequisite to effective communication. Video coding standards define the bitstream syntax, the language that the encoder and the decoder use to communicate. Besides defining the bitstream syntax, video coding standards are required to be efficient, in that they should support good compression algorithms as well as allow the efficient implementation of encoder and decoder.

In this chapter we introduce the video coding standards of the telecommunication standardization sector of the International Telecommunications Union (ITU-T), with the focus on the latest version, H.263. This version is also known as H.263, version 2, or H.263+, as opposed to an earlier version of H.263.

This chapter is organized as follows. Section 1.2 defines what a standard is and the need for standards. It also lists some of the prevalent standards and the organizations involved in developing them. Section 1.3 talks of the fundamental components of video coding standards in general and also some specifics regarding the H.263 standard. The basic concepts of motion compensation, transform coding, and entropy coding are introduced. The section concludes with an overall block diagram of the video encoder and decoder. Section 1.4 is specific to H.263 and describes the optional modes that are available with it. These options are further grouped into options for better picture quality, options for added error resilience, and options for scalabilities. Some other miscellaneous options are also described. There is some discussion on the levels of preferred support and other supplemental information, as well. Section 1.5, the conclusion, includes some general remarks and further sources of information.

1.2 FUNDAMENTALS OF STANDARDS

Multimedia communication is greatly dependent on good standards. The presence of standards allows for a larger volume of information exchange, thereby benefiting equipment manufacturers and service providers alike. It also benefits customers, who now have greater freedom to choose among manufacturers. All in all, standards are a prerequisite to multimedia communication. Standards for video coding are also required for efficiency in the compression of video content. This is because a large number of bits are required for the transmission of uncompressed video data.

The H.263 version 2 standard (1) belongs to a category of standards called voluntary standards. These standards are defined by volunteers in open committees and are agreed upon based on the consensus of all the committee members. They are driven by market needs and try to stay ahead of the development of technologies. H.263, the latest in the series of low bit rate video coding standards developed by ITU-T, was adopted in 1996 (3). It combined the features of MPEG and H.261 (2) (an earlier standard developed in 1990) for very low bit rate coding. H.263, version 2, or H.263+, was adopted in early 1998 and is the currently prevailing standard from ITU-T. This standard is the focus of this chapter and whenever we say H.263 we are referring to H.263 version 2.

Another major organization involved in the development of standards is the International Organization for Standardization (ISO). The ISO and ITU-T have defined different standards for video coding. These different standards are summarized in Table 1.1. The major differences between these standards lie in the operating bit rates and the applications they are targeted for. Each standard allows for operating at a wide range of bit rates; hence each can be used for a range of applications. All the standards follow a similar framework in terms of the coding algorithms, however there are differences in the ranges of parameters and in some specific coding modes. For more detail about ISO standards, see Chapter 2, on MPEG standards.

For a manufacturer to build a standard-compliant codec, it is very important to look at the bitstream syntax and to understand what each layer corresponds to and what each bit represents. This approach is, however, not necessary to understand the process of video coding. To have an overview of the standard, it suffices to look at the coding algorithms that generate the standard-compliant bitstream. This approach emphasizes an understanding of the various components of the codec and the functions they perform. Such an approach helps in un-

Table 1.1   Video Coding Standards Developed by Different Organizations

Standards organization	Video coding standard	Typical range of bit rates	Typical applications
ITU-T	H.261	$p \times 64$ kbit/s, $p = 1, \ldots 30$	ISDN videophone
ISO	IS 11172-2 MPEG-1 Video	1.2 Mbit/s	CD-ROM
ISO	IS 13810-2	4–80 Mbit/s	SDTV, HDTV
ITU-T	H.263	A wide range	PSTN videophone
ISO	CD 14496-2 MPEG-4 Video	24–1024 kbit/s	A wide range of applications
ITU-T	H.26L	<64 kbit/s	A wide range of applications

[a]ITU-T also actively participated in the development of MPEG-2 video. In fact, ITU-T H.262 refers to the same standard and uses the same text as IS 13818-2.

derstanding the video coding process as a whole. This chapter focuses on the second approach.

For transmitting video data over the network, standards other than for video coding are needed. There are several terminal standards for different network environments. For instance, the H.324 standard (4) that defines audiovisual terminals for the public service telephone networks (PSTN) uses H.263 for video coding, H.223 (5) for multiplexing, G.723 for speech coding, and H.245 (6) as the control protocol. H.263 may also be used in other terminal standards, over different networks.

1.3   BASICS OF VIDEO CODING

Video coding not only involves translation to a common language, it also tries to achieve compression by eliminating redundancy in the video data. There are two kinds of redundancy present in video data. The first kind is spatial, while the second kind is temporal. Spatial redundancy refers to the correlation present between different parts of a frame. Removal of spatial redundancy thus involves looking within a frame and is hence referred to as intra coding. Temporal redundancy, on the other hand, is the redundancy present between frames. At a sufficiently high frame rate it is quite likely that successive frames in the video sequence are very similar. Hence, removal of temporal redundancy involves looking between frames and is called inter coding. Spatial redundancy is removed through the use of transform coding techniques. Temporal redundancy is removed through the use of motion estimation and compensation techniques.

1.3.1   Source Picture Formats and Positions of Samples

To implement the standard, it is very important to know the picture formats that the standard supports and positions of the samples in the pictures. The samples are also referred to as pixels (picture elements) or pels. Source picture formats are defined in terms of the number of pixels per line, the number of lines per picture, and the pixel aspect ratio. H.263 allows for the use of five standardized picture formats. These are the CIF (common intermediate format), QCIF (quarter-CIF), sub-QCIF, 4CIF, and 16CIF. Besides these standardized formats, H.263 allows support for custom picture formats that can be negotiated. Details about the five standardized picture formats are summarized in Table 1.2.

The pixel aspect ratio is defined in the recommendations for H.261 as 12:11. From this ratio, it can be seen that all the standard picture formats defined in Table 1.2 cover an area that has an aspect ratio of 4:3.

Each sample or pixel consists of three components: a luminance or Y component and two chrominance or C_B and C_R components. The values of these components are as defined in Reference 7. For example, "black" is represented by $Y = 16$, while "white" is represented by $Y = 235$, while the values of C_B and C_R lie in the range 16 to 240. C_B and C_R values of 128 represent zero color difference or a gray region. The picture formats shown in Table 1.2 define the resolution of the Y component. Since human eyes are less sensitive to the chrominance components, these components typically have only half the resolution, both horizontally and vertically, of the Y component, hence the term "4:2:0 format." Each C_B or C_R pel lies at the center of four neighboring Y pels (Figure 1.1). The block edges can lie in between rows or columns of Y pels.

As mentioned earlier, H.263 allows support for negotiable custom picture formats. Custom picture formats can have any number of pixels per line and any number of lines in the picture. The only constraints applied are that the number of pixels per line should be a multiple of 4 in the range [4, . . . , 2048] and the number of lines per picture should also be a multiple of 4 in the range [4, . . . , 1152]. Custom picture formats are also allowed to have custom pixel aspect ratios, as shown in Table 1.3. These pictures or frames occur at a certain rate to make the

Table 1.2   Standard Picture Formats Supported by H.263

Property	Format				
	Sub-QCIF	QCIF	CIF	4CIF	16CIF
Number of pixels per line	128	176	352	704	1408
Number of lines	96	144	288	576	1152
Uncompressed bit rate (at 30 Hz), Mbit/s	4.4	9.1	37	146	584

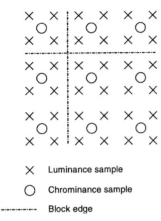

X   Luminance sample

O   Chrominance sample

--------   Block edge

Figure 1.1   Positions of luminance and chrominance samples.

Table 1.3   Different Pixel Aspect Ratios Supported by H.263

Pixel aspect ratio	Pixel width : pixel height
Square	1:1
CIF	12:11
525-type for 4:3 picture	10:11
CIF for 16:9 picture	16:11
525-type for 16:9 picture	40:33
Extended fixed aspect ratio	$m{:}n$, m, and n are relatively prime

video sequence. The standard specifies that all decoders and encoders should be able to use the standard CIF picture clock frequency (PCF). The PCF is 30,000/1001 frames per second for CIF. It is also allowed for decoders and encoders to have custom PCF, even higher than 30 frames per second.

1.3.2   Blocks, Macroblocks, and Groups of Blocks

H.263 uses block-based coding schemes. In these schemes, the pictures are subdivided into smaller units called blocks that are processed one by one, by both the decoder and the encoder. These blocks are processed in the scan order as shown in Figure 1.2.

A block is defined as a set of 8×8 pixels. As the chrominance components are downsampled, each chrominance block corresponds to four Y blocks. The

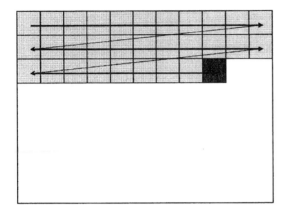

Figure 1.2   Scan order of blocks.

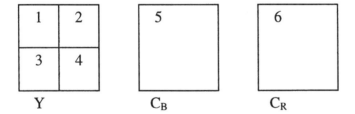

Figure 1.3   Blocks in a macroblock.

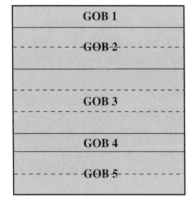

Figure 1.4   Example GOB structure for a QCIF picture.

collection of these six blocks is called a macroblock (MB). A MB is treated as a unit during the coding process.

A number of MBs are grouped together into a unit called a group of blocks (GOB). H.263 allows for a GOB to contain one or more rows of MBs, as shown in Figure 1.4.

The optional slice-structured mode allows for the grouping of MBs into slices, which may have an arbitrary number of MBs grouped together. More details about the slice-structured mode are provided in Section 1.4.2.1.

1.3.3 Compression Algorithms

Compression involves removal of spatial and temporal redundancy. The H.263 standard uses the discrete cosine transform to remove spatial redundancy and motion estimation and compensation to remove temporal redundancy. These techniques are discussed in the subsections that follow.

1.3.3.1 Transform Coding.   Transform coding has been widely used to remove redundancy between data samples. In transform coding, a set of data samples is first linearly transformed into a set of transform coefficients. These coefficients are then quantized and entropy-coded. A proper linear transform can decorrelate the input samples, and thus remove the redundancy. That is a properly chosen transform can concentrate the energy of input samples into a small number of transform coefficients, so that resulting coefficients are easier to encode than the original samples.

The most commonly used transform for video coding is the discrete cosine transform (DCT) (8, 9). Both in terms of objective coding gain and subjective quality, DCT performs very well for typical image data. The DCT operation can be expressed in terms of matrix multiplication:

$$\mathbf{Y} = \mathbf{C}^T \mathbf{X} \mathbf{C}$$

where $\mathbf{X}$ represents the original image block and $\mathbf{Y}$ represents the resulting DCT coefficients. The elements of $\mathbf{C}$, for an 8×8 image block, are defined as follows:

$$C_{mn} = k_n \cos\left[\frac{(2m+1)n\pi}{16}\right] \text{where } k_n = \begin{cases} \dfrac{1}{(2\sqrt{2})} & \text{when } n = 0 \\ \dfrac{1}{2} & \text{otherwise} \end{cases}$$

After the transform, the DCT coefficients in $\mathbf{Y}$ are quantized. Quantization involves loss of information and is the operation most responsible for the compression. The quantization step size can be adjusted based on the available bit rate and the coding modes chosen. Although the intra DC coefficients are uniformly quantized with a step size of 8, a "dead zone" is used while quantizing all other coefficients. This is done to remove noise around zero. The input–output relations for the two cases are shown in Figure 1.5.

The quantized 8×8 DCT coefficients are then converted into a one-dimensional (1D) array for entropy coding. Figure 1.5 shows the scan order used in H.261 for this conversion. Most of the energy concentrates on the low-frequency coefficients, and the high-frequency coefficients are usually very small and are quantized to zero before the scanning process. Therefore, the scan order in Figure 1.6 can create long runs of zero coefficients, which is important for efficient entropy coding, as we discuss next.

The resulting 1D array is then decomposed into segments, with each segment containing some (this number may be zero) zeros followed by a nonzero coefficient. Let an event represent the three values (run, level, last). "Run" represents the number of zeros; "level" represents the magnitude of the nonzero coefficient following the zeros; and "last" is an indication of whether the current nonzero coefficient is the last nonzero coefficient in the block. A Huffman coding table is built to represent each event by a specific codeword (i.e., a sequence of bits). Events that occur more often are represented by shorter codewords, and less frequent events are represented by longer codewords. So, the table is often called a variable-length coding (VLC) table. This coding process is sometimes called "run-length coding." Table 1.4 is an example of the VLC type of table. The transform coefficients in this table correspond to input samples chosen as the residues after motion compensation, which are discussed in section 1.3.3.2.

In Table 1.4, the third column represents the magnitude of the level. The sign bits added at the end of the VLC code takes care of the sign of the level. It

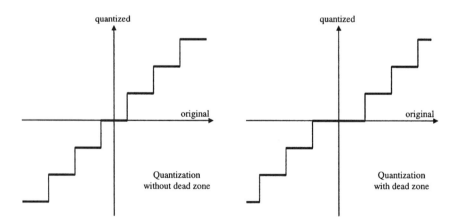

Figure 1.5   Quantization with and without "dead zone."

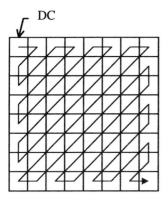

Figure 1.6   Scan order of the DCT coefficients.

Table 1.4   Partial VLC Table for DCT coefficients

LAST	RUN	[LEVEL]	VLC CODE
0	0	1	10s
0	0	2	1111s
0	0	3	0101 01s
0	0	4	0010 111s
0	0	5	0001 111s
0	0	6	0001 0010 1s
0	0	7	0001 0010 0s
0	0	8	0000 1000 01s
0	0	9	0000 1000 00s
0	0	10	0000 0000 111s
0	0	11	0000 0000 110s

can be seen from the table that more frequently occurring symbols (e.g., symbols with smaller magnitudes) are assigned fewer bits than the less frequently occurring symbols. It is reasonable to assume that symbols of smaller magnitude occur more frequently than the large magnitude symbols, because most of the time we code the residue found after motion compensation (discussed in the next section), and this residue does tend to have small magnitudes.

1.3.3.2 Motion Compensation.   Motion compensation involves removing the temporal redundancy present in video sequences. When the frame rate is sufficiently high, there is a great amount of similarity between neighboring frames. It is more efficient to code the difference between frames, rather than the frames themselves. An estimate for the frame being coded is obtained from the previous frame, and the difference between the prediction and the current frame is sent. This concept is similar to predictive coding and differential coding techniques.

Most video sequences contain moving objects, and this motion is one of the reasons for the difference between successive frames. If there were no motion of objects between frames, frames would be very similar. The basic idea behind motion compensation is to estimate this motion of objects and to use this information to build a prediction for successive frames. H.263 supports block-based motion estimation and compensation. Motion compensation is done at the MB level, except in the advanced modes, when it is done at the block level. The process involves looking at every MB in the current frame and trying to find a match for it in the previous frame. Each MB in the current frame is compared to 16×16 areas in a specified search space in the previous frame, and the best matching area is selected. This area is then offset by the displacement between its position and the position of the current MB. This forms a prediction of the current MB. In most cases, it is not possible to find an exact match for the current MB. The prediction area is usually similar to the MB, and the difference or residue between the two is small. Similarly, predictions for all the MBs in the current frame are obtained and the prediction frame is constructed. The residue frame is computed and is expected to have a much smaller energy than the original frame. This residue frame is then coded using the transform coding procedure. More information about motion compensation can be found in References 10 and 11.

The process of motion compensation is highlighted in Figure 1.7, where the gray block on the right corresponds to the current block being coded and the gray area on the left represents the best match found for the current block, in the previous frame. A major part of the encoding process involves finding these best matches or, equivalently, the offsets between the position of the

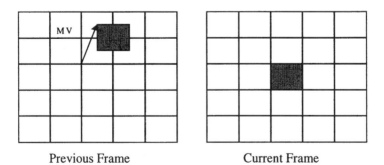

Previous Frame   Current Frame

Figure 1.7   Motion compensation.

best match and the position of the current block. This process of searching for the best matches is called *motion estimation*.

The offsets between the position of the best match and the position of the current MB are called motion vectors. H.263 allows these motion vectors to have nonintegral values. For instance, the motion vector for an MB may have the value (1.5, −4.5), which means that the best match for the current block has pixels that lie at nonintegral positions. All pixels in the previous frame are at integer pixel positions. Hence pixels at nonintegral positions have values that are computed from the original pixel values using bilinear interpolation. The pixel positions and their interpolated values are shown in Figure 1.8.

It is not always possible to find a good match for a particular MB, and when this happens the residue error between the best match and the MB itself may have as much energy as the original MB. For such cases, it is better to not do motion compensation. The encoder has the flexibility to decide for each MB whether it wants to do motion compensation or transform coding. However, in most cases, a saving is accomplished in the bits to code the residue. Besides the residue we also need to send the information regarding construction of the prediction frame to the decoder. This information consists basically of the motion vectors. The decoder can then use these to reconstruct the prediction frame and add to it the residue (this is transform-coded) to obtain the current frame. To avoid a large increase in the bitstream because of these motion vectors, they are also differentially coded. The motion vectors of three neighboring MBs (one to

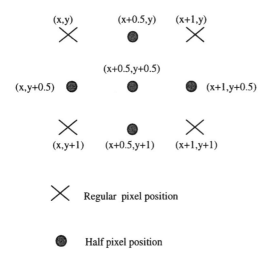

Figure 1.8   Half-pixel positions.

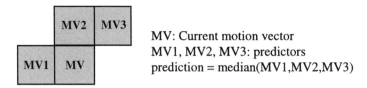

Figure 1.9   Prediction of motion vectors.

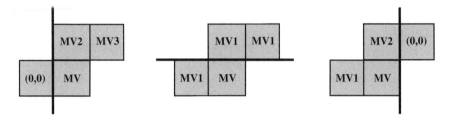

Figure 1.10   Special case motion vector prediction.

the left, one above, and one above right) are used as predictors for the motion vector of the current MB. The prediction is formed by taking the median of these three motion vectors. The prediction error between the actual motion vector and the predicted value in the horizontal direction and the vertical direction is coded as shown in Figure 1.9.

MBs for which the predictors lie outside the picture or GOB boundary are special cases which are handled as shown in Figure 1.10.

Whenever one of the prediction MBs lies outside the picture or GOB boundary, it is replaced by (0,0), when two MBs lie outside, however, they are replaced by the motion vector of the third MB. This is done to avoid having two motion vectors replaced by zeros, in which case the final value obtained after the median operation would be (0, 0). The prediction error in motion vectors is also coded by using a VLC table. Part of such a table is shown in Table 1.5, which indicates that two motion vector difference values correspond to the same codeword. These can be separated by the knowledge that the final decoded motion vector should lie in the range [−16, 15.5]. The exploitation of this fact leads to additional savings in terms of bit rate.

1.3.3.3   Summary.   All the basic techniques just described form part of the baseline options that are specified by H.263. These basic coding algorithms may be put together to form a block diagram representation of the video encoder and

Table 1.5 Part of the VLC Table for
Motion Vector Differences

Vector Difference	Code
–5 or 27	0000 0100 11
–4.5 or 27.5	0000 0101 01
–4 or 28	0000 0101 11
–3.5 or 28.5	0000 0111
–3 or 29	0000 1001
–2.5 or 29.5	0000 1011
–2 or 30	0000 111
–1.5 or 30.5	0001 1
–1 or 31	0011
–0.5 or 31.5	011
0	1
0.5 or –31.5	010
1 or –31	0010
1.5 or –30.5	0001 0
2 or –30	0000 110
2.5 or –29.5	0000 1010
3 or –29	0000 1000
3.5 or –28.5	0000 0110
4 or –28	0000 0101 10
4.5 or –27.5	0000 0101 00
5 or –27	0000 0100 10

decoder, as shown in Figure 1.11. We will discuss other advanced negotiable options in the next section.

Typically, baseline H.263 provides perceptually good quality for simple talking-head sequences at about 400 bytes per frame and sequences with moderate motion at about1000 bytes per frame. In terms of compression ratios, this translates to 100 for low-motion sequences and 40 for moderate-motion sequences.

1.4 NEGOTIABLE OPTIONS

H.263 allows for several advanced negotiable options. At the start of a communication session, the decoder signals the encoder regarding the options it can support. If the encoder also supports those options, they may be turned on. These advanced options are provided for better coding efficiency and error resilience and include some enhancements for scalabilities, as described in Sections 1.4.1.1 to 1.4.1.9.

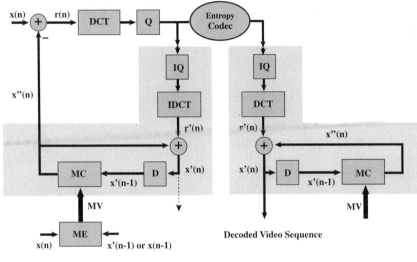

x(n): Current frame   x"(n): Prediction for x(n)   x'(n): Reconstructed Frame

r(n): Residue, x(n)-x"(n)   r'(n): Decoded residue   DCT: Discrete Cosine Transform

MC: Motion Compensation   ME: Motion Estimation   Q: Quantizer

D: Delay   IDCT: Inverse DCT   IQ: Inverse Quantizer

Figure 1.11   Block diagram of encoder and decoder.

1.4.1 Coding Modes for Efficiency or Improved Picture Quality

The modes described in the subsections that follow try to improve either the coding efficiency (by using better coding algorithms) or the quality of the decoded pictures.

1.4.1.1 Unrestricted Motion Vector (UMV) Mode.   In the baseline prediction mode of H.263, all motion vectors are restricted to the picture boundaries. This restriction is removed in UMV mode, and pixels outside the picture boundaries are referred to. Clearly these are not originally defined. Rather, they are obtained through the process of extrapolation. When a pixel referenced by a motion vector lies outside the coded picture area, an edge pixel is used instead. This mode also allows for an extension to the motion vector range. In the baseline mode, motion vectors are restricted to [−16, 15.5]. In the UMV mode, this range is extended to [−31.5, 31.5]. A larger motion vector range is very useful when the scene being encoded is high motion (especially when there is great camera motion) or the frame rate is low. In both cases large amounts of motion can occur between successive frames; hence the best match is likely to be further displaced from the current block, necessitating a large search range.

1.4.1.2   Syntax-Based Arithmetic Coding (SAC).   This option deals with the process of entropy coding and decoding, that is, converting symbols to bits and back. Instead of using the Huffman-like entropy coding VLC tables, the encoder and decoder use arithmetic coding to generate the bitstream. Arithmetic coding is more efficient than the VLC and results in savings in the size of the bitstream. Typically, SAC results in savings of around 10–20% for intra frames and around 1–3% for inter frames. The use of arithmetic coding generates a bitstream different from the VLC-generated bitstream; however, the quality of the reconstructed pictures is the same. Some more information about arithmetic coding can be obtained from Reference 12.

1.4.1.3   Advanced Prediction Mode.   This mode contains two basic features. The first feature supported by this mode is the use of four motion vectors per MB. The second feature supported is overlapped block motion compensation (OBMC). OBMC involves using motion vectors of neighboring blocks to reconstruct a block, thereby leading to an overall smoothing of the image and removal of blocking artifacts. Both these modes are discussed in more detail in the subsections. As in the UMV mode, this mode allows motion vectors to cross picture boundaries. Pixels outside the coded area are obtained by extrapolating, as in the UMV case. The extension of motion vector range, however, is not automatically turned on.

1.4.1.3.1   Four Motion Vectors per Macroblock.   Each luminance block in the MB is allowed to have its own motion vector. This allows greater flexibility in obtaining a best match for the MB. It is now possible to find really good matches for each of the four parts of the MB; hence, when these parts are put together, a much better prediction for the MB is obtained. Having four motion vectors also means that more motion vector data must be sent to the decoder. If the savings in the residue for the MB are offset by the extra bits needed to send the four motion vectors, there is no point in sending four motion vectors. Hence, the encoder needs to be able to intelligently decide whether it wants to send one motion vector or four motion vectors for every MB. With four motion vectors per MB it is no longer possible to use the same scheme as in the baseline case to code the motion vector difference. A new set of predictors is defined in the standard. These are shown in Figure 1.12.

The predictors are chosen such that none of them are redundant. For instance, the choice of MV* as a predictor for the upper left block of the MB probably would make the choice of MV1 redundant. This is because it is quite likely that MV2 and MV*, which come from the same MB, are close together. Hence,

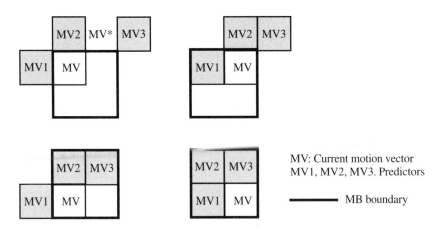

Figure 1.12   Redefinition of motion vector prediction.

the information obtained from MV1 is suppressed by the median operation. Such redundancy is avoided by picking a motion vector from another MB.

1.4.1.3.2 Overlapped Block Motion Compensation (OBMC). Every pixel in the final prediction region for a block is obtained as a weighted sum of three values (13). These values are obtained by using the motion vector of the current block and two out of four remote motion vectors. The remote motion vectors are the motion vectors of the block above, the block below, the block to the left, and the block to the right of the current block. The three values that are linearly combined to get the final pixel value are: (a) the pixel in the previous frame, at a displacement given by the motion vector of the current block, and (b) two pixels in the previous frame, at displacements given by the two remote motion vectors.

The weights are predefined in the standard. The choice of two out of four remote motion vectors is made by the location of the pixel in the current block. Each pixel picks the remote vectors of the two neighboring blocks closest to it. For instance, a pixel in the top left part of the block picks the remote motion vectors as the motion vectors of the blocks above and to the left of the current block, as shown in Figure 1.13.

The overall effect of using the neighboring motion vectors to make a prediction is to smooth the prediction. This reduces blockiness and leads to better predictions, thereby finally resulting in a smaller bitstream.

1.4.1.4   PB Frame Mode.   A PB frame is a unit that is made of two frames, called the P picture and the B picture. The pictures are decoded together and are treated as a single entity. This mode supports three different pictures: the I pic-

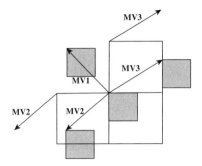

MV1: Motion Vector of current block   MV2: Motion Vector of block to the left

MV3: Motion Vector of block above

Figure 1.13   OBMC for upper left half of block.

ture, the P picture, and the B picture. An I picture is intra-coded, hence is not pre-dicted from any other picture. A P picture is predicted from the previous P pic-ture or from an I picture, like inter-coded frames in the baseline mode. A B picture is so called because parts of it may be bidirectionally predicted. A B pic-ture is obtained by looking at forward motion vectors, backward motion vectors, and delta motion vectors. The forward and backward motion vectors for the B picture are derived from the motion vectors of the P picture. Forward and back-ward motion vectors are calculated such that the motion of a block across the se-quence of P-B-P pictures appears smooth.

For example, consider a block in the P picture that is displaced from the previous P picture by 4 in the horizontal direction. This corresponding B picture block should be displaced by 2 in comparison to the previous P picture and by –2 in comparison to the following P picture, in the horizontal direction. These values correspond to the forward and backward motion vectors. This assumes that the B picture lies exactly between two successive P pictures in time refer-ence, (i.e., if no frames are skipped and the original frames are coded as a se-quence of P-B-P pictures). Another assumption made in the discussion above is that half the motion occurs between the first P picture and the B picture and the remaining half of motion occurs between the B picture and the second P picture. This may not be true. There may be accelerated motion across these frames. The delta motion vectors (Figure 1.14) are introduced to take care of such ac-celeration effects.

The prediction scheme for a B block is shown in Figure 1.15. A scheme like this results in less bit-rate overhead for the B picture. For relatively sim-

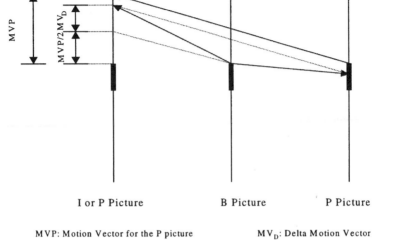

I or P Picture   B Picture   P Picture

MVP: Motion Vector for the P picture MV_D: Delta Motion Vector

Forward motion vector (MVF) = MVP/2 + MV_D Backward motion vector = MVF - MVP

Figure 1.14   Example of use of delta motion vectors for the 1D case.

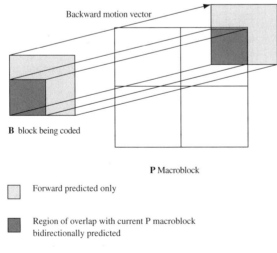

Figure 1.15   B block prediction.

ple sequences at low bit rates, the picture rate can be doubled, with this mode with minimal increase in the bit rate. However, for sequences with heavy motion, PB frames do not work as well as the B picture scheme, as used in MPEG 2. Also, compared with the baseline, the use of PB-frame mode increases the end-to-end delay. Thus this mode may not be suitable for two-way interactive communication.

1.4.1.5 Advanced Intra Coding Mode. This mode attempts to improve the efficiency while coding intra MBs in a given frame using (a) intra block prediction using neighboring intra blocks, (b) a separate VLC for the Intra coefficients, and (c) modified inverse quantization for intra coefficients.

An intra-coded block (the 8×8 DCT block) is predicted from an intra-coded block above or an intra-coded block to the left of it. Special cases are declared when the neighboring blocks are either absent or not intra-coded. First the DC coefficient is predicted from both the block above and the block to the left. Following this, either the first row of the block may be predicted from the first row of the block above, or the first column of the block may be predicted from the first column of the block to the left. This sequence is shown in Figure 1.16.

It is also possible that only the DC coefficient is predicted. The AC coefficients not in the first row or first column are never predicted. This way of predicting tries to exploit the knowledge of whether the block's frequency

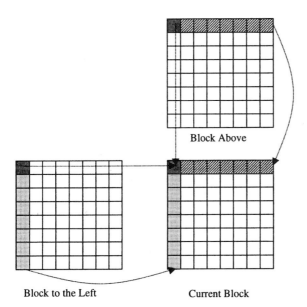

Block Above

Block to the Left   Current Block

Figure   1.16   Neighboring blocks for prediction of DCT coefficients.

components are stronger in the horizontal or vertical direction. If the block
has strong horizontal frequency components, then the first row of AC coefficients is predicted from the block above and all other AC coefficients are predicted as zero.

A similar thing is done with the first column of AC coefficients, when the
block has stronger vertical frequency components. The residue between the predicted coefficients and the actual coefficients is then scanned in different orders.
These different scanning orders, besides the original zigzag scanning, are defined to further exploit this prediction scheme. A horizontal scan is used if the
block has stronger horizontal frequency components; otherwise a vertical scan is
used. These scan orders are shown in Figure 1.17. After the scanning, the array
of coefficients is sent to the entropy encoder. If the prediction is good, there is a
saving in the number of bits for the block.

Besides the prediction introduced above, there are additional improvements available to utilize this prediction. First, an alternate intra VLC table is defined. This table has similar entries as the baseline VLC for intra coefficients, but
the run and the level are interpreted differently. For instance, in this mode intra
DC coefficients are no longer handled separately from the other coefficients. For
example, a value of zero is allowed for the intra DC coefficient, and this leads
only to an increase in the run before the next nonzero coefficient. Second, this
mode allows for an alternate inverse quantization procedure. This is also defined
to take advantage of the fact that we are now coding a residue instead of actual
intra coefficients.

1.4.1.6 Alternate Inter VLC Mode. During the process of inter coding it is
assumed that the residues have significantly less energy than the original blocks.
To take advantage of this property, the VLC tables used to convert these residue

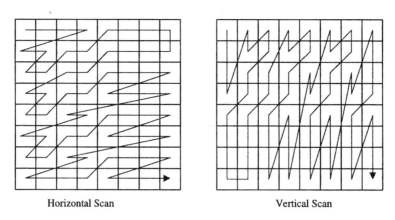

Horizontal Scan   Vertical Scan

Figure 1.17 DCT scanning patterns for advanced intra coding.

blocks or inter blocks are different from the tables for the intra blocks. For instance, inter VLC tables use fewer bits for large runs and low levels, since these symbols occur more frequently. On the other hand, intra VLC tables assign fewer bits to large levels and small runs, since these are the more frequently encountered cases. It is, however, possible for significant changes to occur in the scene, causing inter blocks to have energy comparable to that of the intra blocks. As noted earlier, for this range of values, the intra VLC tables are more efficient. This mode allows the encoder to use the intra VLC for inter blocks so that such cases can be taken care of efficiently.

The encoder is allowed to use the alternate inter VLC mode only when the decoder can deduce that the intra VLC table was used to code these inter block coefficients. The decoder can deduce this information in the following way. While using the inter VLC table to decode an inter block the decoder may encounter illegal values, such as more than 64 coefficients for the block. When this occurs, the decoder can deduce that the intra VLC table was used for the inter block and proceed to decode the block accordingly. The use of different VLC tables in different modes is highlighted in Figure 1.18, where "Table 1" refers to the inter VLC tables, while "Table 2" refers to the intra VLC tables. We can see that in the baseline mode, the AC coefficients for both the inter- and intra-coded blocks use Table 1. The advanced interactive video (AIV) mode allows the encoder to use the intra table for the inter AC symbols for better efficiency in cases of high motion or scene changes, while the advanced interactive compression (AIC) mode allows the encoder to use inter VLC for intra AC coefficients as these are predicted from the neighboring blocks.

1.4.1.7 Modified Quantization Mode. This mode, which modifies the quantizer operation, has four key features. The first feature allows the encoder a greater flexibility in controlling the quantization step size. This allows the encoder greater bit-rate controlling ability. The second feature allows the encoder to use different quantization parameters for chrominance and luminance components. Thus, the encoder can use a much finer step size for the chrominance components, thereby reducing any chrominance artifacts. The third feature extends the DCT coefficient range, so that any possible true coefficient can be represented. The fourth feature tries to eliminate coefficient levels that are very unlikely, thereby improving the ability to detect any errors and also to reduce the coding complexity.

1.4.1.8 Deblocking Filter Mode. The deblocking filter is an optional block edge filter that is applied to I and P frames in the coding loop. This filter is applied to 8×8 block edges to reduce blocking artifacts and improve perceptible picture quality. The selection of this mode requires the use of four motion vectors per MB and an extension of the motion vector range as in the UMV case. The effect of this filtering operation is similar to the effect produced by the

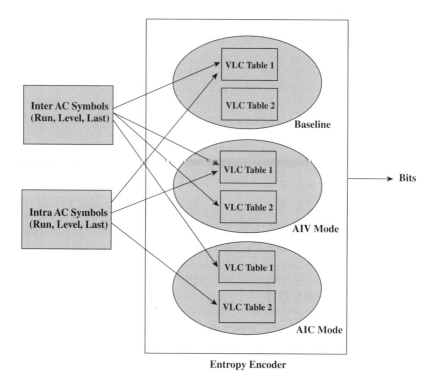

Figure 1.18 Use of different VLC tables for different modes.

OBMC mode described in connection with advanced prediction. Unlike the OBMC, which is done while the prediction frame is being made, this filtering operation is performed on the reconstructed image data.

The deblocking filter operates on sets of four pixel values on a horizontal or vertical line. This is shown in Figure 1.19, where A, B, C, and D are the four pixel values, with A and B belonging to one block (block 1) and C and D belonging to block 2. These four boundary pixels are replaced by four other values (A1, B1, C1, and D1) such that the boundary between blocks 1 and 2 is smoothed. Simplistically, this is done by trying to move the pixel values closer together. All the horizontal filtering for a block is done before any vertical filtering. This filtering operation is limited to the picture or segment boundaries. Special cases arise when some MBs are not coded. On the whole, this filtering operation tries to provide a better quality of decoded pictures by eliminating blockiness in the frame.

1.4.1.9 Improved PB Frame Mode. The PB frames constrain the motion vectors of the B picture to be estimated from the motion vectors of the P picture

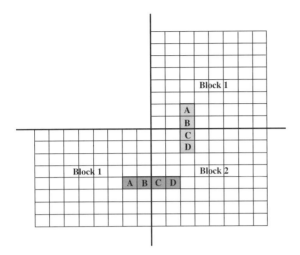

Figure 1.19   Examples of positions of filtered pixels.

part of the same frame. This kind of scheme performs poorly for large or complex motion scenarios when the corresponding prediction, obtained for the B pictures, is not good. This improved mode allows for distinct forward and backward motion vectors. This is different from the PB frame case, when the forward and backward motion vectors were both derived from the motion vector of the P picture, hence were closely related to each other. This allows a better prediction for the B pictures, as in the case with the B frames in MPEG.

There are three different ways of coding a MB of the B picture in the improved PB frame mode. The bidirectional prediction scheme is very similar to what occurs in the regular PB frame mode, with the delta motion vectors set to zero. The forward prediction scheme involves predicting the MB by using only the previous frame as reference. In the backward prediction option, bidirectional prediction is used whenever the backward motion vector points inside the already reconstructed P MB; otherwise, only forward prediction is used. The improved PB frame option tries to allow a greater independence to the prediction of a B picture MB, hence allows for improved performance when there is high or complex motion in the scene.

1.4.2   Enhancements for Error Robustness

The following modes help in increasing error resilience and are of great use if the encoder and decoder must communicate across an unreliable or lossy channel.

1.4.2.1   Slice-Structured Mode.   This is one of the enhancements in the standard to help in improving error resilience. When this mode is turned on, the frames are subdivided into many slices, instead of the regular GOBs. A slice is a group of consecutive MBs in scanning order; the only constraints are that the slice must start at an MB boundary and an MB can belong to exactly one slice. There are two submodes in this mode. In the first, or rectangular slice, submode, the slice is constrained to have a rectangular shape and all slices are transmitted strictly in order. This means that if a slice has MBs that occur before (in terms of the scanning order) the MBs in another slice, it is transmitted before the other slice. In the second submode, the arbitrary slice ordering submode, slices can be transmitted in any order. This grouping of MBs into slices instead of GOBs allows the encoder much flexibility and other advantages, as follows:

1.   It is more convenient to partition the frame into slices rather than into rows of MBs. For instance, the background may be separated from the foreground by grouping MBs appropriately. In fact, different objects in the scene can be partitioned out. In arbitrary slice ordering submode, such objects may be transmitted separately also. This feature is quite useful, especially in applications that call for lip synchronization.
2.   Slices help with error resilience. When combined with the independent segment decoding mode, data dependencies are prevented from crossing slice boundaries. This can help confine errors to slices and prevent them from corrupting the entire frame.
3.   Slice boundaries can be used as resynchronization points in case of bit errors or packet losses. With the GOBs, we send a header every n rows of MBs. This, however, does not translate to uniform spacing of the headers in the bitstream. A uniform spacing of headers in the bitstream may be achieved by grouping the MBs into arbitrary slices, as illustrated in Figure 1.20.

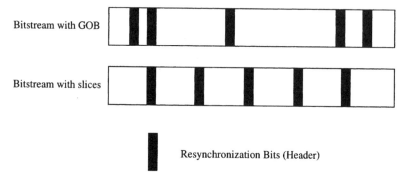

Figure 1.20   Uniform resynchronization points with arbitrary slices.

1.4.2.2 Reference Picture Selection Mode. This option allows for selection of any of the previously decoded frames (within 255 frames of the current frame or, when used with custom picture clock frequency, within 1023 frames of the current frame) as a reference frame to generate the prediction for the current frame. This is very different from the baseline case, when only the frame decoded immediately before the current frame may be used as a reference. This capability of selecting different frames as reference is most useful when the decoder can send information back to the encoder. So, the decoder needs to be able to inform the encoder which frames it received correctly and which frames were corrupted during the transfer. The encoder can then use this information to select as reference only the frames the decoder has acknowledged as received correctly.

This capability of selecting different frames as reference need not be restricted to the frame level. For instance, as shown in Figure 1.21, every GOB of the current frame may be predicted from regions of different reference frames. Thus if a GOB of the previously decoded frame is corrupted, when predicting GOBs of the current frame, which need to use data from that particular GOB, one must select a different frame. This option requires the decoder to use some backward channels to send information to the encoder. (There is a special mode called the *video redundancy coding* mode. In this mode, the decoder does not need to provide this feedback; rather, the encoder encodes multiple representations of the same frame and when the decoder receives adjacent pictures with the same temporal reference, something like a frame number, it should decode the first one and discard all the rest.) The decoder also needs to initially inform the encoder about the amount of memory

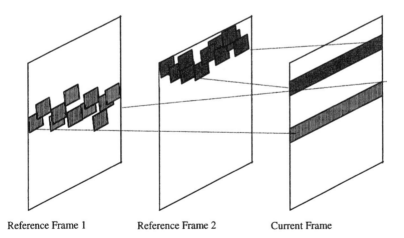

Reference Frame 1   Reference Frame 2   Current Frame

Figure 1.21 GOBs predicted from different reference frames.

it has available. Based on this information, the encoder decides on the maximum number of previously decoded pictures it needs to store and how far back in time a frame can be and still be selected as reference. The information regarding which frame is selected as reference is encoded in the bitstream. There is an increase in the size of the bitstream, and there is an overhead involved in the forward and backward communication between the encoder and decoder. This overhead is tolerated because it leads to a better error resilience. The encoder and the decoder can work together to ensure the quality of the recovered frames, even when they communicate over error-prone networks.

1.4.2.3 Independent Segment Decoding Mode. This mode is another enhancement for improved error resilience. It tries to remove data dependencies across the video picture segment boundaries. A video picture segment may be a slice (only the rectangular slice mode is allowed with ISD) or a number of consecutive GOBs. When this mode is turned on, the segment boundaries are treated as the picture boundaries. So, if this option is selected with the baseline options, each picture segment is decoded independently, as if it were the whole picture. This means that no operation can reference data outside the segment. This option may also be used with options like UMV or advanced prediction, in which case reference is to data outside the segment boundaries. In such cases, one derives data outside the segment boundaries through extrapolation of the segment, as was done in the case of the entire frame.

1.4.3 Scalability-Related Enhancements

If a bitstream is scalable, it allows for the decoding of the video sequence at different quality levels. This is done by partitioning the pictures into several layers. Pictures are partitioned into the base layer (the lowest layer) and enhancement layers. Three different pictures are used for scalability-the B, EI, and EP pictures. Each picture has two numbers associated with it. The first number refers to the layer to which the picture belongs (ELNUM). The second number, the reference layer number, refers to the layer from which the picture was predicted (RLNUM). There are three basic methods of achieving scalability. These are temporal, signal-to-noise ratio (SNR), and spatial enhancements.

Temporal scalability is achieved through the use of bidirectionally predicted B pictures. These B pictures are independent entities, unlike the cases of the PB-frame mode or the improved PB-frame mode, where the B pictures are syntactically intermixed with a successive P or EP picture. Since B pictures are not used as reference for any other pictures, some of them may be dropped without adversely affecting following pictures. Figure 1.22 illustrates the structure of P and B pictures.

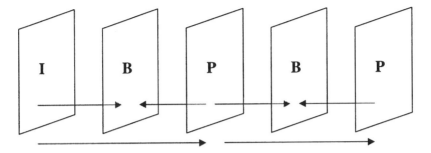

Figure 1.22   B-picture prediction dependencies.

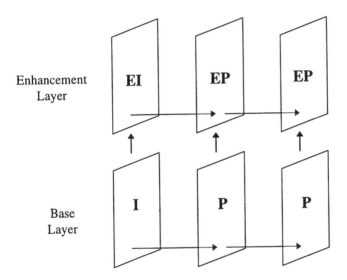

Figure 1.23   Illustration of EI and EP pictures.

During the process of compression, some information about the picture is lost and the encoded picture is not exactly the same as the original picture. The SNR scalability mode allows the codec to send this difference as an enhancement layer, and the presence of this enhancement layer helps in increasing the SNR of the video picture. If the enhancement layer information is predicted only from the layer below, the picture is called an EI picture. Enhancement layer pictures that are predicted from the base layer, as well as the prediction from the previous enhancement layer frame, are called EP pictures. This scheme is shown in Figure 1.23.

Spatial scalability is closely related to SNR scalability, with an additional operation performed before prediction of the enhancement layer pictures. The base layer pictures are interpolated by a factor 2 (i.e., expanded), either in one direction (X or Y) or in both. This interpolated picture is then used as reference for prediction. If the interpolation is done in both directions, then the predicted picture is called the 2D spatial enhancement layer picture; otherwise it is called the 1D spatial enhancement layer picture. This option hence requires the use of custom picture formats and aspect ratios. For example, when a 1D spatial enhancement picture (in the horizontal direction) is built from a QCIF frame, it is of size 352×144, which is not a standard size. All these three methods may be used together also; that is, the standard allows for multilayer scalability. Scalability is very useful for better error resilience support.

1.4.4   Other Enhancement Modes

There are two other modes that are listed in the H.263 standard. These are the reference picture resampling and reduced-resolution update modes.

1.4.4.1   Reference Picture Resampling.   This option allows the resampling of the previously decoded reference picture to create a warped picture that can be used for predicting the future frames. This is very useful if the current picture has a source format different from that of the previously decoded reference picture. Resampling defines the relation between the current frame and the previously decoded reference frame. In essence, resampling specifies the alteration in shape, size, and location between the current frame and the previously decoded reference frame. This resampling is defined in terms of the displacement of the four corners of the current picture area to get to the warped picture area. Four motion vectors are introduced to represent these four displacements. These motion vectors basically describe how to move the corners of the current picture area to map it to the warped picture area. The pixels are assumed to have a unit height and width, and the positions of the centers of the pixels are identified.

Following the position determination, horizontal and vertical displacements are computed for every pixel in the current picture area. These displacements are computed by using the position of the pixel and the four conceptual motion vectors, and they specify the locations of pixels in the warped area. After the location has been determined, bilinear interpolation is used to actually predict the pixel value at that pixel location. This new warped picture area is extrapolated so that the final height and width are divisible by 16. The new warped picture area is used as a reference frame for the current picture. Figure 1.24 describes this. This mode can be used to adaptively alter the resolution of the pictures being coded.

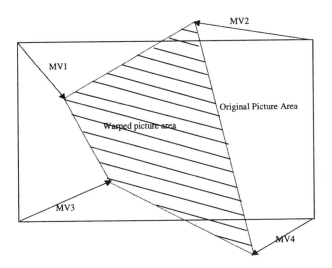

Figure 1.24 Conceptual motion vectors used for warping.

1.4.4.2 Reduced-Resolution Update Mode. This mode allows the encoder to send the residue or update information for a coded frame with reduced resolution, while keeping the finer detail information in the higher resolution reference image. The final frame can be reconstructed at the higher resolution from these two parts without significant loss of detail. Such an option is very useful when coding a very active or high-motion scene. In this mode, MBs are assigned a size 32×32 (correspondingly blocks are 16×16), hence there are one-quarter the number of MBs per picture as before. All motion vectors are estimated corresponding to these new larger MBs or blocks, depending on whether we desire one or four motion vectors for the MB. As against this, the transform-coded residues for each of these 16×16 blocks are thought of as representing an 8×8 area in a reduced resolution frame. The decoder uses the motion vectors corresponding to these large MBs and blocks for motion compensation.

Each of the residue blocks is upsampled to get residues for the higher resolution blocks. These are then added to produce the final-high resolution block. This process is illustrated in Figure 1.25. Since the residue frame is at a lower resolution, the encoder uses a smaller number of bits while encoding it. This means that the bitstream that is sent to the decoder is now smaller. Hence, the reduced-resolution update mode can be used to increase the coding picture rate while maintaining a sufficient subjective quality.

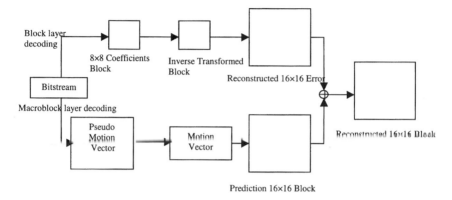

Figure 1.25   Reduced-resolution update block decoding.

1.4.5   Supplemental Enhancement Information Specification

The encoder sends supplemental enhancement information in a special field of the picture layer. It is not necessary for the decoder to have the ability to support these enhanced capabilities. When a decoder does not support these enhanced capabilities, it can just discard this field without affecting the quality of the decoded sequence. This mode differentiates between the decoded image and the displayed image. The displayed image is the image that is currently displayed, while the decoded image is the current image being decoded. Some of the enhanced capabilities require this distinction. For instance one of the options is the freeze picture request, in which case the displayed image is not changed to the successive decoded images unless the option is turned off or a time-out occurs. This means that a particular frame can be held on the display for a specified time while the decoder continues to decode further pictures.

Similarly there are other modes that request partial picture freeze (a particular area is frozen while the rest is updated) or resizing of a frozen partial picture area or release of the partial picture freeze mode. Besides the options to freeze parts of the image, other options allow the current picture to be treated as a snapshot of the video content for external use.

There are other features, among which is the chroma keying information. This option allows the pixels in the decoded pictures to be transparent and semitransparent. If a pixel is defined to be transparent, a background picture is displayed instead of the pixel. This background picture is either a prior reference picture or an externally controlled picture. If a pixel is labeled semitransparent, it is displayed as a blend between the current value and the background pixel value.

The last enhanced capability indicated by the supplemental enhancement information specification mode is the extended function type. This extended function provides a means for ITU to define a larger number of backward-compatible functions later.

1.4.6 Levels of Preferred Mode Support

All the optional modes introduced in Section 1.4.5 are useful; however, not all manufacturers necessarily want to support them all. A set of preferred mode combinations for operation is defined in the standard. Such a definition helps in identifying which combinations of modes are likely to be more widely accepted and also provides a guideline for the order in which modes should be supported in decoders. Manufacturers who make codecs that do not support all optional modes, can thus be assured of being able to communicate with several other codecs at some syntax better than baseline. These preferred mode combinations are grouped into levels based on the effect of each mode on the improvement in subjective video quality, overall delay, and complexity of the codec. A decoder that supports a certain level should be able to support all modes not only in that level, but also in levels below it. Level 1, which is the lowest level, is composed of advanced intra coding mode, deblocking filter, full-frame freeze, and modified quantization. Level 2 includes, in addition, support for unrestricted motion vector mode, slice-structured mode, and reference picture resampling. Level 3, the highest level, includes supporting advanced prediction, improved PB frames mode, independent segment decoding, and alternate inter VLC mode.

1.5 CONCLUSION

This chapter provides a basic overview of the process of video coding in general and the H.263 standard in particular. Through this chapter, we also hope we have conveyed the need for video coding standards. We also state that although standards completely specify the bitstream between encoder and decoder, they allow flexibility in the way the bitstream is produced. For instance, the standard does not specify how motion estimation should be done. Encoders can be optimized in many ways (in terms of speed, quality of decoded video, etc.) without losing standard compliance. Similar to the standard, another document drafted by ITU-T is called Test Model Near-Term (TMN) (14). This and other documents talk about specific encoder algorithms and how to efficiently produce standard-compliant bitstreams. They are, however, only guidelines, hence need not be followed. There is further work being done to develop a third generation of H.263 syntax called H.263++ and H.263L. More information about the H.263 standard and the ongoing efforts is available at the web site for ITU-T (http://www.itu.int)

and from the Video Coding Experts Group via file transfer protocol (ftp://standard.pictel.com/video-site).

REFERENCES

1. ITU-T Recommendation H.263 Version 2. Video coding for low bit rate communication. International Telecommunications Union, Geneva, January 1998.
2. ITU-T Recommendation H.261. Video codec for audiovisual services at p × 64 kbit/s." International Telecommunications Union, Geneva, 1990; revised at Helsinki, March 1993.
3. ITU-T Recommendation H.263. Video coding for low bitrate communication. March 1996.
4. ITU-T Recommendation H.324. Terminal for low bitrate multimedia communication. International Telecommunications Union, Geneva, March 1996.
5. ITU-T Recommendation H.223. Multiplexing protocol for low bitrate multimedia communication. International Telecommunications Union, Geneva, 1995.
6. ITU-T Recommendation H.245. Control protocol for multimedia communication. International Telecommunications Union, Geneva, 1995.
7. ITU-R Recommendation BT.601-5. Studio encoding parameters of digital television for standard 4:3 and wide-screen 16:9 aspect ratios. International Telecommunications Union, Geneva, 1995.
8. N. Ahmed, T. Natarajan, K R Rao. Discrete cosine transform. IEEE *Trans Compute* C-23:90–93, 1974.
9. K R Rao, and P Yip. *Discrete Cosine Transform*. New York: Academic Press, 1990.
10. A N Netravali, J D Robbins. Motion-compensated television coding: Part I. *Bell Syste. Tech. J.* 58(3): 631–670, March 1979.
11. A N Netravali, B G Haskell. *Digital Pictures*. 2nd ed. New York and London: Plenum Press, 1995.
12. I H Witten, R M Neal, J G Cleary. Arithmetic coding for data-compression. Commun. ACM, 30(6):520–540, June 1987.
13. M T Orchard, G J Sullivan, Overlapped block motion compensation—An estimation-theoretic approach. *IEEE Tran. Image Process*, 3(5):693–699, September 1994.
14. Video codec test model, near-term, version 10 (TMN10). Draft 1, Document Q15-D-65 d1. Video Coding Experts Group, April 1998.

2
MPEG Digital Video Coding Standards

Thomas Sikora
Department of Interactive Media–Human Factors,
Heinrich-Hertz Institute for Communication Technology, Berlin, Germany

2.1 INTRODUCTION

Modern image and video compression techniques offer the possibility of storing or transmitting the vast amount of data necessary to represent digital images and video in an efficient and robust way. New audiovisual applications in the fields of communication, multimedia, and broadcasting became possible based on digital video coding technology. Despite the numerous applications for image coding are today, and the manifold different approaches and algorithms, we are only slightly removed from the first hardware implementations and even systems in the commercial field, such as private teleconferencing systems (1,2). However, with the advances in very large scale integration (VLSI) technology, it became possible to open more application fields to a larger number of users, and therefore the necessity for video coding standards arose. Commercially, international standardization of video communication systems and protocols aims to serve two important goals: interoperability and economy of scale. Interworking between video communication equipment from different vendors is a desirable feature for users and equipment manufactures alike. It increases the attractiveness of buying and using video communication equipment because it enables large-scale international video data exchange via storage media or via communication networks. An increased demand can lead to economies of scale—the mass production of VLSI systems and devices—which in turn make video equipment more affordable for a wide field of applications and users.

During the 1980's a number of international video and audio standardization activities started within by consultative committees (CCs) within the International Telecommunications Union (ITU), namely CCITT, followed by CCIR and ISO/IEC (3). The Moving Picture Experts Group (MPEG) was established in 1988 in the framework of the Joint ISO/IEC Technical Committee (JTC 1) on Information Technology with the mandate to develop standards for coded representation of moving pictures, associated audio, and their combinations when used for storage and retrieval on digital storage media with a bit rate at up to about 1.5 Mbit/s. The standard, issued in 1992, was nicknamed MPEG-1. The scope of the group was later extended to provide appropriate MPEG-2 video and associated audio compression algorithms for a wide range of audiovisual applications at substantially higher bit rates not successfully covered or envisaged by the MPEG-1 standard. Specifically, MPEG-2 was given the charter to provide video quality not lower than NTSC/PAL and up to CCIR 601 quality with bit rates targeted between 2 and 10 Mbit/s. Emerging applications, such as digital cable TV distribution, networked database services via asynchronous transfer mode (ATM), digital videotape recording (VTR) applications, and satellite and terrestrial digital broadcasting distribution, were seen as beneficiaries of the increased quality expected to result from the emerging MPEG-2 standard. The MPEG-2 standard was released in 1994.

The MPEG-1 and MPEG-2 video compression techniques developed and standardized by the MPEG group have developed into important and successful video coding standards worldwide, with an increasing number of MPEG-1 and MPEG-2 VLSI chip sets and products becoming available on the market. One key factor for this success is the generic structure of the MPEG standards, supporting a wide range of applications and application-specific parameters. To support the wide range of applications profiles, a diversity of input parameters, including flexible picture size and frame rate, can be specified by the user. In addition, MPEG standardizes only the decoder structures and the bitstream formats, allowing a large degree of freedom for manufacturers to optimize the coding efficiency (i.e., the video quality at a given bit rate) by developing innovative encoder algorithms even after the standards have been finalized.

Anticipating the rapid convergence of the telecommunications, computer, and TV/film industries, the MPEG group officially initiated a new MPEG-4 standardization phase in 1994—with the mandate to standardize algorithms and tools for coding and flexible representation of audiovisual data to meet the challenges of future multimedia applications and applications environments. In particular MPEG-4 addresses the need for universal accessibility and robustness in error-prone environments, high interactive functionality, coding of natural and synthetic data, and high compression efficiency. Bit rates targeted for the MPEG-4 video standard are between 5 and 64 kbit/s for mobile or public service television network (PSTN) video applications and up to 6 Mbit/s for TV/film broadcast applications—and up to hundreds of megabits per second for studio applications. Synthetic coding can operate at a rate as low as 2 kbit/s for suitable video material. The first algorithms for the MPEG-4 standard were adopted by the ISO in July 1999.

This chapter provides an overview of the MPEG video coding algorithms and standards and their role in video communications. It is organized as follows: Section 2.2 reviews the basic concepts and techniques that are relevant in the context of the MPEG video compression standards. Section 2.3 and 2.4 outline the MPEG-1 and MPEG-2 video coding algorithms in more detail. Furthermore the specific properties of the standards related to their applications are presented. Section 2.5 describes the basic elements of the MPEG-4 standard and Section 2.6 addresses the issue of robust transmission in error-prone environments. Section 2.7, discusses the performance of the standards and their success in the market place.

2.2 FUNDAMENTALS OF MPEG VIDEO COMPRESSION ALGORITHMS

Generally speaking, video sequences contain a significant amount of statistical and subjective redundancy within and between frames. The ultimate goals of video source coding are the achievement of bit-rate reduction for storage and transmission by exploring both statistical and subjective redundancies and the encoding of a "minimum set" of information by means of entropy coding techniques. The performance of video compression techniques depends on the amount of redundancy contained in the image data as well as on the actual compression techniques used for coding. With practical coding schemes, a trade-off between coding performance (high compression with sufficient quality) and implementation complexity is targeted. For the development of the MPEG compression algorithms, the consideration of the capabilities of "state-of-the-art" (VLSI) technology foreseen for the life cycle of the standards was most important.

Dependent on the applications requirements, we may envisage "lossless" and "lossy" coding of the video data. The aim of "lossless" coding is to reduce image or video data for storage and transmission while retaining the quality of the original images—the *de*coded image quality is required to be identical to the image quality prior to encoding. In contrast, the aim of "lossy" coding techniques—and this is relevant to the applications envisioned by MPEG-1, MPEG-2, and MPEG-4 video standards—is to meet a given target bit rate for storage and transmission. Important applications comprise transmission of video over communications channels with constrained or low bandwidth and the efficient storage of video. In these applications high video compression is achieved by degrading the video quality—the decoded image "objective" quality is reduced compared to the quality of the original images prior to encoding (i.e., taking the mean squared error between the original and the reconstructed images as an objective image quality criterion). The smaller the target bit rate of the channel, the more highly the video data must be compressed, and, usually, the more coding artifacts become visible. The ultimate aim of lossy coding techniques is to optimize image quality for a given target bit rate subject to "objective" or "subjective" optimization criteria. It should be noted that the degree of image degradation (the objective degradation as well as the amount of visible artifacts) depends on the complexity of the image or video scene as much as on the sophistication of the compression technique—for simple textures in images and low video activity, even simple compression techniques will produce good image reconstruction with no visible artifacts.

2.2.1 The MPEG Video Coder Source Model

The MPEG digital video coding techniques are statistical in nature. Video sequences usually contain statistical redundancies in both temporal and spatial directions. The basic statistical property on which MPEG compression techniques rely is correlation between picture elements (pels), including the assumption of simple correlated translatory motion between consecutive frames. Thus, it is assumed that the magnitude of a particular image pel can be predicted from nearby pels within the same frame (using intra frame coding techniques) or from pels of a nearby frame (using inter frame techniques)[*] Intuitively it is clear that in some circumstances, (e.g., during scene changes of a video sequence), the temporal correlation between pels in nearby frames is small or even vanishes, whereupon the video scene assembles a collection of uncorrelated still images. In this case intra frame coding techniques are appropriate to explore spatial correlation to achieve efficient data compression. The MPEG compression algorithms employ discrete cosine transform (DCT) coding techniques on image blocks of 8×8 pels to efficiently explore spatial correlations between nearby pels within the same image. However, if the correlation between pels in nearby frames is high (i.e., in cases of two consecutive frames having similar or identical content), it is desirable to use inter frame DPCM coding techniques employing temporal prediction (motion-compensated prediction between frames). In MPEG video coding schemes, an adaptive combination of temporal motion-compensated prediction followed by transform coding of the remaining spatial information is used to achieve high data compression (hybrid DPCM/DCT coding of video).

Figure 2.1 depicts an example of intra frame pel-to-pel correlation properties of images, here modeled by using a rather simple, but nevertheless valu-

---

[*]In accordance with the convention introduced in Chapter 1, framing that entails spatial redundancy is designated *intra framing*, and *inter framing* is with reference to temporal redundancy.

INTRA

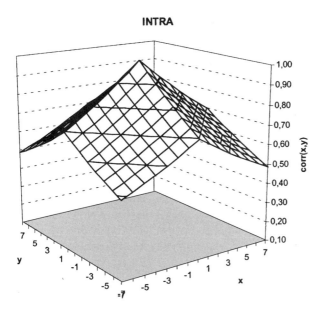

Figure 2.1 Spatial inter element correlation of "typical" images as calculated with an AR(1) Gauss-Markov image model with high pel–pel correlation. Variables x and y describe the distance between pels in the horizontal and vertical image dimension, respectively.

able statistical model. The simple model assumption already inherits basic correlation properties of many "typical" images on which the MPEG algorithms rely, namely, the high correlation between adjacent pixels and the monotonic decay of correlation with increased distance between pels. We will use this model assumption later to demonstrate some of the properties of transform domain coding.

2.2.2 Subsampling and Interpolation

Almost all video coding techniques described in the context of this chapter make extensive use of subsampling and quantization prior to encoding. The basic goal of subsampling is to reduce the dimension of the input video (horizontal dimension and/or vertical dimension) and thus the number of pels to be coded prior to the encoding process. It is worth noting that for some applications video is also subsampled in the temporal direction to reduce frame rate prior to coding. At the receiver, the decoded images are interpolated for display. This technique may be considered to be one of the most elementary compression techniques that also makes use of specific physiological characteristics of the human eye and thus removes subjective redundancy contained in the video data. That is, it takes advantage of the human eye's greater sensitivity to changes in brightness than to chromaticity changes. Therefore the MPEG coding schemes first divide the images into YUV components (one luminance and two chrominance components). Next the chrominance components are subsampled relative to the luminance component with a $Y{:}U{:}V$ ratio specific to particular applications (i.e., with the MPEG-2 standard a ratio of 4:1:1 or 4:2:2 is used).

2.2.3   Motion-Compensated Prediction

Motion-compensated prediction, a powerful tool for reducing temporal redundancies between frames, is used extensively in MPEG-1 and MPEG-2 video coding standards as a prediction technique for temporal DPCM coding. The concept of motion compensation is based on the estimation of motion between video frames: that is, if all elements in a video scene are approximately spatially displaced, the motion between frames can be described by a limited number of motion parameters (i.e., by motion vectors for translatory motion of pels). In this simple example the best prediction of an actual pel is given by a motion-compensated prediction pel from a previously coded frame. Usually both prediction error and motion vectors are transmitted to the receiver. However, encoding one piece of motion information with each coded image pel is generally neither desirable nor necessary. Since the spatial correlation between motion vectors is often high, it is sometimes assumed that one motion vector is representative for the motion of a "block" of adjacent pels. For this purpose images are usually separated into discrete blocks of pels (i.e., 16×16 pels in MPEG-1 and MPEG-2 standards) and only one motion vector is estimated, coded, and transmitted for each of these blocks (Figure 2.2).

In the MPEG compression algorithms, the motion-compensated prediction techniques are used for reducing temporal redundancies between frames; only the prediction error images—the difference between original images and motion-compensated prediction images—are encoded. In general, the correlation between pels in the motion-compensated inter frame error images to be coded is reduced with respect to the correlation properties of intra frames in Figure 2.1 as a result of the prediction based on the previous coded frame.

2.2.4   Transform Domain Coding

Transform coding has been studied extensively during the last two decades and has become a very popular compression method for still image coding and video coding. The purpose of transform coding is to decorrelate the intra or inter frame error image content and to encode transform coefficients rather than the original

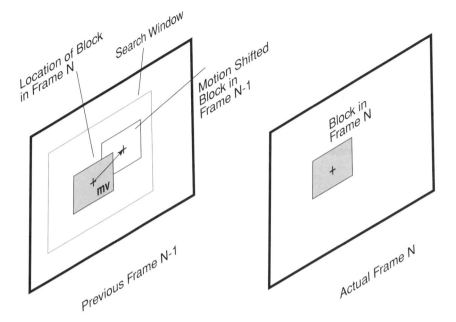

Figure 2.2 Block matching approach for motion compensation: one motion vector (mv) is estimated for each block in the actual frame N to be coded. The motion vector points to a reference block of same size in a previously coded frame $N–1$. The motion-compensated prediction error is calculated by subtracting each pel in a block from its motion-shifted counterpart in the reference block of the previous frame.

pels of the images. To this end, the input images are split into disjoint blocks of pels b (i.e., of size $N \times N$ pels). The transformation can be represented as a matrix operation using an $N \times N$ transform matrix A to obtain the $N \times N$ transform coefficients c based on a linear, separable, and unitary forward transformation:

$$c = A\, b\, A^T$$

Where A^T denotes the transpose of the transformation matrix A. Note that the transformation is reversible, since the original $N \times N$ block of pels b can be reconstructed by using a linear and separable inverse transformation[*]

$$b = A^T\, c\, A$$

---

[*]For a unitary transform, the inverse matrix A^{-1} is identical with the transposed matrix A^T; that is, $A^{-1} = A^T$.

From among many possible alternatives, the discrete cosine transform applied to smaller image blocks (usually 8×8 pels) has become the most successful transform for still image and video coding (5). In fact, DCT-based implementations are used in most image and video coding standards owing to their high decorrelation performance and the availability of fast DCT algorithms suitable for real-time implementations. VLSI implementations that operate at rates suitable for a broad range of video applications are commercially available today.

A major objective of transform coding is to make as many transform coefficients as possible so small that they are insignificant (in terms of statistical and subjective measures) and need not be coded for transmission. At the same time it is desirable to minimize statistical dependencies between coefficients, with the aim of reducing the amount of bits needed to encode the remaining coefficients. Figure 2.3 depicts the variance (energy) of an 8×8 block of intra frame DCT coefficients based on the simple statistical model assumption already discussed in in connection with Figure 2.1. Here, the variance for each coefficient represents

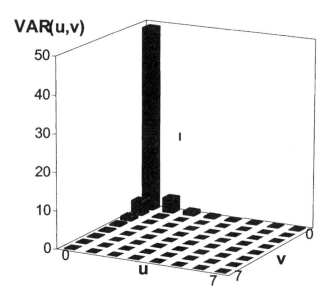

Figure 2.3 The variance distribution of DCT coefficients, "typically" calculated as an average over a large number of image blocks. The variance of the DCT coefficients was calculated based on the statistical model used in Figure 2.1. The horizontal and vertical image transform domain variable within the 8×8 block is u and v, respectively. Most of the total variance is concentrated around the DCT-coefficient ($u = 0$, $v = 0$).

the variability of the coefficient as averaged over a large number of frames. Coefficients with small variances are less significant for the reconstruction of the image blocks than coefficients with large variances. As may be seen from Figure 2.3, on average only a small number of DCT coefficients need to be transmitted to the receiver to obtain a valuable approximate reconstruction of the image blocks. Moreover, the most significant DCT coefficients are concentrated around the upper left corner (low DCT coefficients), and the significance of the coefficients decays with increased distance. This set of circumstances implies that higher DCT coefficients are less important for reconstruction than lower coefficients. Also employing motion-compensated prediction usually results in a compact representation of the temporal DPCM signal in the DCT domain (inter frame). This is the case because the temporal DPCM signal essentially inherits statistical coherency similar to the signal in the intra frame DCT domain (although with reduced energy). Therefore, MPEG algorithms employ DCT coding also for inter frame compression successfully (3,4).

The combination of the two techniques described above—temporal motion-compensated prediction and transform domain coding—can be seen as the key elements of the MPEG coding standards. A third characteristic element of the MPEG algorithms is that these two techniques are processed on small image blocks (of typically 16×16 pels for motion compensation and 8×8 pels for DCT coding). For this reason, the MPEG coding algorithms are usually referred to as hybrid block-based DPCM/DCT algorithms.

2.3 MPEG-1: A GENERIC STANDARD FOR CODING OF MOVING PICTURES AND ASSOCIATED AUDIO FOR DIGITAL STORAGE MEDIA AT UP TO ABOUT 1.5 MBits/s

The video compression technique developed by MPEG-1 covers many applications from interactive systems on CD-ROM to the delivery of video over telecommunications networks. The MPEG-1 video coding standard is thought to be generic. To support the wide range of applications profiles, a diversity of input parameters including flexible picture size and frame rate can be specified by the user. MPEG has recommended a constraint parameter set: every MPEG-1-compatible decoder must be able to support at least video source parameters up to TV size, including a minimum number of 720 pixels per line, a minimum number of 576 lines per picture, a minimum frame rate of 30 frames per second, and a minimum bit rate of 1.86 Mbit/s. The standard video input consists of a noninterlaced video picture format. It should be noted that the application of MPEG-1 is by no means limited to this constrained parameter set.

The MPEG-1 video algorithm has been developed with respect to the JPEG and H.261 activities. It was sought to retain a large degree of commonality with the CCITT H.261 standard so that implementations supporting both standards would be plausible. However, MPEG-1 was primarily targeted for multimedia CD-ROM applications, requiring additional functionality supported by both encoder and decoder. Important features provided by MPEG-1 include frame-based random access of video, fast forward/fast reverse (FF/FR) searches through compressed bitstreams, reverse playback of video, and editability of the compressed bitstream.

2.3.1   The Basic MPEG-1 Inter Frame Coding Scheme

The basic MPEG-1 (as well as the MPEG-2) video compression technique is based on a macroblock structure, motion compensation, and the conditional replenishment of macroblocks. As outlined in Figure 2.4A the MPEG-1 coding algorithm encodes the first frame in a video sequence in intra frame coding mode (I picture). Each subsequent frame is coded using inter frame prediction (P pictures), only data from the nearest previously coded I or P frame can be used for prediction. The MPEG-1 algorithm uses a block-based approach to process the

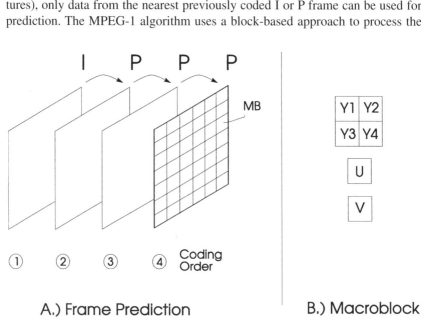

A.) Frame Prediction   B.) Macroblock

Figure 2.4   (A) I pictures (I) and P pictures (P) in a video sequence. P pictures are coded by using motion-compensated prediction based on the nearest previous frame. Each frame is divided into disjoint "macroblocks" (MB). (B) With each macroblock, information related to four luminance blocks ($Y1$, $Y2$, $Y3$, $Y4$) and two chrominance blocks (U, V) is coded. Each block contains 8×8 pels.

frames of a video sequence. Each color input frame in a video sequence is partitioned into nonoverlapping "macroblocks" as depicted in Figure 2.4B. Each macroblock contains blocks of data from both luminance and co-sited chrominance bands - four luminance blocks (Y_1, Y_2, Y_3, Y_4) and two chrominance blocks (U, V), each with size 8×8 pels. Thus the sampling ratio between luminance and chrominance pels $Y{:}U{:}V$ is 4:1:1.

The block diagram of the basic hybrid DPCM/DCT MPEG-1 encoder and decoder structure is depicted in Figure 2.5. The first frame in a video sequence (I picture) is encoded in the intra mode without reference to any past or future frames. At the encoder the DCT is applied to each 8×8 luminance and chrominance block and, after output of the DCT, each of the 64 DCT coefficients is uniformly quantized (Q) . The quantizer step size (sz) used to quantize the DCT coefficients within a macroblock is transmitted to the receiver. After quantization, the lowest frequency DCT coefficient (DC coefficient) is treated differently from the remaining coefficients (AC coefficients). The DC coefficient corresponds to the average intensity of the component block and is encoded by using a differential DC prediction method.* The nonzero quantizer values of the

HYBRID DCT/DPCM CODING SCHEME

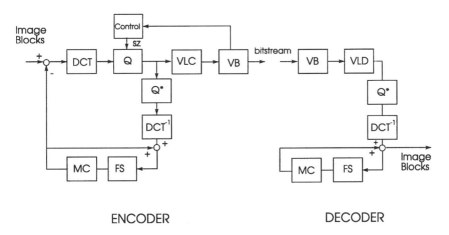

ENCODER   DECODER

Figure 2.5   Block diagram of a basic hybrid DCT/DPCM encoder and decoder structure.

---

*Because there is usually strong correlation between the DC values of adjacent 8×8 blocks, the quantized DC coefficient is encoded as the difference between the DC value of the previous block and the actual DC value.

remaining DCT coefficients and their locations are then "zigzag"-scanned and run-length entropy-coded by means of variable-length code (VLC) tables. The concept of "zigzag" scanning of the coefficients is outlined in Figure 2.6. The scanning of the quantized DCT domain two-dimensional signal followed by variable-length codeword assignment for the coefficients serves as a mapping of the two-dimensional image signal into a one-dimensional bitstream. The nonzero AC coefficient quantizer values (length, ###) are detected along the scan line as well as the distance (run) between two consecutive nonzero coefficients. Each consecutive pair (run, length) is encoded by transmitting only one VLC codeword. The purpose of "zigzag" scanning is to trace the low-frequency DCT coefficients (those containing the most energy) before the high-frequency coefficients.*

For coding P pictures, the previously I- or P-picture frame $N - 1$ is stored in a frame store (FS) in both encoder and decoder. Motion compensation (MC) is performed on a macroblock basis: only one motion vector is estimated between frame N and frame $N - 1$ for a particular macroblock to be encoded. These motion vectors are coded and transmitted to the receiver. The motion-compensated prediction error is calculated by subtracting each pel in a macroblock from its motion-shifted counterpart in the previous frame. An 8×8 DCT is then applied to each of the 8×8 blocks contained in the macroblock followed first by quantization (Q) of the DCT coefficients and then by run-length coding and entropy coding (VLC). A video buffer (VB) is needed to ensure that a constant target bit rate output is produced by the encoder. The quantization step size (sz) can be adjusted for each macroblock in a frame to achieve a given target bit rate and to avoid buffer overflow and underflow.

The decoder uses the reverse process to reproduce a macroblock of frame N at the receiver. After the variable-length words (VLD) contained in the video decoder buffer (VB) have been decoded, the pixel values of the prediction error are reconstructed (Q*, and DCT^{-1} operations). The motion-compensated pixels from the previous frame $N - 1$ contained in the frame store are added to the prediction error to recover the particular macroblock of frame N. By processing the entire bit stream, all image blocks are decoded and reconstructed.

The advantage of using the motion-compensated prediction from the pre-

---

*The location of each nonzero coefficient along the zigzag scan is encoded relative to the location of the previous coded coefficient. The zigzag scan philosophy attempts to trace the nonzero coefficients according their likelihood of appearance to achieve an efficient entropy coding. With reference to Figure 2.5 the DCT coefficients most likely to appear are concentrated around the DC coefficient with decreasing importance. For many images, the coefficients can be traced efficiently by using the zigzag scan.

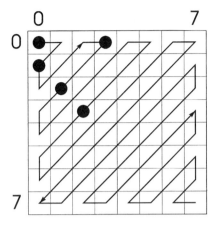

● Non-Zero
DCT-Coefficients

Figure 2.6 "Zigzag" scanning of the quantized DCT coefficients in an 8×8 block; the possible locations of nonzero DCT coefficients are indicated. Only the non zero quantized DCT coefficients are encoded. The zigzag scan attempts to trace the DCT coefficients according to their significance. With reference to Figure 2.3, the lowest DCT coefficient (0, 0) contains most of the energy within the blocks, and the energy is concentrated around the lower DCT coefficients.

viously reconstructed frame $N - 1$ to code video in an MPEG coder is illustrated in Figure 2.7 for a typical test sequence. Figure 2.7A depicts a frame at time instance N to be coded and Figure 2.7B is the reconstructed frame at instance $N - 1$ which is stored in the frame store at both encoder and decoder. The block motion vectors (mv, see also Figure 2.2) depicted in Figure 2.7B were estimated by the encoder motion estimation procedure and provide a prediction of the translatory motion displacement of each macroblock in frame N with reference to frame $N - 1$. Figure 7B depicts the pure frame difference signal [frame $N -$ frame $N - 1$], which is obtained if no motion-compensated prediction is used in the coding process—thus all motion vectors are assumed to be zero. Figure 2.7D depicts the motion-compensated frame difference signal when the motion vectors in Figure 2.7B are used for prediction. It is apparent that in comparison to the pure frame difference coding shown in Figure 2.7C (all motion vectors have zero components), the residual signal to be coded is greatly reduced if motion compensation is used.

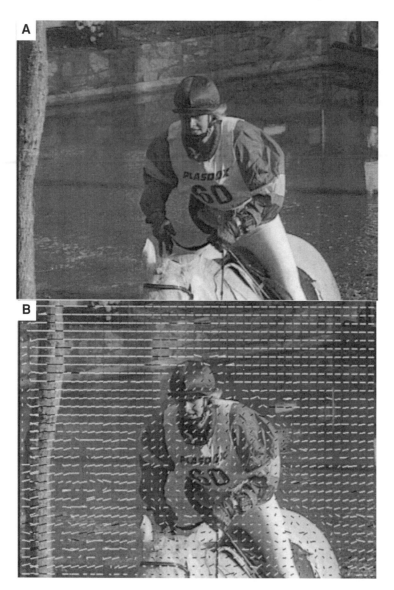

Figure 2.7 (A) Frame at time instance N to be coded. (B) Frame at instance N–1 used for prediction of the content in frame N (note that the motion vectors depicted in the image are not part of the reconstructed image stored at the encoder and decoder). (C) Prediction error image obtained without using motion compensation—all motion vectors are assumed to be zero. (D) Prediction error image to be coded if motion-compensated prediction is employed.

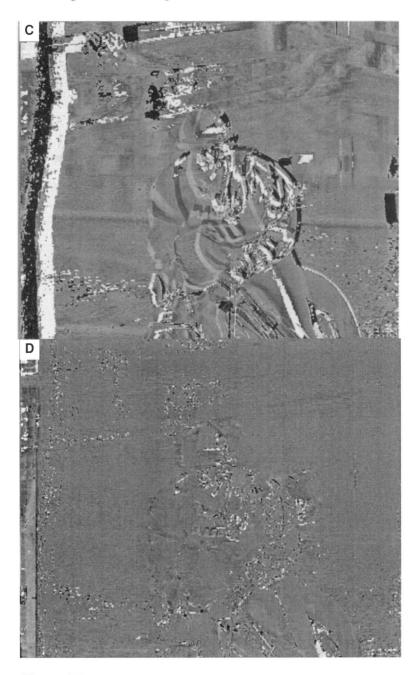

Figure 2.7   (Continued)

2.3.2   Conditional Replenishment

An essential feature supported by the MPEG-1 coding algorithm is the possibility of updating macroblock information at the decoder only if needed—that is, if the content of the macroblock has changed in comparison to the content of the same macroblock in the previous frame. This is known as conditional macroblock replenishment. The key for efficient coding of video sequences at lower bit rates is the selection of appropriate prediction modes to achieve conditional replenishment. The MPEG standard distinguishes mainly between three different macroblock coding types (MB types):

> *Skipped MB:* prediction from previous frame with zero motion vector. No information about the macroblock is coded nor transmitted to the receiver.
>
> *Inter MB:* motion-compensated prediction from the previous frame is used. The MB type, the MB address and, if required, the motion vector, the DCT coefficients, and quantization step size are transmitted.
>
> *Intra MB:* no prediction is used from the previous frame (intra frame prediction only). Only the MB type, the MB address, and the DCT coefficients and quantization step size are transmitted to the receiver.

2.3.3   Rate Control

An important feature supported by the MEPG-1 encoding algorithms is the possibility of tailoring the bit rate (and thus the quality of the reconstructed video) to specific application requirements by adjusting the quantizer step size (sz) in Figure 2.5 for quantizing the DCT coefficients (5,6). Coarse quantization of the DCT coefficients enables the storage or transmission of video with high compression ratios but, depending on the level of quantization, it may result in significant coding artifacts. The MPEG-1 standard allows the encoder to select different quantizer values for each coded macroblock, thus enabling a high degree of flexibility in the allocation of bits in images as needed to improve image quality. Furthermore it allows the generation of both constant and variable bit rates for storage or real-time transmission of the compressed video.

The rate control algorithm used to compress video is not part of the MPEG-1 standard, and it is thus left to the implementers to develop efficient strategies. It is worth emphasizing that the efficiency of the rate control algorithms selected by manufacturers to compress video at a given bit rate heavily impacts the visible quality of the video reconstructed at the decoder.

2.3.4   Specific Storage Media Functionalities

For accessing video from storage media, the MPEG-1 video compression algorithm was designed to support important functionalities such as random access

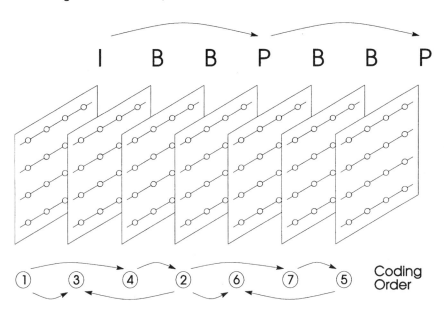

I   B   B   P   B   B   P

① ③ ④ ② ⑥ ⑦ ⑤   Coding
                         Order

Figure 2.8 I pictures (I), P pictures (P) and B pictures (B) used in a MPEG-1 video sequence. B pictures can be coded by using motion-compensated prediction based on the two nearest already coded frames (either I picture or P picture). The arrangement of the picture coding types in the video sequence is flexible to suit the needs of diverse applications. The direction for prediction is indicated.

and fast forward (FF) and fast reverse (FR) playback. To incorporate the requirements for storage media and to further explore the significant advantages of motion compensation and motion interpolation, MPEG–1 introduced the concept of B pictures (bidirectional predicted/bidirectional interpolated pictures). This concept is depicted in Figure 2.8 for a group of consecutive pictures in a video sequence. Pictures of three types are considered: Intra pictures (I pictures) are coded without reference to other pictures contained in the video sequence, as shown earlier (Figure 2.4); I pictures allow access points for random access and FF/FR functionality in the bitstream but achieve only low compression. Interframe predicted pictures (P pictures) are coded with reference to the nearest previously coded I or P picture, usually incorporating motion compensation to increase coding efficiency. Since P pictures are usually used as reference for prediction for future or past frames, they provide no suitable access points for random access functionality or editability. Bidirectional predicted/interpolated pictures (B pictures) require both past and future frames as references. To achieve high compression, motion compensation can be employed based on the nearest past and future P or I pictures. B pictures themselves are never used as references. The user can arrange the picture types in a video sequence with a high degree of flexibility to suit diverse applications requirements. As a general rule, a video sequence coded using I pictures only (I I I I I I . . .) allows the highest degree of random access, FF/FR, and editability, but achieves only low compression. A sequence coded with a regular I-picture update and no B pictures (i.e, I P P P P P P I P P P P . . .) achieves moderate compression and a certain degree of random access and FF/FR functionality. Incorporation of all three pictures types, as depicted, for example, in Figure 2.8 (I B B P B B P B B I B B P . . .), may achieve high compression and reasonable random access and FF/FR functionality, but at the cost of a significantly increased coding delay. This delay may not be tolerable for such applications as videotelephony or videoconferencing.

2.3.5   Coding of Interlaced Video Sources

The standard video input format for MPEG-1 is noninterlaced. However, coding of interlaced color television with both 525 and 625 lines at 29.97 and 25 frames per second, respectively, is an important application for the MPEG-1 standard. A suggestion for coding Recommendation 601 digital color television signals has been made by MPEG-1 based on the conversion of the interlaced source to a progressive intermediate format. In essence, only one horizontally subsampled field of each interlaced video input frame is encoded (i.e., the subsampled top field). At the receiver, the even field is predicted from the decoded and horizontally interpolated odd field for display. The necessary preprocessing steps required prior to encoding and the postprocessing required after decoding are described in detail in the Informative Annex of the MPEG-1 International Standard document (7).

2.4   MPEG-2 STANDARD FOR GENERIC CODING OF MOVING PICTURES AND ASSOCIATED AUDIO

Worldwide MPEG-1 is developing into an important and successful video coding standard, and the number of products available on the market is increasing. A key factor for this success is the generic structure of the standard supporting a broad range of applications and application-specific parameters. However, MPEG continued its standardization efforts in 1991 with a second phase (MPEG-2) to provide a video coding solution for applications not originally covered or envisaged by the MPEG-1 standard. Specifically, MPEG-2 was given the charter to provide video quality not lower than NTSC/PAL and up to CCIR 601 quality. Emerging applications, such as digital cable TV distribution, networked database services via ATM, digital VTR applications, and satellite and terrestrial digital broadcasting distribution, were seen as able to benefit from the increased quality expected to result from the new MPEG-2 standardization phase. Work was carried out in collaboration with the ITU-T SG 15 Experts Group for ATM Video Coding, and in 1994 the MPEG-2 Draft International Standard (which is identical to the ITU-T H.262 recommendation) was released (6). The specification of the standard is intended to be generic—hence the standard aims to facilitate the bitstream interchange among different applications and transmission and storage media.

Basically MPEG-2 can be seen as a superset of the MPEG-1 coding standard and was designed to be backward compatible to MPEG-1 - every MPEG-2-compatible decoder can decode a valid MPEG-1 bitstream. Many video coding algorithms were integrated into a single syntax to meet the diverse applications requirements. New coding features were added by MPEG-2 to achieve sufficient functionality and quality; thus prediction modes were developed to support efficient coding of interlaced video. In addition, scalable video coding extensions were introduced to provide additional functionality, such as embedded coding of digital TV and HDTV, and graceful quality degradation in the presence of transmission errors.

However, implementation of the full syntax may not be practical for most applications. MPEG-2 has introduced the concept of "profiles and levels" to stipulate conformity with equipment not supporting the full implementation. Profiles and levels provide means for defining subsets of the syntax, and thus the decoder capabilities required to decode a particular bitstream. This concept is illustrated in Tables 2.1 and 2.2

As a general rule, each profile defines a new set of algorithms added as a superset to the algorithms in the profile below. A level specifies the range of the parameters that are supported by the implementation (i.e., image size, frame rate, and bit rates). The MPEG-2 core algorithm at MAIN profile features nonscalable coding of both progressive and interlaced video sources. It is expected that most MPEG-2 implementations will at least conform to the MAIN profile at MAIN level, which supports nonscalable coding of digital video with approximately digital TV parameters—a maximum sample density of 720 samples per line and 576 lines per frame, a maximum frame rate of 30 frames per second, and a maximum bit rate of 15 Mbit/s.

2.4.1 MPEG-2 Nonscalable Coding Modes

The MPEG-2 algorithm defined in the MAIN profile is a straightforward extension of the MPEG-1 coding scheme to accommodate coding of interlaced video, while retaining the full range of functionality provided by MPEG-1. Identical to the MPEG-1 standard, the MPEG-2 coding algorithm is based on the general hybrid DCT/DPCM coding scheme as outlined in Figure 2.5, incorporating a

Table 2.1 Upper Bound of Parameters
at Each Level of a Profile

Level	Parameters
HIGH	1920 samples/line 1152 lines/frame 60 frames/s 80 Mbit/s
HIGH 1440	1440 samples/line 1152 lines/frame 60 frames/s 60 Mbit/s
MAIN	720 samples/line 576 lines/frame 30 frames/s 15 Mbit/s
LOW	352 samples/line 288 lines/frame 30 frames/s 4 Mbit/s

macroblock structure, motion compensation, and coding modes for conditional replenishment of macroblocks. The concept of I, P, and B pictures as introduced in Figure 2.8 is fully retained in MPEG-2 to achieve efficient motion prediction and to assist random access functionality. Notice that the algorithm defined with the MPEG-2 SIMPLE profile is basically identical to the one in the MAIN profile, except that no B-picture prediction modes are allowed at the encoder. Thus the additional implementation complexity and the additional frame stores necessary for the decoding of B pictures are not required for MPEG-2 decoders conforming only to the SIMPLE profile.

2.4.1.1 Field and Frame Pictures. MPEG-2 has introduced the concept of frame pictures and field pictures along with particular frame prediction and field prediction modes to accommodate coding of progressive and interlaced video. For interlaced sequences it is assumed that the coder input consists of a series of odd (top) and even (bottom) fields that are separated in time by a field period. Two fields of a frame may be coded separately (field pictures, see Figure 2.9). In this case each field is separated into adjacent nonoverlapping macroblocks and the DCT is applied on a field basis. Alternatively, two fields may be coded together as a frame (frame pictures),in a manner similar to conventional coding of progressive video sequences. Here, consecutive lines of top and bottom fields are

Table 2.2   Algorithms and Functionalities Supported With Each Profile

Profile	Algorithms
HIGH	Supports all functionality provided by the spatial scalable profile plus the provision to support: 3 layers with the SNR and spatial scalable coding modes 4:2:2 *YUV* –representation for improved quality requirements
SPATIAL scalable	Supports all functionality provided by the SNR scalable profile plus an algorithm for Spatial scalable coding (2 layers allowed) 4:0:0 *YUV* representation
SNR scalable	Supports all functionality provided by the MAIN profile plus an algorithm for SNR scalable coding (2 layers allowed) 4:2:0 *YUV* representation
MAIN	Nonscalable coding algorithm supporting functionality for Coding interlaced video Random access B-picture prediction modes 4:2:0 *YUV* representation
SIMPLE	Includes all functionality provided by the MAIN profile and offers an Algorithm for modes but does not support B-picture prediction 4:2:0 *YUV* representation

simply merged to form a frame. Notice that both frame pictures and field pictures can be used in a single video sequence.

2.4.1.2   Field and Frame Prediction.   New motion-compensated field prediction modes were introduced by MPEG-2 to efficiently encode field pictures and frame pictures. An example of this new concept is illustrated in Figure 2.9 for an interlaced video sequence, here assumed to contain only three field pictures and no B pictures. In field prediction, predictions are made independently for each field by using data from one or more previously decoded fields: that is, for a top field a prediction may be obtained from either a previously decoded top field (by means of motion-compensated prediction) or from the previously decoded bottom field belonging to the same picture. Generally the inter field prediction from the decoded field in the same picture is prefered if no motion occurs between fields. An indication of which reference field is used for prediction is transmitted with the bitstream. Within a field picture, all predictions are field predictions.

Frame prediction forms a prediction for a frame picture based on one or

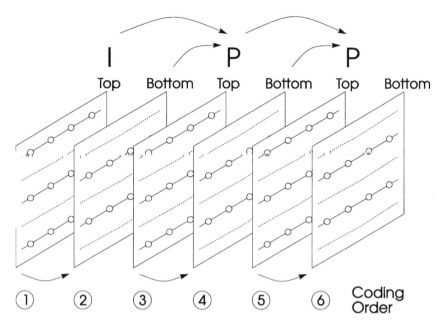

Figure 2.9   The concept of field pictures and an example of possible field prediction. The top fields and the bottom fields are coded separately. However, each
bottom field is coded by means of motion-compensated inter field prediction
based on the previously coded top field. The top fields are coded by means of
motion-compensated inter field prediction based on either the previously coded
top field or the previously coded bottom field. This concept can be extended to
incorporate B pictures.

more previously decoded frames. In a frame picture either field or frame predictions may be used, and the particular prediction mode preferred can be selected
on a macroblock-by-macroblock basis. It must be understood, however, that the
fields and frames from which predictions are made may themselves have been
decoded as either field or frame pictures.

  MPEG-2 has introduced new motion compensation modes to efficiently
explore temporal redundancies between fields, namely the "dual-prime" prediction and the motion compensation based on 16×8 blocks (6). A discussion of
these methods is beyond the scope of this chapter.

2.4.1.3 Chrominance Formats.   MPEG-2 has specified additional $Y{:}U{:}V$
luminance and chrominance subsampling ratio formats to assist and foster applications with the highest video quality requirements. Next to the 4:2:0 format al-

ready supported by MPEG-1, the specification of MPEG-2 is extended to 4:2:2 formats suitable for studio video coding applications.

2.4.2 MPEG-2 Scalable Coding Extensions

The scalability tools standardized by MPEG-2 support applications beyond those addressed by the basic MAIN profile coding algorithm. The intention of scalable coding is to provide interoperability between different services and to flexibly support receivers with different display capabilities. Receivers not either capable or willing to reconstruct the full-resolution video can decode subsets of the layered bitstream to display video at lower spatial or temporal resolution or with lower quality. Another important purpose of scalable coding is to provide a layered video bitstream that is amenable for prioritized transmission. The main challenge here is to reliably deliver video signals in the presence of channel errors, such as cell loss in ATM-based transmission networks or cochannel interference in terrestrial digital broadcasting.

Flexibly supporting multiple resolutions is of particular interest for interworking between high-definition and standard definition television (HDTV and SDTV), in which case it is important for the HDTV receiver to be compatible with the SDTV product. Compatibility can be achieved by means of scalable coding of the HDTV source, and the wasteful transmission of two independent bitstreams to the HDTV and SDTV receivers can be avoided. Other important applications for scalable coding include video database browsing and multiresolution playback of video in multimedia environments.

Figure 2.10 depicts the general philosophy of a multiscale video coding scheme. Here two layers are provided, and each supports video at a different

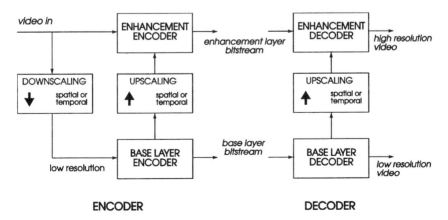

Figure 2.10   Scalable coding of video.

scale; that is, a multiresolution representation can be achieved by downscaling the input video signal into a lower resolution video (downsampling spatially or temporally). The downscaled version is encoded into a base layer bitstream with reduced bit rate. The upscaled reconstructed base layer video (upsampled spatially or temporally) is used as a prediction for the coding of the original input video signal. The prediction error is encoded into an enhancement layer bitstream. If a receiver is not either able or willing to display the full quality video, a downscaled video signal can be reconstructed by decoding only the base layer bitstream. It is important to notice, however, that the display of the video at highest resolution with reduced quality is also possible if only the lower bit rate base layer is decoded. Thus scalable coding can be used to encode video with a suitable bit rate allocated to each layer to meet specific bandwidth requirements of transmission channels or storage media. Browsing through video databases and transmission of video over heterogeneous networks are applications expected to benefit from this functionality.

During the MPEG-2 standardization phase it was found impossible to develop one generic scalable coding scheme capable of suiting all the diverse applications requirements envisaged. While some applications are constricted to low implementation complexity, others call for very high coding efficiency. As a consequence, MPEG-2 has standardized three scalable coding schemes: SNR (quality) scalability, spatial scalability, and temporal scalability, each of which is targeted to assist applications with particular requirements. The scalability tools provide algorithmic extensions to the nonscalable scheme defined in the MAIN profile. It is possible to combine different scalability tools into a hybrid coding scheme. That is, interoperability between services with different spatial resolutions and frame rates can be supported by means of combining the spatial scalability and the temporal scalability tools into a hybrid layered coding scheme. Interoperability between HDTV and SDTV services can be provided *along* with a certain resilience to channel errors by combining the spatial scalability extensions with the SNR scalability tool (8). The MPEG-2 syntax supports up to three different scalable layers.

2.4.2.1 SNR Scalability.

This tool has been primarily developed to provide graceful degradation (quality scalability) of the video quality in prioritized transmission media. If the base layer can be protected from transmission errors, a version of the video with gracefully reduced quality can be obtained by decoding the base layer signal only. The algorithm used to achieve graceful degradation is based on a frequency (DCT domain) scalability technique (6). Both layers in Figure 2.10 encode the video signal at the same spatial resolution. At the base layer, the DCT coefficients are coarsely quantized to achieve moderate image quality at reduced bit rate. The enhancement layer encodes the difference between the nonquantized DCT coefficients and the quantized coefficients from the base layer with finer quantization step size. The method is implemented as a simple and straightforward extension to the MAIN profile MPEG-2 coder and achieves excellent coding efficiency.

It is also possible to use this method to obtain video with lower spatial resolution at the receiver. If the decoder selects the lowest $N \times N$ DCT coefficients from the base layer bitstream, nonstandard inverse DCTs of size $N \times N$ can be used to reconstruct the video at reduced spatial resolution (9,10). Depending on the encoder and decoder implementations, however, the lowest layer downscaled video may be subject to drift (11).

2.4.2.2 **Spatial Scalability.** This tool was developed to support displays with different spatial resolutions at the receiver - lower spatial resolution video can be reconstructed from the base layer. The functionality is useful for many applications including embedded coding for HDTV/TV systems, allowing a migration from a digital TV service to higher spatial resolution HDTV services (6,7,12). The algorithm is based on a classical pyramidal approach for progressive image coding (13,14). Spatial scalability can flexibly support a wide range of spatial resolutions but adds considerable implementation complexity to the MAIN profile coding scheme.

2.4.2.3 **Temporal Scalability.** This tool was developed with an aim similar to that of spatial scalability—steroscopic video can be supported with a layered bitstream suitable for receivers with stereoscopic display capabilities. Layering is achieved by providing a prediction of one of the images of the stereoscopic video (i.e., left view) in the enhancement layer based on coded images from the opposite view transmitted in the base layer.

2.4.2.4 **Data Partitioning.** An additional tool is intended to assist with error concealment in the presence of transmission or channel errors in ATM, terrestrial broadcasting or magnetic recording environments. Because data partitioning can be entirely used as a postprocessing and preprocessing tool in connection with any single layer coding scheme, it has not been formally standardized with MPEG-2 but is referenced in the informative Annex of the MPEG-2 draft document (6). Similar to the SNR scalability tool, the algorithm is based on the separation of DCT coefficients and is implemented with very low complexity compared to the other scalable coding schemes. To provide error protection, the coded DCT coefficients in the bitstream are simply separated and transmitted in two layers that differ in error likelihood.

2.5 MPEG-4 - A STANDARD FOR MULTIMEDIA APPLICATIONS

Anticipating the rapid convergence of the telecommunications, computer, and TV/film industries, the MPEG group officially initiated a new MPEG-4 standardization phase in 1994, with the mandate to standardize algorithms and tools for coding and flexible representation of audiovisual data to meet the challenges of future multimedia applications and applications environments (15,16). In particular MPEG-4 addresses the need for the following:

> *Universal accessibility and robustness in error prone environments.* Multimedia audiovisual data need to be transmitted and accessed in heterogeneous network environments, possibly under severe error conditions (e.g., mobile channels). Although the MPEG-4 standards will be network (physical layer) independent, the algorithms and tools for coding audiovisual data were designed with awareness of network peculiarities.
>
> *High interactive functionality.* Future multimedia applications will call for extended interactive functionalities to assist the user's needs. In particular the flexible, highly interactive access to and manipulation of audiovisual data will be of prime importance. In addition to conventional playback of audio and video sequences, MPEG-4 supports enhanced interactivity to access "content" of audiovisual data with a view to presenting and manipulating/storing the data in a highly flexible way.
>
> *Coding of natural and synthetic data.* Next-generation graphics processors will enable multimedia terminals to present pixel-based audio and video data together with synthetic audio/speech and video in a highly flexible way. MPEG-4 assists the efficient and flexible coding and representation of natural (pixel-based) as well as synthetic data.
>
> *Compression efficiency.* The storage and transmission of audiovisual data requires a high coding efficiency, meaning a good quality of the reconstructed data. Improved coding efficiency, in particular at very low bit rates (<64 kbit/s,) was an important functionality to be supported by the MPEG-4 video standard.

Bit rates targeted for the MPEG-4 video standard are between 5 and 64 kbit/s for mobile or PSTN video applications (17), up to 4 Mbit/s for TV/film broadcast applications, and up to 100 Mbit/s and more for SDTV/HDTV studio applications.

Seven new (with respect to existing or emerging standards) key video coding functionalities have been defined which support the MPEG-4 focus and provided the main requirements for MPEG-4 (16). The requirements cover the main topics related to "Content-Based Interactivity," "Compression," and "Universal Access." The first specification of MPEG-4 was adopted by the ISO in July 1999.

2.5.1 Content-Based Interactivity

In addition to standard MPEG-1- or MPEG-2-like provisions for efficient coding of conventional image or audio sequences, MPEG-4 enables an efficient coded representation of the audio and video data that can be "content based," with the aim of using and presenting the data in a highly flexible way (15,16). In particular MPEG-4 allows the access and manipulation of audiovisual objects in the compressed domain at the coded data level, to assist future multimedia database access applications such as the flexible presentation of image or audio content in the World-Wide Web, computer games, and related applications.

2.5.1.1 Video. The basic concept of the MPEG-4 "content-based" functionality for image/video applications is illustrated in Figure 2.11 for a simple example of an image scene containing a number of video objects: here, the background, several items, and a text overlay. The attempt is to encode the sequence in a way that will allow the user to accomplish the separate decoding and reconstruction of the objects—to assist the presentation and manipulation of the original scene in a flexible way.

The MPEG-4 video coding standard provides an "object-layered" bitstream to assist this functionality. Each object is coded into a separate object bitstream layer. The shape and transparency of the object—as well as the spatial coordinates and additional parameters describing scales and location, such as object zoom, rotation, and translation—are included in the bitstream. The user can either reconstruct the original sequence in its entirety, by decoding all "object layers" and displaying the objects at original sizes and scales and at the original location, as indicated in Figure 2.11A. Alternatively it is possible to manipulate the image sequence by simple operations. For example, in Figure 2.11B some objects were not decoded and used for reconstruction, while others were decoded and displayed subsequently by means of scaling, rotation, or translation.

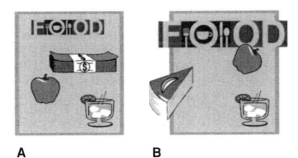

A   B

Figure 2.11 Example of (A) original decoded flexible content-based access and (B) decoded and manipulated objects in MPEG-4 image sequences.

The scaling, rotation, and translation parameters employed for manipulation of the image sequence can be altered in the bitstream by means of simple bitstream editing operations, without the need for further transcoding. In addition, new objects that did not belong to the original scene can be included, or original objects may be neglected. Since the bitstream of the sequence is organized in an "object-layered" form, the inclusion or deletion of objects in the image sequence is performed on the bitstream level by adding/deleting the appropriate object bitstreams—again, without the need for further transcoding.

MPEG-4 can also provide to the user the different video objects with various scales of quality, size, or frame rates to assist the flexible presentation of the data.

2.5.1.2 SNHC. MPEG-4 enables the foregoing capabilities for synthetic (S) and natural (N) audiovisual objects as well as for hybrid (H) coding (C) and representation of natural and synthetic objects. For example, it is possible to allow the coding and generation of text overlays based on graphics primitives. This greatly reduces the number of bits needed to store and transmit text and allows a high degree of flexibility for representing or altering text—for example, it is possible to select various type fonts and sizes for display in Figure 2.11. Other functionalities supported are the efficient coding of computer-animated, texture-mapped wire-grid faces and human bodies.

2.5.2 The MPEG-4 Video Coding Standard

The MPEG-4 video coding algorithms support all functionalities already provided by MPEG-1 and MPEG-2, including the provision to efficiently compress standard rectangular image sequences at varying levels of input formats, frame rates, and bit rates. In addition the content-based functionalities will be assisted. Powerful error resilience functionalities are provided to support streaming and delivery of excellent quality video in error-prone environments, such as over second- and third-generation mobile systems.

A basic classification of the bit rates and functionalities suported by the MPEG-4 video coding algorithm is depicted in Figure 2.12, with the attempt to clusters bit-rate levels versus sets of functionalities and basic applications profiles. At the bottom end a "VLBV core" (VLBV: very low bit rate video) provides algorithms and tools for applications operating at bit rates between 5 and 64 kbit/s, supporting image sequences with lower spatial resolutions (from a few pixels per lines and rows up to CIF resolution) and lower frame rates (ranging from 0 Hz for still images to 15 Hz). The basic application-specific functionalities supported by the VLBV core include (a) conventional VLBV coding of rectangular image sequences with high coding efficiency and high error ro-

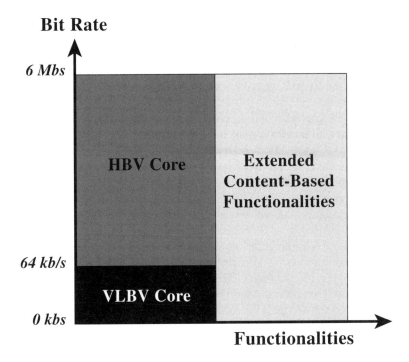

Figure 2.12   Structure of the MPEG-4 video coding standard.

bustness/resilience, low latency, and low complexity for real-time multimedia communications applications, and (b) provisions for "random access" and "fast/forward" and "fast/reverse operations for multimedia database storage and access applications.

The same basic functionalities outlined above are also supported by a higher bit rate video core (HBV core: to bit rates probably around 4–6 Mbit/s) with a higher range of spatial and temporal input parameters up to R.601 resolutions, employing algorithms and tools identical to those for the VLBV core. The reader is referred to References 16 and 17 for a more detailed description of the techniques for the VLBV and HBV cores.

At the heart of the additional "content-based" functionalities is the support for the separate encoding and decoding of content (i.e., physical objects in a scene) as already discussed in connection with Figure 2.11. Within the context of MPEG-4 this functionality—the ability to identify and selectively decode and reconstruct video content of interest—is referred to as "content-based scalability." This MPEG-4 feature provides the most elementary mechanism for interactivity and manipulation with/of content of images or video in the compressed domain without the need for further segmentation or transcoding at the receiver. The extended MPEG-4 algorithms and tools for content-based functionalities can be seen as a superset of the VLBV and HBV cores; thus the tools provided by the VLBV and HBV cores are complemented with additional elements (17).

To enable the content-based interactive functionalities envisioned, the MPEG-4 video standard introduces the concept of video object planes (VOPs), a concept illustrated in Figure 2.13. It is assumed that each frame of an input video sequence is segmented into a number of arbitrarily shaped image regions (video object planes), and each of the regions may possibly cover particular image or video content of interest (i.e., may describe physical objects or content within scenes). In contrast to the video source format used for the MPEG-1 and MPEG-2 standards, the video input to be coded by the MPEG-4 standard is thus no longer considered to be a rectangular region. The input to be coded can be a VOP image region of arbitrary shape, and the shape and location of the region can vary from frame to frame. Successive VOPs belonging to the same physical object in a scene are referred to as video objects (VOs)—a sequence of VOPs of possibly arbitrary shape and position. The shape, motion, and texture information of the VOPs belonging to the same VO is encoded and transmitted or coded into a separate VOL (video object layer). In addition, the bitstream includes relevant information needed to identify each of the VOLs and to discern how the various VOLs are composed at the receiver to reconstruct the entire original sequence. This allows the separate decoding of each VOP and the required flexible manipulation of the video sequence, as indicated in Figures 2.11 and 2.13. Notice that the video source input assumed for the VOL structure either already exists in terms of separate entities (i.e., is generated with chromakey technology) or is generated by means of online or offline segmentation algorithms (18–20).

Notice that MPEG-4 images as well as image sequences are in general considered to be arbitrarily shaped—in contrast to the standard MPEG-1 and MPEG-2 definitions, which encode rectangular image sequences. The MPEG-4 content-based approach can be seen as a logical extension of the conventional MPEG-4 VLBV and HBV core coding approach to image input sequences of arbitrary shape. In particular, if the original input image sequences are not decomposed into several VOLs of arbitrary shape, the coding structure simply degenerates into a single-layer representation, which supports coding of conventional image sequences of rectangular shape.

As illustrated in Figure 2.14, the MPEG-4 video standard supports the coding of rectangular image sequences similar to conventional MPEG-1/2 as well as ITU H.263 baseline coding approaches and involves motion prediction/compensation followed by DCT-based texture coding (21). For the content-based functionalities, where the image sequence input is of arbitrary

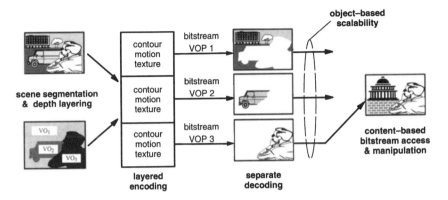

Figure 2.13 The "object-layered" coding approach taken by the MPEG-4 video coding standard.

MPEG-4 VLBV Core Coder

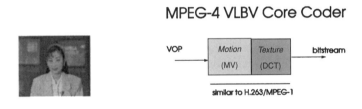

Extended MPEG-4 Coder

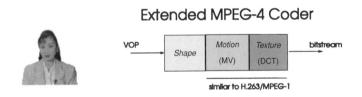

Figure 2.14 MPEG-4 VLBV core and the extended core coder.

shape and location, this approach is extended by also coding shape and transparency information.

2.5.3 The MPEG-4 Sprite Coding Technology

A number of tools that have been standardized within the MPEG-4 video framework attempt to provide higher quality than is available from MPEG-1 and

MPEG-2 as well as additional content-based functionalities for sequences with restricted content. An interesting example is the MPEG-4 "Sprite" prediction (22–24). Sprite coding allows the efficient transmission of background scenes in which changes in the background content are due mainly to camera motion. Thus a static Sprite may be a large still image (i.e., static and flat background panorama) that is transmitted to the receiver first and then stored in a frame store at both encoder and decoder. The camera parameters are transmitted to the receiver for each frame so that the appropriate part of the scene can be mapped (or warped—including zoom, rotation, and translation within the Sprite image) at the receiver for display.

Suppose that for a given video sequence, the content in a scene can be separated into foreground object(s) and a (static) background Sprite. This may be done offline by analysis of the content of a scene prior to coding. Figure 2.15 illustrates the Sprite (background) generation for a video sequence of a tennis match, characterized by high camera motion and texture. One tennis player is moving in front of a background scene. Starting from frame 1, through successive image analysis and with the help of the camera motion, the final Sprite background image is derived in frame 200. Notice that the Sprite generation is not standardized, since it can be seen as a postprocessing tool.

The MPEG-4 Sprite coding technology can be used to code the foreground content and transmit it separately from the receiver. If the background is static, only one frame needs to be transmitted at the beginning of a scene (i.e., frame 200 in Figure 2.15), plus the camera parameters. The receiver composes the separately transmitted foreground and background to reconstruct the original scene. Figure 2.16 illustrates this concept using the example introduced in Figure 2.15. The foreground object tennis player is coded separately from the background as an object of arbitrary shape. The background (Figure 2.16, right) is reconstructed from the Sprite background image in Figure 2.15 stored at the decoder. Only eight motion parameters were transmitted to the receiver to indicate which part of the Sprite is being used under what kind of perspective transformation. Only a few bits are spent for the background information.

The coding gain using the MPEG-4 Sprite technology over existing compression technology appears to be substantial in the foregoing example (depicted in Figure 2.17). Notice, however, that the technique described cannot be seen as a tool that is easily applied to generic scene content. The gain described above can be achieved only if substantial parts of a scene contain regions in which motion is described by simple motion models—and if these regions can be extracted from the remaining parts of the scene by means of image analysis and preprocessing. This certainly is an assumption that can be considered feasible to improve video quality for multimedia database applications, but most certainly not for broadcast applications, where online processing and coding remains a necessity.

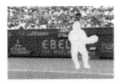

frame 1

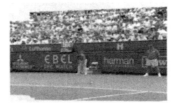

frame 50

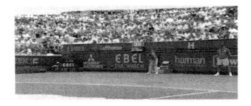

frame 100

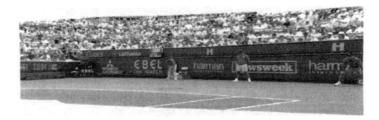

frame 200

Figure 2.15 Sprite background generation.

foreground
flexible 2D—object
with coherent motion

background
rigid 3D—backgound
with global camera motion

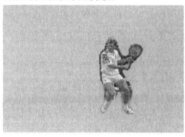
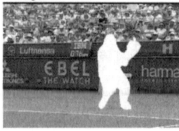

SA—DCT: 12,000 bit/frame
motion: 200 bit/frame
contour: 500 bit/frame

SA—DCT: 7000 bit/frame
motion: 140 bit/frame

=> ca. 320 kbit/s

=> ca. 180 kbit/s

Figure 2.16 Foreground tennis player and background Sprite coded separately.

2.6 ROBUST TRANSMISSION OF MPEG VIDEO IN ERROR-PRONE ENVIRONMENTS

Transmission of compressed video over networks with nonguaranteed quality of service provides many challenges. Efficient video compression algorithms today explore temporal redundancies between images (using predictive coding with motion compensation) to achieve high compression ratios. While on the one hand motion-predictive coding ensures high compression, it also makes the reconstruction at the decoder particularly sensitive to errors introduced during storage or transmission. Even a single bit error or packet loss introduced in a bitstream can result in artifacts visible in the particular reconstructed image (i.e., for video coded in IPPPPP . . . PPI frame mode). Because of the predictive nature of video, this error may propagate over multiple successive P frames until the next intraframe update occurs.

MPEG video compression algorithms were designed with due consideration of error robustness and errors resilience aspects. In particular, the MPEG-2 and MPEG-4 standards define specific error resilience modes that can be used to minimize propagation and reconstruction artifacts of bit or packet errors. The reader is referred to Chapter 8 for a detailed treatment of the topic. Here we outline the basic MPEG modes that address error robustness.

The provisions for error resilience in video coding usually consist of the following aspects.

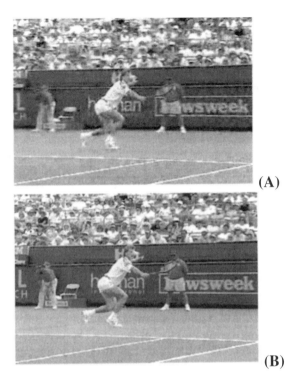

(A)

(B)

Figure 2.17 Sequence coded by means of MPEG-1 (A) and MPEG-4 with Sprite technology (B) at approximately 1 Mbit/s.

Error Detection. To minimize the effects of even a single bit error, it is important to detect quickly that an error has occurred and immediately take steps to prevent degradation of video quality.

Resynchronization. When synchronization between encoder and decoder is lost with the arriving bitstream, the decoder will need to identify the next unique synchronization codeword in the bitstream. MPEG provides unique start codes at various levels of the bitstream (e.g., group-of-pictures start codes, frame start codes, MB-slice start codes) that can be used for such purposes.

Data Recovery. When error detection has occurred and unique start codes are found, encoder and decoder can be resynchronized. It is then desirable to recover as much information as possible from the bitstream (i.e., between the point of loss of synchronization and the point at which resynchronization was regained). For the MPEG-4 standard this is possible by using VLC tables that can be decoded in reversed order.

Concealment. Finally, the impact of any data loss that occurred as a result of errors may be concealed by using correctly decoded information from the same or previous (or future) frames. MPEG coding algorithms provide modes that assist concealment explicitly.

Figures 2.18 and 2.19 illustrate how errors in frames can be concealed. Usually either single MBs or consecutive groups of MBs are corrupted by errors in the transmission path, and no correct information about their content is available to the receiver. However, since MBs in adjacent spatial or temporal locations usually are similar in content, common strategies involve the block replacement of lost content from neighboring MBs. Figure 2.18 depicts spatial interpolation in which the content of the lost MB is concealed with an interpolation of content from blocks above and below. This technique is suitable for I frames that mark the beginning of a video shot. Figure 2.19 illustrates the use of temporal predictive concealment from nearby frames. Lost MBs are either replaced by MBs in the same location in the previous (I, P, or B frame) or from a future (B) frame, or replaced by a motion-compensated prediction of MBs from these frames.

Table 2.3 summarizes MPEG modes that improve robustness of MPEG video in error-prone environments—and help in detecting, synchronizing, and recovering content. The modes are discussed in more detail in the subsections that follow.

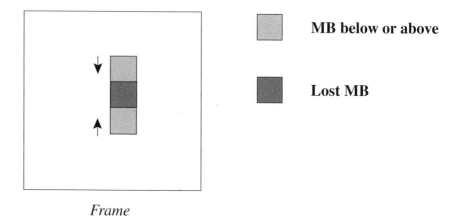

Frame

Figure 2.18   Concealment of a macroblock by means of a spatial concealment technique. Content of a lost MB is concealed by using content from the MB above or below (or both).

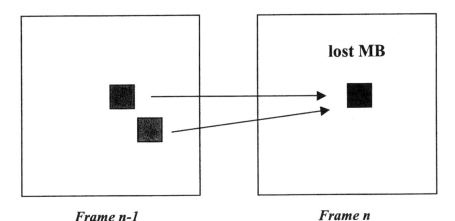

Frame n-1   *Frame n*

Figure 2.19 Temporal concealment: content of a lost MB in frame n is concealed with content from a MB in frame $n-1$. The content of the MB in the same location in frame $n-1$ can be used to replace the lost MB in frame n (suitable for low motion between frames). Alternatively motion vectors in frame n or $n-1$ can be used to perform motion-compensated concealment.

Table 2.3 Error Resilience Modes in MPEG Video Algorithms

	Algorithm[a]		
Error resilience	MPEG-1	MPEG-2	MPEG-4
I-frame update	X	X	X
Intra-MB update	X	X	X
Intra-coded slices			
B-frames	X	X	X
Adaptive MB resynchronization	X	X	X
Layered coding		X	X
Data partitioning		X	X
Separate motion and shape and texture modes		X	
Reversible variable-length codes		X	
Intra-frame motion vectors		X	

[a]X, ; x,

2.6.1   Intra Frame and Intra MB Update

One significant effect of bit or packet errors in video-coded streams is error propagation. In MPEG-coded video streams, this propagation of errors can be restricted to a (suitable) number of successive frames by coding periodically every Nth frame (usually $N = 12$) as an I frame (i.e, I P P P P P P P P P P P I P P . . .). MPEG also allows any arbitrary frame to be coded as an I frame, which provides high flexibility for error resilience purposes. Since I frames usually contain more bits than P or B frames, error robustness is achieved at the expense of reduced compression efficiency.

Alternatively it is possible to encode any MB in a frame as an intra MB (coded without prediction of past or previous frames). This allows periodical or arbitrary intra refresh of MBs instead of full I-frame coding for the same purpose.

2.6.2   B Frames

Coding MPEG video with B frames is particularly suitable in error-prone environments. As discussed above, B frames are not used for predicting content of other frames. Thus errors in B frames will not propagate to other frames, rather artifacts in B frames are visible only for the particular time period of the B frame. That is, coding a sequence in mode I B B P B B P B B P B B I B B P . . . will result in periodic I-frame refresh every 12th frame—and only one-quarter of the frames will be sensitive to error propagation.

A further advantage of B frames is that they usually improve compression efficiency, even in comparison to P frames. Disadvantages are increased coder and decoder complexity as well as increased end-to-end delay (which may be a problem for conversational services, such as videotelephony).

2.6.3   Adaptive MB Resynchronization

MPEG-adaptive MB resynchronization markers provide suitable entities for desynchronizing at various spatial locations in frames. This is particularly of interest if important parts in images are known and must be protected with priority. Figure 2.20 outlines the general MPEG MB syntax for groups of MBs. A header (including resynchronization marker) allows unique identification of the group of MBs. The following bits contain quantization and coding data for each coded block (DCT coefficients, motion vectors, etc.).

Figure 2.21 depicts how resynchronization markers can be allocated by MPEG-1/2 and MPEG-4 standards. While for MPEG-1/2 a marker must always start at the beginning of a row of MBs, MPEG-4 allows flexibility to position markers anywhere in a frame; also, the length of a group of MBs can be between

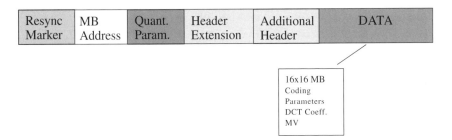

Figure 2.20   General MPEG MB syntax for groups of MBs.

one MB and the total sum of MBs in a frame (one group of MBs per frame). These features provide all the flexibility required to balance high compression efficiency (few markers, fewer bits to code) with high error robustness (many markers, considerable overhead, particularly for low bit rate applications). For the example in Figure 2.21, most of the image content is concentrated at the object. The adaptive MPEG-4 marker approach allows generation of a bitstream that contains markers separated by approximately equal distances in the bitstream (i.e., to suit the size of a video packet for ATM or mobile transmission).

2.6.4   Layered Coding and Data Partitioning: Separate Motion and Texture and Shape Data

Layered coding of video and data partitioning are techniques that aim at separating bits in the bitstream for separate transmission. If a transmission system allows prioritized error protection, the most important information can be transmitted in a separate bitstream layer—and reconstructed with good or even perfect quality. Much interest in the past focused on transmission of MPEG-2 video over ATM networks with two priority levels, the most important information being transmitted with guaranteed quality of service. The residual information is received with a certain error rate and used for improving video quality whenever possible. Similar philosophies are being investigated in the context of mobile transmission systems (see Chapter 8).

MPEG-2 specifies spatial and temporal scalability coding techniques (see above) that can be employed for such purposes. The use of MPEG-2 and MPEG-4 spatial scalability allows the transmission of the base layer (which contains a low spatial resolution or low frequency representation of the video signal) with high priority. The residual information is transmitted in a separate bitstream with lower priority and contains residual information that allows the reconstruction of the video signal with higher spatial resolution or more high-frequency details. The temporal scalability coding technique enables the coding of a base layer

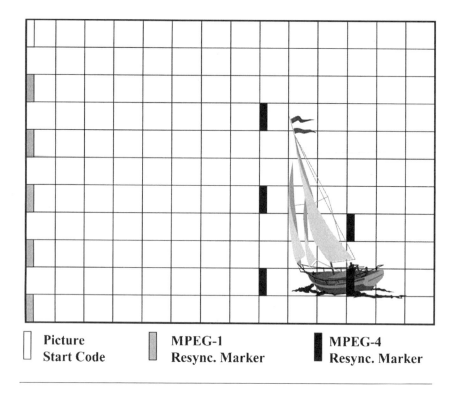

| Picture Start Code | MPEG-1 Resync. Marker | MPEG-4 Resync. Marker |

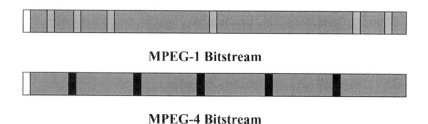

MPEG-1 Bitstream

MPEG-4 Bitstream

Figure 2.21 The MPEG adaptive video packet approach. Resynchronization markers can be allocated flexibly to allow efficient resynchronization after errors have occurred. The MPEG-4 resync markers provide more flexibility for efficient packetization of video.

with reduced temporal resolution, as well as a residual layer with higher temporal resolution details for prioritized transmission. Spatial and temporal scalability techniques can be combined to allow more flexibility for error protection.

The data partitioning approach specified with MPEG-2 is the simplest layered coding technique and is particularly suited for prioritized transmission of video. Data partitioning allows the transmission of the low-frequency DCT coefficients in a base layer and the remaining coefficients in an enhancement layer. If the base layer is sufficiently protected from bit errors or packet loss, excellent error protection is achieved.

In MPEG-4 the data partitioning approach allows the separation of motion and texture data (and additionally the shape data if required) for prioritized transmission of each coded frame. For mobile applications in particular, this can provide excellent protection against transmission errors (see Chapter 8).

2.6.5 Reversible Variable-Length Codes

MPEG-4 reversible variable-length codes provide an excellent means for recovering data in a bitstream. Reversible VLCs can be decoded in reversed order, which allows backward coding of a bitstream. Figure 2.22 illustrates this concept. Usually, when errors occur soon after a resynchronization marker, most of the MBs contained in the group of MBs are lost and cannot be recovered (large areas in an image may be lost). Reversible VLCs allow backward decoding of MBs right to the point at which the error occurred, thus reconstructing much valuable data in many circumstances (see Chapter 8).

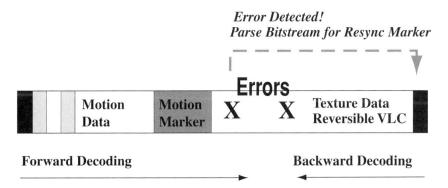

Figure 2.22 Example of data recovery by using backward decoding with reversible VLCs. After an error has been detected, the bitstream is parsed to find the next resynchronization marker. Then the bitstream is decoded backward until unvalid (corrupted) data have been identified.

2.6.6 Intra Frame Motion Vectors

Intra frame motion vectors in MPEG-2 allow the transmission of motion vectors also for I frames. The motion vectors are not used for predictive coding but are specified to ease temporal concealment from I frames in a sequence. If MBs in an I frame are lost, the transmitted intra frame motion vectors can be used to replace these MBs by means of temporal concealment (see Figure 2.19).

2.7 DISCUSSION

International standardization in image coding has made a remarkable evolution from a committee-driven process dominated by telecommunication companies and broadcasters to a market-driven process incorporating industries, telecoms, network operators, satellite operators, broadcasters, and research institutes. With this evolution also, the actual work of the standardization bodies has changed considerably and has evolved from discussion circles of national delegations into international collaborative R&D activities. The standardization process has become significantly faster and more efficient and, for the reason that standardization must follow the accelerated speed of technology development. Otherwise standards might become obsolete before they have been agreed upon by the standardization bodies.

It must be understood that video coding standards necessarily rely on compromises between what is theoretically possible and what is technologically feasible. Standards can be successful in the marketplace only if the cost–performance ratio is well balanced. This is specifically true in the field of image and video coding, where a large variety of innovative coding algorithms exist but may be too complex for implementation with state-of-the-art VLSI technology.

In this respect the MPEG-1 standard provides efficient compression for a large variety of multimedia terminals, affording additional flexibility for random access of video from storage media and supporting a diversity of image source formats. A number of MPEG-1 encoder and decoder chip sets from different vendors are currently available on the market. Encoder and decoder PC boards have been developed from MPEG-1 chip sets. A number of commercial products use the MPEG-1 coding algorithm for interactive CD applications, such as the CD-I product. Software decoding of MPEG-1 video is becoming more and more widespread, with applications in domains like storing and streaming of video on the Internet as well as on desktop PCs.

The MPEG-2 standard is becoming more and more successful because there is a strong commitment from industries, cable and satellite operators, and broadcasters to use this standard. Digital TV broadcasting, pay TV, pay-per-view, video-on-demand, interactive TV, video on DVD and many other future video services are the applications envisaged and to a large extent already on the market. Many MPEG-2 MAIN profile at MAIN level decoder prototype chips are already developed. Single-chip HDTV decoder implementations for MPEG-2 video have been demonstrated.

The world-wide acceptance of MPEG-2 in consumer electronics already has led to large-scale production, making MPEG-2 decoder equipment cheap and therefore also attractive for other related areas, such as video communications and storage and multimedia applications in general.

The scope and potential of the MPEG-4 standard was discussed in the context of future audiovisual multimedia communications environments. The MPEG-4 standard provides tools and algorithms for coding both natural and synthetic video, audio, and speech data, as well as provisions to represent the data at the user's terminal in a highly flexible way. Given the excellent performance at low bit rates and the extraordinary error resilience capabilities of MPEG-4 video, it is expected that the MPEG-4 standard will make a strong initial impact on the Internet, as well as for streaming video over mobile channels. First commercial mass products such as Webcams with real-time MPEG-4 video coders (see Reference 25) have already been introduced to the market. MPEG-4 video software players are supported in standard PC Windows software to allow playback of MPEG-4 video for various applications.

REFERENCES

1. W Chen, and D Hein, Motion compensated DXC system. In Proceedings of 1986 Picture Coding Symposium, Tokyo, April 1986, Vol 2–4, pp 76–77.
2. BR Halhed. Videoconferencing codecs: Navigating the MAZE. Bus Commun Rev, 21, No.(1): 35–40, 1991.
3. R Schäfer, and T Sikora. Digital video coding standards and their role in video communications. Proc IEEE . 83:907–923, 1995.
4. C-F Chen, KK Pang. The optimal transform of motion-compensated frame difference images in a hybrid coder. IEEE Trans. Circuits Syst II: Analog and Digital Signal Processing, September 1963, pp 289–296.
5. N Ahmed, T Natrajan, KR Rao. Discrete cosine transform. IEEE Trans. Comput C-23, (1):90–93, December 1984.
6. ISO/IEC JTC1/SC29/WG11 N0702 Rev. Information technology—Generic coding of moving pictures and associated audio, Recommendation H.262. Draft International Standard, Paris, March 25, 1994.
7. ISO/IEC 11172-2 Information technology—Coding of moving pictures and associated audio for digital storage media at up to about 1.5 Mbit/s—Video. Standards Organization/International Electrotechnical (in German). International Commission, Geneva, 1993.
8. J De Lameillieure, R. Schäfer. MPEG-2 image coding for digital TV. Fernseh Kino Tech 48:99–107, March 1994.

78 Sikora

9. C Gonzales, E Viscito. Flexibly scalable digital video coding. Signal Process Image Commun 5, (1–2), February 1993.
10. T Sikora, TK Tan, K N Ngan. A performance comparison of frequency domain pyramid scalable coding schemes. Proceedings of Picture Coding Symposium, Lausanne, March 1993, pp 16.1–16.2.
11. AW Johnson, T Sikora, TK Tan, KN Ngan. Filters for drift reduction in frequency scalable video coding schemes. Electron Lett 30 (6):471–472, 1994.
12. J De Lameillieure, G Schamel. Hierarchical coding of TV/HDTV within the German HDTVTT project. Proceedings of International Workshop on HDTV, Ottowa, Canada, October 1993, pp 8A.1.1–8A.1.8.
13. A Puri, A Wong. Spatial domain resolution scalable video coding. Proceedings of SPIE Visual Communications and Image Processing, Boston, November 1993.
14. PJ Burt, E Adelson. The Laplacian pyramid as a compact image code. IEEE Trans Commun COM-31:532–540, 1983.
15. L Chiariglione. MPEG and multimedia communications. IEEE Trans Circuits Syst Video Technol 7:5–18, February1997.
16. T Sikora. The MPEG-4 video standard verification model. IEEE Trans Circuits Syst Video Technol 7, (1):19–31, February 1997.
17. T Sikora. MPEG-4 very low bit rate video. Proceedings of IEEE ISCAS Conference, Hong Kong, June 1997.
18. KN Ngan, T Sikora, M-T Sun, eds.Segmentation, description and retrieval of video content. IEEE Trans Circuits Syst Video Technol, special issue, October 1998.
19. KN Ngan, T Sikora, M-T Sun, eds. Representation and coding of images and video. IEEE Trans Circuits Syst Video Technol, special issue, November 1998.
20. AA Alatan, L Onural, M Wollborn, R Mech, E Tuncel and T Sikora. Image sequence analysis for emerging interactive multimedia services—The European COST 211 framework. IEEE Trans Circuits Syst Video Technol 8,(7):797–801, November 1998. special issue on Representation and Coding of Images and Video I.
21. ITU-T Recommendation H.263 Video coding for low bitrate communication.
22. T Sikora, L Chiariglione. MPEG-4 video and its potential for future multimedia services. Proceedings of IEEE ISCAS Conference, Hong Kong, June 1997.
23. M-C Lee, W Chen, CB Lin, C Gu, T Markoc, SI Zabinsky, R Szeliski. A layered video object coding system using Sprite and affine motion model. IEEE Trans Circuits Syst Video Technol 7,(1): 130–145, February 1997.
24. P Kauff, B Makai, S Rauthenberg, U Gölz, JLP DeLameillieure, T Sikora. Functional coding of video using a shape-adaptive DCT algorithm and object-based motion prediction toolbox. IEEE Trans Circuits Syst Video Technol 7(1):81–196, February 1997.
25. T Sikora. MPEG-4 and beyond—When can I watch soccer on ISDN? Proceedings of the Montreux International Television Symposium—Future Technology Forum, Montreux, June 1997.

Part 2
Networks

3
IP Networks

Henning Schulzrinne
*Department of Computer Science and Department of Electrical Engineering,
Columbia University, New York, New York*

3.1 INTRODUCTION

3.1.1 Definition

The Internet is a global collection of autonomously administered packet-switched networks that use the TCP/IP protocols to form a single, virtual network allowing every part to communicate with any other. This chapter provides an overview of the operation of the Internet viewed from the perspective of the rules ("protocols") that govern the exchange of information between elements in the network. For lack of space, we do not cover an equally important aspect, namely, the physical communications infrastructure and how the Internet functions economically and organizationally. Also, we focus on the parts of the Internet architecture that are most relevant to carrying multimedia data and do not discuss protocols used to carry web pages, file transfer, or e-mail, among other more "data"-oriented applications.

The chapter is organized as follows. We begin by describing the role of protocols in the Internet architecture (Section 3.2) and then proceed to summarize the foundational elements of the Internet, several classes of names (Section 3.2.2), and how Internet packets are forwarded from source to destination (Section 3.2.5). Section 3.2.6 discusses the service that the Internet Protocol offers to higher layers, which then leads to a discussion of the current Internet Protocol (Section 3.2.7). Additional transport protocols are covered in Section 3.3.

Given that the two most popular nonnetworked multimedia applications, radio and TV, allow the efficient distribution of content to large groups of receivers, Section 3.4 then focuses on the Internet equivalent, namely, multicast.

The term "quality of service" is generally used to describe predictable network service parameters, sufficient for applications such as audio and video. Sections 3.5 and 3.6 address this areas.

Section 3.7 outlines the overall higher layer architecture for multimedia services, which encompasses protocols for data transport (Section 3.8), control of streaming media (Section 3.9), description of media sessions and capabilities (Section 3.10), initiation and control of sessions (Section 3.11), and the announcement of large-scale radio- and TV-like sessions (Section 3.12).

3.2 INTERNET CONCEPTS AND PROTOCOLS

3.2.1 Terminology

We refer to the algorithms and data structures that describe the interaction of entities as *protocols*. Protocols describe the formats of messages exchanged between elements of the network, the actions taken upon receipt of messages, and the proper way to handle errors. Figure 3.1 shows the Internet protocol hierarchy.

When describing packet networks, it is convenient both to clarify the concepts and to reduce implementation complexity by separating the overall network functionality into *(protocol) layers*. Generally speaking, on the data sender's side, layer N takes blocks of data called *packets** from layer $N + 1$, adds a header, and passes them to layer $N - 1$. The receiver operates in reverse, with layer N taking a packet from layer $N - 1$, stripping it of the layer-N headers, processing the header, and passing the rest to layer $N + 1$. In any layer, a packet thus consists of an initial set of bytes, the *header*, that controls operation of that layer and the remainder of the packet, which is passed unchanged to the next layer, sometimes called the *payload* or simply *data*. Other architectures, such as the ISO Open Systems Interconnection (OSI) (1) or the IBM Systems Network Architecture (SNA) have notions of layering that differ somewhat from the Internet architecture, particularly in the upper layers. Note that the presentation and session layer found in the "classical" seven-layer model (2) do not have general representations in the Internet.

We use "the Internet" (capitalized) to refer to the physical network connecting nodes across the globe and its architecture. The generic term "an internet" (lowercase) describes a system of computer networks that are interconnected but not necessarily publicly accessible. To reduce confusion, it

---

*The first layer above the physical communications layer typically calls these blocks *frames* instead. Sometimes the term derived from the ISO-derived network architecture, *protocol data unit* (PDU) is also used, while application-layer entities are called *messages*.

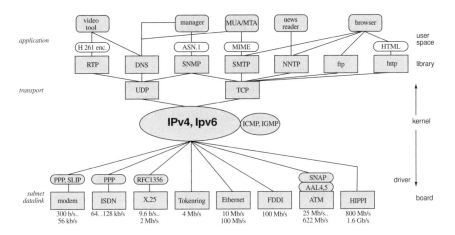

Figure 3.1 The Internet protocol hierarchy.

has become common to use *intranet* to describe an internet that uses the Internet protocols to link networks within an organization.

Within the Internet architecture, the operation of the protocol layers can be roughly defined as follows.

The *physical layer* provides a point-to-point or point-to-multipoint bit transport service over wires, optical fibers, or free space. The description of the physical layer includes electrical or optical characteristics, connectors, and modulation. Common physical layers used within internets include serial lines, wide-area transmission facilities such as those within the time division digital hierarchy (DS-0 through DS-3 running at 56 or 64 kbit/s through 45 Mbit/s), the synchronous digital hierarchy (STS-1 through STS-12, with the integer denoting multiples of about 51 Mbit/s), or the corresponding synchronous optical network (SONET, OC-3 through OC-96) layers. The physical layer sometimes includes *forward error correction,* the addition of redundancy that allows the reconstruction of bits that have been corrupted by the channel.

Within the current Internet, common link speeds range between 14.4 kbit/s and 2.4 Gbit/s, with rates down to 2.4 kbit/s. End-to-end delays can be microseconds in a local network or several hundred milliseconds across a multiple-satellite hop path. Thus, Internet protocols have to operate across six orders of magnitude of speed and delay.

For bit-oriented physical layer technologies that do not have their own link layer, the point-to-point protocol (PPP) is used to delineate groups of bits as packets and to negotiate parameters, such as whether to compress packet headers and payloads.

The *link layer,* or layer 2, provides a point-to-point or point-to-multipoint *packet* service for a relatively small number of nodes. This service may offer the detection of bit errors and sometimes the retransmission of lost or errored packets. The Internet protocols can use just about any link layer, but the most common are the local-area network link layers Ethernet and Tokenring, asynchronous transfer mode (ATM) for both local- and wide-area links, modems (using PPP, see below), and wide-area, point-to-point synchronous links. Some link layers emulate others; for example, there are wireless versions of Ethernet or the ATM LAN emulation mode (LANE).

A network at the link layer (e.g., a single Ethernet) is called a *subnet.* Generally, at the link layer, there is only one path between source and destination, however, some link-layer *switches* for Ethernet and ATM also maintain a map with different paths to destinations and find the shortest one, a process called "routing."

From an Internet viewpoint, link layers are classified into point-to-point, broadcast, and nonbroadcast multiple-access (NBMA) networks. Point-to-point networks have links with only two end points, with most "classical" wide-area links and telephone line modems falling into this category. Broadcast networks can have several nodes attached within the same subnet and allow the sending of a packet simultaneously to all nodes of the network. Ethernet (3), Tokenring, and fiber-distributed data interface (FDDI) (4) are classical examples, with FireWire (IEEE 1394) a more recent addition. (In their original design, broadcast was the natural mode of these networks. In switched versions of these technologies, the switch has to perform the packet replication, but this is invisible to the upper layers.) NBMA networks (5) may have more than two nodes but do not natively support broadcast. ATM and frame relay are the most common examples of NBMA networks.

The *network layer,* or layer 3, carries packets end to end, across multiple subnets. Subnets are connected by *routers,* whose primary function is the forwarding of network-layer packets. A router can connect subnets of the same or different technologies (e.g., a wide-area synchronous link to an Ethernet). The path of packets is determined by *routing protocols.* In the Internet architecture, there is only one network-layer protocol, the Internet Protocol (IP) (6), although there are several versions of this protocol. Version 4 of IP, known as IPv4 or simply IP, is currently used for production traffic on the Internet. Version 6, known as IPv6 or earlier as IPng (7), is being tried out.

The *transport layer,* or layer 4, operates only within the communication end points, the so-called *end systems* or *hosts.* The Internet architecture is built primarily on two transport protocols, User Datagram Protocol (UDP) for unreliable datagram service and the Transmission Control Protocol (TCP) for supplying a reliable, sequenced byte stream service.

Most Internet applications have an additional protocol layer that supports a limited set of applications. Examples of the application layer include SMTP (8) for electronic mail, HTTP (9) for information retrieval in the World-Wide Web, ftp (10) for file transfer, and the Telnet Protocol (11). We discuss application-layer protocols for multimedia transmission and signaling in Section 3.7.

Note that the layering indicated is a rough architecture and is violated quite frequently: layers may recurse; a single layer may contain several protocols; or a protocol may be said to "belong" to more than one layer, depending on one's view of the world. Recursion occurs, for example, when PPP (12), a link-layer protocol, is being run on top of IP as part of so-called layer-two tunneling, with another full protocol stack on top of this. The link layer often has two protocols; for example, ATM has the cell layer and adaptation layer 5 (AAL5). The Real-Time Transport Protocol (RTP) for real time, discussed in Section 3.8, can be viewed either as a second transport-layer protocol on top of UDP or as an application-layer protocol. The media encapsulation within RTP is then either a second transport protocol within RTP or is the actual application protocol. Aside from religious arguments, this distinction is largely unimportant. It matters only in that most applications have to layer on top of either UDP or TCP if they do not want to modify the operating system kernel or standard libraries.

Hosts and routers are collectively referred to as *(network) nodes.* Hosts typically have one network interface and do not forward packets between network interfaces, while routers generally have more than one interface and forward packets between these interfaces. ("Multihomed" hosts have multiple network interfaces, but do not forward packets between them.) Routers implement many of the same upper layer protocols as hosts, such as Telnet for remote access or http for web-based management.

The link layer and the physical layer are largely outside the scope of Internet efforts, except insofar as mechanisms must be defined that describe how the link-layer protocols operate within the Internet architecture. One exception is the point-to-point protocol (PPP) (12), which defines how a continuous bitstream such as provided by a modem or a synchronous optical network (SONET) can be divided into packets.

An *internet* is a collection of packet-switching networks interconnected at the network layer by *routers.*

3.2.2 Names, Addresses, Routes

The Internet follows the terminology of Shoch (1978) (13), who distinguishes *names* that uniquely identify a network object, *addresses* that describe where it is, and *routes* that map a way to reach the object. Binding mechanisms establish a (temporary) equivalence of two names or between a name and an address. In the Internet, we find primarily three types of identifier: link-layer media access control (MAC) addresses, IP addresses, and host names. All three are, with minor (but annoying) exceptions, unique across the Internet. MAC addresses such as Ethernet addresses are 48 bits long, are allocated permanently (typically by the manufacturer of the network interface), and have no naming hierarchy except that network interface card (NIC) vendors assign addresses from blocks delegated to them. An example of a MAC address as commonly written is 8:0:20:72:93:18. In contrast, IP addresses, either 32 bits or 128 bits long, are used for routing, designate network interfaces and are assigned topologically, so that nodes that are within the same subnet or region have IP addresses whose most-significant bits are the same. An example of an IP address, written as four decimal integers, is 132.151.1.35. In many cases, such as dial-up Internet access, a host does not have a permanent Internet address, but rather uses protocols such as the Dynamic Host Configuration Protocol (DHCP) (14) to "lease" a new address each time it is connected to the network. Some organizations that have no packet-level connectivity to the Internet maintain their own private Internet address space, often drawn from address ranges specifically reserved for that purposes. Finally, host names or *domain names* name nodes according to the organization that owns them (see Section 3.2.3).

Protocols exist to map between these three: DNS (Domain Name System) provides a bidirectional mapping between IP addresses and domain names; ARP (Address Resolution Protocol) delivers the MAC addresses belonging to an IP address in a local network; and RARP (Reverse Address Resolution Protocol) maps from MAC addresses back to IP addresses.

3.2.3   The Domain Name System

The most common designation for Internet hosts is the domain name. Since it would not be efficient to have a single entity name several million hosts and track the mapping between domain names and addresses, the naming and mapping are delegated in a multilevel hierarchy. The naming scheme combines both geographical and functional elements. Although the depth of the hierarchy is not limited, the use of two to four levels is most common. A typical naming scheme within larger organizations is *host.suborganization.organization.tld,* such as *mail.cs.columbia.edu.* The most-significant part, labeled "tld" for top-level domain, is either a two-letter country designation (such as "us" for the United States,* "fr" for France, or "jp" for Japan) or a three-letter designation of the type of organization. The three-letter domains are as follow:

.*com:* commercial organizations, independent of geographic location
.*int:* international organizations and entities, such as the ITU

---

*In the United States, the tld "us" is mainly used by state and local governments and their agencies.

.org: nonprofit organizations, mainly in the United States
.net: providers of network-related services (about 46,000)
.edu: U.S. four-year colleges
.mil: U.S. military
.gov: U.S. federal government agencies

A single organization may have the same second-level domain within different top-level domains, such as "att.net" and "att.com." In February 1997, an international advisory panel suggested adding international top-level domains so that organizations whose names are already taken in the crowded .com space can get domain names. This proposal is currently under discussion by the Internet Corporation for Assigned Names and Numbers (ICANN), a new organization responsible for assigning names and numbers in the Internet.

Just as Internet hosts connected to a dial-up Internet service provider typically get only a temporary Internet address (see below), they are assigned a temporary domain name reflecting the dial-in location.

The pseudodomain in-addr.arpa (15) is used to map IP addresses back to domain names. For example, the DNS record 191.19.59.128.in-addr.arpa maps the host with IP address 128.59.19.191 to the host name bart.cs.columbia.edu. This inverse mapping is often used for weak authentication and for providing more descriptive log files.

3.2.4 Internet (IP) Addresses

Internet addresses (also called IP or IPv4 addresses) are currently 32 bits long, to be extended to 128 bits in IPv6. Internet addresses are globally unique (with some local-use exceptions) and are assigned according to topology. They are used for routing and identifying nodes (e.g., for maintaining associations in a transport protocol). IPv4 addresses are usually written as four decimal integers separated by periods, as in 135.1.2.3, while the 128-bit IPv6 addresses are written as eight 16-bit hexadecimal numbers separated by colons and zeros elided (e.g., 1080::::8:800:200C:417A).

Special IPv4 addresses designate the local host (127.0.0.1) itself and broadcast to every host on a local network or a remote network.

It would be unwieldy for every router to maintain a complete list of every host in the Internet: in October 1999 there were 62.3 million. Since IP addresses are assigned topologically, they can be aggregated by exchanging just a common *prefix* of the address. Currently, topology is expressed generally by assigning all customers of a network provider addresses from the same consecutive address range. Aggregation may happen at several levels, so that a router, say, in Chicago, may aggregate all Japanese addresses into one prefix pointing to the West Coast, while the router terminating the transpacific cable may maintain separate routing entries for all the major providers. Routing table entries are matched by longest prefix; that is, a more specific route takes precedence. When describing routing table entries, an n-bit routing prefix is written as "$/n$". In the Internet backbone, n is 22 or smaller.

Traditionally, IP addresses were divided into a network and a host part, with only the network part used for routing within the Internet. The 32-bit address space was divided into "classes," with the division into network and host addresses depending on the address class designated by the first byte, as illustrated in Table 3.1. In addition, segments of address space are set aside for multicast addresses (class D) and reserved for future, unspecified use (class E). (No such use is currently being contemplated.)

The notion of address classes proved to be too rigid, for most organizations fall between needing a class-B and a class-C network. There were too few class-B networks, and assigning several class-C network addresses to each organization would inflate the backbone network routing tables beyond their current size of approximately 50,000. Thus, the current Internet has transitioned to classless interdomain routing (CIDR) (16), where address ranges carry explicit prefix lengths designating the routing-relevant part of the address. A class-C address in the old, "classfull" scheme is equivalent to a/24 address, since 24 bits are used for routing.

The multicast address space, the class-D addresses shown in Table 3.1, are not assigned statically to a particular node, but rather designate groups of receivers within the network, as discussed below (Section 3.4).

As of late 1999, about 45 to 50% of the total available address space below 224.0.0.0 had been assigned, with relatively modest growth in the last few years (17,18).

The IPv4 addressing scheme has a number of architectural problems. If a host moves from one network to another or if a smaller organization changes network providers, the host's IP address changes. Historically, address blocks were given out more or less chronologically, so that despite recent efforts, most IP addresses still cannot be aggregated. Aggregation limits address as-

Table 3.1 Internet Address Classes

Class	Network	Host	First octet	Hosts per network	Nets	Delegated[a]
Class A	8	24	< 128	16×10^6	128	37.5%
Class B	16	16	128 ... 191	65,534	16,384	70.3%
Class C	24	8	192 ... 223	254	2×10^6	65.6%
Class D			224 ... 239		268×10^6	Multicast
Class E			240 ... 255		134×10^6	Reserved

[a] As of October 1999.

signment density, providing the main motivation for the next-generation Internet protocol.

Network nodes that are permanently connected to the Internet (e.g., through a local-area network) are assigned their addresses by the local system administrator from the block of addresses assigned to the subnet. Most computers that utilize dial-up modems to connect to the Internet only "borrow" an address for the duration of their connection by using DHCP (14). This greatly reduces the address space requirement for Internet service providers.

Some organizations also use a range of IP addresses that are not globally unique, drawn from 10.0.0.0/8. Addresses in packets that are exchanged with hosts outside that network are translated to and from a small set of globally unique addresses using a so-called network address (and port) translator (NAT or NAPT) (19). NAPTs are becoming quite common for home networking, for example.

3.2.5 IP Forwarding

Every router and host goes through the same decision process when forwarding a packet received on one of its interfaces or generated by an application, respectively. First, the node checks whether the node named as the IP destination address is attached to the same local network or link by comparing its own network address to that of the packet's recipient. If the proper attachment exists, the node maps the destination address to a link-layer address, using a protocol that depends on the link layer, such as ARP, and sends the packet to that address by wrapping the IP packet in the appropriate link-layer packet. Otherwise, it locates the router along the path to the destination and forwards the packet to that router, again wrapping the IP packet into a link-layer packet, but addressed to the next-hop router.

3.2.6 IP Service Model

The Internet network-layer service model is currently extremely simple: each network packet is logically independent of all others. In other words, no setup of connections (i.e., state shared by routers), is required before data are sent to another network node. This is commonly known as *datagram* or *connectionless* delivery. Packets are transmitted on a best-effort basis; that is, the network makes no guarantees when or indeed whether a packet will arrive at the destination. Packets may also arrive out of order, or they may be duplicated. In IPv4, if a packet is too long for a particular link layer, the network may fragment it into smaller, independent IPv4 packets to be reassembled at the destination. This minimalist service model can be supported by just about any link-layer technology and follows the end-to-end architectural principle (20), but it may make better service available from the lower layers invisible to the Internet applications.

3.2.7 IPv4 Packet Header

Each IP packet consists of a packet header and the *payload* (i.e., the higher layer protocol data). The packet header is at least 20 bytes long, but it may be extended for additional functionality. The complete packet can be up to 65,535 bytes long, including the IP header, most link-layer protocols restrict the maximum packet length to between 1 500 and 8 192 bytes, however, with 1 500 bytes being the most common upper bound. Longer IP packets can be *fragmented* into the maximum transmission unit (MTU) that the link layer can handle. Generally speaking, audio and video applications should not rely on IP-layer fragmentation, since the whole IP packet is lost if one of the fragments does not make it. Thus, fragmentation multiplies the loss probability of the network.

The IPv4 packet header is shown in Figure 3.2. The type-of-service flags govern trade-offs between reliability, throughput, delay, and cost, but are rarely used. [Recently, there has been a great deal of interest in using these bits for providing coarse-grained *differentiated service* classes (21).] Each packet carries an identifier needed for assembling packets from fragments, with fragments indicating their offset into the original packet. The time-to-live (TTL) field limits the number of hops before the packet is discarded. The protocol field indicates the transport protocol the packet needs to be handed to. A simple arithmetic check-

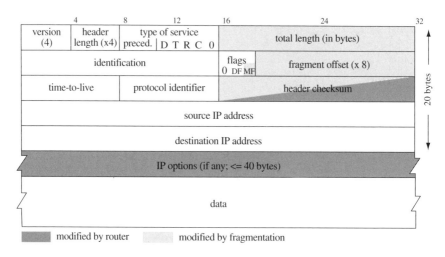

Figure 3.2   The Ipv4 packet header.

sum protects the header, but not the data. As the packet traverses the network, only the TTL and the checksum within the fixed packet header are changed by each router.

IP packets may carry optional blocks of data to support special functionality, particularly for debugging and to enable the source to influence the routing of packets within the network. This form of routing is referred to as *source routing*. *Loose source routing* does no more than prescribe addresses the packet must visit on its way to the destination, with possibly several hops between these addresses. *Strict source routing* enumerates all routers that a packet is allowed to visit; it is rarely used.

The Internet Control Message Protocol (ICMP) (22) is an integral part of any IP implementation and is used to communicate network-level error conditions and information to end systems.

3.3 TRANSPORT PROTOCOLS: UDP AND TCP

While the Internet architecture would in theory allow almost any number of transport protocols, only two are used in practice, namely, the User Datagram Protocol (UDP) for unreliable, connectionless messages and TCP for reliable, connection-oriented stream of bytes (see Table 3.2).

Both protocols support *multiplexing;* that is, they allow several distinct streams of data between two hosts. The streams are labeled by source and destination *port numbers*. Port numbers are 16-bit unsigned integers. Some destination port numbers are allocated to specific common services, registered with the Internet Assigned Numbers Authority (IANA), while other services use some external mechanism to let the communication partners know about the port number. For example, the Hypertext Transfer Protocol (HTTP) has been assigned TCP port number 80, but URLs can indicate any other port number.

Table 3.2 Classification of Internet Service Grades

Characteristic	Without resource reservation		Reserved resources	
	UDP	TCP	UDP	TCP
Packet loss	Yes	No	No	No
Delay bound	No	No	Possible	Possible
Abstraction	Packet	Byte stream	Packet	Byte stream
Ordering	None	Always in order	None	In order
Duplication	Possible	No	Possible	No
Multicast	Yes	No	Yes	No

3.3.1 UDP

The User Datagram Protocol (UDP) (23) offers only minimal services beyond
those provided by the network-layer protocol, namely, multiplexing via port numbers, as discussed above, and a checksum for the data included in the packet. The
packet header format is shown in Figure 3.3. (Recall that IP carries only a checksum for the IP header, not the data.) The checksum is optional, and a sender can set
it to zero if it did not compute it. Omitting the checksum is in almost all cases a bad
idea, but the practice may be useful for multimedia data that can tolerate bit errors.

3.3.2 TCP

The Transmission Control Protocol (TCP) (24) offers a reliable, sequenced byte
stream between two Internet hosts. Reliability is achieved by retransmission of lost
or errored packets and flow control to prevent a fast sender from overrunning a slow
receiver. For efficiency, a sender is allowed to transmit a *window* of data packets before it has to wait for confirmation from the receiver. The window size advertised by
the receiver indicates how much buffer space the receiver has available. In addition,
the sender reduces the window size to take into account network congestion. This
mechanism is the principal means of limiting Internet traffic, allowing the Internet
to encompass link speeds from a few kilobits per second to gigabits per second,
without explicitly configuring the sender application with the minimum available
bandwidth to each receiver. The sender TCP implementation probes for the currently available bandwidth by gradually increasing its transmission window until it
senses packet loss. At that point, it quickly reduces its window (25).

TCP offers a byte-stream service; that is, the receiver may not receive data
in the same units used for transmission. Higher layer mechanisms, such as a simple byte count (26,27), can be used to create "records" or "messages" on top of a
byte stream.

TCP can be used to transmit multimedia data, but it less suited for this task
than UDP if there is an end-to-end delay limit. In principle, TCP would be desirable for some point-to-point multimedia applications, since it can guarantee reli-

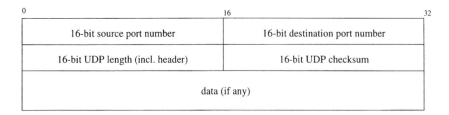

0	16	32
16-bit source port number	16-bit destination port number	
16-bit UDP length (incl. header)	16-bit UDP checksum	
data (if any)		

Figure 3.3   The UDP packet header.

able packet delivery and, from a practical perspective, it is often the only protocol that can traverse corporate firewalls. However, TCP trades reliability for delay. In addition, since TCP enforces in-order delivery, a single lost packet can hold up packets that have arrived after it.

If an application can modify the behavior of a TCP implementation, it would be feasible to improve the TCP delay behavior. An implementation is free to accept out-of-order packets and to acknowledge packets that have not been received, but are excessively delayed. However, the latter behavior may interfere with the TCP congestion control mechanism.

The TCP congestion control mechanism poses an additional problem for multimedia applications that want to use the protocol. Generally, multimedia applications have a bit rate that is given by the content and the audio or video encoding, but TCP's congestion control imposes its own bandwidth limits, with changes on very short time scales. Thus, a sender either has to buffer data, with a gap at the receiver, or drop packets.

3.4 IP MULTICAST

IP multicast allows sender to transmit a single IP packet to multiple receivers. The packet is replicated inside the network, whenever the path to two destinations or groups of destinations diverges. Multicast can be supported in at least three ways: namely, by receivers setting up virtual circuits to senders they would like to receive packets from, by senders including a list of addresses in the packet header (28), and by a radio-like model of host group multicast. Setting up virtual circuits is not currently possible within the Internet, and enumerating all possible receivers in the packet header does not scale to large groups. Thus, the third approach has been implemented in the Internet.

The best analogy to the host group model is that of a radio broadcast system. A user that wants to listen to a radio station tunes to that particular station's frequency. The radio station has no way of knowing that the radio tuned in and does not need to change its transmitter as additional radios tune in. It also does not need to receive in order to send. The same radio frequency can be reused by different stations that are sufficiently far apart. Radios do not know about other radios that are tuned in.

The host group model replaces the radio frequency by an IP address drawn from the range of so-called class-D addresses, 224.0.0.0 to 239.255.255.255. A host that wants to multicast data chooses an address, either using a well-known address registered with IANA* or choosing one randomly, hoping that nobody

---

*Well-known addresses from 224.0.*x.x* are registered as *service*.mcast.net. About 177 services were registered as of November 1999.

else is using it. Receivers subscribe to multicasts by finding out the multicast address, but they do not need to notify the sender or even know where the sender is located. An IP multicast group can have any number of senders and receivers. IP multicast does not depend on the transport protocol, but TCP can clearly not be used. In the future, a distributed equivalent of a frequency allocation service (such as the Federal Communications Commission in the United States) may become available, where transmitters can lease multicast addresses (29).

Unlike in radio, packets clearly should not be distributed to every receiver, regardless of whether it wants to listen to the packets. Rather, in IP multicast, routers discover whether there are any receivers located downstream from their outgoing network interfaces and send copies of the packets only to links with listeners. In addition, the distribution of multicast packets can be limited by setting their time-to-live (TTL) value and by using scoped multicast addresses (30). Scoped multicast addresses limit packet distribution to a single organization or a provider's network. For example, addresses in the 239.192.0.0/14 range are used within an organization, and packets with that destination address are never forwarded beyond the organization's boundary router.

Discovering where members are located is the role of two sets of protocols, namely, a local-area protocol called the Internet Group Management Protocol (IGMP) (31,32) and its IPv6 successor, the Multicast Listener Discovery (MLD) protocol (33) and one of a set of multicast routing protocols.

IGMP and MLD are based on a model that local-area networks have natural multicast support, so that the router connecting the LAN to the Internet does not have to worry about replicating packets. Thus, it simply needs to know whether there are one or more listeners for each group, but it does not matter whether there are one or one thousand. In IGMP and MLD, receivers are periodically asked by a router which multicast groups they are interested in. Each host waits a locally chosen random delay but does not respond if some other host has already declared its membership. To avoid long start-up latencies, if a host joins a group, it sends an unsolicited membership report.

For multicast routing within an autonomous system, two protocols are commonly used: Multicast Open Shortest Path First (MOSPF) (34) and Distance Vector Multicast Routing Protocol (DVMRP) (35,36). Both distribute information about group membership to all routers in a network. In DVMRP, the routing protocol distributes information about the shortest *reverse* path (i.e., from the source to the router). Packets are forwarded only if they come from the interface with the lowest distance to the source. In addition, routers can send *prune* messages to their neighbors to indicate that a particular group is of no interest. If all interfaces of a router are pruned, the router will then forward the prune on any interfaces that multicast packets arrive on. An edge router can also *join* a multicast group again if IGMP indicates local interest. MOSPF floods group membership information, along with link state reachability information.

For interdomain routing, protocols are still in development, since all existing protocols tend to be rather complex. Protocols in current use include Protocol Independent Multicast (PIM), in two flavors, sparse mode (SM) (37) and dense mode (DM) (38). In addition, the Core Base Tree (CBT) protocol (39) has been proposed. All these protocols have in common a reliance on an underlying unicast routing protocol, such as OSPF or the Border Gateway Protocol (BGP), to distribute reachability information. Indeed, PIM-DM is very similar to DVMRP, minus the reverse-path routing. PIM-SM and CBT define a *core,* which is used as the default destination for multicast packets. Packets are then distributed to all receivers in a single tree routed at the core. PIM-SM allows sources to transition to a per-source tree if their data rate warrants it.

Multicast is an active research area, with work being pursued in multicast routing, simplified multicast protocols for single-sender applications, congestion control for multicast, and reliable multicast (40).

3.4.1   Status

All common desktop and server operating systems support multicast reception and sending, but fewer can act as multicast routers. Routers generally support at least some multicast protocols, but such routing is often not enabled by default. Ethernet hubs and switches do not have to be modified to support multicast hubs, and they treat low-end switches as broadcast, while better switches perform "IGMP snooping" (i.e., listen for IGMP membership reports on links and send multicast packets only on links where there are listeners).

Despite hardware and software support, the availability of wide-area multicast in the Internet is currently spotty at best. Often, multicast works within a single company or ISP, but an overlay network called the *Mbone* usually is the only available method for wide-area connectivity, with very marginal quality and reliability in many parts of the Internet.

3.4.2   Additional Information

Additional information about Internet multicast can be found, for example, in books by Thomas (41) and Huitema (42). A number of white papers, including reports on multicast-related developments at recent meetings of the Internet Engineering Task Force (IETF), can be found at http://www.ipmulticast.com/.

3.5   INTERNET QUALITY OF SERVICE

We can classify network services by two principal quality-of-service impairments: delay and packet loss. In addition, packet reordering and duplication sometimes occur, but are less important. We discuss each impairment in turn.

3.5.1   End-to-End Delay

The end-to-end delay is the time elapsed between sending and receiving a packet or a particular byte. Note that the value of delay depends strongly on where it is measured: either at the host's network interface or after mechanisms for loss recovery, such as forward error correction or retransmission, have been applied. End-to-end delay consists of several components. The *propagation delay* depends only on the physical distance of the communications path and to a lesser extent on the communication medium. When transmitted over fiber, coaxial cable, or twisted wire pairs, packets incur a one-way delay of 5 μs/km, while wireless transmission incurs a delay of about 3.3 μs/km. The network path may change during a connection, but this happens rather infrequently in practice (43,44).

The *transmission delay* is the sum of the time it takes the network interfaces to send out the packet. (Even if there are no other packets waiting to be transmitted, routers have to store a complete packet and then forward it. Some Ethernet switches operate in "cut-through" mode, where the header leaves the outgoing interface while the tail end of the packet is still arriving at the incoming interface.) The transmission delay is given by

$$p \sum_{i=1}^{N} \frac{1}{r_i}$$

where p is the packet size and r_i is the link speed of the ith link in a path of N links. For all but modem or wireless links, this delay component is small. Typical wide-area Internet links have OC-12 (622 Mbit/s) speed, so that a maximum-sized packet of 1 500 bytes suffers 20 μs of transmission delay at each hop. In connections across the United States, hop counts of 10 to 15 are typical.*

Note that the transmission delay of a maximum-sized packet also affects the minimum per-hop delay of priority queueing or weighted-fair-queueing scheduling schemes, since a packet always has to wait until a lower priority packet clears the transmission link ahead of it. (Routers do not preempt the transmission of lower priority packets.)

Variable delays are caused by resource contention and link-layer retransmissions. Resource contention can occur either in routers or end system, if the number of packets arriving for a particular outgoing link temporarily exceeds the capacity of that outgoing link. This "queueing delay" depends on the average value and higher order statistical properties of the packet arrival process and, if the

---

*See http://vancouver-webpages.com/net/hops.html or http://www.nlanr.net/NA/Learn/wingspan.html for some data for this topic.

outgoing link is preempted by higher priority streams, the behavior of those higher priority streams. It is unusual to find delays higher than one second in modern Internet paths: since most routers cannot store that much data, packets are dropped rather than delayed if the overload becomes severe.

For some types of access network, bit interleaving and media access resolution can add delay. While one would suspect Ethernet delays as a prime example, most modern Ethernet networks, certainly those dimensioned to carry packet video, are switched Ethernet, where media access contention plays no role. Those Ethernets behave in a manner very similar to routers in terms of delay, with the above-mentioned exception that some Ethernet switches use cut-through rather than store-and-forward packet handling to minimize delays under light load. Cable modems, however, may suffer significant contention delays in the upstream direction (45), that is, from the subscriber to the cable head-end. The delays depend on the media access protocol; currently, the most widely implemented specification for cable modems in the United States is DOCSIS (Data-Over-Cable Service Interface Specification) 1.0, developed by the Packet Cable Consortium. Cable modems following this specification have to contend for upstream bandwidth by sending a request to the cable head-end. The head-end then broadcasts a map with a list of permissions for mini-slots to a subset of the requesters.

Delays vary significantly among cable modems of different types, but average delays of 45 ms and peak delays of 800 ms have been reported,* while others have observed average round-trip delays of around 5 to 6 ms, with peak delays of 200 ms.†

Modem delays are increased by link-layer retransmission (46) from about 127 ms to 167 ms. Similar link-layer retransmissions take place on some high error rate wireless links.

Variable network delays generally are "translated" by continuous-media applications into additional fixed delays. This translation is performed by playout delay buffers. The depth of the playout delay buffer is generally adjusted to reflect the variability in network delay, so that (say) 95 or 99% of all arriving packets are played out, and the remainder are dropped as excessively delayed. Delay adjustment can take place only if either the receiver can adjust its playout rate or there are gaps in the media stream that can be stretched and shortened by the receiver. The latter technique is generally used for packet speech, with the pauses between talkspurts adjusted to reflect changing delay jitter conditions (47–51).

In addition to these network-induced delays, the application and media

---

*Phil Karn, ftp://ftp.isi.edu/end2end, May 1999.
†Sanjay Waghray, personal communications.

coding may add significant additional delays. Details are beyond the scope of this chapter (see Reference 52 for additional material and references), but coding delays may dwarf network delays in many situations. These delays are caused by coding look-ahead as well as operating system and application-layer processing. Coding look-ahead is found in many low-rate audio codecs such as G.729 or G.723.1. Similarly, the MPEG I (intra), P (predictive), and B (bidirectional predicted) frame sequence adds look-ahead delay. The actual processing required for compressing and decoding the audio or video data obviously depends on the speed of the sender and receiver hardware, as well as any other tasks that needs attention, but this time must be less than a frame interval if the host wants to have a chance of keeping up. (For example, if an encoder takes 20% of CPU resources, we can expect the encoding delay to be 20% of a frame interval.) Finally, the operating system itself may add delays: for example, if it copies packets several times between different buffers (53).

Additional end-system delays occur when the receiver has to wait for later packets to reconstruct packet loss (54).

The Internet Protocol Performance Metrics (IPPM) working group within the IETF is defining a set of standardized metrics for important network performance measures. For network round-trip (55) and one-way delay (56), the drafts suggest measuring the median, percentile, and minimum delays. (Mean delays are less useful because they are biased too much by a small number of outliers.) Measuring one-way delays is made difficult by the need for synchronizing sender and receiver clocks and other factors, such as step-function clock adjustments (57). Even for the simpler round-trip measurement, care must be taken that the probe packet does indeed suffer the same delay as the packet of interest. In particular, at 60 bytes, ping packets are often smaller than real application packets and may in addition be treated worse than other packets by certain routers.

3.5.2   Packet Loss

For continuous-media applications, packet loss has two components: the packets that never arrive and those that arrive too late to be useful to the application. Generally, only the former are considered when one is characterizing network paths. While "ping" measurements are most commonly used, it may be preferable to sample path loss with a Poisson process (58,59).

In a network, packets are lost either because they are dropped when a router queue overflows or because a corrupted packet, detected by a link-layer or IP header checksum, is discarded. For all but wireless links with significant bit error rates and no link-layer packet retransmission, packet loss is dominated by buffer overflow.

Continuous-media applications are sensitive not only to the packet loss probability, but also to the correlation of packet losses. For example, bursts of lost packets may defeat forward error correction (60–62), but may on the other hand be less objectionable than spreading the same loss over a larger number of audio or video frames. Since audio and video packets are often closely spaced and small, loss correlation is a more serious issue here than it is with many data applications (63,64).

IPPM defines (65) metrics for loss period lengths and for noticeable losses (i.e., losses separated by less than a threshold of uninterrupted packets). A similar metric is used by Maxemchuk and Lo (66) to evaluate packet audio performance.

3.5.3 Packet Reordering

Under certain conditions, packets may arrive out of order—for example, when packets are inverse-multiplexed over several links to a common destination, if routes change frequently ("route flutter"), or if a router temporarily stops forwarding packets during a routing update and later releases the packets that arrived during the routing update. The likelihood of packet reordering strongly depends on packet spacing, but in general appears to be quite low except for parallel links between pairs of routers. Few studies appear to be available, but Matthews (67) indicates that only 0.03% of packets spaced one second apart were reordered in a 1999 experiment. Paxson (43, p. 233f) indicates that during his experiments in 1995, paths would have widely divergent incidence of packet reordering, ranging from 2.0% of data packets in one data set to 0.26% in another, with, for example, 15% of the packets sent by one site arriving out of order. Packet reordering causes no harm for most continuous-media applications, but it may need to be taken into account for playout delay estimation.

3.5.4 Packet Duplication

On rare occasions, packets are duplicated. This appears to be generally caused by faulty hardware or drivers,* transitions in spanning trees, and other anomalies. It is conceivable that a link-layer retransmission algorithm could generate duplicate packets if the acknowledgment gets lost (43, p. 245). For packet audio, duplicate packets may lead to a volume boost if the content of packets is mixed by sample addition without checking for duplicates. For packet video, duplicate packet appear generally harmless, except that a "dumb" decoder may waste time decoding the same information twice.

---

* Some Ethernet cards have been implicated here.

3.5.5 Connection Refusal

For networks with resource reservation, reservations may be refused by the call admission control (CAC) mechanism if sufficient bandwidth is not available. In the telephone network, call blocking rates of 0.05% are typical. In the Internet, we can further distinguish between the failure of reservations on any link between two or more parties or partial reservation failures, where a reservation on some fraction of links could not be established, so that traffic is handled on a best-effort basis on those links ("partial reservation") (68).

3.5.6 Service Probability

Another important service metric is end-to-end service probability, which can be defined either from the perspective of a single user or from a wider perspective. It indicates the likelihood that a certain site can be reached. However, given that the popularity of destination domains or autonomous systems varies dramatically, it is hard to come up with truly useful measures. IETF Request for Comments 2498 (69) defines instantaneous and "interval–temporal connectivity" for a pair of hosts.

3.5.7 Trade-offs Between Metrics

The most important considerations are bounds on delay, packet loss, and connection refusal. Note that it is impossible, at least in a statistically multiplexed network where the sum of the access speeds exceeds the speed of backbone link, to satisfy all three criteria at the same time. If one wants delay bounds and no packet loss, this implies the need for admission control and thus the possibility of connection refusal. Without connection refusal (i.e., in a best-effort network), an application can trade increased delay for decreased packet loss by requesting retransmissions or adding forward-error correction. Playout buffers can trade increased packet loss for lower delay.

A number of interesting combinations of service qualities are currently not available in the Internet. These include reliable *datagram* transmission for unicast and multicast, as opposed to the reliable byte stream offered by TCP. In particular, a reliable packet protocol may deliver packets to an application out of sequence, without waiting for an earlier packet to be retransmitted. This is desirable for continuous-media applications as well as for Internet telephony signaling. For unicast, the Reliable Datagram Protocol (RDP) (70) was proposed in 1990, but never caught on. There are ongoing efforts to define a protocol [the Multinetwork Datagram Transmission Protocol (MDTP)] within the SIGTRAN and MEGACO IETF working groups. A large amount of recent work (such as that described in References 71–79) has focused on reliable multicast, with different definitions of reliability. For example, it may be sufficient that *almost all* receivers receive all packets, and some receivers may join late or drop out early.

3.6 INTERNET MEASUREMENTS

It is commonly asked whether the Internet can support continuous-media services or what quality of service the Internet offers. It is, unfortunately, about as easy to answer such questions as it is to state how long it takes to travel 10 miles by car—it can be less than 10 minutes, or it can be an hour. However, just as road systems have their bridges and tunnels (and tollbooths in the eastern United States) as classical choke points, there appear to be common conditions that make drastic performance impairments likely. These appear to be access links, connections between different network providers, and international links. The speed of access links determines the monthly cost of the Internet connection for smaller ISPs and organizations, so that there is reluctance to upgrade.

Recently, a number of companies have started to measure and track Internet performance on a continuing basis. These organizations include Keynote Systems Inc., Inverse Network Technology, the Andover News Network, the Advanced Network and Systems Surveyor Project, and Matrix Information and Directory Services. We summarize some of their results.

Internet performance varies somewhat from day to day and significantly more over the length of the day. For example, Keynote Systems reports* that during the workweek, Internet web access is about 10% slower on Fridays, the busiest day, than on Tuesdays, the least busy weekday. A study of European web sites indicates a delay variation of about a factor of 2 between the "fastest" day, Saturday, and the slowest day, Monday. Note, however, that these performance measures include both network and server performance.

The hourly variation in load or delay, however, is significantly less than for telephone traffic. Among other reasons, much of Internet traffic has a human only on one end of the connection (see Figure 3.4), so that people use the Internet later in the evening than they would make phone calls.

Also, Internet access speed depends on the geographic location of the user, with Tampa, San Diego, and New York City faring the worst, experiencing clocking delays up to three times higher than cities such as Kansas City, Boston, and Phoenix.[†]

In June 1999, an average dial-up user could expect a throughput of about 24.9 kbit/s with a 33.6 kbit/s modem, which increased to 30.4 kbit/s for a V.90 (56 kbit/s) modem user.[‡] This effective throughput has slowly increased over the past few years, indicating that the Internet infrastructure has, in general, kept up with demand. [This impression is supported by measurements (80) that indicate

---

*Numbers drawn from week of June 28, 1999, reported at http://www.keynote.com/measures/business/business40.html.
[†] Keynote Systems, week of June 28, 1999.
[‡] Inverse Network Technology study at http://www.inversenet.com/news/pr/19990617.html.

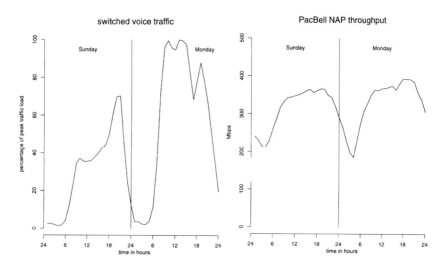

Figure 3.4   Hourly variation of telephone (left) and Internet traffic (right).

that mean latencies decreased by about 30% between January 1994 and January 1996. Long-term quality-of-service statistics for the SuperJANET U.K. academic network show similar behavior (81).]

Personal experience indicates that speeds for a 640/96 kbit/s modem on an asymmetric dial-up subscriber line (ADSL) may reach 480 kbit/s, while the author has never seen a sustained wide-area Internet TCP throughput above 800 kbit/s, even with a lightly loaded T3 line out of Columbia University. Matthews (67) indicates a steadily increasing TCP available bandwidth between U.S. educational institutions that has risen from about 80 kbit/s to about 2.4 Mbit/s between July 1994 and October 1998.

For end-to-end delay and packet loss, there are fewer general industry estimates. However, CWI provides a map showing round-trip times between major U.S. cities (http://www.traffic.cwusa.com/). For example, in July 1999, round-trip times ranged from 7 ms between New York and Washington, D.C. (direct connection) to 85 ms between New York and Los Angeles (six hops). Speed-of-light propagation delay accounts for 3 and 40 ms of those figures, respectively. The Internet Weather Report published by Matrix Information and Directory Services (www.mids.org) measures "ping" delays between Austin, Texas, and a large number of hosts all over the world. A related organization, MIQ Ratings, measures median round-trip latencies for major ISPs from beacons in Austin, Edinburgh (U.K.), Alameda (California), New York, Chicago, and Amsterdam. For example, for July 13, 1999, the best large ISP was measured at a median delay of 49.3 ms, while the worst clocked more than 200 ms, with little difference between daily, weekly and monthly medians. Packet losses in this study range from below 1% to about 7% monthly averages. However, the study shows common carriers that sustain packet losses of close to 20% for the whole day.

The Internet Traffic Report (http://www.internettrafficreport.com) performs similar measurements. Recent data indicate a round-trip time of 213 ms within North America, averaged over one week, with an average loss of 2%; but loss peaks reach 10% several times a day.

The Surveyor Project (82) by Advanced Network and Services (http://www.advanced.org) is measuring *one-way* delays and packet loss between about 50 measuring stations located at universities and research institutes in the United States, Korea, Australia, New Zealand, Singapore, Switzerland, and elsewhere. The measuring stations use a local Global Positioning System (GPS) receiver to achieve microsecond-accuracy absolute clock synchronization. The results indicate that while the median delay does not change significantly over the day, the 90th percentile of delay increases dramatically on many routes between about 6 P.M. and midnight. Tables 3.3 and 3.4 summarize some initial results (82), obtained in November 1998. The authors also found that 5% of the paths with more than 1% loss have highly asymmetric loss, with one direction having loss of more than double the other direction.

The PingER project (http://www-iepm.slac.stanford.edu/pinger/) measures the round-trip time of Internet links. A number of other measurement projects are being undertaken. For example, Bass (83) describes measurements done for Internet access for the U.S. Air Force.

The results summarized so far provide a macro-level description of Internet performance. A number of researchers have looked at more detailed characteristics of performance.

For example, Agrawala and Sanghi (84) describe delay and loss measurements by their autocorrelation function. They observe that most losses, even at packet spacings of just 20 ms, are isolated, with no obvious correlation to packet delay. Like others later, they observed step changes in delay

Table 3.3 Measurements of Internet Loss

		Loss (%)		
	Paths	Entire day	Worst 6 hours	Worst hour
All paths	1084	1.06	1.44	4.88
Intra-U.S.	1060	1.04	1.40	4.79
U.S.-Europe	12	1.39	1.52	5.71
U.S.-New Zealand	10	2.58	4.04	11.15
Europe-New Zealand	2	0.58	1.51	6.97

Source: Ref. 82.

Table 3.4 Percentage of U.S.—U.S. Paths with Losses Greater
than Threshold

| | Paths with losses exceeding threshold (%) | | |
Loss threshold (%)	Entire day	Worst 6 hours	Worst hour
1	34.1	25.7	70.3
2	12.6	16.1	53.9
5	2.2	3.4	32.1
10	0.4	0.6	11.9
20	0.0	0.2	0.5

Source: Ref. 82.

lasting several seconds. Bolot (85) confirms the essentially random nature of packet loss unless the probe traffic consumes a large fraction of the bottleneck bandwidth.

Odlyzko (86) observes that most of the Internet backbone is relatively lightly used, with congestion at the transition points between networks, in particular the "public" NAPs. Some university access links are also subject to congestion, as upgrades may lag behind increased traffic volume.

A number of researchers have measured packet loss and delay for audio. For example, Bolot et al. (87) used frequency distributions of consecutive packet losses and a $D + D^x/D/1/K$ queueing model to describe the loss process on a heavily loaded link between INRIA in southern France and University College, London.

Maxemchuk and Lo (66) measured the loss and delay variation of an intrastate, interstate, and international link, using as a metric "the fraction of time that the signal is received without distortion for intervals of time that are long enough to convey useful speech segments." They measured quality for minimum loss-free intervals (MLFIs) of between 0.5 and 3 seconds and found that as long as single-packet losses are restored, intrastate and interstate connections obtain acceptable quality about 95% of the time, with modest delays of about 200 ms. The international connection, however, is significantly worse, with qualities of 90% acceptable only at delays of above a second.

Yajnik et al. (88) investigate statistical descriptions for loss traces gathered from unicast and multicast connections. They investigate the autocorrelation function and good run and loss run lengths, and check how well losses can be modeled as Bernoulli or two-state Markov chains.

Mukherjee (89) describes the frequency behavior of round-trip ("ping") delay. His results show a shifted gamma distribution for the delay and only modest correlation between loss and delay.

Borella and Brewster (90) attempt to model round-trip delay traces for packets spaced similarly to audio or video packets as a long-range dependent process. While reliably estimating the Hurst parameter turns out to be difficult, the data do indicate long-range dependency. It is not yet clear how this result will influence, for example, the design of playout delay algorithms.

Even though the papers above do not directly address it, behavior for video traffic can be expected to be similar, since the packet spacing of audio and (full-rate) video packets is of the same magnitude, around 30 ms. Compared to audio, video exhibits higher bandwidths and variable packet lengths; these are likely to matter only if video fills a large fraction of the link capacity.

3.7 INTERNET PROTOCOL ARCHITECTURE FOR CONTINUOUS-MEDIA SERVICES

3.7.1 Architecture

While still works in progress, a set of protocols and an architecture for support-ing continuous media services in the Internet are emerging (91). In this architec-ture, a small set of protocols covers both communication and distribution services, as well as their combinations. Generally speaking, we may distinguish three types of protocol (Figure 3.5): media transport, quality-of-service-related protocols, and signaling protocols. Media transport protocols are responsible for carrying the actual media content (i.e., audio and video frames). Figure 3.5 shows RTP, described in Section 3.8, as the standardized IETF protocol for this purpose, but RealAudio and Microsoft currently still use proprietary protocols for their media-on-demand applications.

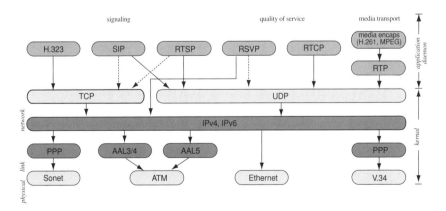

Figure 3.5 Internet multimedia protocol stack.

3.7.2 Quality of Service

We can distinguish protocols for measuring quality of service and those that set
aside network resources to assure subsets of packets of a predictable quality of
service. (We discussed quality-of-service metrics in the Internet in Section 3.5.)
Currently, network management protocols like SNMP allow network managers
to observe aggregate quality measures such as packet loss for all packet streams,
while the Real-Time Control Protocol (RTCP), part of RTP, may be used to monitor end-to-end quality of service for individual continuous-media streams. Multicast has specific extensions to IGMP for reporting on connectivity, packet rates,
and loss (92).

Resources can be managed either per flow or on an aggregate basis (93). A
(micro) flow is "a single instance of an application-to-application flow of packets
which is identified by source address, source port, destination address, destination port and protocol id" (21). The integrated services architecture deals with
flows (as they are called in Reference 21) or microflows, the more recent term,
assuring individual quality of service for each such flow. The integrated services
approach currently defines two services, guaranteed and controlled load, where
the former offers end-to-end bounds on delay, while the latter offers a looser performance notion of assured bandwidth and an experience similar to a lightly
loaded network.

Recently, the "differentiated services" approach has attempted to provide
differing levels of service to a relatively small number of packet classes, where
classes are defined by values of the type-of-service byte in the IP header. Thus,
while there might be thousands of microflows in a given router, one for each
telephone call, say, there would be only a handful of differentiated services "behavior aggregates." A (behavior) aggregate is defined as "a collection of packets
with the same DS [differentiated service] codepoint crossing a link in a particular direction" (21). Depending on the definition of the service, individual microflows within a behavior aggregate may or may not obtain service guarantees.
For example, if all videophone calls are bundled into a single service class, but
there is no admission control into the class, individual calls on certain links may
still suffer packet loss or excessive delay. Thus, to guarantee quality-of-service
levels, even the differentiated-services approach needs a mechanism to monitor
the microflows contributing to the behavior aggregate (94–96). Also, since the
aggregate flow is constrained only by the sum of a large number of leaky buck-
ets, say, delay bounds are, in general, not offered.

3.7.3 Signaling

While the media transport and quality-of-service components are the same for all
continuous-media applications, the signaling differentiates the various applica-

tions involving continuous media. We can roughly divide Internet media applications by whether the media delivery is controlled by the sender or the receiver and by whether the sender and receiver "meet" each other before the sender starts its transmission.

Internet media-on-demand is an example of an application in which the receiver explicitly connects to the sender and the sender starts transmission only with one or more receivers present. Also, receivers can generally control the flow of media (e.g., by pausing the flow).

Internet telephony (97)* is similar, except that the media stream is generally bidirectional and from live sources, so that operations such as "fast forward" do not make sense (much as this would be desirable in some circumstances).

Finally, Internet broadcast dispenses with an explicit per-user establishment of a session. Rather, the sender or a proxy announces the availability of a multicast stream, with receivers tuning in. Note that there may be a network-layer mechanism, namely, IP multicast pruning, that keeps a sender from injecting packets into the wide-area network if nobody is listening; generally, however, the application remains unaware of this.

These three rough categories are represented by different signaling protocols: the Real-Time Stream Protocol (RTSP) for media-on-demand (Section 3.9), SIP (and H.323) for Internet telephony (Section 3.11), and SAP (Section 3.12) for broadcast applications. All three applications require a mechanism to describe the streams making up the multimedia session. Currently, the Session Description Protocol (SDP) (98) is most commonly used, although it is likely that new formats will emerge to address some of the shortcomings of SDP.

While these notions appear to be relatively distinct, there are opportunities to combine them into novel applications. For example, a user may use SIP to invite a friend (presumably) to an Internet broadcast, where neither the caller nor the callee is an active, media-emitting participant. Similarly, SIP may be used to invite somebody to a joint video-watching session, with the RTSP "remote control" being passed back and forth between users.

Also, Internet telephony may well use a media-on-demand control protocol such as RTSP for a voicemail service.

Other signaling protocols, such as for the negotiation of who "has the floor" (i.e., is allowed to send data into a conference) are still being developed.

---

* Following current custom, we use the "Internet telephony" or "IP telephony" (IPtel) even when one term refers to a multimedia stream or a multiparty conference, instead of the more awkward "Internet videotelephony." Internet telephony is also called packet voice or voice-over-IP (VoIP), but these terms appear too limiting to the author.

3.8 THE REAL-TIME TRANSPORT PROTOCOL (RTP) FOR TRANSPORT MULTIMEDIA DATA

Real-time flows such as voice and video streams have a number of common requirements that distinguish them from "traditional" Internet data services:

Sequencing. The packets must be reordered in real time at the receiver, should they arrive out of order. If a packet is lost, it must be detected and compensated for without retransmissions.

Intramedia synchronization. The amount of time between points at which successive packets are to be "played out" must be conveyed. For example, no data is usually sent during silence periods in speech. The duration of this silence must be reconstructed properly.

Intermedia synchronization. If a number of different media are being used in a session, there must be a means to synchronize them, so that the audio that is played out matches the video. This is also known as lip-sync.

Payload identification. In the Internet, it is often necessary to change the encoding for the media ("pay load") on the fly to adjust to changing bandwidth availability or the capabilities of new users joining a group. Some kind of mechanism is therefore needed to identify the encoding for each packet.

Frame indication. Video and audio are sent in logical units called frames. To aid in synchronized delivery to higher layers, it is necessary to indicate to a receiver where a frame begins and ends.

These services are provided by a *transport protocol.* In the Internet, the Real-Time Transport Protocol (99) is used for this purpose. RTP has two components. The first is RTP itself, and the second is RTCP, the Real-Time Control Protocol. Transport protocols for real-time media are not new, dating back to the 1970s (100). However, RTP provides some functionality beyond resequencing and loss detection:

Multicast friendly. RTP and RTCP have been engineered for multicast. In fact, they are designed to operate both in small multicast groups, like those used in a three-person phone call, and in huge ones, like those used for broadcast events.

Media independent. RTP provides services needed for generic real-time media, such as voice and video. Any codec-specific additional header fields and semantics are defined for each media codec in separate specifications.

Mixers and translators. Mixers are devices that take media from several users, mix or "bridge" them into one media stream, and send the resulting stream out. Translators take a single media stream, convert it to another format, and send it out. Translators are useful for reducing the bandwidth requirements of a stream before sending it over a low-band-width link, without requiring the RTP source to reduce its bit rate. This allows receivers that are connected via fast links to still receive high-quality media. Mixers limit the bandwidth if several sources send data simultaneously, fulfilling the function of conference bridge. RTP in-cludes explicit support for mixers and translators.

QoS feedback. RTCP allows receivers to provide feedback to all members of a group on the quality of the reception. RTP sources may use this in-formation to adjust their data rate, while other receivers can determine whether quality-of-service (QoS) problems are local or network-wide. External observers can use it for scalable quality-of-service management.

Loose session control. With RTCP, participants can periodically distribute identification information such as name, e-mail, address, phone number, and brief messages. This provides awareness of who is participating in a session, subject to temporary divergence due to packet loss and the peri-odic nature of RTCP, without maintaining a centralized conference par-ticipant registry. Maintaining conference state in such a distributed fashion is sometimes called loose session control (91).

Encryption. RTP media streams can be encrypted by using keys that are exchanged by some non-RTP method [e.g., SIP or the Session Descrip-tion Protocol (SDP) (98)].

3.8.1 RTP

RTP is generally used in conjunction with the User Datagram Protocol (UDP), but it can make use of any packet-based, lower layer protocol. When a host wishes to send a media packet, it formats the media for packetization, adds any media-specific packet headers, prepends the RTP header, and places it in a lower layer payload. It is then sent into the network, either to a multicast group or uni-cast to another participant.

The RTP header (Figure 3.6) is 12 bytes long. The V field indicates the protocol version. The X flag signals the presence of a header extension between the fixed header and the payload. If the P bit is set, the payload is padded to en-sure proper alignment for encryption.

Users within a multicast group are distinguished by a random 32-bit syn-chronization source SSRC identifier. With an application-layer identifier, it is easy to distinguish streams coming from the same translator or mixer and to as-sociate receiver reports with sources. In the rare event that two users happen to choose the same identifier, one redraws its SSRC.

As described above, a mixer combines media streams from several sources (e.g., a conference bridge might mix the audio of all active participants). In cur-rent telephony, the participants may have a hard time distinguishing who hap-

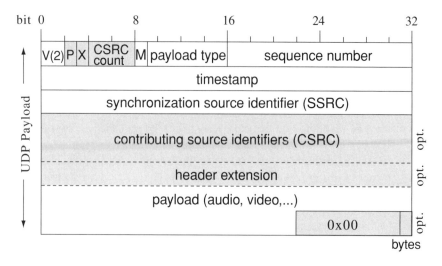

Figure 3.6 RTP fixed header format.

pens to be speaking at any given time. The Contributing SSRC (CSRC) list, whose length is indicated by the CSRC length field, lists all the SSRCs that "contributed" content to the packet. For an audio conference, it would list all active speakers.

RTP supports the notion of media-dependent framing to assist in the reconstruction and playout process. The marker M bit provides information for this purpose. For audio, the first packet in a voice talkspurt can be scheduled for playout independently of those in the previous talkspurt. The bit is used in this case to indicate the first packet in a talkspurt. For video, a video frame can be rendered only when its last packet has arrived. Here, the marker bit is used to indicate the last packet in a video frame.

The label payload type identifies the media encoding used in the packet. The label sequence number increments sequentially from one packet to the next, and is used to detect losses and restore packet order. The timestamp, incremented with the media sampling frequency, indicates when the media frame was generated.

The payload itself may contain headers specific for the media; this is described in more detail below (Section 3.8.3) and in Chapter 13.

3.8.2 RTCP: Control and Management

The Real-Time Control Protocol, RTCP, is the companion control protocol for RTP. Media senders (sources) and receivers (sinks) periodically send RTCP packets to the same multicast group (but different ports) used to distribute RTP packets. Each RTCP packet contains a number of elements, usually a sender report (SR) or a receiver report followed by source descriptions (SDES). Each serves a different function.

Sender reports (SR) are generated by users who are also sending media (RTP sources). They describe the amount of data sent so far, as well as correlating the RTP sampling timestamp and absolute ("wall clock") time to allow synchronization between different media.

Receiver reports (RR) are sent by RTP session participants that are receiving media (RTP sinks). Each such report contains one block for each RTP source in the group. Each block describes the instantaneous and cumulative loss rate and jitter from that source. The block also indicates the last timestamp and delay since a sender report has been received, allowing sources to estimate their distance to sinks.

Source descriptor (SDES) packets are used for session control. They contain the CNAME (canonical name), a globally unique identifier similar in format to an e-mail address. The CNAME is used for resolving conflicts in the SSRC value and to associate different media streams generated by the same user. SDES packets also identify the participant through its name, e-mail address, and phone number. This provides a simple form of session control. Client applications can display the name and e-mail information in the user interface. This allows session participants to learn about the other participants in the session. It also allows them to obtain contact information (such as e-mail and phone) to allow for other forms of communication (such as initiation of a separate conference using SIP). This also makes it easier to contact a user should he, for example, have left his camera running.

A user who is leaving includes a *BYE* message. Finally, *application* (APP) elements can be used to add application-specific information to RTCP packets.

Since the sender reports, the receiver reports, and SDES packets contain information that can continually change, it is necessary to send these packets periodically. If the RTP session participants simply sent RTCP packets with a fixed period, the resulting bandwidth used in the multicast group would grow linearly with the group size. This is clearly undesirable. Instead, each session member counts the number of other session members it hears from (via RTCP packets). The period between RTCP packets from each user is then set to scale linearly with the number of group members. This ensures that the bandwidth used for RTCP reports remains fixed, independent of the group size. Since the group size estimate is obtained by counting the number of other participants, it takes time for each new participant to converge to the correct group size count. If many users simultaneously join a group, as is common in broadcast applications, each user will have an incorrect, and very low, estimate of the group size. The result is a flood of RTCP reports. A backoff algorithm called reconsideration (101) is used to prevent such floods.

3.8.3 Payload Formats

The foregoing mechanisms in RTP provide for services needed for the generic transport of audio and video. However, particular codecs will have additional requirements for information that needs to be conveyed. To support this, RTP allows for payload formats to be defined for each particular codec. These payload formats describe the syntax and semantics of the RTP payload. The particular semantic of the payload is communicated in the RTP payload type indicator field. This 7-bit field is mapped to actual codecs and formats via a binding to names. There are two types of binding: *static* payload types and *dynamic* payload types. The static payload types are established once in an RTP *profile* document (102). For example, payload type 0 designates the μ-law audio codec. Given the limited space available and the continuing development of new codecs, no further static payload type assignments will be made. Instead, applications need to agree, on a per-session basis, about which payload type number corresponds to which payload format. Currently, applications use the range of payload type numbers from 96 to 127 for these dynamic mappings. For example, an application may indicate that it wants to use payload type 120 for an H.263 video codec. Currently, the H.323 signaling protocol and the Session Description Protocol (SDP) (Section 3.10) can convey such RTP-payload-type mappings. Furthermore, anyone can register a name (as long as it has not been used), and procedures are defined for doing so. This allows for RTP to be used with any kind of codec developed by anyone.

RTP media payload formats have been defined for the H.263 (103), H.261 (104), JPEG (105), and MPEG (106) video codecs, and a host of other audio and video encoders are supported with simpler payload formats, defined in the *RTP Profile for Audio and Video Conferences with Minimal Control* (102).

Furthermore, RTP payload formats are being defined to provide some generic services. One format, for redundant audio codings (107), allows a user to transmit audio content using multiple audio codecs, each delayed from the previous, and of a lower bit rate. This allows for lost packets to be recovered from subsequent packets, albeit with a lower quality codec. Another payload format is being defined for parity and Reed Solomon-like forward error correction (FEC) mechanisms, to allow for recovery of lost packets in a codec-independent manner (108). Yet another format is being introduced to multiplex media from multiple users into a single packet (109). This is particularly useful for trunk replacement between Internet telephony gateways, where it can provide a significant reduction in packet header overheads.

For low-speed links, the combined size of IP, UDP, and RTP headers add up to 40 bytes, which may be prohibitively inefficient for low bit rate voice codecs. RTP header compression (110) codes the first- and second-order difference between successive IP/UDP/RTP packets and can often reduce the combined header size to one or two bytes. However, this compression method is sensitive to packet loss and works only across one link-layer hop. Another reason for restricting compression to a single hop is that the receiver has to be able to request resynchronization in case a packet is lost. A requests of this type would add significant delay if used across the Internet.

3.8.4 Resource Reservation

Given the importance of telephony services, we anticipate that a significant fraction of the Internet bandwidth will be consumed by voice and video, that is, RTP-based protocols. Owing to tight delay constraints, IPtel streams are also likely candidates for guaranteed QoS. Unfortunately, existing proposals such as RSVP (111) are rather complex, largely because of features such as receiver orientation and support for receiver diversity that are likely to be of limited use for Internet telephony. We have proposed (112) to dispense with a separate resource reservation protocol altogether and simply use RTCP messages to tell routers along the path to reserve sufficient resources. To determine the amount of bandwidth for the reservation, RTCP sender reports (SR) can be used as is (by observing the difference between two subsequent SR byte counts), or an additional field can be inserted that specifies the desired grade of service in more detail. RTCP messages carrying reservation requests are marked for special handling by a router alert option (113). The receiver reports back whether the reservation was completely or only partially successful.

Similar proposals of simplified, sender-based resource reservation protocols can be found (albeit not using RTCP) in the Scalable Reservation Protocol (SRP) (114).

The issue of reservations for IPtel services has another facet: if a reservation fails, the call can still take place, but using best-effort transport of the audio. This is certainly preferable to a fast-busy signal, where no communications at all are established. This introduces the possibility of removing the admission decision altogether. On each link in the network, sufficient bandwidth for voice traffic can be allocated. Time-honored approaches to telephone network engineering can be used to determine the amount of allocation needed. The remaining bandwidth on links will be used for other services, and for best effort. Incoming packets can be classified as voice or nonvoice. Should them be too many voice connections active at any point in time (possible, since there is no admission control), the extra calls can simply become best effort. Good network engineering can place reasonably low probabilities on such an event, and the use of "spillover" best-effort bandwidth can eliminate admission control to handle these unlikely occurrences.

The mechanism above is generally referred to as part of the class of IP service known as *differentiated services*. These rely on user subscription (to facilitate network engineering) and packet classification and marking at network peripheries. From the discussion above, IPtel is a prime candidate for such a service. In fact, the *premium service* (115) provides almost no delay and jitter for its packets, making it ideal for real-time voice and video.

3.9 REAL-TIME STREAMING PROTOCOL

3.9.1 Purpose

The Real-Time Streaming Protocol (RTSP) (116) is an Internet Proposed Standard for the control of multimedia streams. It allows a client to open a media session consisting of one or more streams, which may be located on a single server or on multiple servers. RTSP is agnostic in the use of network and media protocols; that is, it does not depend on the use of RTP, say, or a particular media format, such as MPEG. (Indeed, RealAudio uses RTSP in it G2 client and server, but chooses stream audio and video data as a proprietary stream format.) The protocol is cognizant of RTP, however, and indications of the initial timestamp and sequence number for the protocol are supported.

RTSP can be used not just for playback, but also to tell a server to record packets from a particular network address, allowing it to serve as a "telephone answering machine" or as a conference recorder.

3.9.2 Syntax

RTSP is similar in syntax to HTTP, the hypertext transfer protocol underlying the World-Wide Web, as well as SIP, the session management protocol described below in Section 3.11. Like HTTP and SIP, RTSP it is a textual protocol, with very similar message syntax. The protocol consists of requests issued by the client and responses returned by the server. However, unlike HTTP, a client may receive a request—for example, to go elsewhere for service (REDIRECT). As in HTTP, requests consist of a request line indicating the method (Table 3.5), the request URL, and the protocol version, followed by a number of parameter-value header lines and then the message body, if any. The message body may contain a "session description," a description of the media streams for the session. While SDP is currently the only commonly used format, others could be defined in the future. Responses are similar, except that the first line indicates the status of the request, with both a three-digit numeric code and a textual response. The first digit of the response indicates the nature of the response, with status codes from 200 to 299 indicating success, 300 to 399 redirection to another server or multiple choices, 400 to 499 client errors such as syntax problems or invalid session

Table 3.5 RTSP Methods

Request	Direction	Description
OPTIONS	S ↔ C	Determine capabilities of server (S) or client (C)
DESCRIBE	C → S	Get description of media stream
ANNOUNCE	S ↔ C	Announce new session description
SETUP	C → S	Create media session
RECORD	C → S	Start media recording
PLAY	C → S	Start media delivery
PAUSE	C → S	Pause media delivery
REDIRECT	S → C	Use another server, please
TEARDOWN	C → S	Destroy media session
SET_PARAMETER	S ↔ C	Set server or client parameter
GET_PARAMETER	S ↔ C	Read server or client parameter

identifiers, and 500 to 599 indicating server problems such as an unimplemented method or server overload.

3.9.3   Relationship to HTTP

RTSP differs from HTTP in a number of respects. For example, while HTTP is currently limited to TCP, RTSP can use either TCP or UDP. When run over UDP, RTSP requests have their own retransmission mechanism to ensure reliability. Also, unlike HTTP, RTSP does not deliver data itself in responses*; rather, it simply sets up a separate, "out-of-band" media stream. Because of that, RTSP, unlike HTTP, has the notion of a *session,* even though requests for a session are not tied to any transport-layer connection. (It is quite possible to start a session from one host and continue it from somewhere else, assuming the server does not disallow this for security reasons. An RTSP session can span many TCP connections or several RTSP sessions can reuse the same TCP connection.)

3.9.4   RTSP Extensions

The protocol is designed to be extensible. New requests methods can be added, and clients can find out which methods a server supports by sending an OPTIONS request. As with any of the HTTP-like protocols, clients and servers may add headers and parameters that consenting applications can process and others

---

*RTSP supports in-band delivery for certain network configurations, such as network address translators (NATs) or firewalls, which allow no other alternative, but this in-band mechanism is not recommended for general use.

may ignore. To make sure that the server understands a particular new header, a client must label the request with a Required header, indicating the name of the extension (not the header). For example, a "Require: edu.columbia.cs.rtspd.ppv" might indicate that the server needs to understand a feature for the Columbia University server having to do with pay-per-view TV, which may consist of a set of new headers or simply new parameters for existing headers. Servers may add new response codes, as long as their class indicates whether the request has succeeded or the nature of the failure.

3.9.5 Timing

As a protocol operating in a best-effort Internet, RTSP needs to hide latency variations. Thus, PLAY requests may contain information about when the request is to be executed, so that they can be staged well ahead, allowing a smooth transition between different media segments. Indeed, a user could send a whole "play list" containing a sequence of requests to create his own virtual "cut" of a movie or sound track.

RTSP offers three types of timestamp for the clock the viewer associates with a program: SMPTE (117), normal play time, and absolute time. RTSP's SMPTE timestamps are the same as those used in TV production and simplify the specification of timing for frame-based codecs. They have the format hours:minutes:seconds:frames:subframes. Normal play time is measured relative to the beginning of the stream and is expressed in hours, minutes, seconds, and fractions of a second. Finally, absolute time corresponds to "wall clock" time and can be used to replay a particular time interval from the recording of a live stream, identified by its original time of occurrence. For example, it might be used with a security camera to play the frames around the time a door alarm was reported.

If a movie is being played in slow motion, the RTSP timestamp rate is also reduced, so that time progresses at a slower pace. Since, however, the RTP timestamp rate remains the same, the frames are rendered at the appropriate rate. (Depending on the implementation, the server may deliver fewer frames per second in that case.) Thus, the media-rendering application does not need to know about the RTSP notion of time, which would be relevant only for, say, an elapsed-time display.

3.9.6 Aggregate and Stream Control

Sessions can be controlled either as an aggregate of all streams (i.e., with a single request) or as individual streams. For example, a movie may consist of several sound tracks in different languages, a video stream, and a stream of subtitles. Each stream has its own transport parameters and is typically delivered to either a different port or a different multicast address. The client issues a DESCRIBE request to obtain a description of the aggregate stream, with each stream within the aggregate identified by a separate URL. Then, the client sets up transport associations via a sequence of SETUP requests. The first SETUP request returns the session identifier, which is then reused when the other component streams within the aggregate are set up. PLAY, RECORD, and PAUSE requests can operate on either the aggregate or the individual stream. PAUSE on the aggregate stream stops the progression of time, while PAUSE on a substream merely stops delivery of that particular stream, while time marches on. A session or stream is destroyed with the TEARDOWN request, thus allowing the server to free up resources. If a server gets too busy or is about to be taken offline, it may ask the client via a REDIRECT request to continue the session elsewhere.

The server may update its session description by sending an ANNOUNCE request to the client, for example, when a live session acquires a new media stream. Mechanisms for obtaining and setting parameter values, GET_PARAMETER and SET_PARAMETER, have been established, but there are currently no well-defined uses for these. One could imagine, for example, using SET_PARAMETER to change the camera angle in a live video session.

3.9.7 Caching

One of the interesting problems for continuous-media content is caching. This is of particular interest because the media streams can be very large, and the somewhat higher cost of producing high-quality material may cause them to be of higher locality than textual or graphical web content. RTSP caching builds on HTTP web caching; it does not cache the response of RTSP requests, however, but rather the media stream itself.

The area of caching for multimedia content remains to be explored, but it differs in some important aspects from web caching. For example, it is likely that a cache may have only parts of a movie, if the previous viewer skipped sections, so that the cache must update itself if a second request comes in. As with web caches, a client may be willing to accept a less desirable version (e.g., last hour's newscast or a lower quality video coding) if it is available locally, to avoid the quality degradation that may be associated with retrieving the material from the original source.

RTSP offers cache control to indicate whether intermediate caching proxies are allowed to deliver cached material rather than forwarding the RTSP request to the origin server. Also, responses can indicate whether proxies are allowed to cache media streams (e.g., if the server wants to restrict caching for reasons of audience estimation or copyright concerns). It is anticipated that many of the mechanisms for retrieval reporting and cache control being discussed for web pages also apply here. Because of the close syntactic relationship between HTTP and RTSP, the same protocol mechanisms can probably be imported into RTSP in the future.

3.10   SESSION DESCRIPTION PROTOCOL (SDP)

The Session Description Protocol (SDP) (98) is a text format for describing multimedia sessions. It is not really a protocol, but rather similar in spirit to a markup language like HTML. SDP can be carried in any protocol, with SIP, RTSP, SAP, HTTP, and e mail being the most common ones. For example, one could link a description of an ongoing video session to a web page, with the SDP stored in a file. The web browser, if suitably configured, would then pass the SDP message to a tool that would in turn invoke the necessary media applications and listen to the session.
SDP can convey the following information.

The type of media (video, audio, shared applications).
The media transport protocol (typically, RTP/UDP/IP, but it could be an ATM virtual circuit).
The format of the media (e.g., H.261 video, MPEG video, G.723.1 audio), with a mapping between encoding names and RTP payload types.
The time and duration of the session, which can be in the future and may span several repetitions at regular intervals or random time instances.
Security information, such as the encryption key for a media session.
Session names and subject information for presentation in "TV Guide"-style session directories.
Human contact information related to a session, so that receivers can find the responsible party if problems develop (e.g., if a session consumes too much bandwidth or has other technical problems). (It can be thought of as the rough equivalent of the FCC-mandated station identification.)

An SDP message consists of a set of global headers describing the session as a whole, followed by a set of media descriptions. Each line consists of a single-character parameter name followed by a list of values. Media descriptions start with an "m=" line and continue until the next "m=" line.

If the session is multicast, SDP conveys the multicast address and transport port to which the source is sending the media stream or expecting to receive data from. For a unicast session, the description indicates where media should be sent to.

SDP was originally designed for multicast sessions, to be distributed via SAP (Section 3.12) to potential listeners. It has since been used in RTSP (Section 3.9) and SIP (Section 3.11) for describing unicast and multicast sessions. Instead of describing streams that are being multicast, in SIP it is used to indicate receiver capabilities.

```
o=- 2890844526 2890842807 IN IP4 192.16.24.202
s=Twister PG-13 (c) Warner Bros.
m=audio 0 RTP/AVP 98
a=rtpmap:98 L16/16000/2
a=control:rtsp://audio.example.com/twister/audio.en
m=video 0 RTP/AVP 31
a=rtpmap:31 MPV
a=control:rtsp://video.example.com/twister/video
```

Figure 3.7 Sample SDP description for an RTSP multimedia session.

One of the benefits of SDP is its simple textual format and its easy extensibility. Attributes can be added for each media type or for the whole session. For example, RTSP adds an attribute for indicating the request URL for controlling the individual media stream.

SDP can describe only an unordered list of media. It cannot currently convey, for example, the information that two audio streams contain the same material, just in different encodings or human languages.

The example in Figure 3.7 shows a session description as it might be used in an RTSP DESCRIBE response for a movie consisting of a video and audio track. The "o=" line identifies the origin of the session description and its version. The "s=" line provides information about the content, while the "m=" lines identify the media, the port, the transport, and the list of supported encodings. The "a=rtpmap" lines map the RTP payload type to an encoding name. (This is necessary because the RTP payload number range is much smaller than the universe of possible encodings.) The "a=control" lines indicate the RTSP request URL.

3.11 SIGNALING: SESSION INITIATION PROTOCOL (SIP)

A defining property of Internet telephony is the ability of one party to signal to one or more other parties to initiate a new call. For purposes of discussing the Session Initiation Protocol, we define a call as an association between a number of participants. The signaling association between a pair of participants in a call is referred to as a connection. Note that there is no physical channel or network resources associated with a connection; the connection exists only as signaling state at the two end points. A session refers to a single RTP session carrying a single media type. The relationship between the signaling connections and media sessions can be varied. In a multiparty call, for example, each participant may have a connection to every other participant, while the media are being distributed via multicast, in which case there is a single media session. In other cases, there may be a single unicast media session associated with each connection. Other, more complex scenarios are possible as well.

An IP telephony signaling protocol must accomplish a number of functions, including the following.

Name translation and user location involve the mapping between names of different levels of abstraction (e.g., a common name at a domain and a user name at a particular Internet host). This translation is necessary to determine the IP address of the host to exchange media with. Usually, a user has only the name or e-mail address of the person with whom communication is desired (e.g., j.doe@company.com). This must be translated into an IP address. This translation is more than just a simple table lookup. The translation can vary based on time of day (so that a caller reaches you at work during the day, and at home in the evening), caller (so that your boss always gets your work number), or the status of the callee (so that calls to you are sent to your voicemail when you are already talking to someone), among other criteria.

Feature negotiation allows a group of end systems to agree on what media to exchange and their respective parameters, such as encodings. The set and type of media need not be uniform within a call, inasmuch as different point-to-point connections may involve different media and media parameters. Many software codecs are able to receive different encodings within a single call and in parallel, for example, while being restricted to sending one type of media for each stream.

Any call participant can invite others into an existing call and terminate connections with some (*call participant management*). During the call, participants should be able to transfer and hold other users. The most general model of a multiparty association is that of a full or partial mesh of connections among participants (where one of the participants may be a media bridge), with the possible addition of multicast media distribution.

Feature changes make it possible to adjust the composition of media sessions during the course of a call, either because the participants require additional or reduced functionality or because of constraints imposed or removed by the addition or removal of call participants.

Two protocols have been developed for such signaling operations, the Session Initiation Protocol (SIP) (118), developed in the IETF, and H.323 (119), developed by the ITU.

3.11.1 SIP Overview

SIP is a client–server protocol. This means that requests are generated by one entity (the client) and sent to a receiving entity (the server), which processes them. Since a call participant may either generate or receive requests, SIP-enabled end systems include a protocol client and server (generally called a user agent server). The user agent server generally responds to the requests based on human interaction or some other kind of input. Furthermore, SIP requests can traverse many *proxy servers,* each of which receives a request and forwards it toward a next hop server, which may be another proxy server or the final user agent server. A server may also act as a *redirect server,* informing the client of the address of the next hop server, so that the client can contact it directly. There is no protocol distinction between a proxy server, redirect server, and user agent server; a client or proxy server has no way of knowing which it is communicating with. The distinction lies only in function: a proxy or redirect server cannot accept or reject a request, whereas a user agent server can. This is similar to the Hypertext Transfer Protocol (HTTP) model of client, origin, and proxy servers. A single host may well act as client and server for the same request. A connection is constructed by issuing an INVITE request, and destroyed by issuing a BYE request.

As in HTTP, the client requests invoke *methods* on the server. Requests and responses are textual, and contain header fields, which convey call properties and service information. SIP reuses many of the header fields used in HTTP, such as the entity headers (e.g., Content-type) and authentication headers. This allows for code reuse and simplifies integration of SIP servers with web servers. Calls in SIP are uniquely identified by a call identifier, carried in the Call-ID header field in SIP messages. The call identifier is created by the creator of the call and is used by all call participants. Connections have the following properties. The *logical connection source* indicates the entity that is requesting the connection (the originator). This may not be the entity that is actually sending the request, since proxies may send requests on behalf of other users. In SIP messages, this property is conveyed in the From header field. The *logical connection destination* contained in the To field names the party who the originator wishes to contact (the recipient). The *media destination* conveys the location (IP address and port) where the media (audio, video, data) are to be sent for a particular recipient. This address may not be the same address as the logical connection destination. *Media capabilities* convey the media that a participant is capable of receiving and their attributes. Media capabilities and media destinations are conveyed jointly as part of the payload of a SIP message. Currently, the Session Description Protocol (SDP) (98) serves this purpose, although others are likely to find use in the future.* SDP expresses lists of capabilities for audio and video and indicates the intended destination of the media. It also allows the scheduling of media sessions into the future and the scheduling of repeated sessions.

SIP defines several methods, where the first three manage or prepare calls

---

*In fact, H.245 capability sets can be carried in SDP for this purpose.

and connections: INVITE invites a user to a call and establishes a new connection; BYE terminates a connection between two users in a call (note that a call, as a logical entity, is created when the first connection in the call is created and is destroyed when the last connection in the call is destroyed); and OPTIONS solicits information about capabilities, but does not set up a connection. STATUS informs another server about the progress of signaling actions that it has requested via the Also header (see below). ACK is used for reliable message exchanges for invitations. CANCEL terminates a search for a user. Finally, REGISTER conveys information about a user's location to a SIP server.

SIP makes minimal assumptions about the underlying transport protocol. It can directly use any datagram or stream protocol, with the only restriction being that a whole SIP request or response has to be delivered in full or not at all. SIP can thus be used with UDP or TCP in the Internet, and with X.25, AAL5/ATM, CLNP, TP4, IPX, or PPP elsewhere. Network addresses within SIP are also not restricted to being Internet addresses, but could be E.164 (GSTN) addresses, OSI addresses or private numbering plans. In many cases, addresses can be any URL; for example, a call can be "forwarded" to a "mailto" URL for e-mail delivery.

3.11.2 Message Encoding

Unlike other signaling protocols such as Q.931 (120) and H.323 (121), SIP is a text-based protocol. This design was chosen to minimize the cost of entry. The data structures needed in SIP headers all fall into the parameter-value category, possible with a single level of subparameters, so that generic data coding mechanisms like Abstract Syntax Notation 1 (ASN.1) (122) offer no functional advantage. Many parameters are textual, so that there is no significant penalty in terms of bytes transmitted.

Unlike the ASN.1 packed encoding rules (PER) (123) and basic encoding rules (BER) (124), a SIP header is largely self-describing. Even if an extension has not been formally documented, as was the case for many common e-mail headers, it is usually easy to reverse-engineer them. Since most values are textual, the space penalty is limited to the parameter names, usually at most a few tens of bytes per request. (Indeed, the ASN.1 PER-encoded H.323 signaling messages are larger than equivalent SIP messages.) Besides, extreme space efficiency is not a concern for signaling protocols.

If not designed carefully, text-based protocols can be difficult to parse owing to their irregular structure. SIP tries to avoid this by maintaining a common structure of all header fields, allowing a generic parser to be written.

Unlike, say, HTTP and Internet e-mail, SIP was designed for character-set independence, so that any field can contain any ISO 10646 character. Since SIP operates on an 8-bit clean channel, binary data such as certificates do not have to be encoded. Together with the ability to indicate languages of enclosed content and language preferences of the requestor, SIP is well suited for cross-national use.

3.11.3 Addressing and Naming

To be invited and identified, the called party has to be named. Since it is the most common form of user addressing in the Internet, SIP chose an e-mail-like identifier of the form *"user@domain," "user@host," "user@IP address,"* or *"phone-number@gateway."* The identifier can refer to the name of the host that a user is logged in at the time, an e-mail address, or the name of a domain-specific name translation service. Addresses of the form *"phone-number@gateway"* designate global switched telephone network (GSTN) phone numbers reachable via the named gateway.

SIP uses these addresses as part of SIP URLs (e.g., sip:j.doe@example.com). This URL may well be placed in a web page, so that clicking on the link initiates a call to that address, similar to a "mailto" (125) URL today.

We anticipate that most users will be able to use their e-mail address as their published SIP address. E-mail addresses already offer a basic location-independent form of addressing, in that the host part does not have to designate a particular Internet host, but can be a domain, which is then resolved into one or more possible domain mail server hosts via Domain Name System (DNS) MX (mail exchange) records. This not only saves space on business cards, but also allows reuse of existing directory services such as the Lightweight Directory Access Protocol (LDAP) [126], DNS MX records (as explained below), and e-mail as a last-ditch means of delivering SIP invitations.

For e-mail, finding the mail exchange host is often sufficient to deliver mail, since users either log in to the mail exchange host or use protocols such as the Internet Mail Access Protocol (IMAP) or the Post Office Protocol (POP) to retrieve their mail. For interactive audio and video communications, however, participants are typically sending and receiving data on the workstation, PC, or Internet appliance in their immediate physical proximity. Thus, SIP has to be able to resolve *"name@domain"* to *"user@host."* A user at a specific host will be derived through zero or more translations. A single externally visible address may well lead to a different host depending on time of day, media to be used, and any number of other factors. Also, hosts that connect via dial-up modems may acquire a different IP address each time.

3.11.4 Basic Operation

The most important SIP operation is that of inviting new participants to a call. A SIP client first obtains an address at which the new participant is to be contacted, of the form *name@domain*. The client then tries to translate this domain to an IP address where a server may be found. This translation is done by trying, in sequence, DNS Service (SRV) records, MX, Canonical Name (CNAME), and finally Address (A) records. Once the server's IP address has been found, the client sends it an INVITE message, using either UDP or TCP.

The server that receives the message is not likely to be the user agent server where the user is actually located; it may be a proxy or redirect server. For example, a server at example.com contacted when trying to call doe@example.com may forward the INVITE request to doe@sales.example.com. A Via header traces the progress of the invitation from server to server, allows responses to find their way back, and helps servers to detect loops. A redirect server, on the other hand, would respond to the INVITE request, telling the caller to contact doe@sales.example.com directly. In either case, the proxy or redirect server must somehow determine the next hop server. This is the function of a *location server*. A location server is a non-SIP entity that has information about next hop servers for various users. The location server can be anything—an LDAP server, a proprietary corporate database, a local file, the result of a finger command, and so on. The choice is a matter of local configuration. Figures 3.8 and 3.9 show the behavior of SIP proxy and redirect servers, respectively.

Proxy servers can forward the invitation to multiple servers at once, in the hope of contacting the user at one of the locations. They can also forward the invitation to multicast groups, effectively contacting multiple next hops in the most efficient manner.

Once the user agent server has been contacted, it sends a response back to the client. The response has a response code and response message. The codes fall into classes 100 through 600, similar to HTTP.

Unlike other requests, invitations cannot be answered immediately, since locating the callee and waiting for a human to answer may take several seconds.

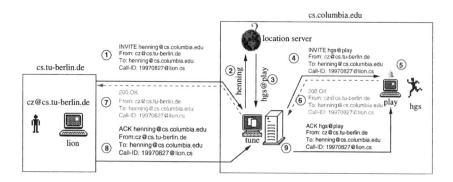

Figure 3.8 SIP proxy server operation.

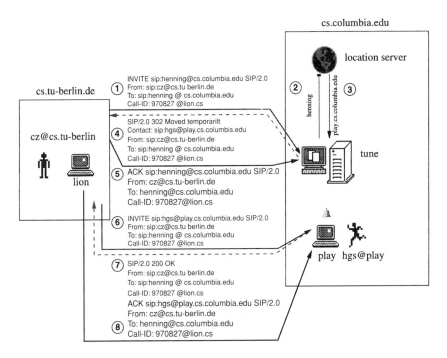

Figure 3.9 SIP redirect server operation.

Call requests may also be queued (e.g., if the callee is busy). Responses of the 100 class (denoted as 1xx) indicate call progress; they are always followed by other responses indicating the final outcome of the request.

While the 1xx responses are provisional, the other classes indicate the final status of the request: 2xx for success; 3xx for redirection; 4xx, 5xx, and 6xx for client, server, and global failures, respectively. 3xx responses list, in a Location header, alternate places at which the user might be contacted. To ensure reliability even with unreliable transport protocols, the server retransmits final responses until the client confirms receipt by sending an ACK request to the server.

All responses can include more detailed information. For example, a call to the central "switchboard" address may return a web page that includes links to the various departments in the company, providing navigation more appropriate to the Internet than an interactive voice response system (IVR).

Since IPtel is still immature, it is likely that additional signaling capabilities will be needed in the future. Also, individual implementations and vendors may want to add additional features. SIP uses the same extension mechanisms as RTSP (Section 3.9.4).

3.11.5 Telephony Services

SIP takes a different approach from standard telephony in defining services. Rather than explicitly describing the implementation of a particular service, it provides a number of elements, namely, headers and methods, to construct services. The two principal headers used are Also and Replaces. When present in a request or response, the Also header instructs the recipient to place a call to the parties listed. Similarly, Replaces instructs the recipient to terminate any connections with the parties listed. An additional method, called STATUS, is provided to allow a client to obtain results about progress of calls requested via the Also header.

These elements, along with the basic SIP components, are easily used to construct a variety of traditional telephony services. *700, 800, and 900* services (permanent numbers, freephone, and paid information services) are, from a call control perspective, simply special cases of call forwarding, governed by a database lookup or some server-specified algorithm. The charging mechanisms, which differ for the three services, are handled by other protocols in an orthogonal fashion. Unlike the case of intelligent networking (IN), the number of such lookups within a call is not limited. Call forwarding services based on user status or preferences similarly require no additional protocol machinery. As a simple example, we have implemented an automatic call forwarding mechanism that inspects a callee's appointment calendar and then forwards the call or indicates a more opportune time to call back.

While *call forwarding* precedes a call, *call transfer* allows a call participant to be directed to connect to a different subscriber. Transfer services include blind and supervised call transfer, attendant and operator services, autodialer for telemarketing, or interactive voice response. All are supported through use of the Also header combined with programmed behavior specific to the particular service. For example, blind transfer is implemented by having the transferring party send the transferred party a BYE containing an Also header listing the transferred-to party.

In SIP, call setup and session parameter modification are accomplished by the same (INVITE) request, as all SIP requests are idempotent.

In an Internet environment, no "lines" are tied up by active calls when media are not being sent. This means that an IP telephone can support an unlimited number of active calls at one time. This makes it easy, for example, to implement call waiting and camp-on.

3.11.6 Multiparty Calls

SIP supports the three basic modes of creating multiparty conferences (and their combinations): via network-level multicast, via one or more bridges (also known as multipoint control units), or as a mesh of unicast connections. Multicast conferences require no further protocol support beyond listing a group address in the session description; indeed, the caller does not even have to be a member of the multicast group to issue an invitation. Bridges are introduced like regular session members; they may take over branches of a mesh through the Replaces header, and the participants need not be aware that there is a bridge serving the conference. SIP also supports conferences through full mesh, also known as *multiunicast*. In this case, the client maintains a point-to-point connection with each participant. While this mode is very inefficient, it is very useful for small conferences for which bridges or multicast service are not available. Full meshes are built up easily using the Also header. For example, to add a participant C to a call between users A and B, user A would send an INVITE to C with an Also header containing the address of B. Mixes of multiunicast, multicast, and bridges are also possible.

SIP can also be used to set up calls to several callees. For example, if the callee's address is a mailing list, the SIP server can return a list of individuals to be called in an Also header. Alternatively, a single address (e.g., sysadmin@acme.com) may reach the first available administrator. Servers can fan out invitation requests, including sending them out via multicast. Multicast invitations are particularly useful for inviting members of a department (product_team@example.com) to a conference in an extremely efficient manner without requiring central list administration.

Multicast invitations also allow a small conference to gradually and smoothly migrate to a large-scale multicast conference without requiring separate protocols and architectures.

3.12 SESSION ANNOUNCEMENT PROTOCOL (SAP)

RTSP (Section 3.9) and SIP (Section 3.11) are designed for one-on-one sessions; in our earlier taxonomy we are thus left to address Internet broadcast sessions. (We use the term "broadcast" in analogy with radio and TV, even though in the Internet context, the continuous media are being distributed only to networks with at least one interested viewer, as described earlier in Section 3.4.)

A viewer can find Internet broadcast multimedia content of interest in several ways: for example, web pages, search engines indexing web pages, or e-mail announcements. However, none of these methods scale well, in that each search request has to be individually answered by a server. Search engines are also less likely to be useful. A search for "Twister" will likely return roughly 122,740 web pages, only one or two of which may contain information about any current broadcasts of the movie. Also, since multicast is usually "scoped" to an administrative domain (see Section 3.4) and may be limited by TTL value to a particular region of the Internet, being able to obtain the session description via a web page does not imply that one could actually receive the media stream. Since the number of concurrent Internet multicasts is limited by the available bandwidth and, for the foreseeable future, on the same order of magnitude as the number of channels in a cable system, it makes sense to multicast announcements about these sessions. This practice also has the advantage that receiving the announcement implies with a high probability that one is able to receive the corresponding media stream, as long as session announcement and media stream have the same origin.

In a multicast session directory, distributed servers periodically send multicast packets containing descriptions of sessions generated by local sources. These advertisements are then received by multicast receivers on a well-known, static multicast address and port (9875). Global-scope advertisements are sent to multicast address 224.2.127.254, while scoped announcements are sent on the highest address within the scope's multicast address range. The advertisement contains information, such as SDP (Section 3.10) to start the media tools needed to partake in the session. The Session Announcement Protocol (SAP) (127) is one such protocol.

With any distributed multicast announcement protocol, there has to be a rate-scaling mechanism so that the overall bandwidth is limited. SAP chooses an overall announcement bandwidth of 4000 bits for a single SAP multicast group. Each announcer listens for other announcements and scales the interval between announcements so that this bandwidth is not exceeded. The minimum interval between announcements is 5 minutes.* This mechanism has the disadvantage that it can take several minutes before a newly started end-user application gains a perspective on the available multicast sessions. (This is a particular problem when end hosts are not permanently connected to the Internet and thus cannot just leave the session directory application running.) Applications typically cache the announcements and may use a SAP proxy cache that captures the announcements to a local web page.

3.13 CONCLUSION

The Internet protocol suite has now the basic ingredients to support streaming audio and video, for both distribution and communication applications. In this chapter, we have seen how applications can build Internet multimedia services without changing the basic IP infrastructure.

---

*It could be argued that the announcement interval should scale with the media bandwidth, but this does not quite work, since announcements are typically sent well ahead of the start of the media session.

However, major challenges remain, both for the protocol foundations and for the operational infrastructure. For example, there currently is no session control protocol that can be used to perform floor control in distributed multimedia conferences. Protocols for sharing computer applications are limited, mostly proprietary, and not well suited for Internet use.

The operational challenges are at least as large. Network reliability and deployment multicast of services with predictable quality-of-service are probably the major hurdles, beyond the need for continuous upgrades in network capacity.

3.14 ACRONYMS

AAL	ATM adaptation layer
APNIC	Asia–Pacific Network Information Center
ARIN	American Registry for Internet Numbers
ARP	Address Resolution Protocol
ASN.1	Abstract Syntax Notation 1
ATM	asynchronous transfer mode
BER	(ASN.1) basic encoding rules
BGP	Border Gateway Protocol
CBT	Core-Based Tree method
DHCP	Dynamic Host Configuration Protocol
DNS	Domain Name System
ftp	file transfer protocol
GSTN	global switched telephone network
HTTP	Hypertext Transfer Protocol
ICANN	Internet Corporation for Assigned Names and Numbers
ICMP	Internet Control Message Protocol
IETF	Internet Engineering Task Force
IGMP	Internet Group Management Protocol
IP	Internet Protocol
ITU	International Telecommunications Union
JPEG	Joint Photographic Experts Group
LANE	LAN (local-area network) emulation
LDAP	Lightweight Data Access Protocol
MDTP	Multinetwork Datagram Transmission Protocol
MLD	Multicast Listener Discovery (protocol)
MOSPF	Multicast Open Shortest Path First (protocol)
MPEG	Motion Pictures Expert Group
NAT	network address translator
NAPT	network address and port translator
NBMA	Nonbroadcast Multiple Access
NFS	Network File System

SAP	Session Announcement Protocol
SDP	Session Description Protocol
SIP	Session Initiation Protocol
SMPTE	Society of Motion Picture and Television Engineers
SMTP	Simple Mail Transfer Protocol
SNMP	Simple Network Management Protocol
TCP	Transmission Control Protocol
TOS	type of service
TTI,	time to live
UDP	User Datagram Protocol
URL	Uniform Resource Locator

ACKNOWLEDGMENT

Jonathan Rosenberg contributed parts of the chapter.

REFERENCES

1. H Zimmermann. OSI reference model—The ISO model of architecture for open systems interconnection. IEEE Trans Communi COM-28: 425–432, 1980.
2. JD Day, H Zimmermann. The OSI reference model. Proceed IEEE 71:1334–1340, December 1983.
3. RM Metcalfe, DR Boggs. Ethernet: Distributed packet switching for local computer networks. Communi ACM 19:711–719, July 1976.
4. J Hamstra. FDDI design tradeoffs. IEEE Computer Society Conference on Local Computer Networks, Minneapolis, MN. October 1988, pp. 297–300.
5. J Heinanen, R Govindan. NBMA address resolution protocol (NARP). Request for Comments (experimental) 1735. Internet Engineering Task Force, December 1994.
6. J Postel. Internet Protocol. Request for Comments (standard) 791. Internet Engineering Task Force, September 1981.
7. S Deering, R. Hinden. Internet Protocol, version 6 (ipv6) specification. Request for Comments (proposed standard) 1883. Internet Engineering Task Force, December 1995.
8. D Crocker. Standard for the format of ARPA Internet text messages. Request for Comments (standard) 822. Internet Engineering Task Force, August 1982.
9. R Fielding, J Gettys, J Mogul, H Frystyk, T. Berners-Lee, Hypertext Transfer Protocol—HTTP/1.1. Request for Comments (proposed standard) 2068. Internet Engineering Task Force, January 1997.
10. J Postel, JK Reynolds. File transfer protocol. Request for Comments (standard) 959. Internet Engineering Task Force, October 1985.
11. J Postel, JK Reynolds. Telnet protocol specification. Request for Comments (standard) 854. Internet Engineering Task Force, May 1983.
12. W Simpson and editor. The point-to-point protocol (PPP). Request for Comments (standard) 1661. Internet Engineering Task Force, July 1994.

13. JF Shoch. Inter-network naming, addressing, and routing. Proceedings on Computer Communications Networks; Computers and Communications: Interfaces and Interactions (IEEE Compcon), Washington, DC, September 1978, pp. 72–79.

14. R Droms. Dynamic Host Configuration Protocol. Request for Comments (proposed standard) 1541. Internet Engineering Task Force, October 1993.

15. PV Mockapetris. Domain names—Concepts and facilities. Request for Comments (standard) 1034. Internet Engineering Task Force, November 1987.

16. V Fuller, T Li, J Yu, K Varadhan. Supernetting: An address assignment and aggregation strategy. Request for Comments (informational) 1338. Internet Engineering Task Force, June 1992.

17. FT Solensky. Ipv4 address space utilization. Web page, Top Layer, October 1999. http://ipv4space.TopLayer.Com.

18. C Huitema. The Internet in October 1999. Web page, Telcordia, Morristown, NJ, October 1999. ftp://ftp.telcordia.com/pub/huitema/stats/

19. P Srisuresh, K Egevang. Traditional IP network address translator (traditional NAT). Internet Draft, Internet Engineering Task Force, November 1998. Work in progress.

20. JH Saltzer, DP Reed, DD Clark. End-to-end arguments in system design. ACM Trans Comput Syst 2:277–288, November 1984.

21. S Blake, D Black, M Carlson, E Davies, Z Wang, W Weiss. An architecture for differentiated service. Request for Comments (informational) 2475. Internet Engineering Task Force, December 1998.

22. J Postel. Internet Control Message Protocol. Request for Comments (standard) 792. Internet Engineering Task Force, September 1981.

23. J Postel. User Datagram Protocol. Request for Comments (standard) 768. Internet Engineering Task Force, August 1980.

24. J Postel. DoD Standard Transmission Control Protocol. Request for Comments 761. Internet Engineering Task Force, January 1980.

25. M Allman, V Paxson, W Stevens. TCP congestion control. Request for Comments (proposed standard) 2581. Internet Engineering Task Force, April 1999.

26. MT Rose and DE Cass. ISO transport services on top of the TCP: Version 3. Request for Comments (standard) 1006. Internet Engineering Task Force, May 1987.

27. P Cameron, D Crocker, D Cohen, J Postel. Transport Multiplexing Protocol (TMUX). Request for Comments (proposed standard) 1692. Internet Engineering Task Force, August 1994.

28. W Livens, D Ooms. Connectionless multicast. Internet Draft, Internet Engineering Task Force, June 1999. Work in progress.

29. S Hanna, B Patel, M Shah. Multicast address dynamic client allocation protocol (MADCAP). Internet Draft, Internet Engineering Task Force, May 1999. Work in progress.

30. D Meyer. Administratively scoped IP multicast. Request for Comments (best current practice) 2365. Internet Engineering Task Force, July 1998.

31. A. Conta and S. Deering. Internet Control Message Protocol (ICMPv6) for the Internet Protocol version 6 (ipv6). Request for Comments (proposed standard) 1885. Internet Engineering Task Force, December 1995.

32. W Fenner. Internet Group Management Protocol, version 2. Request for Comments (proposed standard) 2236. Internet Engineering Task Force, November 1997.

33. S Deering, W Fenner, B Haberman. Multicast listener discovery (MLD) for IPv6. Request for Comments (proposed standard) 2710. Internet Engineering Task Force, October 1999.

34. J Moy. Multicast extensions to OSPF. Request for Comments (proposed standard) 1584. Internet Engineering Task Force, March 1994.

35. D Waitzman, C Partridge, SE Deering. Distance Vector Multicast Routing Protocol. Request for Comments (experimental) 1075. Internet Engineering Task Force, November 1988.

36. T Pusateri. Distance Vector Multicast Routing Protocol. Internet Draft, Internet Engineering Task Force, March 1999. Work in progress.

37. D Estrin, D Farinacci, A Helmy, D Thaler, S Deering, M Handley, V Jacobson, C Liu, P Sharma, L. Wei. Protocol-independent multicast-sparse mode (PIM-SM): Protocol specification. Request for Comments (experimental) 2117. Internet Engineering Task Force, June 1997.

38. S Deering, D Estrin, D Farinacci, V Jacobson, A Helmy, D Meyer, L. Wei. Protocol-independent multicast version 2 dense mode specification. Internet Draft, Internet Engineering Task Force, June 1999. Work in progress.

39. A Ballardie. Core-Based Trees (CBT version 2) multicast routing. Request for Comments (experimental) 2189. Internet Engineering Task Force, September 1997.

40. K. Obraczka. Multicast transport protocols: A survey and taxonomy. IEEE Commun Maga 36:94–102, January 1998.

41. SA Thomas. IPng and the TCP/IP protocols: Implementing the Next-Generation Internet. New York: Wiley, 1996.

42. C Huitema. Routing in the Internet. Englewood Cliffs, NJ: Prentice Hall, 1995.

43. V Paxson. Measurements and analysis of end-to-end internet dynamics. PhD dissertation. University of California, Berkeley, May 1997.

44. V Paxson. End-to-end Internet packet dynamics. SIGCOMM Symposium on Communications Architectures and Protocols, Cannes, France, September 1997.

45. D Sala, JO Limb, SU Khaunte. Adaptive control mechanism for a cable modem MAC protocol. Proceedings of the Conference on Computer Communications (IEEE Infocom) (R. Guerin, ed.), San Francisco, March 1998, p. 8.

46. B Goodman. Internet telephony and modem delay. IEEE Network 13:8–17, May/June 1999.

47. D Cohen. Issues in transnet packetized voice communications. Proceedings of the Fifth ACM/IEEE Data Communications Symposium, Snowbird, UT, September 1977, pp 6-10–6-13.

48. WA Montgomery. Techniques for packet voice synchronization. IEEE J Selected Areas Commun SAC-1:1022–1028, December 1983.

49. H Schulzrinne. Voice communication across the Internet: A network voice terminal. Technical Report TR 92-50. Department of Computer Science, University of Massachusetts, Amherst, July 1992.

50. R Ramjee, J Kurose, D Towsley, H Schulzrinne. Adaptive playout mechanisms for packetized audio applications in wide-area networks. In: Proceedings of the Conference on Computer Communications (IEEE Infocom), Toronto, Canada. IEEE Computer Society Press, pp 680–688. Los Alamitos, CA: June 1994.

51. SB Moon, J Kurose, D Towsley. Packet audio playout delay adjustment: Performance bounds and algorithms. ACM/Springer Multimedia Syst 5: 17–28. January 1998.

52. H Schulzrinne. Operating system issues for continuous multimedia. In: B. Furht, ed. Handbook of Multimedia Computing. Boca Raton, FL: CRC Press, 1998, pp 627–648.

53. C Partridge and S Pink. A faster UDP. IEEE/ACM Trans Networking 1:429–440, August 1993.

54. J Rosenberg, L Qiu, H Schulzrinne. Integrating packet FEC into adaptive voice playout buffer algorithms on the Internet. Proceedings of the Conference on Computer Communications (IEEE Infocom), March 2000.

55. G Almes, S Kalidindi, M Zekauskas. A round-trip delay metric for IPPM. Internet Draft, Internet Engineering Task Force, May 1999. Work in progress.

56. G Almes, S Kalidindi, M Zekauskas. A one-way delay metric for IPPM. Internet Draft, Internet Engineering Task Force, May 1999. Work in progress.

57. V Paxson. On calibrating measurements of packet transit times. Proceedings of the ACM Sigmetrics Conference on Measurement and Modeling of Computer Systems, Madison, WI, June 1998, pp 11–21.

58. V Paxson, G Almes, J Mahdavi, M Mathis. Framework for IP performance metrics. Request for Comments (informational) 2330. Internet Engineering Task Force, May 1998.

59. G Almes, S Kalidindi, M Zekauskas. A one-way packet loss metric for IPPM. Internet Draft, Internet Engineering Task Force, May 1999. Work in progress.

60. EW Biersack. Performance evaluation of forward error correction in ATM networks. Comput Commun Re 22(4), October 1992.

61. GR Pieris, GH Sasaki. The performance of simple error control protocols under correlated packet losses. Proceedings of the Conference on Computer Communications (IEEE Infocom), Bal Harbour, FL, IEEE, April 1991, pp 764–772 (7C.1).

62. J-C Bolot, S Fosse-Parisis, D Towsley. Adaptive FEC-based error control for interactive audio in the Internet. Proceedings of the Conference on Computer Communications (IEEE Infocom), New York, March 1999.

63. H Schulzrinne, JF Kurose, DF Towsley. Loss correlation for queues with single and multiple input streams. Technical Report TR 92-53. Department of Computer Science, University of Massachusetts, Amherst, July 1992.

64. M Yajnik, J Kurose, D Towsley. Packet loss correlation in the MBone multicast network. Proceedings of Global Internet, London, November 1996.

65. R Koodli and R Ravikanth. One-way loss pattern sample metrics. Internet Draft, Internet Engineering Task Force, June 1999. Work in progress.

66. NF Maxemchuk and S Lo. Measurement and interpretation of voice traffic on the Internet. Conference Record of the International Conference on Communications (ICC), Montreal, Canada, June 1997.

67. W Matthews. Monitoring update. ESCC, San Diego, CA, April 1999.

68. P Pan, H Schulzrinne. YESSIR: A simple reservation mechanism for the Internet. ACM Comput Commun Rev 29:89–101, April 1999.

69. J Mahdavi, V Paxson. IPPM metrics for measuring connectivity. Request for Comments (experimental) 2498. Internet Engineering Task Force, January 1999.

70. C Partridge, RM Hinden. Version 2 of the reliable data protocol (RDP). Request for Comments (experimental) 1151. Internet Engineering Task Force, April 1990.
71. L Rizzo, L. Vicisano. A reliable multicast data distribution protocol based on software FEC techniques. Fourth IEEE Workshop on High Performance Communication Systems (HPCS'97), Chalkidiki, Greece, June 1997.
72. S Floyd, V Jacobson, C-G Liu, S McCanne, L Zhang. A reliable multicast framework for light-weight sessions and application level framing. *IEEE/ACM Trans Networking* 5:784–803, December 1997.
73. XR Xu, AC Myers, H Zhang, R Yavatkar. Resilient multicast support for continuous-media applications. Proceedings of the International Workshop on Network and Operating System Support for Digital Audio and Video (NOSSDAV), St. Louis, MO, May 1997.
74. J Nonnenmacher, E Biersack, D Towsley. Parity-based loss recovery for reliable multicast transmission. ACM Comput Commun Rev 27:289–300, October 1997.
75. LW Lehman, S Garland, DL Tennenhouse. Active reliable multicast. Proceedings of the Conference on Computer Communications (IEEE Infocom), San Francisco, March/April 1998, p 581.
76. MP Barcellos, PD Ezhilchelvan. An end-to-end reliable multicast protocol using polling for scalability. Proceedings of the Conference on Computer Communications (IEEE Infocom), San Francisco, March/April 1998, p 1188.
77. C Papadopoulos, G Parulkar, G Varghese. An error control scheme for large-scale multicast applications. Proceedings of the Conference on Computer Communications (IEEE Infocom), San Francisco, March/April 1998, p 1188.
78. J Nonnenmacher, M Lacher, M Jung, E Biersack, G Carle. How bad is reliable multicast without local recovery? Proceedings of the Conference on Computer Communications (IEEE Infocom), San Francisco, March/April 1998, p 972.
79. SK Kasera, J Kurose, D Towsley. A comparison of server-based and receiver-based local recovery approaches for scalable reliable multicast. Proceedings of the Conference on Computer Communications (IEEE Infocom), San Francisco, March/April 1998, p 988.
80. JS Quarterman. Imminent death of the Internet? Matrix News, vol 6, June 1996.
81. AS Induruwa, PF Linington, JB Slater. Quality-of-service measurements on Super-JANET, the U K academic information highway. Proceedings of INET, San Jose, CA, June 1999.
82. S Kalidindi, MJ Zekauskas. Surveyor: An infrastructure for Internet performance measurements. Proceedings of INET, San Jose, CA, June 1999.
83. T Bass. Traffic congestion measurements in transit IP networks. Technical Report TR 97-101. Internet Systems and Services, January 1997.
84. AK Agrawala, D Sanghi. Network dynamics: An experimental study of the Internet. Proceedings of the IEEE Conference on Global Communications (GLOBECOM), Orlando, FL, December 1992, pp 782–786 (24.02).
85. J-C Bolot. End-to-end packet delay and loss behavior in the Internet. Comput Commun Rev 23(4), October 1992.
86. A Odlyzko. Data networks are lightly utilized, and will stay that way. Technical Report. AT&T Labs—Research, Florham Park, NJ, July 1998.

87. J Bolot, H Crepin, A Garcia. Analysis of audio packet loss in the Internet. Proceedings of the International Workshop on Network and Operating System Support for Digital Audio and Video (NOSSDAV), Durham, NH, April 1995, pp 163–174.

88. M Yajnik, S Moon, J Kurose, D Towsley. Measurement and modelling of the temporal dependence in packet loss. Proceedings of the Conference on Computer Communications (IEEE Infocom), New York, March 1999.

89. A Mukherjee. On the dynamics and significance of low frequency components of Internet load. Internetworking: Res Exp 5:163–205, December 1994.

90. MS Borella, GB Brewster. Measurement and analysis of long-range dependent behavior of Internet packet delay. Proceedings of the Conference on Computer Communications (IEEE Infocom), San Francisco, March/April 1998, p 497.

91. M Handley, J Crowcroft, C Bormann, J Ott. The Internet multimedia conferencing architecture. Internet Draft, Internet Engineering Task Force, July 1997. Work in progress.

92. WC Fenner, SL Casner. A "traceroute" facility for IP multicast. Internet Draft, Internet Engineering Task Force, June 1999. Work in progress.

93. R Gurin, H. Schulzrinne. Network quality of service. In I. Foster and C. Kesselman, eds. The Grid: Blueprint for a New Computing Infrastructure. San Francisco: Morgan Kaufmann, 1998.

94. K Nichols, V Jacobson, L Zhang. A two-bit differentiated services architecture for the Internet. Internet Draft, Internet Engineering Task Force, May 1999. Work in progress.

95. X Wang, H Schulzrinne. RNAP: A resource negotiation and pricing protocol. Proceedings of the International Workshop on Network and Operating System Support for Digital Audio and Video (NOSSDAV), Basking Ridge, NJ June 1999, pp 77–93.

96. O Schelen, S Pink. Aggregating resource reservation over multiple routing domains. Proceedings of Fifth IFIP International Workshop on Quality of Service (IwQOS), Cambridge, England, June 1998.

97. H Schulzrinne, J. Rosenberg. Internet telephony: Architecture and protocols—An IETF perspective. Comput Networks ISDN Syst 31:237–255, February 1999.

98. M Handley, V Jacobson. SDP: Session description protocol. Request for Comments (proposed standard) 2327. Internet Engineering Task Force, April 1998.

99. H Schulzrinne, S Casner, R Frederick, V Jacobson. RTP: A transport protocol for real-time applications. Request for Comments (proposed standard) 1889. Internet Engineering Task Force, January 1996.

100. D Cohen. A protocol for packet-switching voice communication. Proceedings of Computer Network Protocols Symposium, Liège, Belgium, February 1978.

101. J Rosenberg, H Schulzrinne. Timer reconsideration for enhanced RTP scalability. Proceedings of the Conference on Computer Communications (IEEE Infocom), San Francisco, March/April 1998.

102. H Schulzrinne. RTP profile for audio and video conferences with minimal control. Request for Comments (proposed standard) 1890. Internet Engineering Task Force, January 1996.

103. C Zhu. RTP payload format for H.263 video streams. Request for Comments (proposed standard) 2190. Internet Engineering Task Force, September 1997.

104. T Turletti, C Huitema. RTP payload format for H.261 video streams. Request for Comments (proposed standard) 2032. Internet Engineering Task Force, October 1996.

105. L Berc, W Fenner, R Frederick, S McCanne. RTP payload format for JPEG-compressed video. Request for Comments (proposed standard) 2035. Internet Engineering Task Force, October 1996.

106. D Hoffman, G Fernando, V Goyal, M Civanlar. RTP payload format for MPEG1/MPEG2 video. Request for Comments (proposed standard) 2250, Internet Engineering Task Force, January 1998.

107. C Perkins, I Kouvelas, O Hodson, V Hardman, M Handley, J-C Bolot, A Vega-Garcia, S Fosse-Parisis. RTP payload for redundant audio data. Request for Comments (proposed standard) 2198. Internet Engineering Task Force, September 1997.

108. J Rosenberg and H Schulzrinne. An RTP payload format for generic forward error correction. Internet Draft, Internet Engineering Task Force, June 1999. Work in progress.

109. J Rosenberg, H Schulzrinne. An RTP payload format for user multiplexing. Internet Draft, Internet Engineering Task Force, May 1998. Work in progress.

110. S Casner, V Jacobson. Compressing IP/UDP/RTP headers for low-speed serial links. Request for Comments (proposed standard) 2508. Internet Engineering Task Force, February 1999.

111. R. Braden (ed), L Zhang, S Berson, S Herzog, S Jamin. Resource ReSerVation Protocol (RSVP)—version 1 functional specification. Request for Comments (proposed standard) 2205. Internet Engineering Task Force, September 1997.

112. P Pan, H Schulzrinne. Yessir: A simple reservation mechanism for the Internet. Technical Report RC 20697. IBM Research, Hawthorne, NY, September 1997.

113. D Katz. IP router alert option. Request for Comments (proposed standard) 2113. Internet Engineering Task Force, February 1997.

114. W Almesberger, J-Y L Boudec, T Ferrari. Scalable resource reservation for the Internet. Proceedings of the IEEE Conference Protocols for Multimedia Systems—Multimedia Networking (PROMS-MmNet), Santiago, Chile, November 1997. Technical Report 97/234, DI-EPFL, Lausanne, Switzerland.

115. K Nichols, V Jacobson, L Zhang. A two-bit differentiated services architecture for the Internet. Internet draft, Bay Networks, LBNL and UCLA, November 1997.

116. H Schulzrinne, A Rao, R Lanphier. Real time streaming protocol (RTSP). Request for Comments (proposed standard) 2326. Internet Engineering Task Force, April 1998.

117. IEC 60461. Time and control code for video tape recorders. International Electrotechnical Commission, Geneva, 1986.

118. M Handley, H Schulzrinne, E Schooler, J Rosenberg. SIP: Session initiation protocol. Request for Comments (proposed standard) 2543. Internet Engineering Task Force, March 1999.

119. ITU-T Recommendation H.323. Packet based multimedia communication systems. Telecommunication Standardization Sector of ITU. International Telecommunications Union, Geneva, Switzerland, February 1998.

120. ITU-T Recommendation Q. 931. Digital Subscriber Signalling system no. 1 (DSS

1)—ISDN user–network interface layer 3 specification for basic call control. Telecommunication Standardization Sector of ITU. International Telecommunications Union, Geneva, March 1993.

121. ITU-T Recommendation H.323. Visual telephone systems and equipment for local area networks which provide a non-guaranteed quality of service. Telecommunication Standardization Sector of ITU. International Telecommunications Union, Geneva, May 1996.

122. ITU-T Recommendation X.680. Abstract Syntax Notation one (ASN.1): Specification of basic notation. Telecommunication Standardization Sector of ITU, International Telecommunications Union, Geneva, December 1997.

123. ITU-T Recommendation X.691. ASN.1 encoding rules - Specification of packed encoding rules (PER). Telecommunication Standardization Sector of ITU, International Telecommunications Union, Geneva, December 1997.

124. ITU-T Recommendation X.690. ASN.1 encoding rules—Specification of basic encoding rules (BER), canonical encoding rules (CER) and distinguished encoding rules (DER). Telecommunication Standardization Sector of ITU. International Telecommunications Union, Geneva, December 1997.

125. L Masinter, P Hoffman, J Zawinski. The mailto URL scheme. Internet Draft, Internet Engineering Task Force, June 1998. Work in progress.

126. M Wahl, T Howes, S Kille. Lightweight directory access protocol (v3). Request for Comments (proposed standard) 2251. Internet Engineering Task Force, December 1997.

127. M Handley, C Perkins, E Whelan. Session announcement protocol. Internet Draft, Internet Engineering Task Force, October 1999. Work in progress.

128. DE Comer. Internetworking with TCP/IP. Vol 1. 3rd ed. Englewood Cliffs, NJ: Prentice Hall, 1995.

129. WR Stevens, TCP/IP Illustrated: The implementation. Vol 2. Reading, MA: Addison-Wesley, 1994.

130. DC Lynch, MT Rose, Internet System Handbook. Reading, MA: Addison-Wesley, 1993.

131. AS Tanenbaum. Computer Networks. 2nd ed. Englewood Cliffs, NJ: Prentice-Hall, 1988.

132. DE Comer, DL Stevens. Internetworking with TCP/IP. Vol 2. Englewood Cliffs, NJ: Prentice Hall, 1991.

133. C Partridge. Gigabit Networking. Reading, MA: Addison-Wesley, 1993.

134. J Crowcroft, M Handley, I Wakeman. Internetworking Multimedia. San Francisco: Morgan Kaufmann, 1999.

4
ATM Networks

Arthur W. Berger*
Lucent Technologies, Holmdel, New Jersey

4.1 INTRODUCTION

Asynchronous transfer mode (ATM) is a technology and suite of standards for high-speed packet networks that uses small, fixed-size packets called cells and provides connection-oriented transfer and a variety of service classes. ATM networks can provide high-speed transmission with low cell loss and low delay variation and thus are well suited for supporting the transport of video. This chapter provides an overview of ATM. Basic concepts are covered, with greater detail given to aspects of most relevance for the transport of video.

As shown in Figure 4.1 the ATM cell is 53 bytes in length and consists of 5 bytes of header followed by 48 bytes of payload into which user information can be placed. ATM is connection oriented in the sense that a connection is first established between a source and destination, and then ATM cells are relayed along the connection, arriving in order at the destination.

As in any connection-oriented packet network, the ATM connection is "virtual" in the sense that a particular portion of a transport facility, such as a time slot, is not dedicated to the given connection, which, would have been the case in a "circuit-switched" connections such as in traditional telephony networks. Various types of connections can be established, providing a variety of service classes, some more suitable for the transport of video than others, as discussed below (see Section 4.7). The virtual connections can be established by signaling protocols for on-demand transport, or, on a slower time scale, can be established by management plane procedures (1–3). The establishment by signaling protocols is analogous to the dialing of a telephone call,

---

Current affiliation: Akamai Technologies, Cambridge, Massachusetts

139

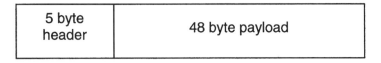

5 byte header	48 byte payload

Figure 4.1   ATM cell.

while establishment via management plane procedures is analogous to private-line service.*

The ATM standards, such as those for signaling, are in recommendations issued by the International Telecommunications Union (ITU) and specifications issued by the ATM Forum. The recommendations of the ITU are approved after the delegates from participating countries have reached a consensus. This process can result in recommendations that lack the specificity that would be desirable for simple, interoperable implementations. Beginning in 1991, the ATM Forum, an industry forum of member companies, began preparing specifications that were based on existing and draft ITU recommendations and were focused on unambiguous implementations. The ATM Forum progressed more quickly in its work than the ITU and began to lead on some topics. To the extent that the ATM Forum and the ITU worked on common topics, individual participants endeavored to obtain consistency between the two bodies, and were largely, but not completely, successful. Except where noted below, the ATM standards reviewed in this chapter are consistent between these two bodies. As a practical matter, one can consider that both the ITU and the ATM Forum specify the standards for ATM, and the distinction between a recommendation and a specification is of little significance.

The ATM standards partition functions of an ATM network into three layers: the physical layer, (and with some redundancy of terminology) the ATM layer, and the ATM adaptation layer. At end points of the ATM connection all three layers are present, while at intermediate nodes, there are just the first two layers, as illustrated in Figure 4.2. The end point of the ATM connection can be the actual end point of the user information transfer, such as a personal computer or a video terminal. Alternatively, the ATM connection may be only a portion of the end-to-end transfer of the user information. For example, the ATM connection may span only the backbone of a given service provider, in which case the end point of the ATM connection would be at a node (a gateway, router, or

---

*From the viewpoint of supporting the transport of video, the mechanism by which an ATM connection is established is not a major concern, and thus owing to limited space is not covered in this overview. The reader interested in signaling and associated topics of addressing and routing can consult the literature discussed in Section 4.9, as well as References 1–3.

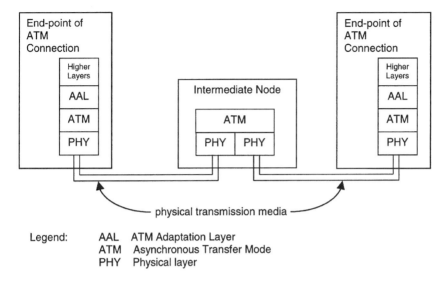

Legend: AAL   ATM Adaptation Layer
            ATM   Asynchronous Transfer Mode
            PHY   Physical layer

Figure 4.2 Protocol stack in ATM networks.

switch) on the path of the information transfer. In either case, at the end point of
the ATM connection, the user information is in some non-ATM format, such as a
file stored in memory, or an Internet Protocol (IP) packet. The ATM adaptation
layer packages, adapts the higher layer information into 48-byte chunks. This
packaged user information is placed into an ATM cell at the ATM layer, which
also associates the cell with a particular ATM connection. The ATM cell is then
processed by the physical layer and transmitted onto the physical transmission
path. At intermediate nodes along the ATM connection, the ATM cell header
needs to be examined to determine the appropriate egress port from the node (the
appropriate next transmission path). At the receiving end point of the ATM connection, the user information is then extracted from the ATM cell and returned to
the higher layer format.

   ATM connections, particularly those that pass through a public network,
are associated with a traffic contract. A traffic contract is part of the service
agreement with the public network provider whereby the provider commits to
meeting specified quality-of-service objectives, given that the ATM cell flow
entering the provider's network is in conformance with the given type of ATM
connection. The present chapter, in the context of an overall introduction to
ATM, gives relatively greater weight to describing these quality-of-service aspects and the types of ATM connections and discusses their applicability for the
transport of video.

4.1.1 Outline of Remainder of Chapter

The physical, ATM, and adaptation layers are briefly described in Sections 4.2, 4.3, and 4.4, respectively, with emphasis on the ATM layer. Section 4.5 then reviews the quality of service that can be provided by ATM networks. Section 4.6 presents the different types of ATM connections, known as "service categories" or "ATM transfer capabilities." Section 4.7 discusses the strengths and weaknesses of the different ATM connections from the viewpoint of transporting encoded video, and Section 4.8 briefly discusses the deployment of ATM in core and access networks. Section 4.9 points the reader to further readings, and Section 4.10 lists the acronyms used in the chapter.

4.2 ATM PHYSICAL LAYER

The ATM physical layer provides the needed functionality to insert and extract ATM cells onto and from physical transmission media, such as fiber, coaxial cable, and twisted copper wires. The ATM physical layer (abbreviated as PHY) has been defined for various interfaces, and Table 4.1 provides a sampling.

The ATM physical layer is divided into two sublayers: the transmission convergence sublayer, and the physical media dependent sublayer; the latter is of less interest for present purposes and, as the name suggests, is concerned with functionality that is dependent on particular media. ITU Recommendation I.432 (4) contains details on the functions of the physical layer, and Onvural (5) provides a more readable presentation, as well as more details than given here.

Table 4.1   Some Physical Interfaces for Which an ATM Physical Layer Is Defined

Physical layer interface	Transmission rate (Mbit/s)	Medium
DS-1 (T-1)	1.544	Coaxial cable
E-1	2.048	Coaxial cable
DS-3 (T-3)	44.736	Coaxial cable
E-3	34.368	Coaxial cable
SDH STM-1, SONET OC-3c	155.52	Fiber
SDH STM-4c, SONET OC-12c	622.08	Fiber
SDH STM- 16c, SONET OC-48c	2,488.32	Fiber
FDDI	100.	Fiber
Raw cells	155.52	Fiber
Raw cells	622.08	Fiber
Raw cells	51.84	Unshielded twisted pair copper wire, UTP-3

4.2.1   Transmission Convergence Sublayer of the ATM Physical Layer

The transmission convergence sublayer accepts cells from the ATM layer and forms a bit-stream for the physical media dependent sublayer, and likewise, accepts a bitstream from the physical media dependent sublayer and passes cells to the ATM layer. Some of the functions of the transmission convergence sublayer are header error control, framing, cell delineation, cell rate decoupling, and cell scrambling.

Header error control (HEC) provides protection from bit errors in the ATM cell header that can occur, primarily during the propagation of the cell between ATM nodes. The HEC can detect and correct one-bit errors and can detect some multiple-bit errors. At the transmitting end, the ATM layer passes to the PHY layer the first four bytes of the cell header, and the 48-byte payload. The transmission convergence sublayer then computes the HEC value, which is placed in the fifth byte of the cell header. At the receiving end, the transmission convergence sublayer checks the integrity of the cell header, and if no errors are detected, passes the ATM cell to the ATM layer.

Framing is used by some physical layers, such as Synchronous Optical Network (SONET) and Synchronous Digital Hierarchy (SDH). A frame consists of overhead bytes and a payload, which of present interest would support the transfer of ATM cells. In the case of SONET and SDH, a frame is generated synchronously, one frame each 125 μs, and the overhead bytes provide a rich functionality for operations, including restoration from network failures, administration, and maintenance. The transmission convergence sublayer is responsible for the generating the appropriate framing structure and for the placement of cells within it.

Cell delineation determines the location of the boundary of an ATM cell in the stream of bits from the physical medium. The receiving end of the ATM connection is the "hunt state" when it is searching for the cell boundary, which occurs at connection start-up, or when the cell boundary is lost—for example, because a burst error has occurred somewhere along the transmission path. A basic search mechanism is to continuously compute the HEC value on 32 contiguous bits and see if it matches with the next 8 bits; if a match occurs, then a candidate cell header, hence a cell boundary, is found, and the receiver moves to the "presync state." If the subsequent *n* presumed cell headers also check out, the receiver presumes that the cell boundary is indeed detected, and declares itself to be in the "sync state." Depending on the physical medium, the byte boundaries may already be known. Also, some framing structures contain a pointer that identifies the location of the cell boundary.

Cell rate decoupling provides a continuous stream of cells to the physical interface, regardless of whether the ATM layer has anything to send. Cell rate decoupling is analogous to the continuous transmission of bits, regardless of whether higher layer information is being conveyed. Most of the physical interfaces in Table 4.1 require that a continuous stream of cells be sent. When no cells are being handed down from the ATM layer, the transmission convergence sublayer itself generates cells, called idle cells. Idle cells have a particular cell header, not used by any other cell, and their the payload contains a particular byte repeated 48 times.

Scrambling ensures that the bitstream contains changes in the bit value sufficiently frequent to permit timing and synchronization to be maintained by the physical medium dependent sublayer. Scrambling avoids the situation of the transmission of many contiguous bits with the same value. Another technique is block coding at the physical medium dependent sublayer, whereby a group of 4 bits, say, is encoded as a 5-bit block.

4.2.2 Physical Medium Dependent Sublayer of the ATM Physical Layer

Some of the functions of the physical medium-dependent sublayer are (a) encoding of bits for transmission, (b) timing and synchronization, and (c) the actual insertion and extraction of the electrical or optical signal to and from the physical medium.

4.3 ATM LAYER

4.3.1 ATM Cell Header

The ATM cell header is 5 bytes in length and has two slightly different, standardized formats depending on the interface. The user–network interface (UNI) is the interface between a public network and an ATM end system, or a public network and a private (enterprise or corporate) network. The other interface, the network–network interface (NNI) (aka as the network–node interface within the ITU), is the interface between two public networks or between two private networks, or between two switches within a public or private network. At the user–network interface, the ATM cell header consists of the following fields:

1. Generic flow control (GFC), 4 bits in length
2. Virtual path identifier (VPI), 8 bits
3. Virtual channel identifier (VCI), 12 bits
4. Payload type (PT), 3 bits
5. Cell loss priority (CLP), 1 bit
6. Header error control (HEC), 8 bits

8	7	6	5	4	3	2	1	Bit Octet
GFC				VPI				1
PI				VCI				2
VCI								3
VCI				PT			CLP	4
HEC								5

Figure 4.3 ATM cell header at the user–network interface (UNI). (From Ref 6.)

The positions of the fields in the cell header are shown in Figure 4.3.*
The ATM cell header at the network–node interface (NNI) is the same as at the UNI, except the GFC field is not present, and instead the VPI field is extended from 8 bits to 12 bits.

The *generic flow control* (GFC) field is generally not used, and the field is set equal to zero. The intent of GFC was for media access control for ATM cells on bus, ring, or star topology customer-premise networks, which are on the "user" side of the user–network interface, and where the network element on "network" side of the UNI had primary control. The GFC protocol procedures are defined in ITU Recommendation I.361 (6).

The *virtual path identifier* (VPI) and the *virtual channel identifier* (VCI) associate the ATM cell with a given connection and enable the multiplexing of many connections on a single transmission path. The VPI and VCI fields are discussed in Section 4.3.2 below. The lowest values of the VPI and VCI fields are reserved for special functions, such as signaling, and operations, administration, and maintenance. See ITU Recommendation I.361 for details (6).

As the name suggests, the *payload type* (PT) field identifies the type of payload in the ATM cell, as well as some additional indications. The 3 bits of the payload type field allow for 8 code points, whose assigned meanings are summarized in Table 4.2.

As shown in Table 4.2, the first four code points are for user-data cells; the next two code points identify cells for operations, administration, and maintenance (OAM): see Recommendation I.610 (7); the seventh code point identifies the resource management cell, which is used for feedback control schemes to mediate contention for resources; and the last code point is reserved. The first

*Material from ITU recommendations is reproduced with prior authorization of the ITU as copyright holder. Complete recommendations can be obtained from: ITU, Place des Nations, CH-1211 Geneva 20, Switzerland. http://www.itu.int/publications.

Table 4.2 Standardized Code Points in the Payload Type Field

Payload type coding	Interpretation
000	User-data cell, congestion not experienced ATM user-to-ATM-user indication = 0
001	User-data cell, congestion not experienced ATM user-to-ATM-user indication = 1
010	User-data cell, congestion experienced ATM user-to-ATM user indication = 0
011	User-data cell, congestion experienced ATM user-to-ATM-user indication = 1
100	OAM F5 segment associated cell
101	OAM F5 end-to-end associated cell
110	Resource management cell
111	Reserved for future VC functions

Source: Ref. 6.

four code points distinguish user-data cells with respect to two independent attributes. The first attribute is the binary "ATM-user-to-ATM-user" indication, where "ATM-user" refers to the protocol layer that is above ATM layer, namely, the ATM adaptation layer (AAL). In particular, this indication is used by AAL type 5 to denote the last cell of a given AAL5 protocol data unit (see below: Section 4.4.3). The second attribute indicates whether the given cell passed through a network element that is or may soon be in congestion. User-data cells are originally transmitted with the PT code point equal to (in binary) 000, or 001. An intermediate network element that is in congestion may change the second bit of the PT field from 0 to 1. This function is called explicit forward congestion indication. See ITU Recommendation I.371 for details (8).

The *cell loss priority* (CLP) bit can be used to distinguish between cells of a given ATM connection with regard to loss priority. Depending on network conditions, cells with the CLP bit set equal to 1 (CLP=1) are subject to discard prior to cells with the CLP bit set equal to 0 (CLP=0) (8). The CLP bit is used, particularly, in the ATM service category called "variable bit rate," as described in Section 4.6.2 below.

4.3.2 ATM Connections: VPCs, VCCs, Label Swapping

The term "ATM connection" applies to both virtual channel connections (VCCs) and virtual path connections (VPCs). In informal usage, "ATM connection" is used for either the unidirectional connection (which supports cells from a given source to a given destination), or the bidirectional connection, which consists of the pair of unidirectional connections, one for each direction of communication.

Formally, "ATM connection" pertains to the unidirectional connection. Since, however, OAM support for the ATM connection requires two-way communication, the unidirectional connections are always established in pairs, even if the user information is passing in only one direction. ATM has a two-level hierarchy of ATM connections, whereby a group of VCCs is supported by a VPC. Figure 4.4 illustrates this hierarchy. Within a transmission path between two ATM nodes, there can be multiple VPCs, and within each VPC there can be multiple VCCs. (This hierarchy does not have to be used, and a VPC can contain a single VCC, in which case the end points of the VPC would coincide with the end points of the VCC.)

This hierarchy has been found to be very useful. (As discussed in Chapter 3 of the present volume, multiprotocol label switching for IP networks extends the idea of a hierarchy to an arbitrary number of levels.) A network service provider may wish to establish VPCs that extend across its network and aggregate VCCs that pass through the provider's network. The network service provider could aggregate based on the service category of the VCC (see Section 4.6). Also, the service provider may be renting capacity to other carriers, in which case the VPCs could be dedicated to the support of a given carrier's VCCs. Likewise, a corporation might establish VPCs through a network service provider to interconnect various building locations of the corporation. The presence of VPCs allows for quicker establishment of signaled (switched) VCCs. The VPCs also enable faster restoration. Although a VPC is often chosen to be a constant rate "pipe," a VPC is not restricted to be so and could be any of the service categories discussed in Section 4.6. For more details on VPCs, see ITU Recommendation E.735 (9).

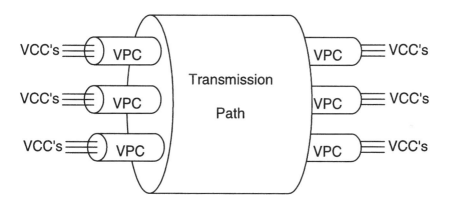

Figure 4.4 Transmission path supports multiple VPCs, which in turn support multiple VCCs.

The virtual channel identifier (VCI) and the virtual path identifier (VPI) in the ATM cell header provide the information needed by ATM nodes to identify the VCC or VPC to which the given cell belongs. For a given ATM connection, the value of the VPI/VCI does not remain constant on all the links the connection passes through. The VPI/VCI is not a destination address. Rather, for a given ATM connection, the value of the VPI/VCI pertains for a given link between two ATM nodes. An intermediate ATM node, upon receiving a cell, can determine from the VPI/VCI the appropriate egress port for this cell and can determine the appropriate value for the VPI/VCI that identifies the given ATM connection on the determined egress link. The ATM node maintains a table that maps the VPI/VCI of an incoming cell to the VPI/VCI to be inserted in the header of the cell upon egress. (With the change in VPI/VCI value, the header error control is recomputed, as discussed in Section 4.2.1.) Thus, the value of the VPI/VCI has local significance— local, that is, to a given transmission path between two ATM nodes. The operation of switching the value of the VPI/VCI at intermediate nodes is called "label switching," or "label swapping," and is also being used in multiprotocol label switching for IP networks.

Figure 4.5 illustrates label swapping in the context of ATM, and shows a VCC originating at end system A and terminating at end system B, and passing through three intermediate network nodes. Between network nodes 1 and 3, the VCC is carried inside a VPC. The particular values for the VPIs and VCIs in Figure 4.5 were chosen arbitrarily and are of interest only to the extent that they are different on different portions of the connections.

Between end system A and network node 1, cells belonging to the given VCC have a VPI=71 and a VCI=63. For each cell that network node 1 receives on a given input port, it examines the value of the VPI/VCI to determine the egress port. In the present example, a cell with VPI/VCI equal to 71/63 is to be forwarded to a network VPC that runs between network nodes 1 and 3. At the egress port of network node 1, this VPC is identified by VPI=37, and the cells of the given connection are identified by VCI=56. Thus, network node 1 replaces, the VPI/VCI value of 71/63 with 37/56. Network node 1 could be transmitting cells of many VCCs on this given VPC. Since the length of the VCI field is 16 bits, in principle this VPC could support 2^{16} VCCs [minus 32, because VCI values 0 through 31 are preassigned or reserved for future functions (6)].

When network node 2 receives a cell on the given input port with VPI=37, network node 2 knows that this VPI is associated with a VPC that continues on to network node 3. Thus, network node 2 does not need to look at or modify the VCIs of cells of this VPC, since network node 2 does not need to be concerned with the individual VCCs this VPC. Network node 2 replaces the VPI value of 37 with the value 96 when it transmits cells of this VPC to network node 3. Net-

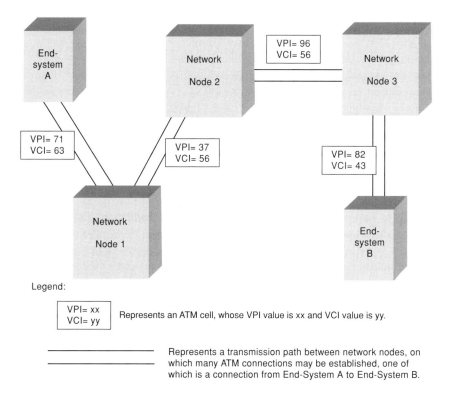

Legend:

VPI= xx
VCI= yy

Represents an ATM cell, whose VPI value is xx and VCI value is yy.

———————————— Represents a transmission path between network nodes, on
———————————— which many ATM connections may be established, one of
which is a connection from End-System A to End-System B.

Figure 4.5 Illustration of label swapping of VPI/VCI values for a given virtual channel connection.

work node 2 does not change the VCI of any of the VCCs within this VPC, and thus the VCI of the given connection remains at 56.

Network node 3 knows that arriving cells with VPI=96 on the given input port are associated with a VPC that ends at network node 3. Thus, network node 3 also examines the VCI, and from its forwarding table, knows that a cell with VPI/VCI = 96/56 should egress on a particular port and should have the VPI/VCI values replaced with 82/43. End system B, upon receipt of cells with VPI/VCI = 82/43, knows that these are cells from end system A.

Quite likely end system B is transmitting cells to end system A on the companion, paired, VCC that runs from B to A. Even if the user data is going in just one direction, control traffic will be present on the reverse connection, such as OAM cells, or cells transporting Transmission Control Protocol (TCP) acknowledgments. In order that each network node can easily associate a VCC with its companion paired VCC, the same values for the VPI and VCI are used, at each segment along the path, for the cells traveling in each direction on this pair of VCCs.

4.3.3 ATM Connections: Point-to-Multipoint

The ATM connections discussed so far have been point-to-point; that is, they have a single source and a single destination. The ATM layer also supports point-to-multipoint connections, which have a single source and multiple destinations. The source end emits one copy of each cell, and each cell is then replicated at nodes within the network. A natural application for point-to-multipoint connections is for video distribution to multiple customers. Point-to-multipoint connections are also used in the emulation of local-area networks (LANs). The ATM Forum has specified a LAN emulation protocol (10), which includes a multicast server called a broadcast and unknown server (BUS). The BUS is connected to all of the LAN emulation clients via a point-to-multipoint VCC, and each LAN emulation client is connected to the BUS via a point-to-point VCC. If a LAN emulation client wishes to send a higher layer packet, such as an IP packet, to all of the clients, it sends the packet to the BUS, which in turns forwards it to all of the clients via the point-to-multipoint VCC. (The BUS needs to transmit all cells associated with a given packet before sending any cells of another packet.) There are many more aspects to LAN emulation; see Reference 10 for details. The ATM Forum has also specified a generalization of LAN emulation that operates across the wide area, across multiple logical IP subnets. This extension is called multiprotocol over ATM (MPOA) (11).

4.4 ATM ADAPTATION LAYER (AAL)

As illustrated in Figure 4.2, the ATM adaptation layer (AAL) is above the ATM layer and below any higher layers. At the transmitting end of an ATM connection, the AAL takes higher layer protocol data units (PDUs), such as IP packets, and segments them into ATM cells; at the receiving end, it does the reverse function of reassembly. In addition, the AAL provides functionality that enhances the service provided by the ATM layer. This additional functionality is tailored to support various classes of service or types of traffic. Thus, multiple AALs have been defined, each tailored to support particular services.

The following sections provide an overview of the different types AAL. For all of the AALs, the functions are divided into sublayers. Standardization has focused on the sublayers designated the segmentation and reassembly (SAR) sublayer, and the common part of the convergence sublayer (CPCS).

4.4.1   AAL Type 1

AAL type 1 (AAL1) supports circuit emulation. As specified in ITU Recommendation I.363.1 (12), the functionality provided by AAL 1 includes the following:

segmentation and reassembly of higher layer information
handling of cell delay variation
handling of cell payload assembly delay
handling of lost or misinserted cells
source clock frequency recovery at the receiver
recovery of the source data structure at the receiver

To provide these functions, AAL1 uses one byte of the 48 byte payload. Thus, 47 bytes per ATM cell are available for the transport of higher layer information. The AAL1 convergence sublayer provides two methods for the support of asynchronous constant bit rate services where the clocks are not locked to a network clock. The two methods are "adaptive clock" and "synchronous residual time stamp," (see Sections 2.5.2.2 and 2.5.1.2 of Reference 12).

4.4.2   AAL Type 2

AAL type 2 (AAL2) is a recently standardized AAL designed for low-rate, delay-sensitive applications that generate short, variable-length packets. A motivating application for AAL2 was low bit rate voice, where the delay to completely fill the payload of an ATM cell with the encoded speech from a single voice source would have degraded performance. Thus, a key attribute of AAL2 is the ability to multiplex higher layer streams onto a single-ATM virtual channel connection (VCC). Up to 255 higher layer streams can be multiplexed on a single VCC, which is possible because AAL2 does not require that each encapsulated packet fit within a single ATM payload; rather, an encapsulated packet can span across payloads. Another key attribute is the ability to handle higher layer packets of variable length, which occur from various encoding schemes. AAL2 is specified in ITU Recommendation I.363.2 (13). A more readable description is provided by Baldwin et al. (14); and Sriram and Wang (15) analyze the performance of AAL2 in the context of supporting voice with bit dropping.

    Although the specification of AAL type 2 was motivated by voice, the specification does not restrict AAL2 to that application. AAL2 is also suitable to encapsulate low bit rate (<64 kbit/s) video streams, such as H.263 or MPEG-4 video encodings, which can have rates in the range of 20 kbit/s, or video encodings originally designed for transport over the current public switched telephone network.

4.4.3 AAL Type 5

AAL type 5 (AAL5) is designed for variable-rate applications that do not require
a timing or synchronization between the source and destination or, if the application does need such synchronization, the application can obtain it by means other
than the AAL. AAL5 supports the nonassured transfer of higher layer PDUs,
where the length of the PDU can be from 1 to 65,535 bytes. AAL5 maintains the
sequence of the user data and can detect transmission errors (16). As discussed in
Section 4.3.1, the "ATM-user-to-ATM-user indication" in the ATM cell header
distinguishes the last ATM cell that segments a given higher layer PDU.

The overhead for AAL5 (other than the "ATM-user-to-ATM-user indication") is placed in the rear of the last ATM cell that segments a given higher layer
PDU. The overhead consists of 8 bytes plus any padding that may be needed to
fill out the payload of the cell. Thus, for example, a 1024-byte higher layer PDU
would be segmented into 22 cells, where the full payload of the first 21 cells is
used for the higher layer PDU, and the 22nd cell contains the remaining 16 bytes
of the PDU, followed by 24 bytes of padding, and finally 8 bytes of AAL5 protocol overhead, called the "common part convergence sublayer (CPCS)–PDU
trailer. This trailer includes a 32-bit cyclic redundancy check and a 16-bit length
field, which is used to determine the end of the user-data PDU (and the start of
any padding) and also to detect any lost or misinserted cells.

4.4.4 AAL Type 3/4

AAL type 3/4 (AAL3/4) was originally defined as two separate AALs: AAL3
was designed for connection-oriented variable-rate services, while AAL4 was
designed for connectionless (i.e., datagram) variable-rate services. It was found
that these two AALs could be combined into a single, harmonized AAL, called
AAL3/4. AAL3/4 provides significantly more functionality than AAL5; in particular, AAL3/4 can multiplex higher layer flows onto a single ATM connection,
but at the expense of greater complexity and of a greater overheard—4 bytes out
of each 48 byte payload. Shortly before the completion of AAL3/4, AAL5 was
proposed and has subsequently gained wide acceptance as providing a better
trade-off of simplicity versus features.

4.5 QUALITY OF SERVICE

An important feature of ATM networks is the performance commitments that
can be provided to connections. The performance commitments can be at the
connection level, such as the delay in establishing the connection or the probability a request for connection establishment is denied. ITU Recommendation I.358 (17) covers performance at the connection level. In addition, and the

focus of greater interest, are performance commitments at the cell level, such as cell loss and delay. Section 4.5.1 summarizes cell-level performance parameters that have been defined, and Section 4.5.2 reviews the associated performance objectives.

4.5.1 Quality of Service and Network Performance Parameters

ITU Recommendation I.356 (18) defines the following cell-level network performance parameters:

1. Cell transfer delay (CTD)
2. Cell delay variation (CDV)
3. Cell loss ratio (CLR)
4. Cell error ratio
5. Cell misinsertion rate
6. Severely errored cell block ratio

The ATM Forum adopts the same parameters and uses the term "quality-of-service" (QoS) parameters (19). The following are informal definitions of the parameters above; precise definitions are given elsewhere (18,19).

Cell transfer delay (CTD) is the delay of a cell between to two reference locations, such as the end points of an ATM connection, or the ingress and egress of a service provider's network. ITU defines the mean transfer delay as the arithmetic average of a specified number of cell transfer delays. The performance objective is in terms of an upper bound on the mean CTD. The ATM Forum defines the maximum cell transfer delay, denoted maxCTD, as a high quantile on the histogram of transfer delays: that is, the probability that the cell transfer delay is greater than this quantile is small.

Heuristically, cell delay variation is the variation in the delay. ITU defines two types of cell delay variation—a "one-point" and a "two-point." The one-point cell delay variation is defined at a single reference location (and thus is relatively easy to measure) and quantifies the variability in the cell arrival times at the reference location with respect to equally spaced, nominal reference times. This notion of delay variation is useful for measuring deviation from the peak cell rate in constant bit rate connections (see below: Section 4.6.1). The two-point cell delay variation is defined with respect to two reference locations and is the difference between the realized CTD and a reference cell transfer delay. The ATM Forum defines a third notion, called the peak-to-peak cell delay variation, which equals the maxCTD minus the fixed portion of the delay, and thus is approximately the difference between the shortest and longest cell transfer delays. ATM Forum's peak-to-peak CDV is essentially the range of the distribution of ITU's two-point CDV, if the reference delay of the latter is taken to be the fixed delay.

The *cell loss ratio* (CLR) is the ratio of the total number of lost cells to the total number of transmitted cells for a population of interest, such as all the cells transmitted on a connection, or on multiple instances of connections with a given end point. The cell loss ratio excludes cells in "severely errored cell blocks," though this may not be followed in some service offerings.

An errored cell is a cell that, although received at a reference location, has its binary content in error. The *cell error ratio* is the ratio of errored cells to received cells.

A misinserted cell is a cell that is received at a downstream reference location on a given connection but was never present on the connection at an upstream reference location. A misinserted cell can occur if bit errors corrupt the VPI/VCI of a cell of a given connection, and the corrupted VPI/VCI happens to be a valid VPI/VCI of another ATM connection sharing the transmission path. In such a case, the first connection experiences a cell loss, and the second connection experiences a misinserted cell. The *cell misinsertion rate* is the number of minsinserted cells observed over a specified time interval.

A cell block is N consecutively transmitted cells of a given connection. A severely errored cell block is a cell block in which more than M errored, lost, or misinserted cells have occurred. The *severely errored cell block ratio* is the ratio of severely errored cell blocks to the total cell blocks for a population of interest.

4.5.2 Quality-of-Service Objectives

ITU Recommendation I.356 (18) includes provisional QoS classes and associated performance objectives. There are currently four QoS classes: stringent class, tolerant class, bilevel class, and "U" (unbounded, or unspecified) class. The QoS class can be selected on a connection-by-connection basis.

The associated performance objectives are stated for a very stressful scenario of a 27,500-kilometer reference connection with 25 nodes and one geostationary satellite hop. Thus, for "typical" connections, the performance objectives may appear to be rather weak. In practice, a service provider offering ATM service would state its own performance objectives.

Three of the QoS parameters, the cell error ratio, the cell misinsertion rate, and the severely errored cell block ratio, are primarily caused by impairments in the physical transmission media and are thus not readily controlled, or selectable, on a connection-by-connection basis (modulo selecting or avoiding routes with particular transmission media). Thus, these parameters are given default values that apply across all classes (except the "U" class, for which no performance objectives are stated). The default values are as follows. The upper bound on the cell error ratio is 4×10^{-6}. The upper bound on the mean cell misinsertion ratio is 1/day. The upper bound on the severely errored cell block ratio is 10^{-4}.

Table 4.3   Provisional Performance Objectives in ITU Recommendation 1.356

	Provisional performance objectives([a])			
QoS class	Upper bound on the mean cell transfer delay	Upper bound on the difference between the upper and lower 10^{-8} quanitles of cell transfer delay	Upper bound on the cell loss probability (regardless of the value of the CLP bit in the cell header)	Upper bound on the cell loss probability for cells with CLP bit = 0
Stringent class	400 ms	3 ms	3×10^{-7}	None
Tolerant class	U	U	10^{-5}	None
Bilevel class	U	U	U	10^{-5}
"U" class	U	U	U	U

[a] U, unspecified, or unbounded.
Source: Ref. 18.

For each of these objectives, as well as those in the sequel, explanatory notes are provided in Recommendation I.356(18).

The remaining three QoS parameters, cell transfer delay, cell delay variation, and cell loss ratio, are influenced by the choice of route and by buffering and scheduling capabilities and policies in network nodes, as well as influenced by physical transmission media. Thus, it is reasonable for a user to be able to select on a per-connection basis objectives for these QoS parameters, from among the objectives supported by the network service provider. In particular, the user can select on a per-connection basis the QoS class, where each class is associated with a unique set of objective values. Table 4.3 summarizes the provisional performance objectives in ITU Recommendation I.356 associated with each QoS class.

4.5.3   Associating QoS Objectives to a Given ATM Connection

Applications that are using an ATM network, such as for the transport of video, can require a certain quality of service from the network. In such cases, when the ATM connection is established, the user application would wish to have certain quality-of-service objectives pertain for that connection. As discussed in Section 4.5.2, QoS parameters that are primarily determined by physical layer impairments, such as cell error ratio, have default values that cannot be selected on a per-connection basis. However, the QoS parameters of cell transfer delay, cell delay variation, and cell loss ratio are affected by the ATM layer, and it is reasonable to select objectives for these QoS parameters on a per-connection basis.

One way for the user application to select the quality-of-service objectives is to choose one of the QoS classes offered by the service provider. This method is supported by the signaling procedures defined by the ITU and the ATM Forum (1–3).

A second way for the user application to select the quality of service objectives is to signal an acceptable value for the cell transfer delay, the delay variation, and/or the cell loss ratio. The user application could do this without needing to know the particulars of the QoS classes offered by the service provider. If the network, or networks, through which the connection would pass can meet the objectives signaled by the user, the connection would be established; otherwise it would be denied, in which case the application could possibly try another carrier, or could modify the requested performance. The ATM Forum UNI and private network–network interface specifications (2,3) support this procedure for the three QoS parameters above, and ITU Recommendation Q.2931 (1) supports this procedure for cell transfer delay. For cell transfer delay and cell delay variation, the signaling message also includes a field for the cumulative impairment. The value in this field is increased as the setup message passes from network to network, or from node to node, including the portion within the end user's network. If the cumulative value becomes greater than the acceptable value, the connection is denied. The user application can also indicate that any value is acceptable (i.e., and thus not a priori impose a limit), and then can learn from the cumulative value what will be the likely performance.

Note that the QoS objectives are probabilistic and need not hold for each realization of a connection. For example, if the cell loss ratio objective is 10^{-6}, then heuristically at least 10^8 cells should be transported to obtain a reasonable measurement; but this is more than a gigabyte of user data and thus may be more than the content transmitted. Service providers state the performance objectives in the context of averaging over multiple connections or over a period of time.

Requesting particular QoS for a connection makes sense for certain types of ATM connections. In particular, setting delay and loss objectives is most pertinent for ATM connections that are "constant bit rate" or "real-time variable bit rate." Both of these types of ATM connections are tailored to support the transport of video. These and other types of ATM connections are the subject of Section 4.6.

4.5.4 Quality of Service and Video

The foregoing material is from the perspective of QoS at the ATM layer. For the transport of video, the QoS the user cares about is the perceived quality of the decoded and displayed video. Unfortunately the relationship between the QoS at the ATM layer and the user's perceived quality of the decoded video is not well understood. However, one can make some fairly obvious, qualitative statements. The end-to-end cell transfer delay objective is important for interactive video applications, where the delay experienced by the user also includes the additional delays in the video end systems. Subjective tests on interactive voice communication have shown that if the delay experienced by the user is no more than 100 ms, the interaction feels normal: that is, the delay is not noticed as an impairment. If the delay reaches 150 ms, some impairment is noticed, at least for a proportion of test subjects. When the delay is as big as 250 ms, as occurs with a geostationary satellite, the interaction can feel quite awkward, particularly for people who tend to start talking before the other talker has completed the sentence. In contrast, for noninteractive video applications, such as playback of stored video, or live broadcast of a sports event or the nightly news, the end-to-end delay objective is not important.

Cell losses cause the loss of a higher layer protocol data unit, such as a transport packet. Thus, cell losses are bad, they will occur, and a natural question is: At what level of cell loss can the decoder still obtain video of good quality? Unfortunately, the question does not have a simple answer, for many factors are pertinent. A cyclic dependency occurs where networking people want to be told by video people "the cell loss objective that the network needs to meet," so they can design and engineer the network appropriately. And the video people want to be told by the networking people "the cell loss objective that the network does meet," so they can design video encoding and decoding algorithms that work well given this level of cell loss. One reference point is that the best (i.e., smallest) cell loss ratio the ATM network can meet is around 10^{-9} to 10^{-10}. This can occur for constant bit rate connections (see Section 4.6), where cell loss occurs only as a result of physical layer impairments.

Although constant bit rate connections are appropriate in some cases, they are not the complete solution, since they are relatively expensive (they inefficiently use network bandwidth) for video traffic that is actually variable rate, where the constant rate of the connection is set equal to peak rate of the video traffic. Thus, additional solutions are sought that make better use of the statistical multiplexing potential of ATM networks and of the inherent variable rate of encoded video, which brings us back to the cycle above. There seems to be some convergence, where cell loss rates in range of 10^{-4} to 10^{-6} are often mentioned. One potentially complicating factor is that cell losses tend to occur in bunches. Thus for a given objective of say 10^{-5}, cell losses tend not to be isolated at roughly one out of every 100,000 cells. Rather, 10 consecutive cells might be lost, with longer intervals of no loss. This bunching of cell losses occurs for an aggregate cell stream, and an individual VCC may indeed experience only isolated cell losses, depending on circumstances and implementation in the network node. Another factor is that the impact of cell loss on the displayed video depends on attributes of the encoding. If there is no interframe dependency, then the impact is confined to a single frame, while with interframe dependency (which has the advantage of enabling significant compression), the impact of cell losses can be quite noticeable.

To deal with cell losses, a possible variation is to make use of the cell loss priority (CLP) bit in the ATM cell header. Here the less significant, lower order, encoded bits would be transmitted in the lower priority CLP=1 cells, while the more significant, higher order encoded bits would be transmitted in the higher priority CLP=0 cells. If the network needs to discard a cell because of congestion at a buffer in a network node, the lower priority CLP=1 cells would be discarded first. Although this provides more flexibility, cell losses of higher priority CLP=0 cells can still occur, and one would still need to establish a cell loss objective for the CLP=0 cells.

Providing objectives on cell delay variation within the ATM network is useful for sizing the build-out delay buffers at the receiving end. The cells that arrive late are equivalent to cells that are lost. Thus, it is sensible to have the performance objective on cell delay variation be as strict as the objective on cell loss (and in the case of layered coding, as strict as the loss objective for the high priority, CLP=0, cells).

4.6 ATM SERVICE CATEGORIES (aka ATM TRANSFER CAPABILITIES)

The ITU and the ATM Forum have defined roughly the same service categories, though with different terminology, which is a source of confusion. Since both terminologies are used, it is worthwhile to be aware of them. Thus, in this paragraph we mention both terminologies and thereafter use the vocabulary from the ATM Forum, which is somewhat more popular. The term "service category" is used by the ATM Forum, while the ITU uses the term "ATM transfer capability." ITU Recommendation I.371 (8) defines four ATM transfer capabilities: Deterministic Bit Rate, Statistical Bit Rate, Available Bit Rate, and ATM Block Transfer. The ATM Forum in the Traffic Management Specification (9) also defines four service categories. The first three are the same as in Recommendation I.371, except the ATM Forum uses "Constant Bit Rate" instead of "Deterministic Bit Rate," and "Variable Bit Rate" instead of "Statistical Bit Rate." The fourth service category defined by the ATM Forum is called "Unspecified Bit Rate." These terms are summarized in Table 4.4.

Although there is some overlap in the features of the service categories and more than one may be suitable for a given application, the set of all service categories is intended to be able to support effectively a wide range of applications. In addition, both the ITU and the ATM Forum are studying additional service categories to supplement the ones already defined. For example, the ATM Forum and

Table 4.4 Comparison of ITU and ATM Forum Vocabularies

International Telecommunications Union	ATM Forum
ATM transfer capability	Service category
Deterministic bit rate	Constant bit rate
Statistical bit rate	Variable bit rate
Available bit rate	Available bit rate
ATM block transfer	—
—	Unspecified bit rate
ATM performance parameters	Quality-of-service parameters

the ITU are expected to complete the definition of the guaranteed frame rate service category, which is an enhancement to unspecified bit rate and provides a minimum cell rate commitment to conforming blocks of cells, called frames (20,21).

Sections 4.6.1 through 4.6.5 provide an overview of the five service categories above. Then Section 4.7 discusses the suitability of the various service categories for transporting video.

4.6.1 Constant Bit Rate

The constant bit rate (CBR) service category is used by connections that request a static volume of bandwidth, which is then available at any time during the lifetime of the connection. The volume of bandwidth is specified by the peak cell rate (PCR).

In practice, the specification of a rate at a location in the network, such as at an interface, needs a second parameter to be well defined. Without this second parameter, it is unclear how strict or loose is the intended meaning. For example, a very strict interpretation would apply to every intercell time, and thus would not allow for any delay variation that might occur in upstream nodes, or (for an absurd example) would prevent the specification any peak rate between 150 and 75 Mbit/s on a transmission path of capacity 150 Mbit/s, since to attain such rates a portion of the cells must be placed in adjacent cell slot times (i.e., back to back), and thus at a rate of 150 Mbit/s. At the other extreme, a very loose interpretation would allow a source to request a peak cell rate of 10 Mbit/s, and then if the source is idle for a minute, it could transmit at 20 Mbit/s for the next minute. Thus, a second parameter is needed to provide a tolerance, or an averaging, over some time scale. The PCR is specified with a tolerance, known as the cell delay variation (CDV) tolerance. The specification is made precise via an algorithm called the generic cell rate algorithm (GCRA), where the PCR and the CDV tolerance are parameters in the algorithm.

The GCRA is shown in Figure 4.6 and is specified by both the ITU (8) and the ATM Forum (19). The GCRA has two parameters, the increment, denoted *I*, and the limit, denoted *L*. When the GCRA is used to define the notion of peak cell rate, the increment *I* is set equal to the reciprocal of the peak cell rate, and the limit *L* is set equal to the CDV tolerance. The GCRA is another name for the leaky-bucket algorithm and for the virtual scheduling algorithm. The latter two, although different in appearance, are isomorphic with regard to the key attribute that for any arriving stream of cells, both algorithms will detect the same cells to be conforming, and consequently the same cells to be nonconforming.

Although often in the literature the "token bank" algorithm is used synonymously with the leaky-bucket algorithm, these two algorithms are not isomorphic in foregoing sense of detecting the same set of cells to be conforming. For

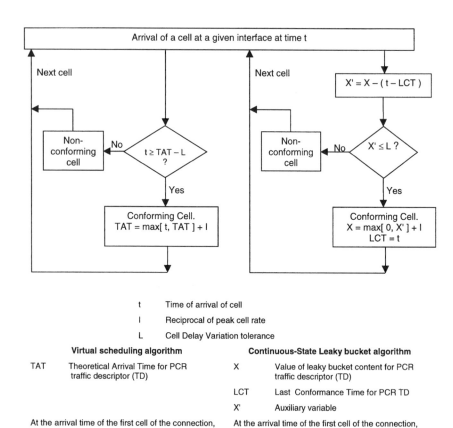

Figure 4.6 Generic cell rate algorithm (From Ref. 8.)

most practical purposes, however, they are close enough that the differences are negligible (see Section 7 of Reference 22). Moreover, a fluid version of the token bank algorithm is isomorphic to the leaky bucket, where conceptually, instead of discrete tokens arriving to the bank, a continuous flow of credit arrives. The GCRA has advantages over another popular algorithm known as the sliding window (23); for a broader perspective on desirable properties for algorithms for traffic descriptors, see Berger (24) and Berger and Eckberg (25).

In the CBR service category the source can emit cells at the PCR, or any lower rate, at any time and for any duration, and the QoS commitments still pertain. A natural QoS to select for a CBR connection is the "stringent" QoS class specified in ITU Recommendation I.356 and summarized in Section 4.5.2 above. A natural service agreement by a network operator would be that if the submitted traffic is conforming to the specified PCR, the network operator commits to a QoS that includes a specified cell loss ratio objective and an end-to-end cell delay variation objective sufficient to support an application relying on circuit emulation.

An obvious application for the CBR service category is to support circuit emulation at a higher layer. However, this is not the only application. With circuit emulation, from the viewpoint of the ATM layer, there is an ongoing stream of cells, nominally spaced at the reciprocal of the PCR. In contrast, the CBR service category supports another type of ATM connection in which the source may emit cells at any rate less than or equal to the PCR, and may emit no cells for periods. An important example is semipermanent connections (leased lines) that may be established for periods of months but whose usage, at the ATM layer, varies during the course of the day. An important special case is a semipermanent user-to-user virtual path connection that is established between two locations of a corporation.

The traffic controls used in the CBR service category include the negotiation of the PCR and the subsequent policing of the submitted cell flow for conformance to the PCR. To obtain the QoS commitment of a tight end-to-end cell delay variation, the network operator needs to isolate the CBR connections from other types of connection. One way network nodes attain this isolation is to serve the CBR connections with higher delay priority than other types of connections.

4.6.2 Variable Bit Rate

In the variable bit rate (VBR) service category, the end system uses standardized traffic parameters to specify, in greater detail than just the peak cell rate, the cell flow that will be emitted on the connection. The standardized traffic parameters are the peak cell rate (PCR), the sustainable cell rate (SCR), and the maximum burst size (MBS). (In addition, associated tolerances are used at public interfaces.) The source may also describe the traffic via the declaration of the "service type" that pertains for the connection (8). Informally, the SCR is thought of as the average rate of a connection. More precisely, the SCR is an upper bound on the average cell rate of the connection, where average cell rate is the total number of cells transmitted divided by the duration of the connection. In the VBR service category, the SCR is always strictly less than the PCR, and often is between a third and a tenth of the PCR. The maximum burst size is the maximum number of cells that may be sent at the peak cell rate and still be conforming to the traffic descriptor.

Conformance to the pair of parameters SCR and MBS is made precise via the generic cell rate algorithm (GCRA): see Figure 4.6. The increment I in the GCRA is set equal to the reciprocal of the SCR. The limit L is determined from the three parameters PCR, SCR, and MBS and is set equal to $L = [MBS - 1][(1/SCR) - (1/PCR)]$. See Section C.4 of Reference 19 for more details. In the context of SCR, the limit L is called the burst tolerance (aka the intrinsic burst tolerance). The MBS, in a somewhat convoluted way, is the second parameter that provides the needed tolerance for the SCR. The traffic parameters are typically static for the duration of the connection, though their values can be renegotiated via signaling or management procedures.

The VBR service category makes use of the cell loss priority (CLP) bit in the ATM cell header. The CLP bit distinguishes between high priority (CLP=0) cells and low priority (CLP=1) cells of a connection. The CLP bit can be set by the source, or, at the request of the user, the network can use the "tagging" feature, whereby for cells submitted with CLP=0 that are not conforming to the SCR/MBS traffic parameters for CLP=0 cells, the network changes the CLP bit to 1. In the VBR service category, three configurations of the traffic parameters along with the CLP bit and the tagging option are specified:

1. The PCR and the SCR/MBS traffic parameters apply to the aggregate of all cells (i.e., regardless of the value of the CLP).
2. The PCR applies to the aggregate of all cells, and the SCR/MBS traffic parameters apply only to CLP=0 cells.
3. The same as configuration 2, except with the tagging option invoked.

When the connection has both CLP=0 and CLP=1 cells, the cells entering the network with CLP=0 can be viewed as the committed portion of the traffic (the QoS commitment includes a specified cell loss ratio for the CLP=0 cells) and the cells entering the network with CLP=1 (or cells tagged by the network as CLP=1) can be viewed as the "at-risk portion" (the cell loss ratio is unspecified for the CLP=1 cells).

To precisely define the three configurations above, again the GCRA was used—once for the PCR and once again for the SCR/MBS. The two GCRAs can put together in multiple ways, all a priori reasonable, but unfortunately inconsistent. This caused some confusion. One way was chosen: cells are first tested with respect to the PCR and then tested with respected to the SCR/MBS, where the specifics of the second test depend on which of the three configurations pertains. Figure 4.7 presents the algorithm for the second configuration: that is, the SCR/MBS only applies to the CLP=0 cells and tagging is not used. The algorithm for the first configuration, wherein the SCR/MBS applies to all cells and not just the CLP=0 cells, is the same as the algorithm in Figure 4.7, except the second decision box (the second diamond) that tests "Cell has CLP=0?" is omitted. And in the last box, the "Conforming cell" box, the text "If arriving cell had CLP=0 then" is also omitted. Likewise, the algorithm for the third configuration is the same as the algorithm in Figure 4.7, except that in the third decision box (the third diamond) the arrow corresponding to "No" does not go to the "Nonconforming cell" box but rather goes to a box wherein the CLP bit is changed to 1, and from which an egress arrow goes to the "Conforming cell" box.

VBR service can be partitioned into real-time and non-real-time subcategories. In the ATM Forum, real-time VBR service is for applications requiring constrained delay and delay variation, as would be appropriate for voice and video applications (19). Non-real-time VBR makes no commitment on delay but does include a commitment on cell loss. Non-real-time VBR service is analogous to frame relay service, which is popular for enterprise networks for connectivity between business locations.

As with CBR, key traffic controls used in the VBR service category include the negotiation of the PCR and SCR/MBS traffic parameters or the declaration of the service type and the subsequent policing of the submitted cell flow. In addition, the connection admission control (CAC) policy used in VBR enables the network operator to attain a statistical multiplexing gain, versus a CAC policy that allocates the PCR to the connections, while still meeting QoS commitments. Many such CAC policies are possible, and the choice is at the discretion of the network operator. A network operator could choose a conservative policy that is based on the worst-case traffic allowed by the PCR and SCR/MBS traffic parameters of the new and the established connections. Less conservative policies could use measurements of traffic of currently established connections and/or historical measurements of previous VBR connections. The historical measurements could be used to determine and/or validate stochastic models of the source traffic, and these models in turn could be used by the CAC policy. A popular concept is effective bandwidth, where the variable-rate connection is viewed as having a constant rate, its effective bandwidth, that in some sense captures the stress the connection places on network resources. For example work on CAC see References 26–29.

4.6.3 Available Bit Rate

The available bit rate (ABR) service category is designed for applications that can adapt their information transfer rate based on feedback information from the

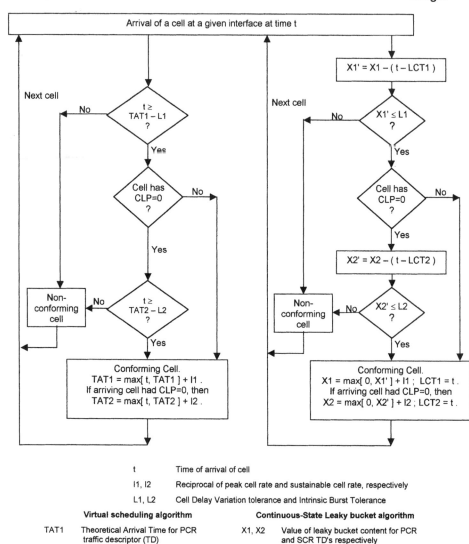

t	Time of arrival of cell
I1, I2	Reciprocal of peak cell rate and sustainable cell rate, respectively
L1, L2	Cell Delay Variation tolerance and Intrinsic Burst Tolerance

Virtual scheduling algorithm		**Continuous-State Leaky bucket algorithm**	
TAT1	Theoretical Arrival Time for PCR traffic descriptor (TD)	X1, X2	Value of leaky bucket content for PCR and SCR TD's respectively
TAT2	Theoretical Arrival Time for SCR traffic descriptor (TD)	LCT1, LCT2	Last Conformance Times for PCR and SCR TD's respectively
		X1', X2'	Auxiliary variables
At the arrival time of the first cell of the connection, TAT1 = TAT2 = t.		At the arrival time of the first cell of the connection, X1 = X2 = 0 and LCT1 = LCT2 = t.	

Figure 4.7   Genetic cell rate algorithm for peak cell rate on aggregate CLP = 0 + 1 cell flow and for sustainable cell rate on CLP=0 cell flow. (From Ref. 8.)

network; the feedback information is conveyed in a special control cell, called the resource management (RM) cell. The RM cell is distinguished from user cells via the payload type field in the ATM cell header (see Table 4.2 above). In the ABR service category, the RM cell provides the source with an indication of the currently available bandwidth for the connection. Closed-loop traffic controls are a basic feature of this service category.

In ABR, a source will specify a PCR and a minimum cell rate, where the latter may be zero. The bandwidth available for the connection may become as small as the minimum cell rate. The network commits to a QoS specified on the cell loss ratio, given that the cell flow is conforming at public interfaces, which will be the case if the source and destination follow a specified reference behavior in response to receiving a RM cell. The network also makes the relative assurance that for connections that share the same path, no connection shall be arbitrarily discriminated against nor favored. The generic cell rate algorithm (GCRA) is again used to determined conformance, though in a dynamic form where the increment parameter I varies over time to follow the currently allowed cell rate on the connection; see Reference 19 or 30 for details. As a rough summary of the ABR control procedures, a source determines the current bandwidth available for the connection by periodically emitting RM cells. Some of the fields of the RM cell, in particular the congestion-indication bit, the no-increase bit, and/or the explicit-rate field, are modified at network nodes to indicate to the source a revised allowed rate. When the destination receives the RM cell, the destination sends the RM cell back to the source (on the companion connection in the reverse direction). When the source receives the RM cell, the source updates the allowed sending rate, based on the information in the RM cell. There are many more aspects to the control; see References 19 and 30 for the complete specification and Fendick (31) for a more readable summary.

4.6.4 ATM Block Transfer

The ATM block transfer (ABT) service category introduces the concept of a block of cells that is delineated by RM cells. The ABT service category transports complete blocks with low cell loss and low cell delay variation, comparable to that from the CBR service category. In a typical case, a higher layer protocol data unit would be packaged as an ATM block, though an ATM block may also contain multiple higher layer data units. In the ABT service category bandwidth is allocated on a block-by-block basis. Two service categories within ABT are defined. In ABT with delayed transmission, the source sends an RM cell to request a rate at which to transmit cells of a block, called the block cell rate, and then the source waits for a response RM cell from the network before sending the block of user data. In ABT with immediate transmis-

Table 4.5 Summary of ATM Service Categories

Attribute	ATM Service Category					
		VBR				
	CBR	Real-time	Non-real-time	ABR	UBR	ABT
Cell loss ratio	Specified[a]	Specified[a]	Specified[a]	Specified[b]	Unspecified	Specified[c]
Cell transfer delay and delay variation	Specified	Specified	Unspecified	Unspecified[d]	Unspecified	Specified
Peak cell rate	Specified	Specified	Specified	Specified[e]	Specified[d]	Specified
SCR/MBS	Not applicable	Specified	Specified	Not applicable	Not applicable	Specified[f]
Real-time control via RM cells	No	No	No	Yes	No	Yes

[a] For CBR and VBR, the cell loss ratio may be unspecified for CLP=1 cells.
[b] Cell loss ratio is minimized for sources that adjust their cell flow in response to control information.
[c] For conforming blocks, the cell loss ratio is comparable to that for CBR. Block loss ratio is specified.
[d] Peak cell rate is not subject to CAC and UPC procedures.
[e] Represents the maximum rate at which the source may ever send. The momentary maximum allowed rate is subject to control information.
[f] SCR specified for ATM Blocks.
Source: Copyright © 1996, The ATM Forum.

sion (ABT/IT), a user wishing to transmit an ATM block sends an RM cell followed by the user-data cells. If a network node along the connection cannot support the requested rate, the request is denied, and in the case of ABT/IT the cells of the block may be discarded. At connection establishment the user may negotiate a sustainable cell rate traffic descriptor to obtain a guaranteed bandwidth for the connection. In the ABT service category, the SCR is at the block level, as opposed to the cell level as in VBR. Again, the generic cell rate algorithm is used to define conformance at public interfaces, where the increment parameter I varies over time to track the current block cell rate. Again, there are many more aspects to ABT, and References 8 and 30 provide a complete specification.

In the ABT framework, resource allocation within the network is block oriented: resources needed for the transfer of an ATM block are dynamically allocated on a block basis. The network operator engineers resources and implements a connection admission control policy to keep the probability that a request is denied within a specified level. At this time, ABT has not been broadly implemented.

4.6.5 Unspecified Bit Rate

The unspecified bit rate (UBR) service category is intended for delay-tolerant applications. In contrast to ABR, UBR does not use a feedback traffic control mechanism. However, such mechanisms may be operating at a layer above the ATM layer, such as the transmission control protocol (TCP) running on top of the internet protocol (IP), which in turn is running over a UBR connection. Although the network operator may engineer resources to support UBR connections, the specification of UBR does not include QoS commitments on cell loss or cell delay. UBR can be viewed as a simple cell relay service analogous to the common term "best-effort service." The PCR traffic parameter is negotiated for a UBR connection because it may identify a physical bandwidth limitation of the application or of a link along the path of the connections. However, the PCR is not necessarily policed by the public network. Network nodes that support UBR connections would need to isolate in some fashion the non-UBR connections (if present) from the UBR connections. In addition, a desirable feature would be some isolation of each UBR connection from the other UBR connections. This could be accomplished via weighted fair queueing and buffer management schemes.

4.6.6 Summary of ATM Service Categories

Table 4.5 is based on Table 2-1 Reference 19 and is expanded to include the ABT service category specified in by I. 371 (8).

4.7 SUITABILITY OF ATM SERVICE CATEGORIES FOR TRANSPORTING VIDEO

Any of the five service categories above could be used to support the transport of video—some more effectively than others.

To begin with the least likely candidate: although the unspecified bit rate (UBR) service category provides no loss or delay guarantees, if the network is lightly loaded, the loss and delay will indeed be low. Just as Ethernet LANs can support some types of video, since LANs are typically lightly loaded, so too could a UBR VCC, in a similarly lightly loaded network. Of course, if many video transmissions are attempted, the assumption of light load would be violated. A UBR VCC, like any VCC, has the desirable attribute of delivering the transmitted bits in order. Also, a UBR VCC places few requirements on the video system—no need to shape the encoded bits to a traffic descriptor, or to react to control messages (resource management cells) from the network.

In contrast, a CBR VCC is similar to a circuit-switched connection, or private line, in traditional public telephone networks. Thus, a CBR VCC is a natural choice for transporting constant-rate encoded video, where the peak cell rate of the CBR VCC is chosen to match the bit rate of the encoded video. Besides duplicating traditional private-line service, a CBR VCC has the additional flexibility that the requested rate can be whatever is appropriate for the source, and is no longer constrained to the rather coarse granularity of traditional services. Also, a CBR VCC can be used to transport variable-rate encoded video, given that the maximum bit rate of the video is no more than the capacity of the CBR VCC. Moreover, the maximum bit rate can be reduced via smoothing of the encoded video over a few frame times. The smoothing could be done in the encoder's buffer, or at the ATM level at the beginning of the ATM connection, or, as a service to the user, at the ingress to a service provider's network. However, using a CBR VCC for variable-rate video leads to a relatively inefficient use of the bandwidth. The remaining three service categories offer solutions for transporting variable-rate video while obtaining greater efficiency of network resources, compared with using a CBR VCC.

The real-time VBR service category was defined to support voice and video applications. The specifics of how video transport can effectively use real-time VBR connections have attracted a good deal of research interest. For a recent review see Lakshman et al. (32). A simple, natural idea is for the encoder to hold the quantizer step size constant, to eliminate the encoder buffer, and to transmit the encoded video as soon as possible to reduce delay in the end system. Unfortunately, it is difficult to select values a priori for sustainable cell rate and maximum burst size such that the flow of emitted cells is indeed conforming. If the video is prerecorded, as in a playback application, then an offline computation can be done to determine the appropriate traffic parameters. There is a continuum of choices. For each value of the SCR that is between the average and peak bit rates of the video, there is a minimum value for the MBS for which the video transmission would be conforming. However these parameters are fairly "loose" in the sense that if the network operator were to use them for connection admission control, the network resources would be inefficiently used, leading, in principle, to higher prices for the transport of the video. Some improvement is obtained if, prior to transmission, the encoded video is smoothed in some fashion over a time scale of a few frame times; see Reference 33 for an illustrative study.

Video and real-time VBR connections are better matched to one another if the video encoder knows the traffic descriptor of the ATM connection and suitably adapts the encoding. Heuristically, one can think of the leaky-bucket algorithm for the SCR/MBS traffic parameters as a virtual extension to the physical encoder buffer. The video terminal emits cells and keeps track of the resulting state of the leaky bucket (which corresponds to the content in a virtual buffer: "virtual" because the cells are not actually being buffered). When the leaky bucket is close to being filled, the video terminal begins to physically buffer encoded bits, and thus allows the state of the leaky bucket to decrease. When the physical buffer is getting full, the encoder can adjust the encoding (e.g., by increasing the quantizer step size). Various authors have proposed particular schemes that have additional desirable properties such as controlling the end-to-end delay (including the delay in the end systems), maintaining the quality of the video, and creating traffic streams that enable efficient use of network resources. For recent examples, see Hsu et al. (34), Hamdi et al. (35), and the literature cited in Reference 32.

The ATM Block Transfer (ABT) service category can also be used for the transport of variable-rate video. The basic idea would be that the source would request a block cell rate that is currently needed, say on a scene-by-scene basis, or possibly a frame-by-frame basis. Of course, the source would need to determine what should be the requested rate. This is relatively straight-forward if the encoding is already completed, such as with stored (playback) video. The rate could also be determined in real time based on the current buffer occupancy. If ABT with delayed transmission is used, the source needs to wait for an acknowledgment before transporting (if the request is for a higher rate), which might be preferable to ABT with immediate transmission, which entails the risk that transmitted cells will be discarded if the requested rate is not granted. To have an assurance that a requested rate would be granted, the ABT connection should be established with the block-level SCR. Given that the source stays within the SCR, requested rate changes, in particular requests to increase the rate, would be granted. Of course, there is the issue of determining the appropriate choice for the SCR.

The ABR service category was originally defined for non-real-time data applications. However, the feedback information on the rate that the network can currently support, combined with a minimum cell rate can be used by a video encoder to good effect. For illustrative schemes on this theme see Lakshman et al. (36) and Duffield et al. (37). And in particular see Chapter 10 of the present volume, which pursues this theme in detail.

4.8   WHERE IS ATM?

Regarding Figure 4.2, we mentioned that the end point of the ATM connection may or may not be at the user's end system. Currently ATM is mainly deployed in the backbone network of service providers, as well as within large interconnection points, called network access points, between Internet service providers. Even when the ATM network is within the backbone, and does not extend to the end systems, ATM can be used to transport video. A given ATM connection could be used to transport the aggregate video traffic between two backbone nodes. The ATM connection might reasonably be a CBR or a real-time VBR connection. Multiple video streams could be put on one VCC, or each video stream could be put on its own VCC, and the aggregate carried as a VPC across the backbone. The ATM network does not need to know that the user data is actually encoded video, but only that the given packets are to be transported on ATM connections with specified QoS objectives, particularly with regard to delay variation and loss.

If the ATM connection did extend to the end system, the video encoding and the ATM connection could be tailored for each other. For real-time VBR connections, the various shaping, buffering, and encoding procedures referenced in Section 4.7 could be used. For ABR connections, the video encoder could also exploit feedback information from the network.

ATM could begin to become popular in end systems in conjunction with higher speed access to the Internet from the home and business. One of the contending technologies for Internet access is asymmetric digital subscriber line (ADSL), which uses the current telephone wires and operates at speeds up to a few megabits per second in the direction toward the end system and at speeds of some hundreds of kilobits per second in the direction from the end system. The asymmetry in the bandwidths takes advantage of the asymmetry in traffic load for typical user applications of web browsing. One variant of ADSL is being developed by the Universal ADSL Working Group and is called Universal ADSL (U-ADSL). Designed for easy and early deployment, U-ADSL supports speeds up to 1.5 Mbit/s to the home and 512 kbit/s from the home. U-ADSL has been standardized in ITU Recommendation G.992.2 (38), in which the support of ATM is a requirement. On the software front, Microsoft has announced that its Windows 2000 Professional software and the next major release of NT Server will support ATM. Sun Microsystems already provides ATM network interface cards running at speeds of 155 and 622 Mbit/s. Some telephone companies have begun to offer ADSL service, and some of the major personal computer manufacturers have ADSL modems available. A detailed discussion of running ATM over ADSL is provided by Kwok (39).

4.9 FURTHER READING

This chapter has provided a basic introduction to ATM networks. References were given to source material, which mainly consists of ITU and ATM Forum documents. Although this material constitutes the primary source, it was not written to be explanatory or educational, and thus is not particularly readable for someone who is not already knowledgeable in ATM (and sometimes even prior expertise does not help). If the reader is inclined to learn more about ATM, there is a wealth of secondary source material in the form of readable textbooks. The following is a somewhat arbitrary sampling—all provide a good, overall introduction and summary of ATM.

A recent book, published in 1999, is by Ginsberg (40), who focuses on internetworking and services and includes a discussion of MPLS. Black has written a three-volume series on ATM, the first covering the foundations of broadband networks (41), the second on signaling (42), and the third on internetworking (43). Handel, Huber, and Schroder provide a thorough and readable treatment (44). Onvural also provides thorough coverage and has a focus on performance issues (5). McDyson and Spohn include a discussion of ATM hardware, software and end systems (45). A classic text, revised in 1995, is by Prycker (46). For readers having a particular interest in topics of traffic characterization, connection admission policies, and network design, an excellent text is the one edited by Roberts, Mocci, and Virtamo (26). Kwok focuses on ATM in access networks to the home and business, including multicasting of video (39).

ACRONYMS

AAL	ATM adaptation layer
ABR	available bit rate
ABT	ATM block transfer
ADSL	asymmetrical digital subscriber line
ATM	asynchronous transfer mode
B-ISDN	broadband integrated services digital network
BUS	broadcast and unknown server
CAC	connection admission control
CBR	constant bit rate

CDV	cell delay variation
CDVT	cell delay variation tolerance
CLR	cell loss ratio
CPCS	common part of the convergence sublayer
CTD	cell transfer delay
DBR	deterministic bit rate
DSL	digital subscriber line
GCRA	generic cell rate algorithm
GFR	guaranteed frame rate
HEC	header error control
IP	Internet Protocol
ITU	International Telecommunications Union
LAN	local-area network
maxCTD	maximum cell transfer delay
Mbit/s	10^6 bits per second
MBS	maximum burst size
MPLS	multiprotocol label switching
MPOA	multiprotocol over ATM
NNI	network–network interface, or network–node interface
OAM	operations, administration, and maintenance
PCR	peak cell rate
PDU	protocol data unit
PHY	physical layer
PT	payload type
QoS	quality of service
RM	resource management
SAR	segmentation and reassembly
SBR	statistical bit rate
SCR	sustainable cell rate
SDH	synchronous digital hierarchy
SONET	synchronous optical network
TCP	transmission control protocol
TD	traffic descriptor
U-ADSL	universal asymmetric digital subscriber line
UBR	unspecified bit rate
UNI	user–network interface
UTP	unshielded twisted pair
VBR	variable bit rate
VCC	virtual channel connection
VCI	virtual channel identifier
VPC	virtual path connection
VPI	virtual path identifier

REFERENCES

1. ITU-T Recommendation Q.2931. Broadband integrated services digital network (B-ISDN)–Digital subscriber signalling system no. 2 (DSS 2)–User–network interface (UNI)—Layer 3 specification for basic call/connection control. International Telecommunications Union, Geneva February 1995.
2. ATM Forum ATM User–network interface (UNI) signalling specification, version 4.0. ATM Forum Technical Committee, July 1996.
3. ATM Forum private network–network interface specification, version 1.0 (PNNI 1.0). ATM Forum Technical Committee, April 1996.
4. ITU-T Recommendation I.432. B-ISDN user network interface specification. International Telecommunications Union, Geneva, August 1996.
5. R Onvural, Asynchronous Transfer Mode Networks, Performance Issues. Norwood, MA. Artech House, 1995.
6. Recommendation I.361. B-ISDN ATM Layer specification. International Telecommunications Union, Geneva, November 1995.
7. ITU-T Recommendation I.610. B-ISDN operations and maintenance principles and functions. International Telecommunications Union, Geneva, November 1995.
8. ITU-T Recommendation I.371. Traffic control and congestion control in B-ISDN. International Telecommunications Union, Geneva, May 1996.
9. ITU-T Recommendation E.735. Framework for traffic control and dimensioning in B-ISDN. International Telecommunications Union, Geneva, May 1997.
10. ATM Forum, LAN emulation over ATM specification, version 1.0. ATM Forum Specification, January 1995.
11. ATM Forum, Multi-protocol over ATM specification, version 1.0. ATM Forum Specification, July 1997.
12. ITU-T Recommendation I.363.1. B-ISDN ATM adaptation layer specification: Type 1 AAL. International Telecommunications Union, Geneva, August 1996.
13. ITU-T Recommendation I.363.2, B-ISDN ATM adaptation layer specification: Type 2 AAL. International Telecommunications Union, Geneva, September 1997.
14. JH Baldwin, BH Bharucha, BT Doshi, S Dravida, S Nanda. A new ATM adaptation layer for small packet encapsulation. Bell Labs Tech J 2:111–131, 1997.
15. K Sriram, YT Wang. Voice over ATM using AAL2 and bit dropping: Performance and call admission control. IEEE J Selected Areas Commun 17:18–28, 1999.
16. ITU-T Recommendation I.363.5. B-ISDN ATM adaptation layer specification: Type 5 AAL. International Telecommunications Union, Geneva, August 1996.
17. ITU-T Recommendation I.358. Call processing performance for switched virtual channel connections in a B-ISDN. International Telecommunications Union, Geneva, June 1998.
18. ITU-T Recommendation I.356. B-ISDN ATM layer cell transfer performance. International Telecommunications Union, Geneva, May 1996.
19. ATM Forum Traffic management specification, version 4.0. ATM Forum Technical Committee, April 1996.
20. H Heiss. QoS results for the GFR ATM service. In: P Key, D Smith, eds. Teletraffic

Engineering in a Competitive World, Proceedings of the 16th International Teletraffic Congress. Amsterdam: Elsevier, 1999, pp 227–236.

21.   (a) R Guerin J Heinanen. UBR+ service category definition. ATM Forum contribution 96-1598, December 1996. (b) R Guerin, J Heinanen. UBR+ enhancements. ATM Forum contribution 97-0015, February 1997.

22.   AW Berger, W Whitt. The Brownian approximation for rate-control throttles and the G/G/1/C Queue. Discrete Event Dyn Syst 2:7–60, 1992.

23.   AW Berger, W Whitt. A comparison of the sliding window and the leaky bucket. Queueing Syst 20:117–138, 1995.

24.   AW Berger. Desirable properties of traffic descriptors for ATM connections in a broadband ISDN. In: J Labetoulle, JW Roberts, eds. The Fundamental Role of Teletraffic in the Evolution of Telecommunications Networks, Proceedings of the 14th International Teletraffic Congress. Amsterdam: Elsevier, 1994, pp 233–242.

25.   AW Berger, AE Eckberg. A B-ISDN/ATM traffic descriptor and its use in traffic and congestion controls. Proceedings of GLOBECOM, Phoenix, AZ, 1991, pp 266–270.

26.   J Roberts, U Mocci, J. Virtamo, eds. Broadband Network Traffic, Performance Evaluation and Design of Multiservice Networks. Berlin: Springer-Verlag, 1996.

27.   FP Kelly. Notes on effective bandwidths. In: FP Kelly, S Zachary, I. Ziedins, eds. Stochastic Networks. Oxford: Claredon Press, 1996, pp 141–168.

28.   EW Knightly, NB Shroff. Admission control for statistical QoS: Theory and practice. IEEE Network 13(2):20–29, March 1999.

29.   AW Berger, W Whitt. Extending the effective bandwidth concept to networks with priority classes. IEEE Commun Mag 36:78–83, 1998.

30.   ITU-T Recommendation I.371.1. Traffic control and congestion control in B-ISDN, conformance definitions for ABT and ABR. International Telecommunications Union, Geneva, June 1997.

31.   K Fendick. Evolution of controls for the available bit rate service. IEEE Commun Mag 34:35–39, 1996.

32.   TV Lakshman, A Ortega, AR Reibman. VBR video: Tradeoffs and potentials. Proc IEEE 86:952–973, 1998.

33.   AR Reibman, AW Berger. Traffic descriptors for VBR video teleconferencing over ATM networks. IEEE/ACM Trans Networking 3:329–339, 1995.

34.   CY Hsu, A Ortega, AR Reibman. Joint selection of source and channel rate for VBR video transmission under ATM policing constraints. IEEE J Selected Areas Commun 15:1016–1028, 1997.

35.   M Hamdi, JW Roberts, P Rolin. Rate control for VBR video coders and broadband networks. IEEE J Selected Areas Commun 15:1040–1051, 1997.

36.   TV Lakshman, PP Mishra, KK Ramakrishnan. Transporting compressed video over ATM networks with explicit rate feedback control. Proceedings of IEEE Infocom 1997, Kobe, Japan, 1997, pp 38–47.

37.   NG Duffield, KK Ramakrishnan, AR Reibman. SAVE: An algorithm for smoothed adaptive video over explicit rate networks. IEEE/ACM Trans Networking 6:717–728, 1998.

38.   ITU-T Recommendation G.992.2. Splitterless asymmetrical digital subscriber line (ADSL) transmissions. International Telecommunications Union, Geneva, COM 15-R 27-E, determined for approval October 1998.

39. T Kwok. ATM: The New Paradigm for Internet, Intranet and Residential Broadband Services and Applications. Englewood Cliffs, NJ Prentice Hall, 1998.
40. D Ginsberg. ATM Solutions for Enterprise Internetworking. Harlow, UK: Addison-Wesley, 1999.
41. UD Black. ATM: Foundations for Broadband Networks. Vol I. Englewood Cliffs, NJ: Prentice Hall, 1996.
42. UD Black. ATM: Signaling in Broadband Networks. Vol II. Englewood Cliffs, NJ: Prentice Hall, 1997.
43. UD Black. ATM: Internetworking. Vol III. Englewood Cliffs, NJ: Prentice Hall, 1997.
44. R Handel, MN Huber, S Schroder. ATM Networks Concepts Protocols Applications. Harlow, UK: Addison-Wesley, 1998.
45. DE McDyson, DL Spohn. ATM Theory and Application. New York: McGraw-Hill, 1995.
46. MD Prycker. Asynchronous Transfer Mode: Solution for Broadband ISDN. Hempstead, UK: Prentice Hall, 1995.

5
Wireless Systems and Networking

Li Fung Chang
AT&T Labs–Research, Red Bank, New Jersey

5.1 INTRODUCTION

The cellular industry has enjoyed tremendous growth since its introduction in the early 1980s. In particular, after worldwide deployment of the all-digital second-generation wireless systems, it opened up markets not only for traditional voice service but also for data services, such as facsimile transmission or short message services. Although uptake of the wireless data has yet been achieved, it is believed that with the explosive subscription rate of the Internet services, end users will eventually demand that such services be made available on the Internet at any time and in any place. Furthermore, the demand of the traditional voice services in some markets has reached the saturation point. It is in the best interest of the wireless service providers to offer value-added wireless data services to boost the revenue and to retain/attract subscribers. To offer a cost-effective multimedia service, the air interface needs to be able to support data rates higher than the existing second-generation rate (i.e., 9.6 or 13 kbit/s). In addition, the entire wireless infrastructure must migrate from voice-centric circuit-based network status to packet-based data-centric network status. The applications also need to adapt to the time-varying unstable, low-bandwidth wireless channel. With advances in technology, increased spectrum availability, and the development of innovative algorithms for applications such as low bit rate video and image compression schemes, a cost-effective wireless multimedia service will be available in the near future.

This chapter offers readers with a background in video a road to understanding the basic designs of wireless systems and networks. We start with an overview of wireless system characteristics, including channel impairments and various multiple-access schemes. The intent is to provide readers with the basic

concept of the cause of wireless channel impairments and to present related statistics to facilitate more research activities in the field of low bit rate video over
wireless channels. The representative third-generation air interface is then briefly
discussed, together with its individual attributes. Where possible, there is comparison with its second-generation counterpart. Wireless/mobile ATM, the Internet mobility management protocol (Mobile IP), the packet-based general packet
radio services (GPRS), and the infrastructure approach of the CDMA2000 and
Wideband CDMA are described. Finally, the challenges of optimized video
codec for wireless environments are presented.

5.2 OVERVIEW OF WIRELESS SYSTEM CHARACTERISTICS

5.2.1 Propagation Characteristics

In radio communications, the signals transmitted over the radio channel are subject to two types of signal variation, namely, small- and large-scale signal variations (1,2). Factors affecting the large-scale signal variations include path
attenuations due to the distance between the transmitter and the receiver, terrain
obstructions, antenna height, and so on. The impacts of these factors on the receiving signal cannot be mathematically analyzed and are mostly resolved by
measurements or experimental data.

Unlike propagation in free space, where a signal is attenuated by 20 dB per
distance decade (i.e., the distance exponent is -2), it has been shown experimen-
tally that when one or both antennas are in the proximity of the ground and
within the ground clutter (i.e., below the treetops, power lines, housetops, etc.),
the distance dependence is about a factor of 3.5–4. Measurements done in the
800 to 900 MHz band in the urban area, in large buildings, and in residential areas have also indicated that the local mean signal is a log-normal distributed random variable with a mean that varies with distance. This type of signal variation,
excluding the effect of path attenuation, is called shadow fading.

The small-scale signal variations are due to multipath signal propagation.
Between each transmitter/receiver pair, many scattered or reflected signals result
from signal reflections from walls, ceilings, or other objects, leading to multipath
signal propagation. The signals in each path may have different time delays and
may encounter different path attenuations. Thus, the multipath propagation
medium introduces time delay spread and amplitude fluctuations on the received
signal.

Instantaneous signal amplitude fluctuations are due to the additions of the
multipath signals. The effect of multipath propagation on the amplitude of the received signal can be explained simply through Figure 5.1, which shows two distinct propagation paths between the transmitter and the receiver. Typically there

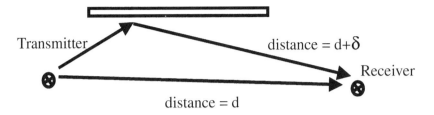

Figure 5.1   Diagram of two-path propagation.

are many more paths, but for simplicity we consider just the two paths shown. If the difference in path length between the two paths is half a wavelength, which at 2 GHz is 3 in., then the signals will exactly cancel, causing a deep fading condition. However, if the receiver, the transmitter, or the reflecting object in Figure 5.1 is moved only a few inches, the phase relationship between the two received signals can easily change. As a result, the two signals may be received in phase, resulting in an upfaded condition. In the typical case, the statistics of the received signal amplitude fit a Rayleigh distribution (3,4), and the phase of the received signal is uniformly distributed between 0 and 2π. That is, if r (the received signal amplitude) is a Rayleigh random variable, then the probability density function of r is:

$$p(r) = \frac{r}{\sigma^2} \exp\left(-\frac{r^2}{2\sigma^2}\right)$$

where σ is the root-mean-square (rms) value of the received signal envelope.

Note that the duration and rate of change of the signal due to this type of fading is dependent on the speed of the transmitter, the receiver, and the environment. Errors occur in bursts when the received signal envelope fades below some noise-related threshold and the length of the erroneous bursts depends on the time spent in a fade. For example at a carrier frequency of 2 GHz, if the user is traveling at a speed of 1 ft/s or about 0.7 mph, the signal is relatively stationary during a period of, say, 5 or 10 m. Therefore, if the signal is in a fade, the length of the erroneous burst can be as long as 10 ms. However, for a user traveling at a speed of 88 ft/s or 60 mph, the signal strength would vary quite rapidly during a burst duration and the effect would be random errors.

Figure 5.2 shows the multipath fading variation over a distance of about 20 ft for a 2 GHz signal from the two orthogonal antennas, namely, vertically and horizontally polarized antennas. Note that in this figure the Rayleigh fading as measured on a vertically polarized antenna is independent of the Rayleigh fading as measured on a colocated horizontally polarized antenna. When the signal was quite unusable at one antenna, the other antenna received a very strong signal.

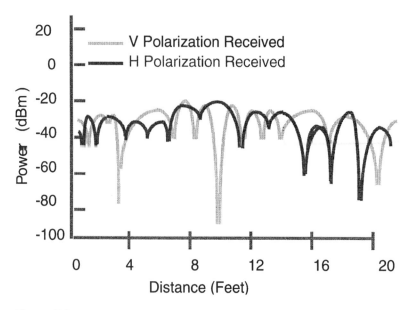

Figure 5.2 Received signal power from two antennas.

Thus by using two antennas and choosing the best received signal, one can improve the overall received signal quality substantially. This technique, called antenna diversity, is a well-known means of mitigating the effect of multipath fading. Note that the independence of the two antennas can be achieved in other ways—for example, by using two identical antennas separated by about half a wavelength, or 3 in. at 2 GHz.

Time delay spread can degrade system performance by causing intersymbol interference (ISI). ISI leads to an irreducible bit error rate for typical modulation schemes [e.g., BPSK, QPSK, QAM, etc. (5,6)]. The impairment caused by ISI is usually called *frequency-selective fading* (since from a frequency domain point of view, the time dispersion of the transmitted signal causes certain frequency components in the received signal spectrum to have higher gains than others).

Figure 5.3, which explains the cause of ISI in a simple diagram, illustrates the effect of multipath delay spread. In this figure, which could represent the propagation environment of a modest-sized auditorium, a small warehouse, or an open office area, the dimensions are 50 ft × 100 ft. If a base station is located in a corner as shown and a portable environment is located only 50 ft away, the difference in path length between the reflected and direct signal would be about 150 ft. Therefore, the reflected signal would be delayed by about 150 ns (since the

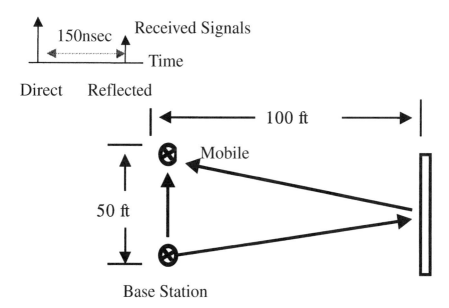

Figure 5.3   Received signal at the mobile due to multipath delay spread.

speed of light is roughly equivalent to 1 ft/ns). If the radio channel symbol rate is 500 kilosymbols/s, then the symbol duration is 200 ns. Therefore the reflected signal is delayed by 75% of a symbol. In other words, adjacent symbols are over-lapping by 150 ns or 75% of their total duration. Thus the signal is interfering with itself. This creates a condition called the irreducible bit error rate. Even if the ratio of signal to noise plus outside interference is excellent, the error rate cannot be improved because of this self-interference.

The effect of multipath delay spread varies from environment to environment and can be characterized by a power delay profile $p(t)$. Some measured power delay profiles in mobile (3,7) and portable (8,9) radio environment have been documented. One important parameter in the frequency-selective fading channel is the width of the power delay profile, normally called the root-mean-square (rms) delay spread τ, defined as the square root of the second central moment. The rms delay spread of a radio channel limits the maximum transmission rate of a digital system. Typically, the rms delay spread ranges from a few tenths of a microsecond to several microseconds from portable to mobile propagation environments. In mobile propagation environments, where the rms delay spread significantly degrades system performance, techniques such as channel equalization (10) (i.e., picking up a "main signal" and canceling the echoes) or the use of a Rake receiver (11), which takes the advantage of the entire multipath, may be employed to combat the effect of multipath delay spread. In the portable propagation environment (short transmission range, in-building, low antennas), the multipath delay spread is generally a few tenths of a microsecond. In this case, the system can support reasonable transmission rates (a few hundreds kilobits per second to 1 Mbit/s) without equalization. Antenna diversity deployed as a defensive measure to mitigate the effects of Rayleigh fading can also improve the delay spread tolerance by a factor of 2.5.

Readers who are interested in acquiring a more detailed understanding of radio propagation and mitigation techniques are encouraged to read Rappaport's book (12).

5.2.2 Multiple-Access Schemes/Duplexing Techniques

The duplexing method is crucial to overall system design in two-way (full-duplex) transmission systems. In systems using time division duplexing (TDD), the uplink (portables to base) and the downlink (base to portables) data are transmitted together on the same radio frequency channel but at different times. That is, the uplink and downlink transmissions are operated at the same carrier frequency in ping-pong fashion as illustrated in Figure 5.4.

TDD requires only one frequency band; however, the transmission rate in each direction is only half the radio channel rate. The uplink performance of a TDD system with asynchronous base station transmissions is very sensitive to the height and power difference between the portable and the base, since uplink interferences come not only from the cochannel portables but also from cochannel base transmissions. In general, for systems employing TDD, time synchronization among base stations is required to maintain good system performance and frequency reuse efficiency (because higher frequency reuse needs to be adopted to mitigate the interference caused by the asynchronous uplink/downlink transmissions among base stations).

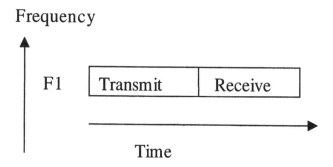

Figure 5.4   Time division duplex.

Frequency division duplex (FDD) uses a pair of frequencies for uplink and downlink transmission separately, as shown in Figure 5.5. Thus it requires two distinct frequency bands. However, it gives complete freedom for the transmitter and the receiver to operate independently. FDD avoids the need for base station synchronization, since base stations receive and transmit at different frequencies; one base's transmission will not interfere with another base's reception. Most of the second-generation digital wireless systems, such as the Global System for Mobile (GSM) for pan-European vehicular digital cellular mobile radio, CdmaOne (North America digital cellular radio system), and the IS-136 system employed FDD to avoid strong interbase station interference.

In addition to the duplex method, the multiple-access scheme plays a major role in the engineering of wireless systems. In general there are three multiple-access technologies: frequency division–multiple access (FDMA), time division–multiple access, and spread spectrum–multiple access (SSMA).

In an FDMA communication system, radio spectrum is divided into nonoverlapping frequency segments where each user is assigned to an exclusive frequency segment for communicating with the base station, as demonstrated in Figure 5.6a. At the receiver, a band-pass filter is used to filter out signals carried in each frequency channel. Thus after receiver filtering, the individual user signal will be recovered (Figure 5.6b). An FDMA system is a one-channel-per-carrier system; multiple radio receivers are required for implementing antenna diversity. In FDMA systems, simultaneous use of multiple frequency segments or a flexible bandwidth assignment scheme must be implemented to accommodate various transmission rates.

In a time division–multiplex access (TDMA) system, users communicating with the same base station transmit data on the same carrier frequency but at

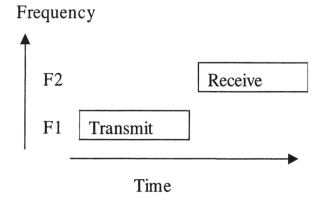

Figure 5.5   Frequency division duplex.

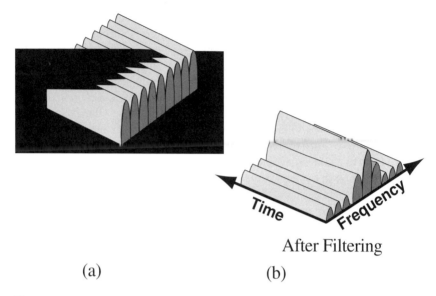

After Filtering

(a)   (b)

Figure 5.6   Frequency division multiple access (a) before and (b) after filtering.

different times. The transmission time is segmented into frames, and each frame is further divided into time slots. A user with a transmission rate equivalent to the time slot duration (i.e., basic transmission rate) uses that time slot in every frame to communicate with the base station. Figure 5.7 illustrates the concept of the TMDA/FDMA. In Figure 5.7a an available spectrum is divided into three frequency bands called carriers. For each carrier, a TDMA frame is further divided into three time slots (time axes); therefore, each carrier can carry three users at the basic transmission rate. At the receiver, with proper timing and carrier recovery, the user signal is obtained. (Figure 5.7b shows the received signal for the user assigned carrier 2 and time slot 2.) For subrate transmission, a time slot is shared by two (half-rate) of four (quarter-rate) users, and each individual user communicates with the base station by using the sharing time slot in every other frame (half-rate) or every fourth frame (quarter-rate), respectively. For a multiple basic rate transmission, time slot aggregation (multiple time slots per frame) is used to carry the user information.

In commercial TDMA systems (e.g., GSM, IS-136), other functions (e.g. assessing the quality of other frequency channels, interference measurement, etc.) are performed during the time that a subscriber is not transmitting or receiving. A TDMA system requires frame/time slot synchronization and guard times shared among various users.

Code division multiple access (CDMA), as shown in Figure 5.8, is based

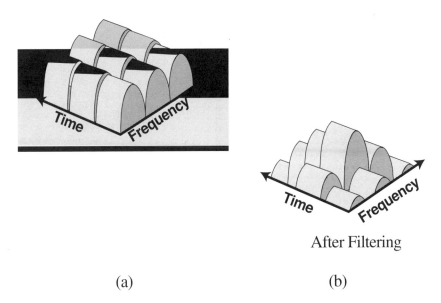

After Filtering

(a)   (b)

Figure 5.7   Time division multiple access (a) before and (b) after filtering.

on spread-spectrum technology. In a CDMA communication system, a unique binary spreading pseudorandom code (PN code) is assigned for each call to each user, and all active users share the same frequency spectrum at the same time (Figure 5.8a). The signal of each user is separated from the others at the receiver by using a correlator keyed with the associated selected binary spreading code (Figure 5.8b). Since all users share the same frequency spectrum, all other users' signals contribute to the interference level in the system. Power control is essential in a CDMA system, where the near–far problem arises (transmitters near a receiver generate overwhelming interference relative to those far from the receiver). If power control can be performed *perfectly,* the overall interference for the weakest users can be minimized. As a result, CDMA system capacity in terms of the number of simultaneous users that can be handled in a given system bandwidth can be maximized. With proper design, CDMA is more robust in the multipath delay spread environment than the other access schemes because of the use of the multiple PN correlators at the receiver to provide path diversity (if PN correlators can capture all the signal power from each individual delay path). CDMA also does not need frequency coordination among all the base stations.

The choice of different access/duplex technologies for a wireless communications system is determined by the service environments and the applications contemplated. For various wireless communications environments,

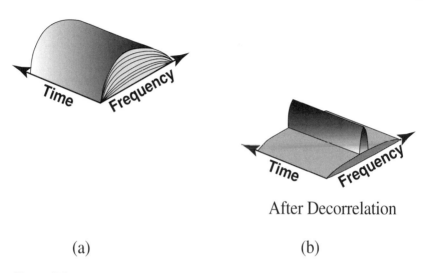

After Decorrelation

(a)   (b)

Figure 5.8   Code division multiple access before and after despreading.

some technology compromises are required with respect to such issues as complexity, quality, coverage area, capacity, and spectrum efficiency (13).

5.3   WIRELESS NETWORKS

5.3.1   First- and Second-Generation Wireless Systems

The first-generation wireless systems introduced in the 1980s, are designed for local or national coverage and primarily for voice services. They are overlay networks with the fixed infrastructure. Some of these early systems, such as AMPS in North America, TACS in United Kingdom, and NMT in Nordic countries, are mutually incompatible. They all use analog frequency modulation for speech transmission, and in-band signaling for control information between terminals and the rest of the network during a call. In addition, most of the mobility management functions are network-controlled. For example, in a handover the mobile switching center (MSC) assembles measurement information on the signal strength received at several neighboring base stations from the mobile and decides when the mobile should tune to a different base station.

Since the introduction of first-generation wireless systems, demand has continuously exceeded expectation. To meet the demand for wireless access, and to enlarge the range of applications, the "all-digital" second-generation systems were deployed in early 1990s. The second-generation digital wireless systems are designed to solve the capacity problem associated with the first-generation wireless systems. In addition, a pan-European system with full international roaming and handoff is in demand in Europe to eliminate incompatibility among the first-generation systems. The GSM system was therefore developed and deployed in Europe to serve this purpose. In fact, GSM has been deployed worldwide, and today 50% of the users of the second-generation systems are GSM subscribers.

Figures 5.9 and 5.10 illustrate network reference models (NRM) for the North America ANSI-41 system and the European GSM system to support wide-area roaming and handoff for voice and short message services. Note that the major difference between the two NRMs is in the base station and the base station controller (BSC). In ANSI-41, functions of BSC, which provides control and radio resource management to the mobile units, are colocated within the mobile switching center (MSC), whereas in GSM architecture BSC is separated from MSC to handle radio resource related management functions.

In Figures 5.9 and 5.10, interfaces between different network entities are labeled. For example, the interface between BS/BSC and MSC is the "A" interface, the interface between MSC and the home location register (HLR) is the "C" interface, and so on. In these architectures, an MSC is the switching and signaling interface between the mobile stations and the fixed network.

The MSC performs normal ISDN switching and call control functions as well as cellular network specific functions such as handover of calls, interworking and adaptation between mobile and ISDN communication services, and remote control of the wireless access network. The BS, BSC, and the MSC

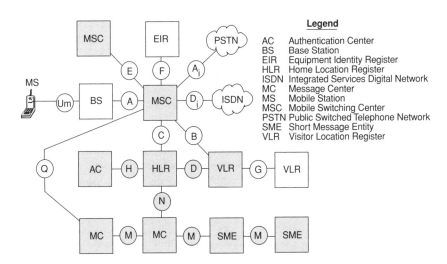

Figure 5.9 ANSI-41 network reference model.

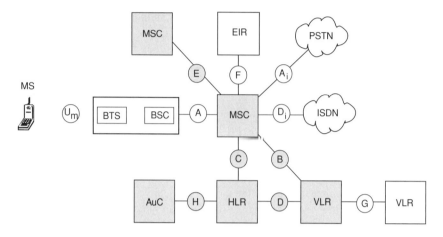

Figure 5.10 GSM 900/DCS 1800 network reference model.

together form the wireless access network. The signaling network consists of databases called home and visitor location registers (HLR and VLR, respectively), which provide mobility management functions. An HLR contains the user service profile and subscriber location information. The location information is the information of the VLR and the MSC that the mobile station is currently attached to. The location information is maintained via a registration process initiated by the subscriber whenever it moves into a new location area. A VLR is a local database in charge of one or more location areas. It maintains temporary copy of selected subscriber information. The HLR and VLR may or may not be located within MSC. They may serve one or more MSCs. An MSC communicates with HLRs and VLRs across the signaling system 7 (SS7) (14) network.

The authentication center (AC, or AuC) provides authentication functions used to verify and validate a mobile station's identity and manages encryption and authentication keys, by means of standard signal processing algorithms. AC functionality can be deployed internally or externally to HLR. The equipment identity register (EIR) provides for storage of mobile equipment related data (e.g., mobile station electronic serial numbers and status). The message center (MC) has the ability to store and forward short messages (for short message services) to subscribers and supports both mobile-originated and mobile-terminated short message delivery.

The access networks of second-generation wireless systems can be classified into high-tier and low-tier systems. The high-tier system is designed for high-mobility vehicular services and has characteristics such as the following:

large base station antenna heights via tower mounting, high transmission
power
larger coverage area (e.g., several miles)
complex receiver design (e.g., forward error correction coding, interleaving, equalizer for combating radio link impairments)
voice bit rates around 8–13 kbit/s

In North America, several high-tier systems are in service now. IS-95 (CdmaOne) is a CDMA-based standard. IS-136 is a TDMA-based standard. PCS-1900 is a derivative of GSM that is also based on TDMA. In the GSM network, all the interfaces (air interface, interface between base stations and the MSC, the MSC and the signaling network, etc.) are standardized. This gives GSM cellular service providers greater flexibility in configuring their networks and obtaining equipment from various manufacturers. Table 5.1 summarizes the characteristics

Table 5.1   Air Interface Characteristics[a] of IS-136, GSM, and IS-95

Attributes	IS-136	GSM	IS-95
Multiple access	TDMA	TDMA	CDMA
Duplex	FDD	FDD	FDD
Channel spacing	30 kHz	200 kHz	1.23 MHz spreading bandwidth
Frame duration	40 ms	4.615 ms	20 ms (speech frame)
Number of time slots/frame	6	8	N/A
Modulation	$\pi/4$ shifted, differentially encoded QPSK	GMSK	Uplink: Walsh noncoherent modulation; downlink, QPSK
Channel coding	Rate 1/2, memory 5 convolutional and 7-bit CRC codes	Rate 1/2, memory 4 convolutional and 7-bit CRC codes	Rate 1/2 downlink; rate 1/3 uplink convolutional codes with memory 8
Interleaving depth	40 ms	40 ms	20 ms
Speech code rate	13 kbit/s	13 or 6.5 kbit/s	8 or 13 kbit/s
Transmission rate	48.6 kbit/s	270.8 kbit/s	1.23 mchip/s
Adaptive equalizer	Mandatory	Mandatory	Not required
Handoff	Mobile assisted	Mobile assisted	Mobile-assisted soft and softer handoff
Short message services	Yes	Yes	Yes

[a] CRC, mean shift keying; QPSK,; GMSK, Gaussian quadrature phase shift keying.

of these three air interface technologies. Some details such as modulation schemes and channel coding are provided for completeness but are not covered further here.

Low-tier systems (15) are targeted for low-speed pedestrian and indoor usage. Some of the characteristics of a low-tier system are small, inexpensive base stations for pole or wall mounting, large number of base stations and small coverage area per base station, low transmit power and small batteries for mobile terminals, and wireline-quality voice service (32 kbit/s).

PACS, DECT, and PHS are TDMA-based, low-tier systems. PACS is a low-tier standard in the United States and can be used for both indoor and outdoor environments. DECT, a pan-European standard, was designed to offer voice services in the indoor environment (residential, wireless PABX, local loop). PHS, which has been deployed in Japan, has some similarity to PACS. Both are designed as wireless access systems for integration into the fixed network and for indoor and outdoor usage. The major differences between PACS and PHS are the use of frequency division duplex versus time division duplex and 2.5 ms versus 5 ms frame structures. CT2 and CT2+ are the only low-tier systems using frequency division–multiple access. CT2 can support only outgoing calls (i.e., no paging capability). CT2+ is an enhanced version of CT2 with incoming call capability and a dedicated channel for control signaling. CT2 was the first low-tier system to be deployed; because of its limited one-way calling capability and limited coverage, however, the deployment was not very successful.

5.3.2 Third-Generation Wireless Systems

The development of third generation (3G) systems is targeted to provide high-speed packet data services in addition to offering higher capacity for the voice services. The focus on offering high-speed wireless packet data services reflects the expectation that the growth of wired multimedia applications will need to be extended over the wireless link to meet the demand for multimedia services that are available at any time and in any place. Furthermore, the design of 3G systems also contains the following objectives: to offer smoother interconnecting between different networks, environments, and so on, to encourage the convergence of disparate systems and wireless access technologies, and to provide global roaming. Today, different networks and wireless transmission technologies are used to offer services such as paging, interactive messaging, and voice services. It will be more efficient and cost-effective to integrate these services and to converge these disparate systems to offer convenience services to consumers. Today's second-generation systems allow only limited roaming, since there are different systems operating at different frequencies in different parts of the world. It will be highly desirable to offer global roaming so that users can have wireless access anywhere in the world, from the same terminal. Objectives of the 3G systems were initially defined in the European RACE (Research for Advanced Communications in Europe) program (16) and in the Future Public Land Mobile Telecommunications System (FPLMTS) program of the International Telecommunication Union (ITU) which evolved to the initiative called IMT-2000.

In 3G, subscribers will be able to use the same terminal indoors and outdoors, in residential and in business settings, at high speed and at low speed. The same terminal will be used for multimedia services. In addition to terminal mobility, the system is expected to provide personal mobility. Personal mobility implies that a user carrying a personal subscription identity (personal telecommunication number) rather than a terminal can access services from any terminal, whether it is in a fixed or wireless communications network. When a caller dials this number, it is the network's responsibility to route the call to the terminal of the subscriber's choice. Intelligent network functionality will play a crucial role in support of this feature.

As mentioned above, one of the design objectives of the 3G system is to provide variable-rate services for different propagation environments (e.g., indoor, outdoor, pedestrian, vehicular). Because of this objective, in IMT-2000 radio transmission technologies (RTT) for terrestrial access, the bearer capability requirements are divided into three basic categories: indoor, outdoor-to-indoor and pedestrian, and vehicular. Table 5.2 summarizes the minimum bearer capability requirements in these environments.

Several radio transmission technologies are designed to meet these requirements. Section 5.3.3 offers a brief overview of the 3G wireless access systems that are designed to support high-speed packet data services with features such as link adaptation for variable data rates, bandwidth-on-demand, and independent asymmetric uplink downlink radio resource assignment.

Table 5.2 Minimum Bearer Capability in Different Environments

	Environment[a]		
Capability	Indoor	Outdoor-to-indoor and pedestrian	Vehicular
Speech	32 kbit/s, BER $\leq 10^{-3}$	32 kbit/s, BER $\leq 10^{-3}$	32 kbit/s, BER $\leq 10^{-3}$
Circuit-switched data	2 Mbit/s, BER $\leq 10^{-6}$	384 kbit/s, BER $\leq 10^{-6}$	144 kbit/s, BER $\leq 10^{-6}$
Packet-switched data	2 Mbit/s, BER $\leq 10^{-6}$, exponentially sized packets, Poisson arrivals	384 kbit/s, BER $\leq 10^{-6}$, exponentially sized packets, Poisson arrivals	144 kbit/s, BER $\leq 10^{-6}$, exponentially sized packets, Poisson arrivals

[a] BER, bit error rate.

5.3.3 Emerging Air Interface Approaches for Packet Data Services

We now focus on three key technologies, namely, enhanced data rates for GSM evolution (EDGE), CDMA2000, and wideband CDMA (WCDMA).

5.3.3.1 Edge. EDGE is an air interface technology evolving from GSM to provide higher data rate services (17–20). EDGE is designed to operate on the infrastructure of GSM and (general packet radio services (GPRS) to provide high-speed end-to-end packet data services. EDGE was proposed to Standard Subcommittee TR45.3 of the Telecommunications Industry Association (TIA) as an evolution of IS-136 toward higher data rate services and was accepted by TR45.3. Preliminary design of EDGE is adopted by TR45.3 and is included as part of the UWC-136 (universal wireless communications 136), namely "136 HS" (136 high speed) for outdoor/vehicular application.

The basic concept of EDGE is to employ a higher level modulation scheme per radio time slot than GMSK modulation, currently used in the GSM system. In addition, dynamic multi-time-slot allocation and link adaptation are used in EDGE to provide data rates between 64 and 384 kbit/s. Table 5.3 summarizes the physical layer designs of EDGE and GSM.

Note that the modulation scheme for EDGE has been changed from the original proposed quaternary-offset-QAM (Q-O-QAM), binary-offset-QAM (B-O-QAM) to 8-PSK, to take advantage of the better performance of the 8-PSK at

Table 5.3 Comparison of the Physical Layer Designs of EDGE and GSM

Attributes	GSM	EDGE
Frame Structure	TDMA, 8 time slots/frame, 4.62 ms frame duration	Same as GSM
Modulation (downlink)	GMSK, 1 bit/symbol	8-PSK, 3 bits/symbol
Modulation (uplink)	GMSK	8-PSK and GMSK
Payload/burst	114 bits	346 bits
Gross rate/time slot	22.8 kbit/s	69.2 kbits/s
Channel spacing	200 kHz	200 kHz
Time slot assignment	Fixed, single	Dynamic, up to 8 time slots
Link adaptation	No	Yes (8 classes)
Handover	Mobile-assisted hand over (MAHO)	MAHO for transparent mode; cell reselection for packet data operation
Channel coding	Rate 1/2 convolutional code with memory 5	Rate 1/3 convolutional code with memory 6 and different puncturing patterns

the higher data rates, the same symbol rate as GMSK, and compatibility between UWC-136 and EDGE. Both 8-PSK and GMSK modulation schemes are included for the uplink to provide mobile subscriber units with a smooth evolution path from GSM to EDGE.

In current EDGE for handover, a cell reselection algorithm is used in packet data operation. In this case MS measures the received signal strength indicator (RSSI) of serving cell and neighbor cells, and the best cell having the highest priority class is selected. Link adaptation uses channel coding with coding rate ranging from 1, 3/4, 2/3, to 1/2 to accommodate a wide range of C/I variation. The design also supports asymmetrical data traffic loading by providing different link adaptations and different numbers of time slots in uplinks and downlinks.

Currently, ETSI standard committee is working on refining the EDGE common air interface that meets the requirements from both GSM and IS136 communities (e.g., smooth evolution, compatibility, etc.).

5.3.3.2 WCDMA. Wideband CDMA is under joint development by the European Telecommunications Standards Institute (ETSI) and (ARIB) and has been proposed jointly by these bodies as one of the IMT-2000 wireless access technologies (20,21). It is a wideband, spread-spectrum radio interface that uses code division multiple access (CDMA) technology. Like IS-95 CDMA system, WCDMA has many similar features such as the use of RAKE receivers to suppress multipath delay spread impairment and power control to resolve the near–far problem. Among the new features considered in the WCDMA system design are different spreading factors to support variable-rate bearer services, reference pilot symbols for coherent detection, and asynchronized base stations. In WCDMA, variable-rate transmissions are possible by changing the spreading factor from 256 to 4; the rate can vary on a 10 ms frame basis. Furthermore, multiple variable services can be time-multiplexed on one variable-rate physical channel or code-multiplexed on different variable-rate physical channels. This approach can be used to vary the bit rate on a frame-by-frame basis without any explicit resource allocation and negotiation. WCDMA also introduces a synchronization channel (SCH) in the downlink for MS to perform cell search. In this way, inter-BS synchronization can be avoided. The SCH consists of two subchannels, the primary and secondary SCH. The MS first uses primary SCH to acquire slot synchronization to the strongest base station. It then uses secondary SCH to find frame synchronization, identify the code group of the found base station, and identify its scrambling code. After the scrambling code has been found, cell-specific information can be detected via the cell broadcast channel.

For packet data transmission, a dual-mode packet transmission scheme is used that can take place either on a common fixed-rate channel or on a dedicated channel. For short infrequent packets, the common packet transmission channel is used, to avoid the overhead required for maintaining the dedicated channel. For common-channel packet transmission, only open-loop power control is in operation. Dedicated-channel packet transmission is normally in operation for the transmission of a sequence of packets. A dedicated channel needs to be set up via random-access request. In this mode of operation, closed-loop power control will be used. Table 5.4 summarizes the features and characteristics of this technology.

5.3.3.3 CDMA2000. CDMA2000 is under development in TIA Subcommittee TR-45.5 (22). It is an evolution of the TIA/EIA-95B family of standards for the IMT-2000 radio transmission technology. TIA/EIA-95B is an enhanced version of the IS-95 system with higher data rate operation (e.g., up to 76.8 kbit/s for rate set 1 and 115.2 kbit/s for rate set 2). It can achieve a higher data rate by allowing a maximum of eight codes (one for fundamental channel and up to seven to supplemental channels) to a subscriber. For CDMA2000, key characteristics include coherent pilot-based reverse radio interface, fast forward and reverse power control, data rates from 1.2 kbit/s to 2 Mbit/s, support of a wide range of radio frequency channel bandwidths, and transmitter diversity.

In the CDMA2000 forward link design, two types of forward link are considered, namely, multicarrier and direct spread. For the multicarrier configura-

Table 5.4 WCDMA Features and Characteristics

Feature or characteristic	Value or description
Frame duration	10 ms
Number of time slots	16 (time slot duration= power control period)
Duplexing	FDD (outdoor), TDD (indoor)
Modulation	QPSK (downlink), BPSK (uplink)
Channel bit rate (FDD)	32×2^k kbit/s (downlink), 16×2^k kbit/s (uplink), $k = 1,10$
Channel bit rate (TDD)	512 kbit/s
Spreading factor	Variable, ranging from 4–256
Spreading bandwidth	5 MHz (10 MHz, 20 MHz available for FDD)
Chip rate	4.096 M chip/s (8.192 M chip/s, 16.384 M chip/s available for FDD)
Power control	1.6 kHz for FDD, 100 Hz for TDD
Power control step size	0.25–1.5 dB for FDD, 2 dB for TDD
Inter-BS synchronization	FDD, not required; TDD, required
Handover	MAHO (mobile-assisted handoff)
Multirate/variable-rate scheme	Variable spreading factor + multicode

tion, multiple 1.25 MHz radio frequency channels are overlaid with the multiple TIA/EIA-95B 1.25 MHz carriers to provide services to both CDMA2000 and TIA/EIA-95B mobile subscribers. For the direct spread configuration, data are spread directly over a $N \times 1.25$ MHz spectrum, where $N = 3, 6, 9$, or 12. In the CDMA IS-95 design, the reverse (uplink) link employs noncoherent demodulation using a 64-ary Walsh code. Consequently, the system suffers 2–3 dB capacity loss because of the noncoherent demodulation. In the CDMA2000 uplink design, pilot channels are used to enable coherent demodulation and thus improve uplink performance.

Transmitter diversity is employed in the downlink (forward link) to reduce the required transmitter power per channel, thus increasing forward link capacity. For the multicarrier configuration, antenna diversity is used. For the direct spread configuration, orthogonal transmit diversity (OTD) is used. For OTD, coded bits are split into two bit-streams, spread by different orthogonal codes and transmitted via separate antennas. Thus orthogonality between two data streams is maintained.

In the TIA/EIA-95B system, open-loop power control is used in the forward link. To compensate for the inaccuracies in open-loop power control, fast closed loop power control is used in the CDMA2000 on the forward link dedicated channels with 800 updates per second. Frame duration of 5 and 20 ms are supported in the CDMA2000 for control information on the fundamental and dedicated control channels. The shorter frame for the control information enables the system to react to the burst nature of the data transmission. For packet data transmission, similar to WCDMA, both dedicated channel and packet channel approaches are employed.

Table 5.5 summarizes some of the key differences between TIA/EIA-95 B and CDMA2000.

Table 5.5 IS-95 Versus CDMA-2000

Characteristic	TIA/EIA-95 B	CDMA2000
Frame duration	20 ms	20 or 5 ms
Duplexing	FDD	FDD, TDD
Uplink modulation	64 orthogonal (Walsh)	Pilot coherent
Channel bit rates	1.2–19.2 kbit/s	1.2 kbit/s to 2 Mbit/s
Spreading bandwidth	1.25 MHz	$N \times 1.25$ MHz, $N = 1, 3, 6, 9, 12$
Downlink power control	Slow open loop	800 Hz closed loop
High data rate support	Multiple codes	Variable spread
Transmitter diversity	No	Yes
Low-latency 5 ms control frame	No	Yes

5.3.4   Wireless/Mobile ATM

The development of wireless/mobile ATM is motivated by the potential effectiveness and efficiency that integrating broadband cell-based technologies with emerging wireless access may bring for the future broadband wireless multimedia services. Anticipated benefits include the use of ATM transport as the single platform to support multiple services, extension of the bandwidth-on-demand feature from the wired network to the wireless network (this is especially desirable for the wireless medium where the bandwidth is scarce), and the advent of a single transport for both data and signaling traffic. Most importantly, from the users' perspective, it could potentially offer an extension of the quality of service (QoS) from the wired broadband network to users of portable equipment, wherever they might be.

However, many incompatibilities between wireless and ATM need to be resolved before the true wireless ATM concept can be deployed. For example, ATM is designed for a fixed network with the expected bit error rates around 10^{-10}. The wireless medium typically encounters time-varying bit error rates as high as 10^{-2}, and users are not fixed. The ATM cell is designed for bandwidth-rich environments, where each cell carries a 5-byte overhead (per 53-byte cell), whereas in a wireless network extra wireless-specific headers are required for each cell. Thus, the amount of overhead per cell over the bandwidth-hungry wireless medium may not be acceptable. Another issue is the maintenance of QoS during handoff. For a wireless environment, a session may need to be handed off to another base station (which may be connected to a different ATM switch) coverage area when the received signal quality is below the system's set threshold. Determining how to reconnect the session and maintain its QoS after handoff is a major challenge. Solutions such as compressed ATM cells over the air, a new medium access control protocol, handoff rerouting algorithms, QoS negotiation, and QoS designed for the wireless medium have been proposed and published. Readers who are interested in these topics are referred to References 23 and 24.

In the industry, "wireless ATM" implies sending ATM cells or ATM-like cells over wireless links, and "mobile ATM" refers to wireless access to ATM networks. Wireless ATM is intended to provide seamless extension of ATM capabilities to wireless users. Mobile ATM is to provide a unified transport medium for both data and signaling traffic over the ATM transport, and the focus is on the design of the ATM transport to support mobility management, that is, handoff and location management.

A wireless ATM working group was formed in the ATM Forum in June 1996 to develop specifications to facilitate the use of ATM technology for a broad range of wireless network access scenarios, both private and public. The group does not focus on the designs of the radio physical layer and data link control layer. Instead, it concentrates on the network architecture alternatives and signaling protocol development. A WATM reference architecture has been developed by the WATM Working Group of the ATM Forum. The architecture supports the following configurations.

Fixed wireless access to the ATM network without mobility support. This is the simplest scenario to provide wireless access to the ATM network. In this configuration, all the network components and the end-user devices are fixed. Therefore there is no need for the ATM network to support end-user mobility. A wireless link simply provides transport between the fixed end user and the network. This scenario can provide service to fixed wireless LANs.

Wireless ATM mobile end users. In this scenario, the mobile end user communicates with the edge ATM switch called end-user mobility-enhanced ATM switch (EMAS) directly or via an access-point (AP). The EMAS supports handoff and location management. Figure 5.11 illustrates the reference architecture for this scenario. Most of the efforts in the WATM

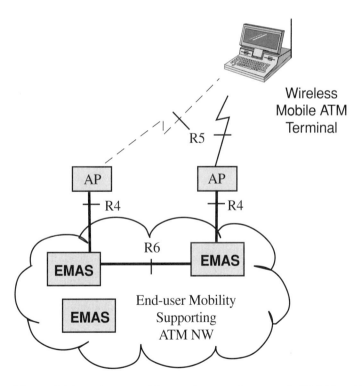

Figure 5.11 Reference architecture for network support for WATM mobile end users.

working group are devoted to this scenario. Signaling protocols to support different handoff scenarios such as intra-AP, intra-EMAS, and inter-EMAS were developed. The protocols are similar to those developed for the cellular networks except that each ATM connection is associated with an acceptable grade of QoS between the end user and the network. During handoff, the new base station receiving the handoff probably will have a user load different from that of the old base station, which negotiates the traffic contract. Therefore, to support ATM handoff, a mechanism to renegotiate the QoS parameters of an ongoing connection must be developed. The approach for location management is very similar to the one used for mobile IP, which is discussed in Section 5.3.5. Basically, all devices have two addresses, end-system ID and routing ID. In static wired systems, these addresses are the same. In mobile systems, they are different. That is, the end-system ID remains constant while the routing ID changes as the mobile device changes its network point of attachment. When the mobile moves, it informs its location server in its home network about its current point of attachment via a registration process.

Mobile switches. This scenario can support both fixed and mobile end users. In either case, the end user first establishes a connection to the mobile switch, which will then establish connections to the fixed network, either directly or via satellites. An example of the service environment for this scenario is the implementation of a wireless ATM network onboard a commercial flight.

Wireless ad hoc networks. This scenario considers that a wireless ad hoc network connects to a mobility-enhanced ATM switch directly or via an access point. A node in the ad hoc network can forward the wireless ATM packets from one wireless ATM radio to another. The service environment can be in a business conference environment where laptop PCs gather and form an ad hoc network.

PCS (personal communication services) access to the WATM network. In this scenario, the end users are PCS terminals. PCS technologies include second- and third-generation access systems. This is the only scenario in which the ATM cells are not transmitted over the air; instead, they are terminated either at the BSC or at the MSC. The mobility-supporting fixed ATM network is used to route traffic to the proper PCS BS, BSC, or MSC via an interworking function (IWF), whose major functionality is to perform protocol conversion between ATM network and the PCS network. IWF can be colocated with the BSCs or MSCs. Figure 5.12 illustrates the reference architecture of this scenario.

There are many research activities (23–25) and prototypes (26,27) in wireless ATM. Most of the research publications and all the prototype systems (e.g., a

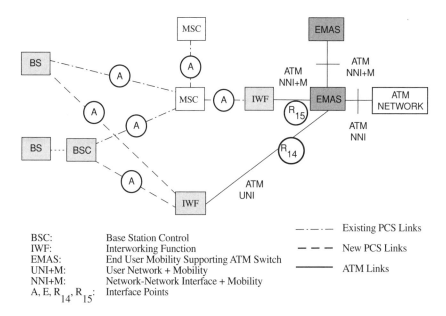

BSC: Base Station Control
IWF: Interworking Function
EMAS: End User Mobility Supporting ATM Switch
UNI+M: User Network + Mobility
NNI+M: Network-Network Interface + Mobility
A, E, R$_{14}$, R$_{15}$:   Interface Points

Figure 5.12   Reference architecture of PCS interworking with the ATM transport.

wireless LAN environment with > 2 Mbit/s information rates and limited coverage) are for the wireless customer premises network. The takeoff of the end-to-
end wireless ATM depends strongly on the success of ATM/B-ISDN in the wired
network, on spectrum availability, and on marketplace demand. Its future is uncertain, however, it can be predicted with confidence that mobile ATM or the
scenario of wireless access to the ATM transport will play a major role in the
third-generation backbone network. In fact, in Europe the third-generation Universal Mobile Telecommunications System (UMTS) overall system architecture
has been standardized to include WCDMA as the UMTS terrestrial radio access
(UTRA) technique, and ATM as the transport between UTRA network and the
edge of the core network. The architecture of the UMTS is quite similar to that
of the PCS access to the ATM transport discussed in the ATM Forum. The detailed interface design, protocol stacks, and functions of various network entities
are undergoing standardization in ETSI. The architecture of UMTS will be described in Section 5.3.5.4.

5.3.5   Wireless IP

As the number of Internet subscribers increases, the demand for wireless access for Internet applications becomes ever more apparent. Technologies to

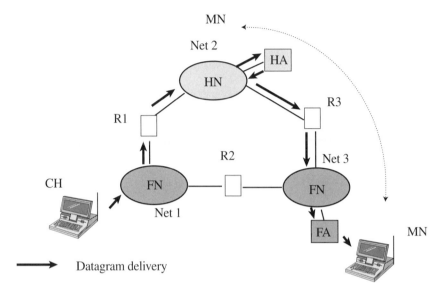

Figure 5.13   Datagram delivery on basic mobile IP.

support high-speed wireless access to the Internet are actively pursued by both industry and standards committees. Packet-based air interface developments such as CDMA2000, EDGE, and WCDMA described earlier are examples of such efforts.

Although the existing wireless data networks such as CDPD, RAM, and Metricom provide Internet services, only limited Internet applications can be offered over these networks because the systems have such low throughput (≤ 19.2 kbits/s). To provide wireless subscribers with full scope of the Internet services such as web browsing and Internet video/audio entertainment, the PCS/cellular core network architecture is migrating to packet/cell-based architecture. For wide-area wireless IP services, EDGE/IS-136 TDMA and IS-95-based CdmaOne systems have taken a similar migration path from circuit-switched architecture to packet-switched architecture. In GSM/EDGE/IS-136, the GPRS network architecture has been considered to be the core network, where the diversion of the packet traffic is handled via a packet control unit (PCU). The data packets are routed to an IP-based backbone and then to the public Internet. While in CdmaOne, the packet traffic is routed off the base station (BS) or the base station controller (BSC) via either an external or an integrated interworking function (IWF) unit. GPRS network uses PCS-like protocols for mobility management, whereas CdmaOne employs the Mobile Internetworking Protocol

(Mobile IP) originally designed for mobility management within wireless local-area networks for wireless IP services. In the rest of this section, we briefly discuss mobile IP, GPRS, CdmaOne, IP-based core networks, and UMTS networks.

5.3.5.1 Overview of Mobile IP. Mobile IP (28) specifies architectures and mechanisms to provide continuous network connectivity to mobile nodes, while providing transparent access to the "net." Mobile IP permits a mobile host to use a permanent IP address regardless of which subnetwork it attaches to. It achieves this through a packet readdressing approach, registration to the mobile agent, and encapsulation to forward datagrams to the mobile host at its current location in the network. The basic mobile IP has been standardized in the Internet Engineering Task Force (IETF) to provide IP mobility support to users (29). The IETF is the protocol engineering, development, and standardization arm of the Internet Architecture Board (IAB).

Mobile IP addresses user mobility problem in turns of a routing problem. Two mobility agents, home agent (HA) and foreign agent (FA), are introduced. A home agent is a router attached to the mobile node's (MN) home network, which

> maintains current location information for the mobile node (MN)
> intercepts datagrams destined to the MN
> encapsulates these datagrams and forwards the encapsulated IP packets to the MN while the MN is away from its home network
> performs authentication for the MN

The MN's home address identifies the mobile's home network and does not change with the location of the MN in the network. When a mobile is away from its home network, it is assigned a temporary care-of address (COA), which changes as the mobile changes its point of attachment to the network. A foreign agent is a router in an MN's visited network, it provides routing services to the MN while registered, detunnels datagrams to the MN, and may serves as default router for the registered MN. Key functions of Mobile IP are agent discovery, mobile registration, and datagram delivery.

5.3.5.1.1 Agent Discovery. A mobile station becomes aware of the mobility agents that serve it in its home and visited network by exchanging messages for agent discovery with the agents. Agent discovery messages, such as agent advertisement and agent solicitation, are extensions of the Internet Control Message Protocol (ICMP) (30) router discovery messages defined for fixed hosts in the Internet. A mobility agent transmits periodic advertisements that are broadcast or multicast to mobile stations. If a mobile station has not received agent advertisements, it can explicitly request information about the agents present in the network through agent solicitation. The mobility agents in the network that receive the solicitation reply with a unicast advertisement.

5.3.5.1.2 Mobile Registration. A home agent is made aware of the current location of the mobile stations it serves through mobile registration. Registration is required when the MN detects a change in network connectivity, when the FA serving it has rebooted, or when the lifetime for the current registration is nearing expiration. On receiving an agent advertisement, if the MN discovers that it is at home, it explicitly deregisters with its HA. The HA deletes all bindings for the MN from its mobility binding table. The MN behaves like a stationary IP node. It uses the Address Resolution Protocol (ARP), Reverse ARP (RARP), or other well-known mechanisms to make itself known to the network. If a mobile node determines that it is in a foreign network, it obtains a care-of address. The COA could be associated with the IP address of the FA or a temporary address assigned to the MN via some other means, such as by a Dynamic Host Configuration Protocol (DHCP) server. The MN then informs its home agent of its current mobility binding, which associates the home address of the mobile to its current care-of address.

5.3.5.1.3 Datagram Delivery. Datagram exchange between an MN and a host on the Internet is illustrated in Figure 5.13. When the MN is located in its home network, it sends and receives IP datagrams like an ordinary stationary IP node. When the MN is visiting a foreign network, all IP datagrams destined to the mobile station are routed through its HA. This process of routing IP datagrams through the HA is called *triangular routing*. Mobile IP packets are encapsulated within IP datagrams and tunneled between the HA and the FA. At the FA, packets are decapsulated and delivered to the MN. Datagrams originated by the MN are routed directly to the destination by means of standard IP routing. If the FA is the mobile station's default router, IP datagrams are sent to the FA, which routes them to the destination host. The HA is not involved in datagram delivery from the MN, unless an MN desires location privacy. In such a case, the MN can choose to send encapsulated IP datagrams originated by it to its HA. The HA decapsulates and delivers the packet.

Mobile IP has been discussed in the IETF and other standards committees such as the ETSI UMTS working group to evaluate its applicability to provide wide-area mobility management for the future wireless packet systems. Some of the concerns are as follows.

Agent discovery. Mobile IP relies on agent advertisement or solicitation messages to detect the MN's movement into a foreign network. These messages are network-layer messages. For wireless networks that provide routing area information or location area information in the system control channel, the agent discovery or solicitation messages are redundant and shall not be sent over the air. Consequently, when the MN performs a cellular routing area update or a location area update, the network needs to be able to perform mobile IP registration on behalf of the MN if necessary.

Registration delay. Mobile IP registration request and reply messages are carried over UDP and routed to the HA, which may be many hops away from the visited network. The delay involved in this process may not be acceptable for some real-time data services.

Authentication. The authentication of the MN is performed at the HA in the Mobile IP protocol design. This may result in significant registration delay when the MN moves from one subnet to another within the same domain of the foreign network.

Dynamic IP address versus static IP address. Mobile IP assumes that the MN has a static IP address (home address) that uniquely identifies the MN. Since IP address space is limited, it is desirable to assign the IP address to the MN dynamically. Mobile IP needs to be modified to work with dynamic home addresses.

Triangle routing. In RFC2002, the datagrams are routed to the HA and then tunneled to the foreign network. This is a very inefficient way to route packets generated from a source that is in the same foreign network as the MN. It may be more efficient to designate a temporary HA in the foreign network. When the MN moves to a different point of attachment within the foreign domain, the temporary HA remains the anchored point for registration update, authentication, and packet delivery.

Mobile IPv4 with route optimization and Mobile IPv6 could solve the concern of triangle routing and some of the security issues. However, a protocol or algorithm still needs to be developed to reduce registration delay, and to enable interworking of such functions as mobile IP signaling and radio system location management signaling, for mobile IP to support wide-area mobility. In ETSI, work on the convergence of mobile IP and a PCS mobility signaling protocol is ongoing. In the IETF, the Mobile IP working group is also addressing these problems. It is believed that mobile IP service is essential to provide future wireless voice over IP or other real-time video applications over wide areas.

5.3.5.2 GPRS (General Packet Radio Service) Network.

General packet radio service (GPRS) (31–34) is a new packet data service introduced in the GSM phase 2 standard. The system consists of the packet wireless access network and the IP-based backbone and is designed to provide access to packet data networks such as X. 25 or the public Internet. The basic GPRS wireless access network offers a payload bit rate ranging from 9 to 21.4 kbit/s (single time slot), while the enhanced GPRS wireless access technology (i.e., EDGE) will provide bit rates ranging from 8.8 to around 59.2 kbit/s. In the rest of this section, we focus on the network aspect of the GPRS system.

Figure 5.14 shows the logical architecture of GPRS. Two network entities are introduced in the original GSM architecture, they are the serving GPRS support node (SGSN) and the gateway GPRS support node (GGSN). The SGSN is

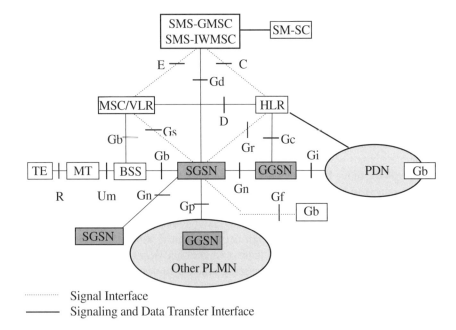

Signal Interface
Signaling and Data Transfer Interface

SMS-GMSC: Short Message Service-Gateway Mobile Switching Center
SM-SC: Short Message Service Center   IWMSC; Inter-Working MSC
PLMN: Public Land Mobile Network
TE: Terminal Equipment
MT: Mobile Terminal

Figure 5.14   GPRS logical architecture.

at the same hierarchical level as the MSC; it keeps track of individual MSs' location and performs security functions and access control. The GGSN provides interworking with external packet-switched networks and is connected with
SGSNs via an IP-based GPRS backbone network. GGSN contains the routing
information for the attached GPRS users and controls the dynamic Packet Data
Protocol (PDP) address assignment if the address is not provided by the GPRS
attached users during the PDP context activation process. The interface between
the SGSN and the MSC/VLR is to enable MSC/VLR to send voice paging messages to the SGSN and have SGSN page users who subscribe to both GPRS and
GSM services. The interface between GGSN and the HLR enables the GGSN requesting subscribe location information from the HLR if needed.
     GPRS is designed to support QoS negotiation for different service classes. A
subscriber's QoS profile includes information such as precedence (high, normal, or

low priority), delay, reliability (in terms of probability of data loss, missequence, corruption, etc.), and throughput (maximum bit rate, mean bit rate). Table 5.6 shows the specification of the delay classes defined in the current GPRS standard, where SDU is the service data unit. As can be seen from this delay specification, the current GPRS standard does not support real-time QoS. The GPRS-related standards committees are working to modify the GPRS MAC protocol and other related protocols to support real-time services such as packet voice over GPRS.

The data transmission plane used in GPRS (Figure 5.15) consists of a layered protocol structure providing user information transfer. Because GPRS is designed to support both X.25 and IP data, the GPRS backbone network is not fully optimized for IP. In the GPRS backbone, the GPRS Tunneling Protocol (GTP) is designed to support multiprotocol packets to be tunneled among GPRS support nodes, which are all IP-capable nodes. It is also used to carry GPRS signaling messages among GPRS service nodes (GSNs). As shown in Figure 5.13, IP packets that arrive at the GGSN must be encapsulated into GTP packets, then into UDP packets, and encapsulated again into IP packets for routing among GSNs. The destination GSNs must perform the reverse process to recover the IP packet. Consequently, GTP creates a certain amount of inefficiency in supporting pure IP services. Note that among the GSNs within the GPRS backbone network, Internet Protocol (IPv4 or IPv6) is used for routing user-data and control signaling.

Between the SGSN and MS, the Subnetwork-Dependent Convergence Protocol (SNDCP) is performed to map network-level characteristics onto the characteristics of the underlying network. SNDCP also provides multiplexing of multiple layer 3 messages onto a single virtual logical link connection. The logical link control (LLC) layer is above the MAC layer and provides a logical link between SGSN and MS. SNDCP layer packets, GPRS mobility management

Table 5.6 GPRS Delay Classes: Maximum Values

	Delay(s)			
	128-Octet SDU size		1024-Octet SDU size	
Delay class	Mean transfer delay	95th-Percentile delay	Mean transfer delay	95th-Percentile delay
1. (Predictive)	<0.5	<1.5	<2	<7
2. (Predictive)	<5	<25	<15	<75
3. (Predictive)	<50	<250	<75	<375
4. (Best effort)[a]	U	U	U	U

[a] U, unspecified.

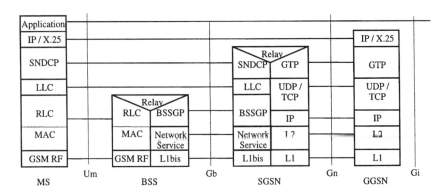

GTP   GPRS Tunnelling Protocol
SNDCP   Sub-network Dependent Convergence Protocol
BSSGP   Base Station System GPRS Protocol
LLC   Logical Link Control
RLC   Radio Link Control

Figure 5.15   GPRS data transmission plane.

signaling packets, and packets from short message services are multiplexed onto the LLC layer. In the design, LLC is independent of the underlying radio interface protocols to accommodate alternative GPRS radio solutions with minimum changes to the network subsystem. The Base Station System GPRS Protocol (BSSGP) conveys routing- and QoS-related information, which is transported by the network service (NS) layer between BSS and SGSN. Between the BSS and the MS, the radio link control (RLC) function provides a reliable radio-solution-dependent link, and the medium access control (MAC) controls the access procedures for the radio channel, respectively.

Three MS classes, A, B, and C, are defined in GPRS to serve different needs of various market segments. Class A represents the high-end MS, it can support GSM circuit calls and GPRS packet services concurrently. Class B supports GSM circuit calls and GPRS packet services sequentially; that is, class B does not support simultaneous traffic. Class-C terminals support only GPRS service. The first deployment of the GPRS network will be for the class-B terminal; in Europe, GPRS-based services will be offered in 2000 or 2001 for class-B terminal services.

There are some concerns of the role of GPRS in Europe beyond 2002. This is because GPRS promises packet data services with traffic rates from several kilobits per second (single time slot assignment) to possibly 144 kbit/s (multi–time slot assignment), which is in the low end of the UMTS service that are expected to be deployed around 2002 and 2003. However, for the UMTS system to provide continuous coverage, many base stations must be deployed. This is because UMTS offers a bit rate ranging from several hundred kilobits per second to 2 Mbit/s, and consequently the cell size will be relatively small (no more than several hundred feet) compared to the GSM or GPRS cell size (several miles) owing to its high transmission rate. Therefore, these two services will be able to coexist. Because of the cost of UMTS most probably will be deployed for islandlike coverage (picocell), while GPRS services will be used to provide wide-area packet data services. Furthermore, the enhanced GPRS backbone network has also been recommended as the core network to support the UMTS terrestrial access network (UTRAN), with WCDMA as the access technology. Hence it is expected that GPRS will be widely deployed not only to provide GSM packet data services but also to serve as the backbone for the future UMTS system in Europe.

5.3.5.3 CdmaOne Backbone Architecture.

In contrast to EDGE and GPRS, the packet-based infrastructure for CDMA2000 is not well developed. The high-level architecture is illustrated in Figure 5.16. In this architecture, circuit data traffic is routed off to the router via the MSC and interworking functions, whereas data traffic is routed off the BSC via the interworking function directly to the router. The interworking function (IWF) provides information conversion for one or more network entities. Note that two types of packet data service are supported. Type 1 packet data service provides packet data connections based on

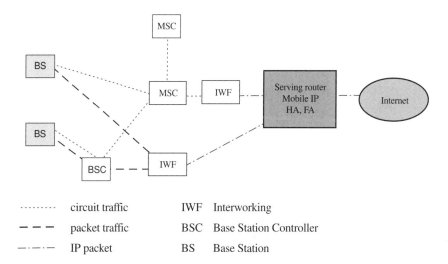

⋯⋯⋯	circuit traffic	IWF	Interworking
— — —	packet traffic	BSC	Base Station Controller
—⋅—⋅—	IP packet	BS	Base Station

Figure 5.16   Architecture of the CdmaOne/CDMA2000.

Internet and ISO standard protocol stacks, while type 2 packet data service provides packet data connection based on CDPD protocol stacks. Mobile IP is proposed to handle mobility management of type 1 packets within the wireless access network, to enable possible integration with the wired Internet services. The CdmaOne community has not yet agreed on an industry standard for the interface between the IWF and the router and its related protocol stack. As discussed in Section 5.3.5.1, the Mobile IP has its shortcomings. The CdmaOne community must develop solutions to extend this protocol to address issues such as security, efficiency, and delay.

Figure 5.17 illustrates the layer functions of CdmaOne/Cdma2000. Packet data applications are encapsulated into TCP/UDP and further into IP packets. A

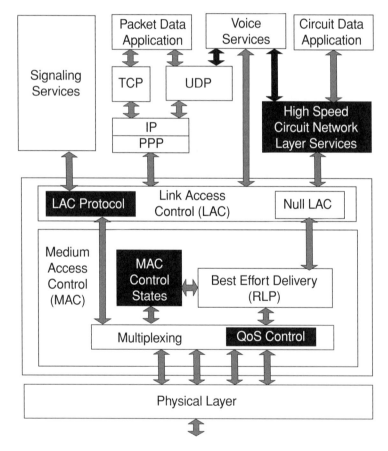

Figure 5.17 Layer functions of the CdmaOne/Cdma2000.

point-to-point link access control protocol is used to control link status and to establish links between MS and IWF. The link access control (LAC) layer manages point-to-point communications over the radio interface and provides reliable transmission of signaling control information and packet data information over the air link. To provide backward compatibility with the TIA/EIA-95-B (enhanced version of IS-95, i.e., TIA/EIA-95) protocol stack, null LAC is included as an option to support ordinary voice services. The medium access control (MAC) layer consists of functions such as MAC control states, QoS control, resource allocation between competing services and competing mobile stations, and multiplexing of information from multiple services onto available physical channels.

5.3.5.4 UMTS Network Architecture. Universal Mobile Telecommunications Systems (UMTS), the third-generation system under standardization by ETSI, is envisioned to provide efficient support for voice, data, and multimedia services. The air interface for the UMTS Terrestrial Radio Access Network (UTRAN) is WCDMA. The UTRAN consists of two major functional subnetworks, as shown in Figure 5.18. The radio access subnetwork provides interworking between the wireless access system and the wired access infrastructure. The core network provides interworking between the access subnetwork and the various core networks. Note that the architecture presented in Figure 5.18 is one of the architectures in which the GPRS core network serves as the core network for the packet data traffic. Other options for the core network are also possible. The radio network control (RNC) element provides overall management of

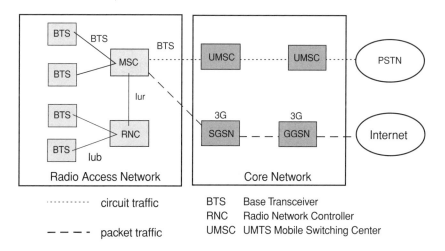

Figure 5.18 Architecture of the UMTS network.

UTRAN resources and interacts with the core network via signaling messages to provide service (circuit oriented and packet oriented) to subscribers. The RNC performs radio connection control and soft handover control. Radio connection control includes service multiplexing, link-layer QoS control, and mapping logical service channels onto WCDMA code channels.

Note that in the current phase of the UMTS standard, ATM transport is selected for the Iub, Iur, and Iu interfaces. Furthermore, the ATM adaption layer 2 (AAL2) has been selected as the preferred ATM adaptation layer for voice transmission (partially filled ATM cells are allowed for the low radio frame rate) and the ATM adaptation layer 5 (AAL5) has been selected for data transmission.

5.4   VIDEO APPLICATIONS OVER WIRELESS NETWORKS

The increase in wireless system capacity ($\leq$ 144-kbit/s for third-generation systems in a wide area), innovative low bit rate video coding techniques, as well as the standardization work in MPEG-4 have made possible interactive mobile multimedia services and applications. However, interactive real-time services such as multimedia conferencing including audio, video, and data applications, will set stringent technical challenges for the underlying systems.

It is clear that video compression techniques are crucial in making wireless video transmission feasible. In the past few years, quite a few papers (35) have been presented on the design and trade-offs on video over wireless channels. Chapter 12 of this book presents a comprehensive investigation of the performance and trade-offs of video over wireless using well-known error control mechanisms. It is clear that the "best" compression algorithm for wireless video transmission will likely be quite different from the one chosen for the present compression standards. Compression algorithms for wireless video communications need to consider the following issues that pertain to the PCS system, namely: delay, portability of the terminal (i.e., minimum computation power), and robustness to the radio channel impairments.

The conventional approach for designing a digital communications system is to optimize the source coder and channel coder separately. If the video coder is to be optimized separately from the channel coder for the wireless environments, the design of the video coder requires following features:

> Scalable video compressing rate (ranging from 10 to several hundred
> kbit/s) to be adaptive to the variations of the wireless channel quality.
> Most of the third-generation wireless systems are designed with link
> adaptation capability. That is, when the channel is of excellent quality
> (e.g., low interference, free from multipath fading, good location, etc.),
> the physical channel link rate can be adjusted to several tens of kilobits
> per second (e.g., with EDGE, around 60 kbit/s payload per time slot).

When the channel is in poor condition, the bit rate can be as low as 8.8 kbit/s. A wavelet-based video codec (36) may be a potential solution. However, the sensitivity of this type of the video coder to the adaptation delay due to wireless link variations requires further investigation.

Robustness to the transmission errors so that the loss of video synchronization of hierachical picture format or false symbol decoding can be minimized. A highly optimized video coding algorithm normally sacrifices its robustness to transmission errors. Very low bit rate coding techniques proposed elsewhere (37,38) rely on joint estimation and prediction. If the estimated objects are in error, the impact of these errors on the estimation results has not been studied.

Minimum end-to-end delay to improve the visual quality. The delay estimation of the present chosen standard includes mainly the video signal processing delay of the compression technique. For wireless transmission, extra delay is likely to result from error recovery techniques (e.g., error detection plus an automatic repeat request protocol) and privacy/authentication algorithms employed in the system. (Authentication is needed to ensure that service is not obtained fraudulently; the privacy of the communication is provided to avoid eavesdropping, since the radio channel is more susceptible to eavesdroppers than the wireline channel.) Therefore, for a given visual quality criterion, the allowable delay budgeted for the compression/decompression technique designed for wireless applications must be less than that of the wireline transmission.

Capability of handling missing frames intelligently to avoid noticeable degradation of the video quality. In a wireless system, a subscriber may move or the channel quality may deteriorate. Under these conditions, the session will be routed to a different base station. During this channel handoff process, the radio link may be momentarily interrupted. Therefore, the video codec should be designed to handle missing frames intelligently, so that appearance of jerky motion can be avoided during the handoff (typically lasting from 20 ms to several seconds).

An alternative approach is to adopt combined source coding and channel coding (39,40) in the system. The basic concept is that different features of the digital signal to be transmitted may have different error protection needs stemming from the characteristics of the source coding algorithm. For example, the coding process may result in certain bits having more "significance" than others; in that case, the more significant bits should be more heavily coded. In addition, error-correcting coding can be further made to adapt to the channel error conditions by using side information containing channel state. This technique has been adopted in the third-generation air interface design. For example, a rate-compatible punctured convolutional code has been selected in EDGE, to achieve this purpose (41).

The design of a high-quality, low-delay, low-complexity video codec for personal communications is a challenging task. Several factors influence the design, such as the multiple access scheme, or the duplexing method that is to be employed in the system. Of course, one critical point in the design is securing robustness to radio channel errors. In this chapter, we did not intend to solve the problem; instead, we considered two different approaches. For either approach, one should always bear in mind that asymmetric compression/decompression schemes that require minimum operations and circuitry at the portable are highly desirable. This results in minimum power consumption by the portable unit and leads to a successful personal communications terminal for multimedia services.

5.5 SUMMARY

Second-generation all-digital wireless access systems offer higher capacity, lower cost, and wider national/global roaming than the first-generation analog systems. The third-generation packet-based air interface design together with the packet/cell-based core network further promises potential cost-effective future wireless multimedia services. The packet-based core network will be a vital part of the future wireless network. It not only utilizes the maximum network capacity by packet multiplexing but also is compatible and interoperable with the Internet. Although the wireless channel is a very harsh environment for real-time data applications, the intelligent third-generation packet air interface and protocol designs and rate adaptation in the application will make interactive wireless multimedia services possible.

This chapter presents brief descriptions of the wireless networks ranging from wireless channel impairments to emerging/future air interface design to various wireless core networks to key design issues on video over wireless networks. The materials presented in this chapter are by no means complete. However, the intention is to provide readers with the current trends in wireless networking. We hope the information will provide readers a good start in conducting research in the area of video coding for wireless communications.

REFERENCES

1.   WC Jakes. Microwave Mobile Communications. New York: Wiley, 1974.
2.   WCY Lee. Mobile Communications Engineering. New York: McGraw-Hill, 1982.
3.   DC Cox, RP Leck. Distributions of multipath delay spread and average excess delay for 910-MHz urban mobile radio paths. IEEE Trans Antennas Propagat AP-23:206–213, March 1975.
4.   PA Bello. Characterization of randomly time-variant linear channels. IEEE Trans Commun Syst CS-11:360–393, December 1963.

5. JB Anderson, SL Lauritzen, C Thommesen. Statistics of phase derivatives in mobile communications. Proceedings of the IEEE Videotechnology Conference, May 20–22, 1986.

6. JC-I Chuang. The effects of time delay spread on portable radio communications channels with digital modulation. IEEE J Selected Areas Commun SAC 5:879–889, June 1987.

7. DC Cox, RP Leck. Correlation bandwidth and delay spread multipath propagation statistics for 910 MHz urban mobile radio channels. IEEE Trans Commun COM-23:1271–1280, November 1975.

8. DMJ Devasirvatham. Time delay spread measurements of wide-band radio signals within a building. Electron Lett 20:950–951, November 1989.

9. DMJ Devasirvatham. Time delay spread and signal level measurements of 850 MHz radio waves in building environments. IEEE Trans Antennas Propagat 34:1300–1305, November 1986.

10. SUH Qureshi. Adaptive equalization. Proc. IEEE 73:1349–1387, September 1985.

11. GL Turin, Introduction of spread-spectrum antimultipath techniques and their application to urban digital radio. Proc. IEEE 68:328–353, March 1980.

12. TS Rappaport. Wireless Communications—Principles and Practice. Englewood Cliffs, NJ: Prentice Hall, 1996.

13. DC Cox. Wireless network access for personal communications. IEEE Commun Mag 30:96–115, December 1992.

14. AR Modarressi, RA Skoog. Signaling System No. 7 (SS7): A tutorial. IEEE Commun Mag 28:19–20, 22–35, July 1990.

15. IEEE Communications Magazine. Special issue on Wireless Personal Communications. Vol 33, January 1995.

16. J Rapeli. UMTS: Targets, system concept, and standardization in a global framework. IEEE Pers Commun Mag 2(1):20–28, February 1995.

17. TR-45 proposed RTT transmission (UWC-136). TR45.3/98.04.06.07. Telecommunications Industry Association, 1998.

18. A. Furuskar et al. EDGE: Enhanced data rates for GSM and TDMA/136 evolution. IEEE Pers Commun Mag 6(3):56–66, June 1999.

19. EDGE—Evaluation of 8-PSK. ETSI SMG 2, Tdoc SMG2WPB 108/98. European Telecommunications Standards Institute, 1998.

20. Hayes. IMT-2000 radio transmission technology candidate. T1P1.1/98-081R1. American National Standards Institute.

21. F. Oversjo et al. Frames multiple access mode 2—wideband CDMA. Proceedings of the IEEE Personal, Indoor Mobile Radio Conference, Helsinki, Finland, September 1997, pp 42–46.

22. The CDMA2000 ITU-R RTT candidate submission. TR45.5/98.04.03.03. Telecommunications Industry Association, 1998.

23. IEEE Communication Magazine. Introduction to mobile and wireless ATM. vol 35, November 1997.

24. IEEE Journal on Selected Areas in Communications. Special issue on Wireless ATM. Vol 15, January 1997.

25. D Raychaudhuri, ND Wilson. ATM-based transport architecture for multiservices

wireless personal communication networks. IEEE J Selected Areas Commun 12(8):1402–1414, October 1994.

26. D Raychaudhuri et al. WatMnet: A prototype wireless ATM system for multimedia personal communications. IEEE J Selected Areas Commun 15(1):83–95, January 1997.

27. J Mikkonen, J Kryus. The magic WAND (wireless ATM network demonstrator): A wireless ATM access system. Proceedings of the ACTS Mobile Summit, 1996, pp 165–175.

28. CE Perkins. Mobile IP—Design Principles and Practices. Reading MA: Addison-Wesley, 1998.

29. CE Perkins. IP mobility support. Request for Comments 2002. Internet Engineering Task Force Network Working Group, October 1996.

30. S Deering. ICMP router discovery messages. Request for Comments 1256. Internet Engineering Task Force September 1991.

31. C Bettstetter, H Vogel, H Vogel, J Eberspacher. GSM phase 2+, general packet radio service, GPRS: Architecture, protocols, and air interface. IEEE Communications Survey. http://www.comsoc.org/pubs/surveys, third quarter, 1999.

32. G Brasche et al. Concepts, services, and protocols of the new GSM phase 2+ general packet radio service. IEEE Commun Mag 35:94–104, August 1997.

33. ETSI, GSM 03 64 v6.0.0. Digital cellular telecommunications system (phase 2+); general packet radio service (GPRS); overall description of the GPRS radio interface. European Telecommunications Standards Institute, 1998.

34. ETSI, GSM 03 60 v5.0.0. Digital cellular telecommunications system (phase 2+); general packet radio service (GPRS); service description. European Telecommunications Standards Institute, 1997.

35. N Farber, B Gilrod. Extensions of ITU-T Recommendation H.324 for error-resilient video transmission. IEEE Commun Mag 36(6):120–128, June 1998.

36. JY Tham, S Ranganath, AA Kassim. Highly scalable wavelet-based video codec for very low bit-rate environment. IEEE J Selected Areas Commun, 16(1):12–27, January 1998.

37. Y-C Li, Y-C Chen. A hybrid model-based image coding system for very low bit-rate coding. IEEE J Selected Areas Commun 16(1):28–41, January 1998.

38. S-C Han, JW Woods. Adaptive coding of moving objects for very low bit rates. IEEE J Selected Areas Commun 16(1):56–70, January 1998.

39. DJ Goodman, C-E Sundberg. Combined source and channel coding for matching the speech transmission rate to the quality of the channel. Bell Syst Tech J 62(7):2017–2036, September 1983.

40. RV Cox, J Hagenauer, N Seshadri, C-E Sundberg. A sub-band coder designed for combined source and channel coding. Proceedings of the International Conference on Accoustics, Speech, and Signal Processing, New York, April 1988, pp 235–238.

41. J Hagenauer. Rate-compatible punctured convolutional codes (RPCU codes) and their applications. IEEE Trans Commun. 36(4):389–400, April 1988.

Part 3
Systems for Video Networking

6

Error Concealment for Video Communication

Qin-Fan Zhu
*Department of Engineering, Convergent Networks, Inc.,
Lowell, Massachusetts*

Yao Wang
*Department of Electrical Engineering, Polytechnic University,
Brooklyn, New York*

6.1 INTRODUCTION

As mentioned in the preceding chapters, various channel/network errors can result
in damage to or loss of compressed video information during transmission or storage. Because very high compression has typically been applied to the compressed
bitstream, any such damage will likely lead to objectionable visual distortion in the
reconstructed signal at the decoder. Depending on many factors such as source coding, transport protocol, and the amount and type of information loss, the distortion
introduced can range from momentary degradation to a completely unusable image
or video signal. Hence it is necessary for the decoder to perform error concealment
to minimize the observed distortion through any possible means. Fortunately or unfortunately, owing to various constraints such as coding delay, implementation
complexity, and need for availability of a good source model, a compressed video
bitstream still possesses a certain degree of statistical redundancy, despite the
tremendous research effort that has been devoted to achieving the best compression
gain. In addition, the human perception system can tolerate a limited degree of signal distortion. These factors can be exploited for error concealment at the decoder.
Through error concealment, the decoded signal presented to the observer can be
made much less visually objectionable. Therefore, it is both necessary and possible
to perform error concealment at the decoder when transmission errors occur.

Error concealment belongs to the general problem of image recovery or restoration. However, because errors are incurred at the compressed bit level, the resulting error patterns in the pixel domain are very peculiar, and special measures are usually needed to handle such errors. The use of prediction and variable-length coding (VLC), although leading to high coding efficiency, makes the compressed video stream extremely sensitive to transmission errors. On the one hand, with predictive coding, the reconstruction error in a single sample will affect all the samples that are directly or indirectly predicted from it. On the other hand, the use of VLC makes it impossible to decode received bits following a single-bit error until a special synchronization codeword is encountered. To contain the error effect, various measures can be taken in the encoder to make the compressed stream more error resilient, at the expense of a certain degree of coding gain and/or complexity. A simple measure is to add synchronization codewords periodically, so that a bit error will have only limited effect. Upon detection of a synchronization codeword, the decoding process can be restored. Another measure is to limit the extent of prediction, both spatially and temporally, so that the effect of a transmission error will be confined within a small spatial/temporal segment. More substantial coverage on error-resilient coding is provided in Chapter 8. Here we assume that synchronization codewords are inserted periodically within a picture and that the prediction loop is periodically reset–for example, by means of an I frame—so that a bit error or packet loss will cause damage to only a confined region in a picture, usually several rows of macroblocks.

Depending on the frequency of synchronization codewords, transport packet size, and bit rate, a damaged region can range from part of a macroblock to an entire picture. For high bit rate transmission over small packet size as in asynchronous transfer mode (ATM), a lost packet may damage only part of a macroblock or several adjacent macroblocks. In this case, a damaged block is typically surrounded by multiple undamaged blocks in the same frame. We refer to approaches that rely on these undamaged neighbors for concealing a damaged block as error concealment techniques in the spatial domain. On the other hand, for low bit rate application over relative large packet sizes (e.g., 128 kbit/s over IP networks), the loss of a packet is likely to damage a big portion or even the entire picture. Under such situations, we have to rely on the previous video frame for concealment of the damaged image part. Techniques in this category are said to be error concealment in the temporal domain. Obviously, information from previous frames can also be incorporated even if neighboring blocks are available in the same frame. Therefore, in practice, error concealment is typically implemented as a combination of techniques of these two kinds.

We begin this chapter by describing several techniques to perform error detection, which is necessary to find out whether a transmission error has occurred and if so the position of the error. The spatial and temporal domain error concealment techniques are covered in Sections 6.3 and 6.4, respectively. As part of the temporal domain techniques, we also discuss estimation of coding modes and motion vectors. In Section 6.5, we consider the problem of certain data that are not lost but arrive at a time later than the desired decoding time. We describe a technique that can stop the propagation of reconstruction errors from previous frames immediately upon the receipt of the delayed information. Because of space limitations, we consider only methods that have been developed for video coders by means of block-based motion compensation and transform coding [discrete cosine transform (DCT)], which is the underlying core technology in all standard video codecs (1–3).

With such a coder, a video frame is divided into macroblocks, which consist of several blocks. There are typically two coding modes at the macroblock level. In the intra mode, each block is transformed by using block DCT and the DCT coefficients are quantized and coded with variable-length coding. In the inter mode, a motion vector is found which specifies its corresponding prediction macroblock in its previous frame, and the macroblock is described by this motion vector and the DCT coefficients of the prediction error blocks. For a more extensive coverage of various coding standards, readers are referred to Chapters 1 and 2.

6.2   ERROR DETECTION

Before any error concealment technique can be applied at the decoder, it is necessary to find out whether a transmission error has occurred, and if so, where. In this section, we describe the most popular and effective techniques for performing error detection, and show how these techniques are used in practical video communication systems and standards. We divide these techniques into two categories: those performed at the transport coder/decoder and those performed at the video decoder.

6.2.1   Error Detection at Transport Level

When a compressed video bitstream is transmitted from a video encoder to a decoder, a transport protocol is normally used to wrap the video bitstream to facilitate the integrity of the transmission. When the underlying network is packet-based, such as an ATM network or an IP network, a header is added to each transport packet so that error detection can be achieved. The most popular and effective way is to include a sequence number field in each packet's header field. For consecutive transmitted packets, the sequence numbers should be also consecutive when no packet loss occurs. So when the receiver finds a sequence number discontinuity between two consecutively received packets, this signals a packet loss. This method has been employed in many practical systems including the H.323 (4) and H.324 (5) systems. In H.323, the video bitstream is packetized into realtime transport protocol (RTP) packets, and the sequence number is located in the RTP header (6). In H.324, the sequence number is located in the H.223 (7) adaptation layer 3 (AL3) header.

For circuit-switched communication, error detection at the transport level is typically achieved by using forward error control (FEC) (8). In networks of this type, transmission errors usually occur as random bit errors. To detect such errors, the compressed video bitstream is typically segmented into small pieces normally called frames. Then error correction encoding is applied to each frame. At the decoder, error correction decoding is employed to detect and possibly correct some bit errors. For example, H.223 uses FEC for both the multiplex packet header and payload to detect errors in the header and payload, respectively (7). In the ITU-T H.320-based systems (9,10), the raw bitstreams coded in either H.261 or H.263 are framed with an 18-bit FEC field in each frame for error detection. As shown in Figure 6.1, the compressed video bitstream is partitioned into segments of 492 bits each. Then each segment is preceded with 1 framing bit and 1 fill bit, and followed by 18 FEC bits. The resulting group of 512 bits is normally referred to as an FEC frame. The framing bits of consecutive FEC frames have to follow a predefined pattern: 00011011. At the beginning of a communication session, operation is performed at the receiver or any intermediate network node when video processing is desired, such as in a multipoint control unit (MCU) or gateway, to search for such a pattern for at least 24 FEC frames. During the course of communication, this framing pattern is monitored in a sliding window fashion. When the pattern is broken, the FEC framing mis-

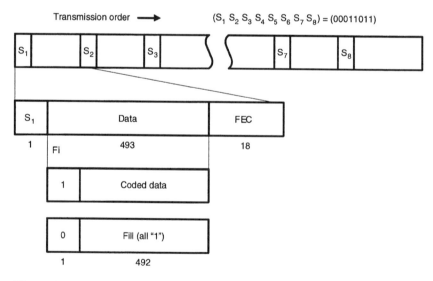

Figure 6.1 H.320 video FEC framing.

alignment is declared. If the misalignment results from bit errors for the framing bits, the decoder can automatically regain the frame alignment without performing any special error recovery operation. However, if the misalignment is caused by other problems, the FEC framing search must be performed again just as at the beginning of a communication session. The 18 FEC bits at the end of each frame can be used to assure the integrity of the video bits contained in the frame. When the decoder receives an FEC frame, the FEC is calculated from the received payload bits; if the resulting FEC is different from that at the end of the frame, the frame is declared damaged.

6.2.2   Error Detection in Video Decoder

When there is no transport level present, or transport information is not readily available, error detection can also be accomplished at the video source decoder stage. First, at the VLC decoding level, the property of VLC coding can be used as a means of detecting transmission errors. In almost all cases, the VLC being used is not a complete code; that is, not all the possible codewords are legitimate codewords. Hence once a video decoder has detected a codeword that is not in its decoding table, a transmission error is declared. For illustration, Figure 6.2 is the VLC table for the macroblock addressing (MBA) in H.261. In decoding the MBA, the following codewords are not included in the table and should be used as a means for error detection: 0000 0000 1, 0000 0000 01, 0000 0000 001, 0000 0000 0001, 0000 0000 0000 1, 0000 0000 0000 01, 0000 0000 0000 001. Second, the decoded symbols after VLC decoding can also be used

MBA	Code		MBA	Code		
1	1		17	0000	0101	10
2	011		18	0000	0101	01
3	010		19	0000	0101	00
4	0011		20	0000	0100	11
5	0010		21	0000	0100	10
6	0001	1	22	0000	0100	011
7	0001	0	23	0000	0100	010
8	0000	111	24	0000	0100	001
9	0000	110	25	0000	0100	000
10	0000	1011	26	0000	0011	111
11	0000	1010	27	0000	0011	110
12	0000	1001	28	0000	0011	101
13	0000	1000	29	0000	0011	100
14	0000	0111	30	0000	0011	011
15	0000	0110	31	0000	0011	010
16	0000	0101 11	32	0000	0011	001
			33	0000	0011	000
			MBA stuffing	0000	0001	111
			Start code	0000	0000	0000 0001

Figure 6.2   H.261 MBA addressing Huffman codes table.

for error detection. When there is no transmission error, the decoded samples should be in their valid domain according to the video coding syntax. For example, if the decoded quantization step size is outside its normal value range (1–31 for H.261 and H.263), or there are more decoded DCT coefficients than the maximum number of coefficients (e.g., 64 for an 8 × 8 DCT transform coder), a transmission error has been detected.

Finally, error detection can be accomplished in the pixel domain. The inherent characteristics of natural image signals render differences between most adjacent pixels relatively small. Hence after decoding, the difference between adjacent blocks can be computed. When a difference measure exceeds a predetermined threshold, a transmission error has been detected. This difference measure has been implemented in both the frequency and the pixel domain. For example, Mitchell and Tabatabai (11) describe the detection of damage to a single DCT coefficient by means of examining the difference between the boundary pixels in a block and its four neighbor blocks. At the decoder, four separate difference vectors are formed by taking the differences between the current block and its adjacent blocks over the 1-pixel-thick boundary in the four respective directions. Then a one-dimensional DCT is applied to these difference vectors. If any of these vectors has a dominant coefficient, it is declared, after some statistic test, that one coefficient* has been damaged. In addition, the position of the damaged coefficient is also estimated. In the approach of Leou and coworkers (12,13), the average intersample difference (AID) is computed for every block. If the AID of a block is greater than that of its neighboring blocks by a threshold, that block is declared corrupted. Note that error detection in the pixel domain requires significant processing power, since the foregoing operations must be applied to every decoded block. In practice, this method needs to be applied only to blocks declared as "questionable" by other means. The nature of VLC coding prevents the first two methods described in this section from detecting the errors immediately. For example, when a random bit error happens, the error detector at either the VLC level or the decoded symbol level may fail to detect it until several blocks after the actual error position. Hence the last method can be applied backward from the detected error position until a "good" block is reached.

Because of transmission errors, the number of decoded blocks may be different from the number of encoded blocks. Typically in video coding, synchronization codewords are inserted at certain predefined spatial locations within a picture. In H.261 and H.263, they are located at the beginnings of groups of blocks (GOBs) or slices. Often, some header information is included after each synchronization codeword such that the number of blocks between two adjacent

---

* This scheme assumes that at most one coefficient is damaged. In the event that multiple coefficients are damaged, the algorithm detects and corrects only the coefficient that has the largest error.

synchronization codewords is known to the decoder. Hence it is easy to find out whether the currently decoded segment has a wrong number of blocks. If this is the case, an error is declared and the position of the erroneous blocks can be determined in the pixel domain by using the method described in the preceding paragraph. Note that this method would not be applicable to streams coded by means of MPEG-4 because the synchronization codewords are inserted in the compressed bitstream at equally distant points in terms of the number of bits, rather than the number of blocks (14) (also see Chapter 9).

Generally, error detection at the transport level by using header information and/or FEC is more reliable and requires less processing complexity, albeit at the expense of additional channel bandwidth. As mentioned, however, in some situations there is no transport information available for error detection. Hence error detection must be fulfilled at the source decoder. In addition, such error detection does not add any overhead bits.

6.3 SPATIAL DOMAIN ERROR CONCEALMENT

As mentioned in Section 6.1, there exists significant spatial redundancy in natural image and video signals. Figure 6.3 shows the histogram of the interpixel difference between adjacent pixels for a natural scene image. The interpixel difference is defined as the average of the absolute difference between a pixel and its four neighboring pixels in both the horizontal and vertical directions. It shows clearly that for most pixels, this difference is very small. This property has been

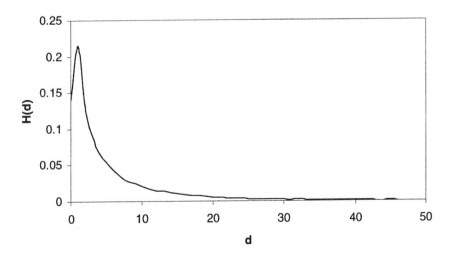

Figure 6.3 Histogram of pixel difference for a natural scene image, STUDENT.

exploited to perform error concealment. In this section, we describe several techniques to perform error concealment in the spatial domain. These techniques can be used to conceal errors in both still image and video transmission. We first present a direct interpolation method in the pixel domain. Then we show how the error concealment task can be formulated and solved through an optimization approach. Later we describe an error concealment technique based on the method of projection onto convex sets (POCS).

6.3.1 Spatial Domain Interpolation

The most straightforward way to perform error concealment is to interpolate a damaged block from its neighbor blocks, assuming they are not damaged. Aign and Fazel proposed such a method, which interpolates pixel values within a damaged macroblock from its four 1-pixel-wide boundaries (15). Two variations of this method were proposed to interpolate the pixel values. In the first variation, a damaged $2N \times 2N$ macroblock is interpolated as four separate $N \times N$ blocks. Each pixel within a block is interpolated from two pixels in its two nearest boundaries outside the damaged macroblock as shown in Figure 6.4a. Hence for a $2N \times 2N$ macroblock, the upper left $N \times N$ block is interpolated from the N pixels in the upper exterior boundary and N pixels in the left exterior boundary. The interpolation procedure can be described as follows:

$$b_1(i,k) = \frac{d_T b_{L2}(i,N) + d_L b_{T3}(N,k)}{d_L + d_T}$$

$$b_2(i,k) = \frac{d_T b_{R1}(i,1) + d_R b_{T4}(N,k)}{d_R + d_T}$$

$$b_3(i,k) = \frac{d_B b_{L4}(i,N) + d_L b_{B1}(1,k)}{d_L + d_B}$$

$$b_4(i,k) = \frac{d_B b_{R3}(i,1) + d_R b_{B2}(1,k)}{d_R + d_B}$$

$$(1)$$

where $i, k = 1, 2, \ldots, N$.

In the second variation, the whole damaged macroblock is treated as one entity (Figure 6.4b). A pixel in the macroblock is interpolated from the four macroblock boundaries as follows:

$$mb(i,k) = \frac{1}{d_L + d_R + d_T + d_B}[d_R mb_L(i,2N) + d_L mb_R(i,1) + d_B mb_T(2N,k) + d_T mb_B(1,k)]$$

where $i, k = 1, 2, \ldots, 2N$.

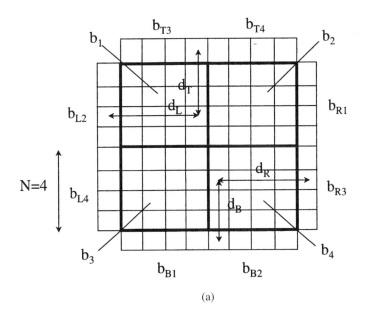

(a)

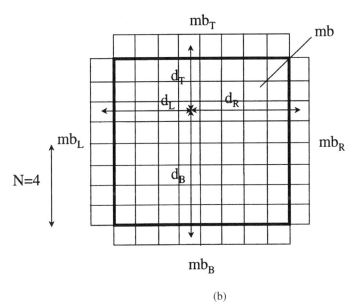

(b)

Figure 6.4 Pixel domain interpolation: (a) block-based and (b) macroblock-based.

6.3.2 Maximally Smooth Recovery

The maximally smooth recovery approach makes use of the smoothness property of most video signals through energy minimization (16). To estimate the intensity value of a damaged pixel, the method requires the difference between this value and the intensity values of its neighboring pixels to be small, so that the resulting estimated image is as smooth as possible. The method formulates the estimation problem as an optimization problem: finding the optimal estimate of the lost coefficients from the available information such that a smoothness measure is maximized (or, more precisely, a roughness measure is minimized).

Let $\tilde{\mathbf{a}}_r$ represent the subvector containing the correctly received coefficients in a damaged block, and $\hat{\mathbf{a}}_l$ be the subvector to be estimated for the lost coefficients. Further, let $\mathbf{T}_l$ and $\mathbf{T}_r$ be the submatrices composed of the basis vectors of the DCT transform corresponding to the entries of $\hat{\mathbf{a}}_l$ and $\tilde{\mathbf{a}}_r$, respectively. Then the reconstructed image block can be described by

$$\hat{\mathbf{f}} = \mathbf{T}_r \tilde{\mathbf{a}}_r + \mathbf{T}_l \hat{\mathbf{a}}_l \tag{2}$$

To determine $\hat{\mathbf{a}}_l$, we require that the reconstructed image block be as smooth as possible. This is accomplished by minimizing a smoothness measure, given by:

$$\psi(\mathbf{a}_l) = \frac{1}{2}\left[\left(\left\|\mathbf{S}_w\hat{\mathbf{f}} - \mathbf{b}_w\right\|^2 + \left\|\mathbf{S}_e\hat{\mathbf{f}} - \mathbf{b}_e\right\|^2 + \left\|\mathbf{S}_n\hat{\mathbf{f}} - \mathbf{b}_n\right\|^2 + \left\|\mathbf{S}_s\hat{\mathbf{f}} - \mathbf{b}_s\right\|^2\right)\right]$$
$$= \frac{1}{2}\left[\left(\hat{\mathbf{f}}^T\mathbf{S}\hat{\mathbf{f}} - 2\mathbf{b}^T\hat{\mathbf{f}} + c\right)\right] \tag{3}$$

The expression on the right is essentially a weighted sum of squared pixel-wise differences in different directions, minimization of which forces the pixels to be connected smoothly with each other within the block and with boundary pixels outside the block. The matrices $\mathbf{S}_w$, $\mathbf{S}_e$, $\mathbf{S}_n$, and $\mathbf{S}_s$ are used to apply the desired amount of smoothing between every two adjacent samples in the directions west, east, north, and south, respectively. The vectors $\mathbf{b}_w$, $\mathbf{b}_e$, $\mathbf{b}_n$, and $\mathbf{b}_s$ are composed of the pixels on the 1-pixel-wide boundaries outside the block in these four directions. Figure 6.5 shows two examples of how the spatial smoothness measure is formed for an 8×8 block. An arrow indicates that a pixel difference is included between the two pixels. In Figure 6.5a the smoothing constraint is applied only along the block boundary. It has been found that if only the DC coefficient is lost, applying smoothing along the boundary alone can yield satisfactory results. Figure 6.5b shows a stronger smoothing constraint, which is effective for all loss cases including the case when only the DC is lost. Note that the second smoothness measure requires not only that the pixels along the boundary of the damaged block be smoothly connected to the neighboring blocks, but also that the pixels within the recovered block be smoothly connected to each other. In addition, this interior smoothness constraint is formulated such that information

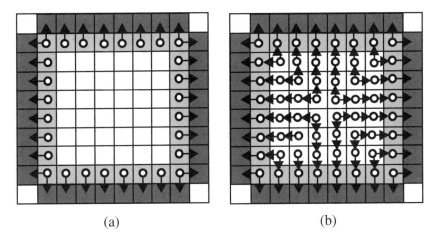

(a)   (b)

Figure 6.5 Illustration of two smoothing constraints. (Figure 1 in Ref. 16. ©1993 IEEE.)

from four neighboring blocks can be effectively propagated into the triangle within the damaged blocks. Another smoothness measure can be constructed, which has four arrows connecting each pixel within the damaged block to its four neighboring pixels. It was found that this pattern will oversmooth the interior of the recovered block and that it lacks the directional smoothness advantage of that shown in Figure 6.5b. The optimal solution $\hat{a}_{opt}$, which minimizes the smoothness measure in Eq. (5), is given by:

$$\hat{a}_{opt} = \left(\tilde{T}^r \, S\tilde{T}_t \right)^{-1} \tilde{T}_t^r \left[\mathbf{b} - \, S\tilde{T}_r \tilde{a}_r \right] \tag{4}$$

Note that the solution above essentially consists of two linear interpolations in the spatial and frequency domains from the boundary vector **b** and the received coefficient subvector $\tilde{a}_r$, respectively. It can maintain the information from the received coefficients, while enforcing the reconstructed image to be as smooth as possible. When all the coefficients are lost in a damaged block, the solution reduces to spatial interpolation only.

In the foregoing work, the first-order smoothness criterion was employed to reconstruct a lost block. Second-order smoothness criteria have also been investigated (17). A combined quadratic variation and Laplacian operator can reduce the blurring across strong edges, which cannot be well recovered with the first-order smoothness measure. The images reconstructed by using this second-order measure are visually more pleasing than those obtained with the first-order measure presented here, with sharper edges that are smooth along the edge directions. To further improve the reconstruction quality, an edge-adaptive smoothness measure can be used, so that variation is minimized along the edges but not across the edges. Several techniques have been developed along these lines (18). This approach requires the detection of edge directions for the damaged blocks. This is a difficult task, and a mistake can yield noticeable artifacts in the reconstructed images. The method using the second-order smoothness measure is in general more robust and can yield satisfactory images at lower computational cost.

6.3.3 Projection onto Convex Sets Method

The projection onto convex sets (POCS) algorithm has been studied for various image recovery and restoration problems. In this method, appropriate convex sets and their associated projections are first identified and defined. Then an iterative projection operation is applied to the convex sets, and the POCS algorithm guarantees that this iterative process eventually converges to a point in the intersection set of all the convex sets. This convergence point is the final solution for the signal to be recovered or restored.

This method was proposed by Sun and Kwok to restore a damaged image block in a block transform coder (19). The convex sets are derived by requiring a recovered block to have a limited bandwidth either isotropically (for a block in a smooth region) or along a particular direction (for a block containing a straight edge). With this method, a combined block is formed by including eight neighboring blocks with the damaged block. First, the Sobel operator is used to apply an edge existence test to this combined block. The block is classified either as a monotone block (i.e., with no discernible edge orientations) or as an edge block. The edge orientation is quantized into one of the eight directions, equally spaced in the range of 0 to 180°. Then two projection operators are applied to the combined block, as shown in Figure 6.6. The first projection operator implements a band-limitedness constraint, which depends on the edge classifier output. If the block is a monotone block, the block is subjected to an isotropic band-limitedness constraint, accomplished by an isotropic low-pass filter. On the other hand, if the block classifier output is one of the eight edge directions, a band-pass filter is applied along that direction. The filtering operation is implemented in the Fourier transform domain. The second projection operator implements a range constraint and truncates the output value from the first operator to the range of [0,255]. The values of pixels in the edge blocks that are correctly received are maintained.

The two projection operations just described are applied alternatively until the block does not change any more under further projections. It is found that 5–10 iterations usually suffices when a good initial estimate is available. Figure 6.7 shows peak signal-to-noise ratio (PSNR) curves for a video sequence called

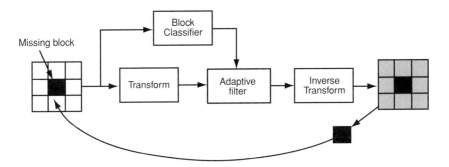

Figure 6.6 Adaptive POCS iterative restoration process. (Figure 6 in Ref. 19. ©1995 IEEE.)

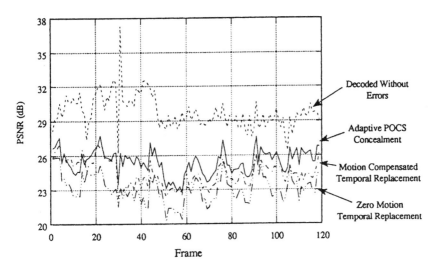

Figure 6.7 PSNR comparison on the sequence BASKETBALL. (Figure 10 in Ref. 18. ©1995 IEEE.)

BASKETBALL reconstructed with this scheme, a method using motion-compensated temporal replacement, and a copying algorithm, respectively. The latter two methods are described in the next section.

6.3.4 Bitstream Domain Error Correction

In the techniques described thus far in this section, it has been assumed either that a block is completely damaged or that the positions of the damaged coefficients are known. The first assumption is true if the transport level discards an entire "questionable" data unit instead of passing it to the video decoder. The second assumption is true if the quantized DCT coefficients from an image block are partitioned into multiple bands and are transported within different data units. However, in many practical video transmission systems, neither of these assumptions holds. The video decoder may receive a damaged transport data unit where error detection can be accomplished at either transport or source coder level, as mentioned in Section 6.2. Under such conditions, if the transmission error is caused by a few bit errors, there are better ways to conceal the corrupted blocks. For example, the pixel domain error detection method can be used to identify the first "real" corrupted block. Then a sequence of bit inversions can be performed and the bitstream from the corrupted block to the next synchronization codeword can be redecoded (12). The result of each iteration is measured by a smoothness measure similar to that shown in Figure 6.5. Note that in this method, if the transmission error is caused by a single bit error, a lossless recovery can be potentially obtained.* On the other hand, the computational complexity of this method increases exponentially with the number of bit errors to be corrected. Because the number of bits in error is typically unknown when a transmission error is detected, this method can work only when the number of error bits is below a predetermined threshold.

6.4 TEMPORAL DOMAIN ERROR CONCEALMENT

In Section 6.3 we presented error concealment techniques that exploit the spatial smoothness property of natural image/video signals. For video signal, there exists significant statistical redundancy between adjacent video frames in the temporal domain in additional to the redundancy within each frame in the spatial domain. This redundancy has been exploited in the design of video compression systems. By the same token, this redundancy can also be used in error concealment for video transmission. In this section, we describe several techniques in this category.

6.4.1 Motion-Compensated Prediction/Interpolation

One simple way to exploit the temporal correlation in video signals is by replacing a damaged macroblock by the spatially corresponding macroblock in the previous frame. This method is widely referred to as the copying algorithm. Although this method is very simple to implement, it can produce adverse vi-

---

* By lossless error recovery, we mean that when the damaged block is recovered, it is exactly the same as the decoded block, subject to only quantization errors.

sual artifacts in the presence of gross motion. Significant improvement can be obtained by replacing the damaged macroblock with the motion-compensated block (i.e., the block specified by the motion vector of the damaged block). Because of its simplicity, this method has been widely used. In fact, the MPEG-2 standard allows the encoder to send the motion vectors for intra-coded macroblocks, so that these blocks can be recovered better if they are damaged during transmission. It has been found that the use of motion-compensated error concealment can improve the PSNR of reconstructed frames by 1 dB at a cell loss rate of 10^{-2} for MPEG-2-coded video (20). This approach, however requires knowledge of the motion information, which is not available in all circumstances. When the motion vectors are also damaged, they need to be estimated from the motion vectors of the surrounding macroblocks, and incorrect estimates of motion vectors can lead to large errors in reconstructed images. Another problem with this approach occurs when intra mode was used to code the original macroblock and the coding mode information is damaged. Then concealment with this method can lead to catastrophic results in situations such as a scene change. Recovery of motion vectors and coding modes is discussed in Section 6.4.7.

A more sophisticated and complex motion-compensated prediction was proposed in 1998 by Chu and Leou (13). For each damaged block, the following candidate concealment blocks are first found from spatially neighboring blocks that are undamaged or had been concealed:

1. The motion-compensated blocks obtained with the motion vectors of its neighboring blocks
2. The motion-compensated blocks obtained with the average or median of the motion vectors of its neighboring blocks
3. The average and median of the blocks obtained in set 1.
4. All its undamaged/concealed neighboring blocks
5. The average and median blocks of the blocks obtained in set 4.

Then for each candidate block, a measure of the smoothness within this candidate block, and between this block and its spatial and temporal neighbors, is evaluated. The candidate block with the smallest error function (i.e., most smooth) is selected as the concealment block.

Up to this point, we have assumed that only past frames are available for concealment of damaged blocks in the current frame. When processing delay is not a stringent parameter in the underlying application, motion-compensated interpolation can also be used for error concealment. In this case, both past and future frames can be used for interpolating a damaged block. Because more neighboring information is available, the performance of the interpolation method is expected to be better than that obtained with prediction only.

6.4.2   Spatial–Temporal Smoothing

We now extend the smoothing technique presented in Section 6.3.2 for application to video transmission (21). In addition to requiring that a concealed block be smoothly connected to its spatial neighbors, we attempt to make the concealed block similar to its motion-compensated temporal neighbor. To achieve this, we extend our smoothness measure to include both spatial differences and temporal differences. Let f_p be the vector consisting of pixels in the motion-compensated block (this vector is set to zero for an intra-coded block). Then the reconstructed prediction error and the original image block can be described by:

$$\hat{e} = T_r \tilde{a}_r + T_l \hat{a} \quad \text{and} \quad \hat{f} = \hat{e} + f_p \tag{5}$$

The smoothness measure is given by:

$$\psi(a_l) = \frac{1}{2}\left[w\left(\hat{f}^t \hat{S} \hat{f} - 2 \hat{b}^t \hat{f} + c \right) + (1-w)\hat{e}^t\hat{e} \right] \tag{6}$$

The first term is the same as that in the still image case, and the second term is the energy of the error vector, minimization of which enforces a smooth transition between corresponding regions in adjacent frames. The weighting factor w controls the relative contribution of the spatial and temporal smoothing constraints and is chosen according to the expected degrees of spatial and temporal smoothness in the damaged block. This information can be derived from the coding mode (intra/inter, motion compensation or not, etc.) and other available information. For intra-coded blocks, a larger w should be used to emphasize the spatial smoothness constraint. On the other hand, for blocks coded in the motion-compensated mode, a smaller w should be used to emphasize the temporal smoothing. When $w \neq 0$, the optimal solution $\hat{a}_{opt}$ is given by:

$$\hat{a}_{opt} = \left(\frac{1-w}{w} I + T_l^t S T_l \right)^{-1} T_l^t \left[b - S f_p - \left(S - \frac{1-w}{w} I \right) T_r \tilde{a}_r \right] \tag{7}$$

Note that the solution above essentially consists of three linear interpolations, in the spatial, temporal, and frequency domains, from the boundary vector **b,** the prediction block $\mathbf{f}_p$, and the received coefficient subvector $\tilde{a}_r$, respectively. It can maintain the information from the received coefficients, while enforcing the requirement that the reconstructed image be as smooth as possible. When all the coefficients are lost in a damaged block, the solution reduces to spatial and temporal interpolation only. When $w = 0$, the optimal solution reduces to that of the motion-compensated prediction method described in Section 6.4.1. On the other hand, with w set to 1, only spatial correlation is used, as in the method of Section 6.3.2. Figure 6.8 shows the PSNR curves for video sequences reconstructed from the foregoing smoothing technique and the copying algorithm.

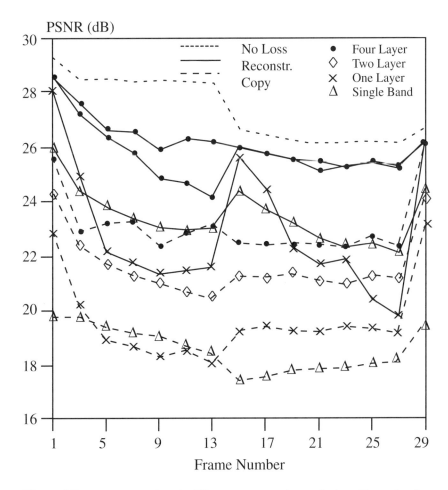

Figure 6.8 PSNR comparison for different reconstruction methods and layered coding. (Figure 7 in Ref. 21. ©1993 IEEE.)

6.4.3 Temporal Estimation of Blocks with Missing Motion Vectors

In Sections 6.4.1 and 6.4.2 we assumed that the motion vector of a damaged block either is available or can be estimated by using the motion vectors from the neighboring blocks. Now we describe a technique that estimates a damaged block directly without estimating the motion vector (22). Because motion vectors are estimated over quite large macroblocks (16×16 for most video coding standards and algorithms), motion vectors of adjacent macroblocks may not produce a reliable estimate for the missing motion vector of the damaged block. To overcome this problem, we consider four 8 × 8 blocks in the macroblocks adjacent to the damaged macroblock, shown in Figure 6.9a as $u1$, $u2$, $l1$, and $l2$, are considered. First, for each of these blocks, a motion vector is estimated and its corresponding 8 × 8 block in the previous frame is determined. The motion vector is found by means of an exhaustive search in an area equal to the size of a macroblock around the center of its motion-compensated block in the previous frame. For each corresponding block identified, a surrounding macroblock is determined, labeled **U1, U2, L1,** and **L2** (cf. Figure 6.9b). The final estimated macroblock is a weighted average of these macroblocks:

$$\hat{p} = w_{u1}\mathbf{U1} + w_{u2}\mathbf{U2} + w_{l1}\mathbf{L1} + w_{l2}\mathbf{L2} \tag{8}$$

The weights w_{u1}, w_{u2}, w_{l1}, and w_{l2} are chosen so that the sum of the squares of interpixel differences along the left and upper boundaries of the macroblock is minimized.

The solution by the foregoing method can lead to visible blockiness along the boundaries of the concealed macroblock. To enhance the algorithm, the boundary smoothness measure can be modified to be a weighted sum of the original squared error and the number of boundary pixels whose interpixel difference is greater than a threshold. The main idea behind this scheme is to preserve image continuity inside the macroblock and across the macroblock boundaries. Al-

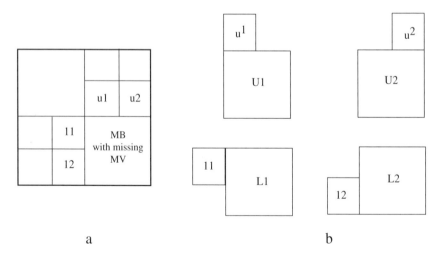

a   b

Figure 6.9 (a)Macroblock with missing motion vector and its surrounding blocks. (b) Motion-compensated macroblocks corresponding to each of the 8 × 8 blocks (Figure 1 in Ref. 22. ©1998 IEEE.)

though this method does not require the estimation of the missing motion vector from that of the adjacent macroblocks, motion estimation for the four 8×8 blocks involves very high implementation complexity.

A similar method is proposed to conceal a damaged block with overlapped-block motion compensation (OBMC) (23), which was introduced in video coding to reduce the blocking effect. In this method, the motion vector is first estimated using the so-called side match distortion (SMD), which is basically the same as the smoothness measure shown in Figure 6.5a. The difference is that SMD uses the absolute difference between adjacent pixels, whereas the smoothness measure uses the square between adjacent pixels. The estimated motion vector is chosen such that the resulting motion-compensated block possesses the minimum SMD. Then the damaged $N \times N$ block is divided into four $N/2 \times N/2$ subblocks. Each subblock is synthesized by a weighted average of three predicted subblocks: one according to the estimated motion vector, the second according to the motion vector of the horizontally neighboring $N \times N$ block, and the third according to the motion vector of the vertically neighboring $N \times N$ block.

Figure 6.10 shows the position of the selection of motion vectors for the four subblocks. The weighting matrices used for the OBMC are the same as those used in H.263 Annex F (2). Figure 6.11 compares PSNR performance for three different error concealment methods. The first method, which is referred to as temporal extrapolation, is the same as the copying algorithm. The second method, labeled "side match," is the motion compensation prediction method with the motion vectors estimated by minimizing the SMD as mentioned above. The curve labeled "Proposed" is the one in which OBMC was used. It can be seen that the OBMC method produces the best performance.

6.4.4 Using Motion Field Interpolation for Error Concealment

Instead of using one motion vector for coding of an entire image block, motion field interpolation (MFI) (also known as mesh-based motion estimation) uses different motion vectors for each pixel to model nontranslational motion such as rotation and scaling. The motion vector for each pixel is interpolated from the motion vectors at several control points, and then motion compensation is applied to each pixel separately. This technique can be used for error concealment where the motion vectors from adjacent blocks are used as the control point motion vectors (24). A bilinear MFI (BMFI) is performed as follows:

$$V(x,y) = \frac{(1-x_n)V_{\mathbf{L}} + x_n V_{\mathbf{R}} + (1-y_n)V_{\mathbf{T}} + y_n V_{\mathbf{B}}}{2}$$

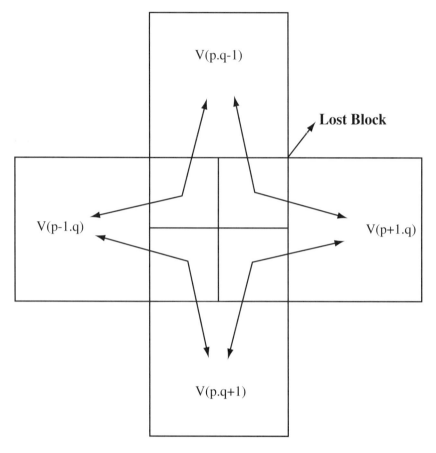

Figure 6.10   Selection of motion vectors for overlapped motion compensation (Figure 1 in Ref. 23. ©1997 IEEE.)

where $\mathbf{V}_L$, $\mathbf{V}_R$, $\mathbf{V}_T$, and $\mathbf{V}_B$ are the motion vectors of the blocks to the left, to the right, above, and below the current block, and x_n and y_n are defined as follows:

$$x_n = \frac{x - x_L}{x_R - x_L} \quad \text{and} \quad y_n = \frac{y - y_T}{y_B - y_T}$$

where x_L and x_R, are the x coordinates of the left and right borders, and y_B and y_T are the y coordinates of the bottom and top borders of the current block, respectively.

Because the motion field is not stationary, the method above may cause severe degradation when the motion within the damage block is purely transla-

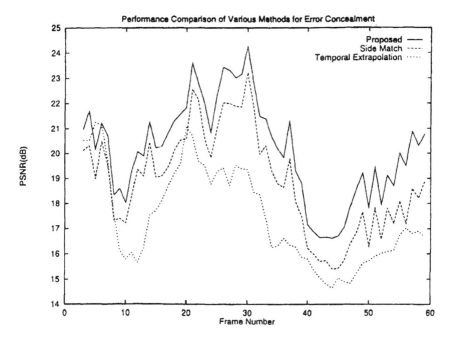

Figure 6.11   PSNR comparison of three error concealment methods (Table tennis at 10 f/s). (Figure 4 in Ref. 23. ©1997 IEEE.)

tional. To mitigate this effect, Al-Mualla et al. have proposed (24) the use of the average of the foregoing method and motion-compensated prediction as described in Section 6.4.1. Figure 6.12 shows the PSNR curves for several algorithms at different block loss rates for the FOREMAN sequence. In the figure, TR stands for temporal replacement, which is the same as the copying algorithm. AV stands for average vector, which uses a motion vector that is the average of the motion vectors from surrounding blocks to perform motion-compensated prediction. The curve labeled with BMSMD (boundary match side match distortion) represents the motion-compensated prediction method by means of motion vectors with the minimum SMD mentioned in Section 6.4.3. It shows that the combined method, which uses the average of the MFI and motion-compensated prediction as the error concealment for a damaged block, outperforms all the other methods at different block loss rates.

6.4.5   Error Concealment for Layered Coding

Layered coding, which is the topic of the next chapter, has been proposed for achieving both transmission scalability and error resilience, among other

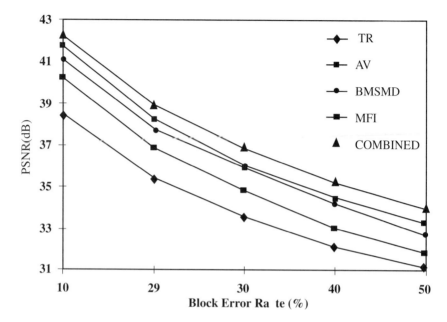

Figure 6.12 Comparison among different algorithms (Figure 1 in Ref. 24.)

objectives. When used for the purpose of error resilience, the more important information, such as the coding mode, motion vectors, and low-frequency DCT coefficients, is transported with a higher degree of error protection, and the less important information, such as the high-frequency DCT coefficients, is transported with less error protection. When the high-frequency coefficients are lost, they are typically set to zero and normal decoding is performed. Hence as long as the base layer is not damaged, a reconstructed signal with reduced quality will be obtained. Instead of simply setting the high-frequency components to zero, Kieu and Ngan showed that using the high-frequency component from the motion-compensated macroblock in the previous frame can improve the reconstructed picture quality (25). It is assumed that the base layer is delivered without error. When the enhancement layer is damaged, for each damaged macroblock, its motion-compensated macroblock is formed and the DCT is applied to the blocks within the macroblock. The resulting high-frequency DCT coefficients are then merged with the base layer DCT coefficients of the damaged blocks in the current frame and the inverse DCT is applied to the combined blocks to form an error-concealed macroblock.

6.4.6   Multiframe-Based Error Concealment

The techniques presented thus far in this section conceal damaged blocks from only one preceding frame. In addition, the use of motion compensation causes errors produced during concealment of a block to still propagate into the following frames. Now we consider error concealment achieved by employing information from multiple frames.

First, information from multiple frames preceding the current frame can be used for error concealment. For example, when the previous frame is itself seriously damaged, a damaged block in the current frame can be concealed by using the frame preceding the last frame. Vetro et al. (26) assume that the motion is uniform from frame to frame, and they multiply the motion vector or the estimated motion vector of the damaged MB in the current frame by 2 to obtain the motion-compensated concealment block from the frame preceding the last frame. Their result (26) shows that significant improvement can be obtained when seriously damaged frames are not used for error concealment in their following frames. In fact, multiple frames can be stored at the decoder for error concealment. When a block is lost, its trace (i.e., motion trajectory) can be estimated from the past motion vectors and a more accurate estimate of the damaged block can be obtained by using the estimated motion trace.

Yu et al. (27) extended the use of multiple frames, as well as an overlapped block transform, for error concealment. Instead of using the typical nonoverlap transform, this scheme relies on an overlapping block transform, where 9×9 blocks are used for DCT with one pixel overlapping along the edges. The overlapping coding structure permits the use of multiple frame buffers to generate the relationship between pixels in a damaged frame. This relationship is used to form a convex set. Together with the other two convex sets, the standard POCS operations are applied. Very good simulation results were presented (27). We do not describe this method in more detail here because it cannot be applied to a typical video coder by means of a nonoverlapping transform. In addition, in this scheme, intentional concealment redundancy has been injected in the source coding stage to improve the performance of error concealment when a transmission error occurs. This technique falls into a more general category of error concealment techniques called forward error concealment, described elsewhere (28).

6.4.7   Recovery of Motion Vectors and Coding Modes

In the techniques described so far, we have assumed that the coding mode and motion vectors are correctly received. If the coding mode and motion vectors are also damaged, they must be estimated. Based on the same assumption about spatial and temporal smoothness, the coding mode and motion vectors can be similarly interpolated from those in spatially and temporally adjacent blocks.

The coding mode for a macroblock can take three different values in a video coder. The first mode is intra, which does not use any temporal prediction for coding a macroblock. This is used for all macroblocks in an intra-coded frame (normally referred to as an I- frame). It can be also used for coding macroblocks in an inter-coded frame when no close match is found in the previous frame for motion-compensated prediction. In the second mode, which is normally referred to as skipped, the decoder simply copies the corresponding macroblock (equivalent to have a zero motion vector) in the previous frame. In the third mode, a nonzero motion vector is transmitted to enable motion compensation in the decoder.

There are several ways to estimate the coding mode. The simplest way is to always use intra mode and estimate the DCT coefficients of the damaged block (21). This method can prevent any catastrophic effect when a wrong coding mode is used. Consider a block that is coded in the intra mode because of a scene change. If we use its corresponding block in the previous frame as an estimate, the result will be completely wrong. However, such a method is in general overly conservative. Because temporal prediction is predominantly used in video coding, a better technique is to interpolate the coding mode of a damaged macroblock from that of the adjacent blocks. Figure 6.13 shows a simple scheme for estimating coding mode for MPEG2 (29). For example, for an MB in a B frame, if the MB above has a mode "Forw" (i.e., using forward motion estimation), and the MB below has a mode "Back" (i.e., using backward motion estimation), the

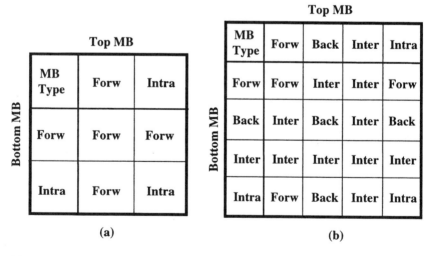

(a)   (b)

Figure 6.13   Estimation of coding mode for MPEG-2: (a) P frame and (b) B frame (from Ref. 29. ©1993 IEEE.)

estimated mode of this MB is "Inter." In a more sophisticated scheme proposed for H.263 (30), the missing coding mode COD_p of a damaged block is estimated from the coding mode cod_i (i = 1, . . . , 8) of its eight surrounding macroblocks as follows:

$$COD_p = \begin{cases} 1 & \text{if } \sum_{i=1}^{8} cod_i \geq 5 \\ 0 & \text{else} \end{cases}$$

where cod_i is preset to 0.5 if the corresponding macroblock itself is damaged, or to 1 otherwise. When the resulting COD_p is 1, the estimated coding mode is uncoded and the damaged macroblock is concealed by the copying algorithm. When the resulting COD_p is 0, the estimated coding mode is further refined as follows: if two of the surrounding macroblocks are coded as intra, the estimated coding mode is intra. Otherwise, the coding mode is motion-compensated prediction.

For estimating lost motion vectors, the following methods have been proposed: (a) simply setting the motion vectors to zero, which works well for video sequences with relatively small motion, (b) using the motion vectors of the corresponding block in the previous frame, (c) using the average of the motion vectors from spatially adjacent blocks, and (d) using the median of motion vectors from the spatially adjacent blocks (31). Typically, when a macroblock is damaged, its horizontally adjacent macroblocks are also damaged; hence the average or mean is taken over the motion vectors above and below. It has been found that the last method produces the best reconstruction results (31,32). Another method (33) goes one step further. It essentially selects among the four methods above, depending on which one yields the least boundary matching error. This error is defined as the sum of the variations along the one-pixel-wide boundary between the recovered macroblock and the one above it, to its left, and below it, respectively. It is assumed that these neighboring macroblocks were reconstructed previously, and for the damaged macroblock, only the motion vector is missing. In the event that the prediction error for this macroblock is also lost, then for each candidate motion vector, the boundary matching error is calculated by assuming that the prediction error of the damaged macroblock is the same as the top macroblock, the left one, the one below, or zero. The combination of motion vector and prediction error that yields the smallest boundary matching error is the final solution. It was shown that this method yields better visual reconstruction quality than the four earlier methods.

6.5 ERROR RECOVERY WITH OUT-OF-ORDER DECODING

In Sections 6.3 and 6.4 we described techniques that conceal damaged image blocks by using the smoothness property of natural images/video signals. In this section, we present a technique that is motivated by a different consideration. It attempts to exploit information that is normally discarded by a receiver to achieve lossless error recovery.* In packet video, to keep the end-to-end delay under a preset value, packets with delay that is beyond the dejitter-buffering time will normally be discarded at a video decoder. This excessive delay may have resulted from traffic congestion in the network and/or retransmission time when retransmission is applied for recovering lost or damaged video data. In fact, the additional delay introduced by retransmission has been the main reason that most real-time applications do not consider retransmission to be a means for error recovery. The technique presented in this section was developed for overcoming the foregoing problems (34,35).

With this technique, we still decode video packets that arrive at the receiver out of the order, and merge the newly decoded information with a previously decoded but corrupted video sequence, so that lossless recovery is achieved. Figure 6.14 illustrates the idea with a simple one-dimensional signal. Assume that the original signal is coded with a simple predictor, which uses the previous sample as the prediction for the current sample. Let f_i and Δf_i be the reconstructed and prediction error values at time i. Then $f_i = f_{i-1} + \Delta f_i = f_1 + \Sigma_{j=2}^{i} \Delta f_j$. So when Δf_3 arrives at the receiver later than its allocated time, we use an error-concealed value $\hat{f_3} = f_2 + \Delta \hat{f_3}$ as the replacement of the decoded value for presentation. Because of error propagation due to predictive coding, all subsequent samples will have an error of $\Delta \hat{f_3} - \Delta f_3$ if Δf_3 is not used when it arrives at sample time 5. On the other hand, if we use Δf_3 after it has arrived at the decoder at sample time 5 and correct the decoded value $\hat{f_5}$ by adding $\Delta f_3 - \Delta \hat{f_3}$ into $\hat{f_5}$, we will reproduce the same f_5 as if Δf_3 had been correctly received at time 3. From this point on, all sample values will be identical to those encoded at the encoder, hence a lossless recovery is achieved.

The idea above can be applied to video coding because motion-compensated prediction is a linear operator at the picture level. This can be proved as follows: arrange an image as a one-dimensional vector and construct the prediction vector of the current frame as the multiplication of a prediction matrix and the previous frame vector. Let $\mathbf{z}_r$ be a vector consisting of reconstructed values of all pixels in frame r, and $\mathbf{P}_r$ represent the predictor at time r, which depends on the motion vectors of the current frame. The predicted vector at time r based on the reconstructed vector at time $r - 1$ can be written as $\mathbf{P}_r(\mathbf{z}_{r-1}) = \mathbf{P}_r \mathbf{z}_{r-1}$. The elements in each row of the prediction matrix $\mathbf{P}_r$ are determined by the coding mode and the motion vectors of the corresponding pixel. For example, if a pixel is inter-coded without motion compensation, the diagonal element will be 1 and the remaining elements in that row will be 0. If a pixel is coded with motion-com-

---

* See the footnote on loss/less error recovery in Section 6.3.4.

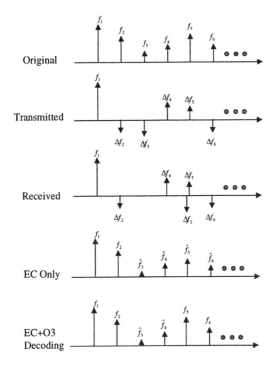

Figure 6.14   Illustration of one-dimensional out-of-order (O3) decoding for error concealment.

pensated prediction, the positions and values of the nonzero elements in that row will be determined by the motion vector. If the motion vector is an integer, only one entry has a nonzero value (being 1) in each row. On the other hand, if the motion vector is fractional, several entries are nonzero, with values equal to the bilinear interpolation coefficients. Although the following derivation is done only for first-order predictors, it also holds for predictors with order greater than 1.

Let $\mathbf{y}_r$ be a vector consisting of prediction errors of all pixels in frame r. Without transmission errors, the output at sample time r is:

$$\mathbf{z}_r = \mathbf{y}_r + \mathbf{P}_r(\mathbf{z}_{r-1}) \tag{9}$$

where $\mathbf{z}_{r-1}$ is the decoded vector at sample time $r-1$. The linearity of the predictor means that $\mathbf{P}_r(\mathbf{z}_1 + \mathbf{z}_2) = \mathbf{P}_r(\mathbf{z}_1) + \mathbf{P}_r(\mathbf{z}_2)$. Assume that the reconstructed vector is correct up to time $r-1$ and that, at time r, transmission errors cause damage in either the prediction error vector or the motion vectors (consequently $\mathbf{P}_r$). Let $\hat{\mathbf{y}}_r$ and $\hat{\mathbf{P}}_r$ be the concealment vector and predictor used. Then the concealed output at sample time r is:

$$\hat{\mathbf{z}}_r = \hat{\mathbf{y}}_r + \hat{\mathbf{P}}_r(\mathbf{z}_{r-1}) \tag{10}$$

Let d be the delay in sample time between the data damage and retransmission arrival. Then from sample time $r + 1$ to $r + d$, reconstructed outputs at the decoder will be:

$$\hat{\mathbf{z}}_{r+1} = \mathbf{y}_{r+1} + \mathbf{P}_{r+1}(\hat{\mathbf{z}}_r)$$

$$\hat{\mathbf{z}}_{r+2} = \mathbf{y}_{r+2} + \mathbf{P}_{r+2}(\hat{\mathbf{z}}_{r+1})$$

$$= \mathbf{y}_{r+2} + \mathbf{P}_{r+2}(\mathbf{y}_{r+1}) + \mathbf{P}_{r+2}(\mathbf{P}_{r+2}(\hat{\mathbf{z}}_r))$$

$$= \mathbf{y}_{r+2} + \mathbf{P}_{r+2}(\mathbf{Y}_{r+1}) + \mathbf{P}_{r+1,r+2}(\hat{\mathbf{z}}_r) \tag{11}$$

$$\vdots$$

$$\hat{\mathbf{z}}_{r+d} = \mathbf{y}_{r+d} + \mathbf{P}_{r+d}(\mathbf{y}_{r+d-1}) + \ldots + \mathbf{P}_{r+1,r+d}(\hat{\mathbf{z}}_r)$$

where the following notation has been used for the multistage linear predictor for brevity:

$$\mathbf{P}_{r+1,r+d}(\mathbf{x}) = \mathbf{P}_{r+d}(\mathbf{P}_{r+d-1}(\mathbf{P}_{r+d-2}(\ldots \mathbf{P}_{r+1}(\mathbf{x})\ldots))) \tag{12}$$

Similarly, the following relation can be derived for the output sample vector $\mathbf{z}_{r+d}$ when there is no transmission error:

$$\mathbf{z}_{r+d} = \mathbf{y}_{r+d} + \mathbf{P}_{r+d}(\mathbf{y}_{r+d-1}) + \ldots + \mathbf{P}_{r+1,r+d}(\mathbf{y}_r) + \mathbf{P}_{r,r+d}(\mathbf{z}_{r-1}) \tag{13}$$

Thus the correction error vector to be added into $\hat{\mathbf{z}}_{r+d}$ to recover $\mathbf{z}_{r+d}$ is:

$$\mathbf{c}_{r+d} = \mathbf{z}_{r+d} - \hat{\mathbf{z}}_{r+d}$$

$$= \mathbf{P}_{r,r+d}(\mathbf{z}_{r-1}) + \mathbf{P}_{r+1,r+d}(\mathbf{y}_r) - \mathbf{P}_{r+1,r+d}(\hat{\mathbf{z}}_r)$$

$$= \mathbf{P}_{r+1,r+d}(\mathbf{P}_r(\mathbf{z}_{r-1})) + \mathbf{P}_{r+1,r+d}(\mathbf{y}_r) - \mathbf{P}_{r+1,r+d}(\hat{\mathbf{z}}_r) \tag{14}$$

$$= \mathbf{P}_{r+1,r+d}(\mathbf{P}_r(\mathbf{z}_{r-1}) + \mathbf{y}_r - \hat{\mathbf{z}}_r)$$

$$= \mathbf{P}_{r+1,r+d}(\hat{\mathbf{s}}_r)$$

Therefore, after the arrival of the retransmitted information for $\mathbf{y}_r$ and $\mathbf{P}_r$, we can generate the correction error vector above and add it to the reconstructed vector at time $r + d$. From this point on, the decoder output will be identical to that without any transmission error.

Note that if no prediction is used (i.e., $\mathbf{P}_i = \mathbf{0}$) when any of the sample vectors are encoded from time $r + 1$ to $r + d$, there is no need to perform signal correction at time $r + d$, since the error propagation stops at the sample vector that is coded without prediction. Furthermore, if it is found that no prediction was used to encode the vector at sample time r after receipt of the retransmitted information, the correction vector $\hat{\mathbf{s}}_r$ is simplified to the following form as a result of $\mathbf{P}_r = \mathbf{0}$:

$$\hat{s}_r = y_r - \hat{z}_r \tag{15}$$

The multistage predictor $\mathbf{P}_{r+1,r+d}$ can be obtained by means of two methods. In the first scheme, the linear predictor operation is accumulated at each sample time from $r + 1$ to $r + d$. Therefore, upon receiving the retransmitted information at sample time $r + d$, the operator $\mathbf{P}_{r+1,r+d}$ is ready to be used to generate the correction error vector $\mathbf{c}_{r+d}$. However, in some cases, this procedure may be quite complicated to implement. In the second scheme, nothing is done during the time from $r + 1$ to $r + d$ except to save all the linear predictors $\mathbf{P}_i$, $i = r + 1, \ldots, r + d$. After receipt of the retransmitted information, the vector $\hat{s}_r$ is first formed and then all the linear predictors $\mathbf{P}_{r+1}, \ldots \mathbf{P}_{r+d}$ are sequentially applied to $\hat{s}_r$ to obtain c_{r+d}.

In the foregoing discussion, we have treated the entire image as one big vector. In practice, one can process one macroblock at a time. This is possible because in most codecs, the macroblock is the basic unit for prediction. It is difficult to trace the motion-compensated predictor on the fly when fractional motion compensation is used, since one pixel will contribute to the prediction of several pixel positions in the next frame (each with a fractional weight). If only integer pixel motion compensation is used in the codec (e.g., H.261 without the loop filter), however, it is possible to form the multistage predictor on the fly. The advantage of tracing the predictor lies in the reduced memory required to store the predictor information and the reduced processing time at frame $r + d$ when the retransmitted packet is received at the decoder. To simplify the description below, all operations are described on a pixel basis instead of on a macroblock basis. For example, $y_i(m,n)$ represents the prediction error signal for pixel (m,n) in frame i.

Tracing the prediction of a pixel is equivalent to summing the motion vectors along its route from the start frame to the end frame. During this process, if a pixel is coded in intra mode, the error propagation stops. In this case, instead of storing the sum of the motion vectors, a flag G is stored. A frame buffer is created to store the motion vectors for each pixel from frame $r + 1$ to $r + d$. Each element in the buffer consists of the x- and y-direction motion vectors. In frame r, the buffer is initialized as follows: if pixel (m,n) is undamaged, then $p_x(r,m,n) = G$; otherwise $p_x(r,m,n) = p_y(r,m,n) = 0$. From frame i, where i is from $r + 1$ to $r + d$, the motion vector sums for each pixel are traced as follows:

1. If pixel (m,n) in frame i is intra-coded, then $p_x(i,m,n) = G$;
2. Else if the corresponding pixel in the previous frame has a G flag, [i.e., $p_x(i - 1,m + v_y(i,k),n + v_x(i,k)) = G$], then $p_x(i,m,n) = G$, where $v_x(i,k)$ and $v_y(i,k)$ are the motion vectors in the horizontal and vertical directions for macroblock k in frame i, which contains pixel (m,n);
3. Else accumulate the motion vector sums:

    $p_x(i,m,n) = p_x(i - 1,m,n) + v_x(i,k)$
    $p_y(i,m,n) - p_y(i - 1,m,n) + v_y(i,k)$

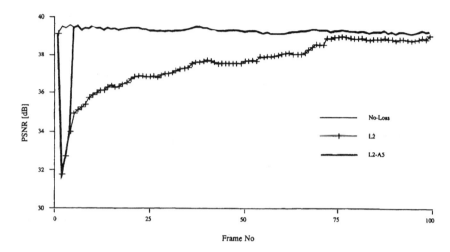

Figure 6.15 PSNR comparison of the Salesman sequence with 20% loss at frame 2 and the retransmission arrival at frame 5 (Figure 3 in Ref. 35. ©1996 IEEE.)

Upon the arrival of the retransmission information, the correction error signal for each pixel is generated as follows:

1. If $p_x(r + d,m,n) = G$, then $c(r + d,m,n) = 0$;
2. Else if pixel $[m + p_y(r + d,m,n),n + p_x(r + d,m,n)]$ was intra-coded in frame r, then $c(r + d,m,n) = y[r,m + p_y(r + d,m,n),n + p_x(r + d,m,n)] - \hat{z}(r,m,n)$;
3. Otherwise,

$$c\,(r - d,m,n) = y[r,m + p_y\,(r + d,m,n),n + p_x\,(r + d,m,n)] - \hat{z}\,(r,m,n) + z\,[r - 1,m + v_y\,(r,k) + v_y\,(r + d,m,n),n + v_x\,(r,k) + p_x\,(r + d,m,n)]$$

In summary, the method described here can achieve lossless recovery except for the time between the information loss and the arrival of the out-of-order packet. During that interval, any postprocessing error concealment techniques described in the last two sections can be applied to the damaged regions to generate a concealed video signal. Figure 6.15 compares three PSNR curves, which correspond to no information loss, error concealment only, and the method described in this section. It is assumed that 20% of the ATM cells of frame 2 are lost, and their retransmission arrives at frame 5.

6.6   SUMMARY AND CONCLUSION

All error concealment techniques recover lost information by making use of some a priori knowledge about the image/video signals, primarily the temporal and spatial smoothness property. In the maximally smooth recovery technique presented here, an isotropic smoothness measure is used everywhere. This is not appropriate near image edges, where smoothness should be enforced along the edges but not across them. To overcome this problem, one should adapt the smoothness (or roughness) measure based on the local image patterns. Several techniques have been developed along these lines (18). Another approach entails using alternating projections onto convex sets determined by smoothness constraints along different directions, which is the essence of the POCS method. Depending on the local image pattern, the constraints can be varied from block to block. This method is computationally more intensive than the optimization approach because it requires many iterations, although it generally gives more accurate results. The interpolation method can be considered to be a special case of the optimization method if only boundary pixels in adjacent blocks are used, and if the interpolation coefficients are derived by maximizing the smoothness measure. In fact, the solution of the optimization problem presented in Eq. (3) represents the reconstructed block as a combination of spatial, temporal, and frequency domain interpolations.

The reconstruction methods reviewed here are for transform-based coders that use nonoverlapping transforms. Error concealment techniques have also been developed for other coding methods, including subband (36–38), LOT (39–41), and Walsh transform (42). Fuzzy logic has also been used to recover high-frequency components, which cannot normally be recovered by the smoothing and interpolation methods presented in this section (43).

Although most error concealment techniques concentrate on estimation of either transform coefficients or pixel data directly, proper estimation of coding mode and motion vectors also plays a very importance role. This is due to the heavy use of motion-compensated prediction in video coding. In addition, coding mode and motion vectors are typically carried together with transform coefficients in the same transport data unit. Although simple interpolation can be applied to estimating the damaged coding mode and motion vectors, better estimates can be achieved with more frame buffers and adaptive estimation mechanisms such as global motion estimation. With the continuing trend of reduced memory cost and increasing processing power, we can expect that more algorithms will be developed along these lines. The out-of-order decoding method described in Section 6.5 is an example. Although the method appears to require more storage space and processing complexity, the effect of achieving almost lossless recovery is worthwhile for certain applications where avoiding delay is one of the most stringent requirements. This method will gain in importance when packet-based networks have become the platform for integrated transport of both time-insensitive data and time-sensitive voice and video signals.

Finally, we note that performing error concealment at the decoder is only one way to enhance the robustness of a video system to transmission errors. The video encoder can also play an important role by embedding a controlled amount of redundancy in the compressed stream, so that the stream is less susceptible to errors, or concealment of errors at the decoder is easier. Another dimension for error control is at the channel coder and transport layer control. These topics are covered in Chapters 9–13 of this book.

REFERENCES

1. ITU-T Recommendation H.261. Video codec for audiovisual services at $p \times 64$ kbits. International Telecommunications Union, Geneva, 1993.
2. ITU-T Recommendation H.263. Video coding for low bitrate communication. International Telecommunications Union, Geneva, 1998.
3. ISO/IEC DIS 13818-2. Information technology—Generic coding of moving pictures and associated audio information—Part 2: Video. 1994.
4. ITU-T Recommendation H.323. Visual telephone systems and equipment for local area networks which provide a non-guaranteed quality of service. International Telecommunications Union, Geneva, 1998.
5. ITU-T Recommendation H.324. Terminal for low bitrate multimedia communication. International Telecommunications Union, Geneva, 1995.
6. ITU-T Recommendation H.225.0. Media stream packetization and synchronization on non-guaranteed quality of services lANs. International Telecommunications Union, Geneva, 1996.
7. ITU-T Recommendation H.223. Multiplexing protocol for low bitrate multimedia communication. International Telecommunications Union, Geneva, 1995.
8. S Lin, DJ Costello. Error Control Coding: Fundamentals and Applications. Englewood Cliffs, NJ: Prentice-Hall, 1983.
9. ITU-T Recommendation H.221. Frame structure for a 64 to 1920 kbit/s channel in audiovisual teleservices. International Telecommunications Union, Geneva, 1993.
10. ITU-T Recommendation H.320. Narrow-band visual telephone systems and terminal equipment. International Telecommunications Union, Geneva, 1993.
11. OR Mitchell, AJ Tabatabai. Channel error recovery for transform image coding. IEEE Trans Commun 29:1754–1762, December 1981.
12. Y-H Han, J-J Leou. Detection and correction of transmission errors in JPEG images. IEEE Trans Circuits Syst Video Technol 8(2):221–231, April 1998.
13. W-J Chu, J-J Leou. Detection and concealment of transmission errors in H.261 images. IEEE Trans Circuits Syst Video Technol 8(1):248–258, February 1998.
14. ISO/IEC 14496-2. Information technology—Coding of audio-visual objects: Visual. March 1998.
15. S Aign, K Fazel. Temporal and spatial error concealment techniques for hierarchical MPEG-2 video codec. Proceedings of Globecom'95, 1995, pp 1778–1783.
16. Y Wang, Q-F Zhu, L Shaw. Maximally smooth image recovery in transform coding. IEEE Trans Commun 41(10):1544–1551, October 1993.
17. W Zhu, Y Wang, Q-F Zhu. Second-order derivative-based smoothness measure for error concealment in DCT-based codecs. IEEE Trans Circuits Syst Video Technol 8(6):713–718, October 1998.

18. W Kwok, H Sun. Multi-directional interpolation for spatial error concealment. IEEE Trans Consumer Electron 39(3):455–460, August 1993.
19. H Sun, W Kwok. Concealment of damaged block transform coded images using projections onto convex sets. IEEE Trans Image Process, 4(4):470–477, April 1995.
20. R Aravind, MR Civanlar, AR Reibman. Packet loss resilience of MPEG-2 scalable video coding algorithms. IEEE Trans Circuits Syst Video Technol, 6(5):426–435, October 1996.
21. Q-F Zhu, Y Wang, L Shaw. Coding and cell loss recovery for DCT-based packet video. IEEE Trans Circuits Syst Video Technol, 3(3):248–258, June 1993.
22. S Shirani, F Kossentini, R Ward. Reconstruction of motion vector missing macroblocks in H.263 encoded video transmission over lossy networks. Proceedings of IEEE ICIP'98, 1998, pp 487–491.
23. M-J Chen, L-G Chen, R-M Weng. Error concealment of lost motion vectors with overlapped motion compensation. IEEE Trans Circuits Syst Video Technol, 7(3):560–563, June 1997.
24. ME Al-Mualla, N Canagarajah, DR Bull. Error concealment using motion field interpolation. Proceedings of IEEE ICIP'98, 1998, pp 512–516.
25. LH Kieu, KN Ngan. Cell-loss concealment techniques for layered video codecs in an ATM network. IEEE Trans Image Process 3(5):666–677, September 1994.
26. A Vetro, H Sun, Y-K Chen, SY Kung. True motion vectors for robust video transmission. Proceedings of SPIE Visual Communications and Image Processing, San Jose, CA, January 1999, pp 230–240.
27. G-S Yu, MM-K Liu, MW Marcellin. POCS-based error concealment for packet video using multiframe overlap information. IEEE Trans Circuits Syst Video Technol, 8(4):422–434, August 1998.
28. Y Wang, Q-F Zhu. Error control and concealment for video communication, a review. Proc IEEE 86(5):974–997, May 1998.
29. H Sun, K Challapali, J Zdepski. Error concealment in digital simulcast AD-HDTV decoder. IEEE Trans Consumer Electron 38(3):108–117, August 1992.
30. J Lu, ML Liou, KB Letaief, JC-I Chuang. Error resilient transmission of H.263 coded video over mobile networks. Proceedings of IEEE ISCAS'98 4:502–505, 1998.
31. P Haskell, D Messerschmitt. Resynchronization of motion compensated video affected by ATM cell loss. Proceedings of ICASSP'92, San Francisco, March 1992, vol III, pp 545–548,
32. A Narula, JS Lim. Error concealment techniques for an all-digital high-definition television system. SPIE Proceedings on Visual Communications and Image Processing, Cambridge, MA, 1993, pp 304–315.
33. W-M Lam, AR Reibman, B Liu. Recovery of lost or erroneously received motion vectors. Proceedings of ICASSP'93, Minneapolis, April 1993, vol V, pp 417–420.
34. Q-F Zhu. Device and method of signal loss recovery for realtime and/or interactive communications. US Patent 5,550,847, August 1996.
35. M Ghanbari. Postprocessing of late cells for packet video. IEEE Trans Circuits Syst Video Technol 6(6):669–678, December 1996.
36. SS Hemami, RM Gray. Subband-coded image reconstruction for lossy packet networks. IEEE Trans Image Process, 6(4):523–539, April 1997.

37. Y Wang, V Ramamoorthy. Image reconstruction from spatial subband images and its applications in packet video transmission. Signal Process: Image Commun 3(2/3):197–229, June 1991.

38. G Gonzalez-Rosiles, SD Cabrera, SW Wu. Recovery with lost subband data in overcomplete image coding. Proceedings of ICASSP'95, Detroit, 1995, vol II, pp 1476–1479.

39. P Haskell, D Messerchmitt. Reconstructing lost video data in a lapped orthogonal transform based coder. Proceedings of ICASSP'88, Albuquerque, NM, April 1990, pp 1985–1988.

40. KH Tzou. Postfiltering for cell loss concealment in packet video. SPIE Proceedings on Visual Communications and Image Processing, Philadelphia, November 1989, pp 1620–1627.

41. D Chung, Y Wang. Multiple description image coding using signal decomposition and reconstruction based on lapped orthogonal transforms. IEEE Trans Circuits Syst Video Technol 9(6):895–908, September 1999.

42. WC Wong, R Steele. Partial correction of transmission errors in Walsh transform image coding without recourse to error correction coding. Electron Lett May 1978, 298–300.

43. X Lee, Y-Q Zhang, A Leon-Garcia. Information loss recovery for block-based image coding techniques—A fuzzy logic approach. IEEE Trans Image Process, 4(3):259–273, March 1995.

7
Layered Coding

Mohammed Ghanbari
*Department of Electronic Systems Engineering, University of Essex,
Colchester, England*

7.1 INTRODUCTION

Video networking in a heterogeneous (IP, ATM, mobile, etc.) environment demands video services of varying spatiotemporal and quality fidelity. Establishing
a framework that allows various video classes to interoperate and new services
to evolve will offer significant advantages in both the effective utilization of network resources and the customer satisfaction. This approach of enabling video
layers to interwork is a concept espoused by *layered* coding, and the ability to
represent an image or sequence of images in a hierarchical data structure would
facilitate such a concept.

Layered video coding, also called *scalable* coding, was originally proposed by the author to increase the robustness of video codecs against packet
(cell) loss in ATM networks (1). At the time (late 1980s), H.261 was under development and it was clear that purely interframe-coded video by the proposed
method was very vulnerable to loss of information. The idea was that the codec
should generate two bit-streams, one carrying the most vital video information
the *base layer*, and the other carrying the residual information to enhance the
quality of the base layer image, the *enhancement layer*. In the event of network
congestion, only the less important enhancement data should be discarded, and
the space made available for base layer data. Such a methodology had an influence on the formation of ATM cell structure, to provide two levels of priority for
protecting base layer data (2). This form of two-layer coding is now known as
SNR scalability in the standard codecs, and currently a variety of new two-layer
coding techniques exist. They now form the basic scalability functions of the
standard video codecs such as MPEG-2 for high-quality video internetworking,

H.263+/MPEG-4 for mobile applications, and still image coding with JPEG-2000 (3–6).

The concept of layered representation of data has now been extended to other nontelecommunication applications. For example, hierarchical representation of the bitstream provides the opportunity to extract a video (an image) of preferred quality of choice from a single bitstream, such as that of MPEG-2. A form of layered representation, used in MPEG-4, provides the opportunity for users to interact with data, following their objects of interest (5).

In this chapter we look at three general methods of layered coding techniques. Although conceptually they have similarities, these days they have found different applications:

> *Pyramidal coding.* Representation of pictures in pyramids, either in the pixel or transform domain. Although this method to some extent resembles spatial scalability, because of its historical importance and applications to coding of still images, it deserves some consideration.
> *Scalability in the standard video codecs.* This type of layering, perhaps the most widely used method, was adopted in the standard codecs such as MPEG-2, H.263+, and MPEG-4.
> *Wavelet-based coding.* The nature of wavelet-transformed images is such that layers of subimages are generated. Since the introduction of efficient method for coding of wavelet coefficients with the *embedded zero tree* (7), this method of coding has attracted some interest. Wavelet-based coding has currently been adopted as the scalable coding method for the still image coding option mode of MPEG-4 and the still image encoder, JPEG-2000.

7.2 PYRAMIDAL CODING

Recursive decimation and interpolation of an image can reconstruct a pyramidal structure of image. "Pyramid" in this context refers to a data structure that provides successively condensed information of an image. Such coding schemes are referred to as *pyramidal coding*. In this regard, the picture at the top of the pyramid, sometimes called the *apex* picture, gives the minimum acceptable picture resolution. Other levels of the pyramid reconstruct images of higher quality by including additional information about the picture fidelity. The information to be added to each layer is generally marginal (depending on the number of layers), such that the presence or absence of a layer can alter picture quality only marginally. As one moves toward the bottom of the pyramid, the importance of the added information becomes less significant.

From the video networking point of view, this type of data structure has an interesting property. For example, in the event of network congestion, less important data from the bottom levels, in order, can be dropped and room made available to the upper level data as well as the apex picture at the top of the pyramid. In doing so, one can reconstruct images of varying quality, depending on the network resources.

In this section I present two methods of pyramidal image coding. The first method describes the Laplacian pyramid introduced by Burt and Adelson (8), which is the classical representation in pyramidal coding. This will serve as an introduction to the concepts and ideas of pyramidal coding. The second technique involves the principles of transform coding by means of discrete cosine transforms, where the DCT coefficients are ordered in a pyramidal structure for more efficient data compression (9).

7.2.1 The Laplacian Pyramid as an Image Coder

In *Laplacian pyramid coding* (LPC), two distinct types of pyramid are generated: the Gaussian pyramid and the Laplacian pyramid, as shown in Figure 7.1. For data reduction, all the levels of the Laplacian pyramid are quantized and coded.

The Gaussian pyramid is generated by recursive filtering and subsampling of the original image, G_0. The low-pass filtering and subsequent downsampling can be represented by a *reduce* operator:

$$G_{k+1} = \text{reduce}(G_k) \tag{1}$$

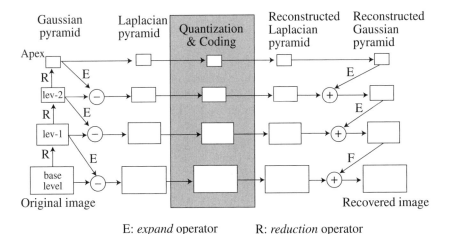

E: *expand* operator   R: *reduction* operator

Figure 7.1   The Laplacian pyramid coding and decoding.

where a higher level is a reduced version of its immediate lower level. When stacked on top of each other, the images form a data structure that assumes the shape of a pyramid. This pyramidal structure creates a set of multiresolution images, G_k, for $k = 0, \ldots, N$, where G_0 resides at the bottom level of the pyramid and G_a, the *apex* image, at the top. Each Gaussian image then shows the original image in a different spatial scale: the higher the level, the coarser the scale. Depending on the type of low-pass filter used and the subsampling procedure, many variations are possible. The Gaussian pyramid representation put forth by Burt and Adelson (8) uses a separable filter that has an approximately Gaussian shape origin, hence its name.

The Laplacian pyramid is a set of difference images, which are constrained to yield a perfect reconstruction of the original image. Pyramidal image reconstruction is performed from coarse to fine, and the idea is to reconstruct the whole Gaussian pyramid staring from the apex and finishing with the original at the bottom level.

The decimation process of Eq. 7.1, *reduce*, which generated G_{k+1} from G_k, throws away information and so is irreversible. This means that additional information in the form of an error signal must be supplied by the Laplacian pyramid, L_k, such that, when it is added back to G_{k+1}, a lower level of the Gaussian pyramid without any distortions is generated: that is,

$$G_k = L_k + \text{expand}(G_{k+1}) \tag{2}$$

Here the *expand* operation is complementary to the *reduce* operation. That is, the Gaussian image is enlarged in both horizontal and vertical directions and is interpolated to its lower-level image size. The interpolation is such that when Eqs. (1) and (2) are combined, the lower level Gaussian pyramid is reconstructed. Thus, the Laplacian pyramid is generated by:

$$L_k = G_k - \text{expand}\{\text{reduce}(G_k)\} \tag{3}$$

This process is recursively continued until the original picture at the bottom of the pyramid has been reconstructed. This is in fact lossless coding.

For lossy coding, the set of error images (Laplacian pyramid), $L_0, L_1 \ldots$, L_N are quantized and coded, as shown in Figure 7.1. Note that $L_N = G_N$, because there is no G_{N+1} image to serve as the predictor for G_N. Decoding starts from $L_N = G_N$, and the subsequent quantized Laplacian images, L_i, after expansion, are added to the previous decoded Gaussian images, to reconstruct the current one.

7.2.1.1 Subband Decomposition. The Gaussian pyramid may be perceived as a set of low-pass filtered versions of the original image. The first-level image of the Laplacian pyramid has an essentially high-pass character, while the other levels, except the apex, are band-pass versions. The effective bandwidth of these band-passed images decreases from level to level of the pyramid, while the center frequency of the passband is reduced by an octave each time. This process of dividing an image into different frequency bands is referred to as subband decomposition. Pyramidal coding thus implicitly embodies subband decomposition and may be viewed as a variant of subband image coding. However, typical subband image coders employ explicitly designed band-pass filters.

In the coding of each band or each decimated image of the pyramid, the sensitivity of the human visual system to contrast perturbations at various bands can be considered. It is well accepted that the observer's sensitivity increases toward lower spatial frequencies; hence more bits per pixel are assigned in this range. These additional bits contribute little to the overall image bit rate because the sample densities at these levels are low (i.e., smaller image sizes). On the other hand, the relative insensitivity of the human visual system to noise at higher spatial frequencies, corresponding to the densely sampled lower level images of the pyramid, could be exploited to significantly reduce the overall bit rate.

7.2.2 DCT Pyramid

In the Laplacian pyramid, each error image L_i is normally coded by means of a differential pulse code modulation (DPCM) technique. Owing to the pixel-to-pixel coding nature of DPCM, this limits the coding efficiency. For higher compression, one may use the discrete cosine transform. However, rather than applying DCT on the Laplacian pyramids, one can generate a DCT pyramid and code the pyramids of coefficients directly.

Fundamental to the technique of manifesting DCT within a pyramidal data structure is the ability to perform decimation and interpolation in the transform domain. To decimate an image that is segmented into sample blocks of size $N \times N$ pixels by a ratio of M/N, where $M < N$, an $(N \times N)$-point forward DCT is applied, followed by an $(M \times M)$-point inverse DCT using the lower order coefficients (10). Decimation via this procedure is realizable because a different set of basis vectors is used during the synthesis transform. Both integer and noninteger ratios of M/N are possible. This process is hereafter denoted by $N{\rightarrow}M$.

It should be noted that the normalizing term of the DCT transform pair for $N{\rightarrow}M$ is N. This is to ensure that the DC level is synthesized correctly. Central to the design of decimators is the need for a filtering operation to minimize aliasing artifacts. The removal of bands in orthogonal transforms provides implicit filtering. This filtering process can be analyzed by deriving its equivalent impulse response in a familiar time-invariant form (10). A decimation ratio of 2 can be implemented via $4{\rightarrow}2$, $8{\rightarrow}4$, or $16{\rightarrow}8$.

In the study of decimation/interpolation via the DCT domain, two observations were made (9). First, for a given decimation ratio of M/N, the number of equivalent filter tap coefficients is determined by N. Second, the number of side lobes in the impulse response is determined by M independently of N. For a given decimation ratio, a larger N will demand a larger value of M. This in turn will provide a wider window for the impulse response, which will approximate toward the ideal brick-wall filter function. Experimental observations have indicated that to minimize aliasing effects, the value of M should be greater or equal to 2. The adequacy of such filtering in DCT decimation has also been found to be acceptable by Vandendorpe (11). A sensible choice of N and M can be made to minimize ringing and aliasing defects.

DCT decimation and interpolation can be exploited to code images in a hierarchical order. The success of this technique is in the segmentation of each block of transform coefficients for different purposes. A set of predictors, consisting of the lower frequency coefficients, is employed to convey the analog function of the signal. The high correlation between pixels of natural images causes most of the image's energy to be concentrated at lower frequencies. The remaining higher frequency coefficients are virtually negligible, and discarding them during the decimation process will not cause significant loss of picture information. Coarse quantization of these coefficients will, however, result in a significant bit-rate reduction (9).

The DCT decimation process effectively decomposes an image into two distinct components. They are a low-passed decimated image and a set of high-passed DCT coefficients. Successive decimation generates the pyramid data structure. Each image in the series of the decimated images is filtered by a weighting function based on a cosine summation (10); hence, it is called the *cosine pyramid*. The hierarchy set of error signals, which are essentially the remaining DCT coefficients, is named the *DCT pyramid*. The image coding technique introduced here results in data compression by encoding the DCT pyramid, as illustrated in Figure 7.2. At each level of the pyramid, every block of $N \times N$ pixels is DCT coded. The corner set of $M \times M$ transform coefficients is then inverse-transformed to form a higher level of the cosine pyramid. The remaining coefficients are quantized and coded. For efficient coding, these coefficients are zigzag-scanned (similar to H.261, runs of zeros and indexes of levels) and are variable-length-coded (VLC) (12). In the scanning process, the lower set of the coefficients designated for the higher layer is omitted. Finally, the apex level, which is the final decimated image, is simply DCT-coded because there is no predictor available.

To decode the image, the apex image is reconstructed from the DCT coefficients of this level. The picture in the next level of the pyramid is reconstructed by $M \times M$ DCT transformation of the reconstructed apex picture and then padding the coefficients of the *reversed-L-shaped* blocks at this level before taking the inverse $N \times N$ ($N > M$) DCT, as shown in Figure 7.2. Iterating this process leads to the final reconstructed image.

It has been observed that coefficients designated for coding tend to be clus-

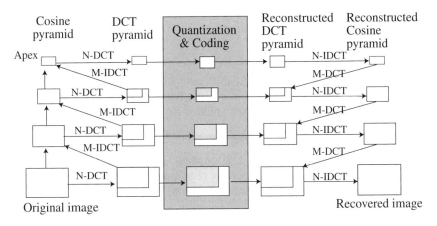

Figure 7.2 A four-level DCT pyramid encoder decoder.

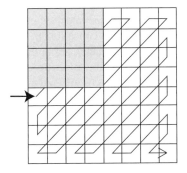

Figure 7.3 Zigzag scanning of the reversed l-shaped AC coefficients.

tered in the top right or bottom left part of the reversed L-shaped blocks. They correspond to blocks featuring vertical or horizontal details. The zigzag scanning has, however, been retained because the possible gain in using appropriate scanning classes to optimize the *runs* of *zeros* was offset by the side information required. Figure 7.3 shows the zigzag scanning of the reversed-L-shaped part of the AC coefficients.

7.2.2.1 Subband Decomposition. The Gaussian and Laplacian pyramids use filtering and subsampling operations to decimate a lower spatial resolution layer that then serves as a predictor in the image recovery process. Spatial redundancy is removed by encoding the uncorrelated prediction error. Iterating this procedure on the decimated layer would produce a hierarchical set of low-passed images and band-passed prediction errors. When the number of levels in the pyramid is large, the coding area approaches to 4/3 of the picture size:

$$1 + \frac{1}{4} + \frac{1}{16} + \frac{1}{64} + \frac{1}{256} + \cdots = \frac{4}{3} \qquad (4)$$

On the contrary, the DCT pyramid does not increase the coding area. It is similar in concept to the hierarchical splitting of image in subband or wavelet transform coding, where the number of transform coefficients is the same as the number of pixels (13). In wavelet transform coding, an image is separated into four bands, followed by iterative division of the baseband as shown in Figure 7.4a. The DCT pyramid follows a filter bank parallel-splitting approach with finer separation being applied hierarchically on the base band. The band-splitting procedure indicated in Figure 7.4b is, however, executed on a block basis with the exploitation of the correlation of the lower frequency components between adjacent blocks through the hierarchy of the pyramid.

The DCT pyramid thus implicitly embodies subband decomposition, in as much as each subsequent decimation on a filtered image generates a batch of band-passed DCT coefficients. The effective bandwidth of these bands decreases from level to level of the pyramid, decided by a factor that is controlled by the decimation rate. Both integer and noninteger factor band divisions are possible when the DCT decimation technique is used.

Quantization and coding of each band of the pyramid can be adapted to reflect the sensitivity of the human observer to contrast perturbations at that band. Since again, the observer's sensitivity increases toward lower spatial frequencies, more bits per pixel are required. However, because of the lower sample densities at these levels (i.e., smaller image sizes), the overall bit rate is not seriously inflated. The relative insensitivity of the human visual system to noise at

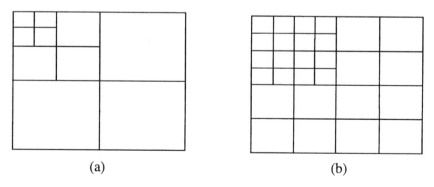

(a)   (b)

Figure 7.4   A hierarchical bandwidth splitting in (a) wavelet and (b) DCT pyramid.

higher spatial frequencies corresponding to the densely sampled lower layers of the pyramid could be exploited to significantly reduce the overall bit rate. The DCT pyramid is similar to wavelet transform coding in that a higher or lower level of a pyramid can be quantized with a larger quantization distortion. Moreover, since each level of the pyramid contains a certain spatial frequency, coding of any significant coefficients from these levels retains the significance of that band. Images are thus coded via a strategy of coarser quantization of the higher frequency bands, which dominate the overall coding area, and finer quantization of the lower bands, which dominate the image rendition properties of the code.

Figure 7.5 shows the PARROT image with a resolution of 704×576 pixels coded with a five-level DCT pyramid. The reconstructed picture with all five levels present is almost subjectively transparent, with a bit rate of 0.25 bit/pixel and objective quality of 39.2 dB, as detailed in Table 7.1. Loss of data from layer 1,

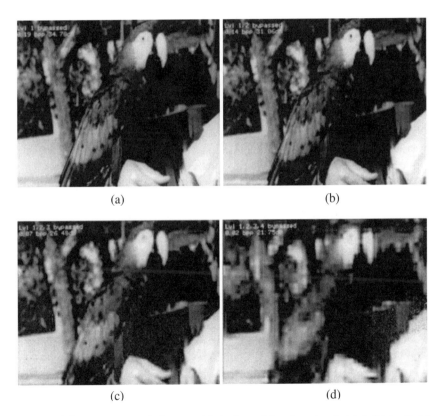

                    (a)   (b)

                    (c)   (d)

Figure 7.5   Reconstructed pictures with the loss of data from levels (a) 1, (b) 1 + 2, (c) 1 + 2 + 3, and (d) all levels except the apex.

Table 7.1 Reconstruction Data for the Images in Figure 7.5

Layers received	Bipicture (kbit)	Bipixel	Discard rate (%)	Quality (dB)
Apex = 5	8.1	0.02	92	21.75
4 + 5	28.4	0.07	72	26.48
3 + 4 + 5	56.8	0.14	44	31.06
2 + 3 + 4 + 5	77	0.19	24	34.78
All	101.4	0.25	0	39.2

which accounts for almost 24% of the overall bit rate, although the quality is degraded by 4.4 dB, hardly affects the subjective quality as seen in Figure 7.5a. Even loss of layers 1 and 2 does not degrade the subjective quality of the image significantly. The picture starts to degrade with the loss of data from the three bottom layers, but this accounts for 72% of the data. Loss of data from all the layers except the apex, which is about 92% of the generated bits, gives a poor quality picture. Nevertheless this is far better than the result that would be obtained if 92% of the data from a nonlayered coded image were lost.

7.3 SCALABILITY IN THE STANDARD CODECS

The scalability tools defined in the standard codecs of MPEG-2, H.263+, and MPEG-4 are designed to support applications beyond that supported by the single-layer video. Among the noteworthy applications areas addressed, depending on the type of codec, are video telecommunications, video on *asynchronous transfer mode* (ATM) networks, video over mobile networks, interworking of video standards, and video service hierarchies with multiple spatial, temporal, and quality resolutions. Depending on the type of application, the main purpose is either to improve picture quality against the channel constraints or to provide facilities for users to choose video quality of their own preference.

In scalable video coding, it is assumed that given an encoded bitstream, decoders of various complexities can decode and display appropriate reproductions of the coded video. A scalable video encoder is likely to have increased complexity compared to a single-layer encoder. However, the standard provides several different forms of scalability that address nonoverlapping applications with corresponding complexities. The basic scalability tools offered are: *data partitioning, SNR scalability, spatial scalability*, and *temporal scalability*. Moreover, combinations of these basic scalability tools are also supported by and are referred to as *hybrid scalability*. In the case of basic scalability, two layers of video, the *base layer* and the *enhancement layer* are allowed, whereas hybrid scalability supports more layers.

Details of these methods of scalability are given in Sections 7.3.1 to 7.3.5. In the descriptions, the scalable codec is often referred to MPEG-2, which was the first standard codec to define scalability. Section 7.3.6 describes the scalability methods used in the H.263+ codec.

7.3.1 Data Partitioning

Data partitioning is a tool intended for use when two channels are available for the transmission and/or storage of a video bitstream, as may be the case in ATM networks, terrestrial broadcasting, magnetic media, and so on. Data partitioning in fact is not a true scalable coding, rather it is a means of dividing the bitstream of a single-layer nonscalable DCT-based codec into two parts or two layers. The first layer comprises the critical parts of the bitstream (e.g., headers, motion vectors, lower order DCT coefficients), which are transmitted in the channel with the better error performance. The second layer is made of less critical data (e.g., higher DCT coefficients) and is transmitted in the channel with poorer error performance. Thus, since the critical parts of a bitstream are better protected, degradations to channel errors are minimized. Data from neither channel may be decoded on a decoder that is not intended for decoding data-partitioned bitstreams. Even with the proper decoder, data extracted from the second-layer decoder cannot be used unless the decoded base layer data are available.

A block diagram of a data-partitioning encoder is shown in Figure 7.6. The single-layer encoder is in fact a nonscalable MPEG-2 video encoder that may or may not include B pictures.

At the encoder, during the quantization and zigzag scanning of each 8×8 DCT coefficient, the scanning is broken at the *priority break point* (PBP), as shown in Figure 7.7. The base layer bitstream is taken to be first part of the scanned, quantized coefficients after variable length coding, with the other

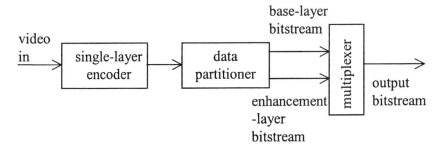

Figure 7.6   Block diagram of a data-partitioning encoder.

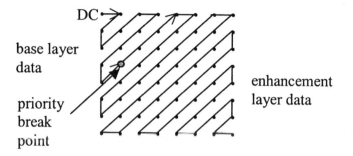

Figure 7.7   Position of the priority break point in a block of DCT coefficients.

overhead information (motion vectors, macroblock types, addresses, etc., including the priority break point PBP). The remaining scanned and quantized coefficients plus the end-of-block (EOB) code constitute the enhancement layer bitstream. Figure 7.7 also shows the position of the priority break point in the DCT coefficients.

The base and the enhancement layer bitstreams are then multiplexed for transmission into the channel. For prioritized transmission such as ATM networks, each bitstream is first packetized into high- and low-priority cells, and the cells are multiplexed. At the decoder, from knowledge of the position of PBP, a block of DCT coefficients is reconstructed from the two bitstreams. Note that PBP indicates the last DCT coefficient of the base layer. Its position at the encoder is determined based on the portion of channel rate from the total bit rate allocated to the base layer.

It should be noted that since the encoder is a single-layer interframe coder, then at the encoder both the base and the enhancement layer coefficients are used at the encoding prediction loop. Thus reconstruction of picture from the base layer only can result in a mismatch between the encoder and decoder prediction loops. This causes *picture drift* on the reconstructed picture: that is, lost enhancement data accumulate at the decoder and appear as *mosquito-like* noise. Picture drift occurs in P and B pictures, since they are predicted from reference pictures. Also, I pictures reset the feedback prediction; hence they clean up the drift. The more frequent the I pictures, the less picture drift, is experienced, but this improvement comes at the expense of higher bit rates.

It should be noted that in the event of loss from the enhancement layer, picture is made of the base layer data only. Since the enhancement layer comprises the high-frequency coefficients, the picture will be blurred in the areas of enhancement data loss. As the base layer bit rate is reduced, the degree of picture fuzziness increases. This type of distortion is to some extent tolerable. The main problem at this low bit rate is picture blockiness, to which the human eye is very sensitive. In data partitioning, blockiness is due to the reconstruction of some macroblocks from only the DC and/or from a few AC coefficients. To ease blockiness artifacts, several AC coefficients need to be included at the base layer. Hence one of the limitations in data partitioning is the need for a high allocated bit rate to the base layer.

In summary, data partitioning, the simplest kind of scalability, has no extra complexity over the nonscalable encoder. Although the base picture suffers from picture drift and may not be usable alone, the enhanced (base layer plus the enhancement layer) picture with occasional losses is quite acceptable. This is due to normally low loss rates in most networks (e.g., $< 10^{-4}$), such that the loss area is cleaned up by I pictures before the accumulation of loss becomes significant, (14).

7.3.2 SNR Scalability

SNR scalability is a tool intended for use in video applications involving telecommunications for multiple-quality video services (i.e., video systems with the common feature that a minimum of two layers of video quality are necessary). SNR scalability involves generating two video layers of same spatiotemporal resolution but different video qualities from a single video source such that the base layer is coded by itself to provide the basic video quality and the enhancement layer is coded to enhance the base layer. When added back to the base layer, the enhancement layer regenerates a higher quality reproduction of the input video. Since the enhancement layer is said to enhance the *signal-to-noise ratio* (SNR) of the base layer, this type of scalability is called SNR. Alternatively, as we will see later, SNR scalability could have been called *coefficient amplitude* scalability or *quantization noise* scalability.

Figure 7.8 shows the block diagram of a two-layer SNR scalable encoder. First, the input video is coded at a low bit rate (lower image quality), to generate the base layer bitstream. The difference between the input video and the decoded output of the base layer is coded by a second encoder, with a higher precision, to generate the enhancement layer bitstream. These bitstreams are multiplexed for transmission over the channel. At the decoder, decoding of the base layer bitstream results in the base picture. When the decoded enhancement layer bitstream is added to the base layer, the result is an enhanced image. The base and the enhancement layers may either use an identical encoder at both layers, or different ones. For example, the MPEG-1 standard can be used for the base layer and MPEG-2 for the enhancement layer.

It may appear that the SNR scalable encoder is much more complex than the data-partitioning encoder. The former requires at least two nonscalable encoders, whereas data partitioning is a simple single-layer encoder, and partitioning is just carried out on the bitstream. The fact is that if both layer encoders in

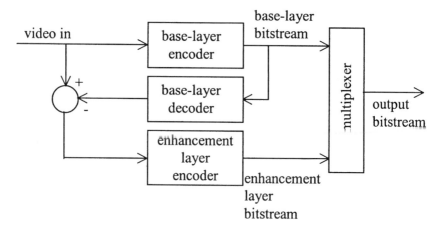

Figure 7.8   Block diagram of a two-layer SNR scalable coder.

the SNR coder are of the same type (e.g., both nonscalable MPEG-2 encoders), the two-layer encoder can be simplified.

In Figure 7.9, which represents a simplified nonscalable MPEG-2 of the base layer (15), the differences between the input pixels block X and their motion-compensated predictions Y are transformed into coefficients $T(X - Y)$. These coefficients after quantization can be represented with $T(X - Y) - Q$, where Q is the introduced quantization distortion. The quantized coefficients after the inverse DCT (IDCT) reconstruct the prediction error. They are then added to the motion-compensated prediction to reconstruct a locally decoded pixel block Z.

Thus after transform coding, the interframe error signal $X - Y$ becomes

$$T(X - Y) \tag{5}$$

and after quantization, a quantization distortion Q is introduced to the transform coefficients. Then Eq. (5) becomes

$$T(X - Y) - Q \tag{6}$$

After the inverse DCT the reconstruction error can be formulated as follows:

$$T^{-1}[T(X - Y) - Q] \tag{7}$$

where T^{-1} is the inverse transformation operation. Because transformation is a linear operator, the reconstruction error can be written as follows:

$$T^{-1}T(X - Y) - T^{-1}(Q) \tag{8}$$

Also, the orthonormality of the transform, where $T^{-1}T = 1$, permits the simplification of Eq. (8) to

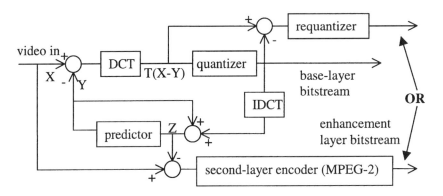

Figure 7.9 A DCT-based base layer encoder.

$$X - Y - T^{-1}Q \tag{9}$$

When this error is added to the motion-compensated prediction Y, the locally decoded block becomes

$$Z = Y + X - Y - T^{-1}(Q) = X - T^{-1}(Q) \tag{10}$$

Thus according to Figure 7.9, what is coded by the second-layer encoder is

$$X - Z = X - X + T^{-1}(Q) = T^{-1}(Q) \tag{11}$$

that is, the inverse transform of the base layer quantization distortion. Since the second-layer encoder is also a DCT-based encoder, DCT transformation of $X - Z$ in Eq. (11) would result in

$$T(X - Z) = TT^{-1}(Q) = Q \tag{12}$$

where again the orthonormality of transform is employed. Thus the second-layer transform coefficients are in fact the quantization distortions of the base layer transform coefficients, Q. For this reason the codec can also be called *coefficient amplitude* scalability or *quantization noise* scalability unit.

Therefore the second layer of an SNR scalable encoder can be a simple requantizer, as shown in Figure 7.9, without much more complexity than a data-partitioning encoder.

The only problem with this method of coding is that since normally the base layer is poor, or at least worse than the enhanced image (base plus the second layer), the prediction used is not good. A better prediction would be a picture of the sum of both layers, as shown in Figure 7.10. Note that the second layer is still encoding the quantization distortion of the base layer.

In this encoder, the motion compensation, variable-length coding of

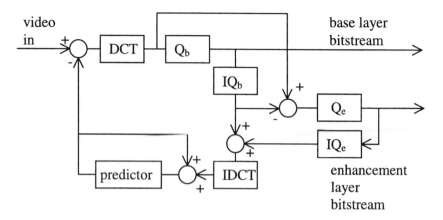

Figure 7.10   A two-layer SNR scalable encoder with drift at the base layer.

both layers and the channel buffer have been omitted for simplicity. In the figure Q_b and Q_e are the base and the enhancement layer quantization step sizes,
respectively. The quantization distortion of the base layer is requantized with
a finer precision $Q_e < Q_b$, and after the inverse quantization is fed back to the
prediction loop, to represent the coding loop of the enhancement layer. Now
compared to data partitioning, this encoder requires only a second quantizer,
an inverse quantizer, and two adders, and the complexity is not extremely
great.

  Note the tight coupling between the two layer bitstreams. For freedom
from drift in the enhanced picture, both bitstreams should be made available to
the decoder. For this reason, this type of encoder is called an SNR scalable encoder with no drift in the enhancement layer. If the base layer bitstream is decoded by itself, then loss of differential refinement coefficients will cause the
decoded picture in this layer to suffer from picture drift. Again, the drift only appears in P and B pictures; I pictures reset the distortion and drift is cleaned up.

  For applications characterized by the occasional loss of information in the
enhancement layer, parts of the picture have base layer quality, and other parts
the quality of the enhancement layer. Therefore picture drift can be noticed in
these areas.

  If drift-free pictures are required at both layers, the coupling between the
two layers must be loosened. Applications such as simulcasting of video with
two different qualities entail such a requirement. One way to prevent picture
drift is not to feed back the enhancement data into the base layer prediction
loop. In this case the enhancement layer will be intra-coded, resulting in a very
high bit rate.

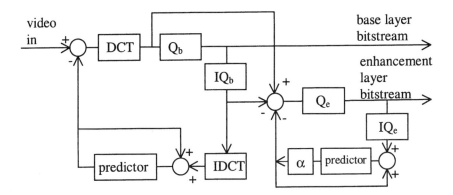

Figure 7.11 A two-layer SNR scalable encoder with no drift at the base and enhancement layers.

    To reduce the second-layer bit rate, the difference between the input to and the output of the base layer (see Figure 7.8) can be coded by another encoder (e.g., H.261) (16). However, here we need two codecs, and the situation is much more complex than data partitioning. To reduce the complexity, we need to code only the quantization distortion. One method is to use a leaky prediction in the enhancement layer prediction loop, as shown in Figure 7.11.

    In this case the prediction in the second layer would be a proportion: (α) for the interframe loop and ($1 - \alpha$) from the intraframe. Our investigations with H.261-type two-layer coding have shown that optimum bit rate versus picture drift can be achieved for $\alpha = 0.9$–0.95 (16). Now, since data in the prediction loop are the transform coefficient quantization distortions, motion compensation must be performed in the frequency domain (17).

    Note that even if these methods of coding can reduce the second-layer bit rate, coding of the base layer is still not as efficient as it would be if both layers were fed to the coding loop. For this reason, this type of encoder is not part of the SNR scalability in the MPEG-2 standard. The standard recommends only the SNR scalability that is compatible with Figure 7.10. Thus picture drift at the base layer is expected to be reduced by more frequent I pictures, which reset the drift. In fact, in practice this is the case, where for most MPEG-2 applications, an I picture is transmitted every half-second. Thus this negligible drift, combined with the normally lower quality base layer pictures, is not very disturbing at all.

    Coarser quantization at the base layer means that some parts of the picture are blocky, as was the case in data partitioning. However, since any significant coefficient can be included at the base layer, the base layer picture of this encoder, unlike that of data partitioning, does not suffer from loss of high-frequency information. Experimental results show that picture quality of the base layer of SNR scalable coder is much superior to that of data partitioning, especially at lower bit rates (18). This is because, at lower base layer bit rates, data partitioning can retain only DC and possibly one or two AC coefficients. Reconstructed pictures with so few coefficients are very blocky.

7.3.3 Spatial Scalability

Spatial scalability involves generating two spatial resolution video streams from a single video source such that the base layer is coded by itself to provide the basic spatial resolution and the enhancement layer employs the spatially interpolated base layer as prediction to code the full spatial resolution of the input video source (19). The base and the enhancement layers may use either both the coding tools in the MPEG-2 standard or the MPEG-1 standard for the base layer and MPEG-2 for the enhancement layer, or even an H.261 encoder at the base layer and MPEG-2 encoder at the second layer. However, although these types of layering are theoretically possible, there are some practical constraints in their usage. For example, MPEG-1 is normally used with noninterlaced video, while in MPEG-2 video is interlaced with several modes of motion prediction. Similarly, in H.261 motion vectors not only are not defined for noninterlaced video, but they also take integer values (20). Hence in practice both layers should be MPEG-2 compatible. Such compatibility also provides some common operations between the two layers, simplifying the encoder (similar to the SNR scalable encoder).

Use of MPEG-2 for both layers achieves a further advantage by facilitating interworking between video coding standards. Moreover, spatial scalability offers the flexibility in choice of video formats to be employed in each layer. The base layer can use source input format (SIF) or even lower resolution pictures at 4:2:2, 4:2:0 or 4:1:1 formats, while the second layer can be kept at CCIR-601 with a 4:2:2 format. Like the other two scalable coders, spatial scalability is able to provide resilience to transmission errors because the more important data of the lower layer can be sent over channels with better error performance, while the less critical enhancement layer data can be sent over a channel with poorer error performance.

Figure 7.12 shows a block diagram of a two-layer spatial scalable encoder. An incoming video is first spatially reduced in both the horizontal and vertical directions to produce a reduced picture resolution. For 2:1 reduction, normally a CCIR-601 video is converted into an SIF image format (21). This requires lowpass filtering of the input images and then selecting alternate pixels in the horizontal and vertical directions of the scanning line. The filters for the luminance and chrominance color components are the 7- and 4-tap filters, respectively. The

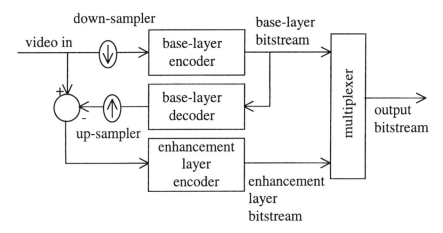

Figure 7.12   Block diagram of a two-layer spatial scalable encoder.

SIF image sequence is coded at the base layer by an MPEG-1 or MPEG-2 standard encoder, generating the base layer bitstream. The bitstream is decoded and upsampled to produce an enlarged version of the base layer decoded video at CCIR-601 resolution. The upsampling is carried out by inserting zero-level samples between the luminance and chrominance pixels, and interpolating with the 7- and 4-tap filters (21). An MPEG-2 encoder at the enhancement layer codes the difference between the input video and the interpolated video from the base layer. Finally, the base and enhancement layer bitstreams are multiplexed for transmission into the channel.

If the base and the enhancement layer encoders are of the same type (e.g., both MPEG-2), they can interact. This is not only to simplify the two-layer encoder, as was the case for SNR scalable encoder, but also to make the coding more efficient. Consider a macroblock at the base layer. Because of the 2:1 picture resolution between the enhancement layer and the base layer, the base layer macroblock corresponds to four macroblocks at the enhancement layer. Similarly, a macroblock at the enhancement layer corresponds to a block of 8×8 pixels at the base layer. The interaction would be in the form of upsampling the base layer block 8×8 pixels into a macroblock of 16×16 pixels, and using it as a part of the prediction in the enhancement layer coding loop.

Figure 7.13 shows a block of 8×8 pixels from the base layer that is upsampled and combined with the prediction of the enhancement layer to form the final prediction for a macroblock at the enhancement layer. In the figure the base layer upsampled macroblock is weighted by w and that of the enhancement layer by $1 - w$. More details of the spatial scalable encoder are shown in Figure 7.14.

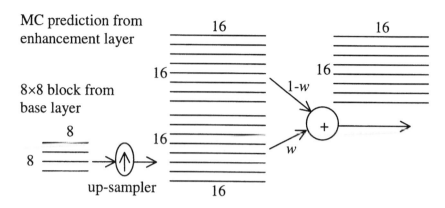

Figure 7.13   Principle of spatiotemporal prediction in the spatial scalable encoder.

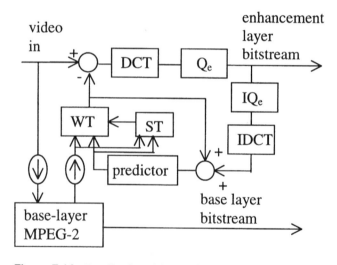

Figure 7.14   Details of spatial scalability encoder.

The base layer is a nonscalable MPEG-2 encoder, where each block of this encoder is upsampled, interpolated, and fed to a *weighting table* (WT). The coding elements of the enhancement layer are shown without the motion compensation, variable-length code and the other coding tools of the MPEG-2 standard. A *statistical table* (ST) sets the weighting table elements. Note that the weighted base layer macroblocks are used in the prediction loop, which will be subtracted from the input macroblocks. This part is similar to taking the difference between the input and the decoded base layer video and coding their differences by a second layer encoder, as illustrated in the general block diagram of this encoder (Figure 7.12).

Note that since in spatial scalability picture size is one quarter the original size, the almost one-quarter of the bit rate allocated to the base layer would be sufficient to code the base layer pictures at almost identical quality to the base plus the enhancement layer. Upon comparing the base layer picture quality of this method with that of data-partitioning and SNR scalable coders, it can be understood that the base layer picture is almost free from blockiness, but still some of very high frequency information is missing. Note that the base layer picture can be used alone without picture drift. This was not the case for the data-partitioning and SNR scalable encoders. However, the price paid is that this encoder is made up of two MPEG-2 encoders and is more complex than the data-partitioning and SNR scalable encoders. A similar complexity ratio can be expected from respective decoders.

7.3.4 Temporal Scalability

Temporal scalability is a tool intended for use in a range of diverse video applications from telecommunications to HDTV. In such systems, migration to higher temporal resolution systems from lower temporal resolution systems may be necessary. In many cases, the lower temporal resolution video systems are either the existing systems or less expensive early-generation systems. The more sophisticated systems may be introduced gradually.

Temporal scalability involves partitioning of input video frames into layers, in which the base layer is coded by itself to provide the basic temporal rate and the enhancement layer is coded with temporal prediction with respect to the base layer. The layers may have either the same or different temporal resolutions, which, when combined, provide full temporal resolution at the decoder. The spatial resolution of frames in each layer is assumed to be identical to that of the input video. The video encoders of the two layers may not be identical. The lower temporal resolution systems may decode only the base layer to provide basic temporal resolution, whereas more sophisticated systems of the future may decode both layers and provide high temporal resolution video while maintaining interworking capability with earlier generation systems.

Since in temporal scalability the input video frames are simply partitioned between the base and the enhancement layer encoders, the encoder need not be more complex than a single-layer encoder. For example, a single-layer encoder may be switched between the two base and enhancement modes to generate the base and the enhancement bitstreams alternately. Similarly a decoder can be reconfigured to decode the two bitstreams alternately. In fact the B pictures in MPEG-1 and MPEG-2 provide a very simple temporal scalability that permits encoding and decoding alongside the anchor I and P pictures within a single codec. I and P pictures are regarded as the base layer, and the B pictures become the enhancement layer. Decoding of I and P pictures alone will result in the base pictures with low temporal resolution, and when added to the decoded B pictures, the temporal resolution is enhanced to its full size. Note that since the enhancement data do not affect the base layer prediction loop, both the base and the enhanced pictures are free from picture drift.

In Figure 7.15, the block diagram of a two-layer temporal scalable encoder is shown. A temporal demultiplexer (demux) partitions the input video into the base and enhancement layers input pictures. For a 2:1 temporal scalability as shown, the odd-numbered pictures are fed to the base layer encoder and the even-numbered pictures become inputs to the second-layer encoder. The encoder at the base layer is a normal MPEG-1, MPEG2, or any other encoder. Again for greater interaction between the two layers, either to simplify encoding or to make it more efficient, both layers may employ the same type of coding scheme.

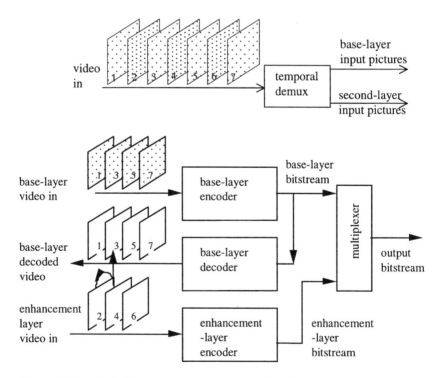

Figure 7.15   Block diagram of a two-layer temporal scalable encoder.

At the base layer, the lower temporal resolution input pictures are encoded in the normal way. Since these pictures can be decoded independently of the enhancement layer, they do not suffer from picture drift. The second layer may use predictions from the base layer pictures, or from its own picture, as shown for frame 4 in the figure. Note that at the base layer, some pictures might be coded as B pictures, using their own previous, future, or interpolated values as predictions, but it is essential that some pictures be coded as anchor pictures. On the other hand, in the enhancement layer, pictures can be coded at any mode. Of course, for greater compression, at the enhancement layer, most if not all the pictures are coded as B pictures. These B pictures have the choice of using past, future, or their interpolated values, from either the base or the enhancement layer.

7.3.5 Hybrid Scalability

Scalable encoders are allowed to combine individual scalabilities such as spatial, SNR, or temporal scalability to form hybrid scalability for certain applications. If two scalabilities are combined, then three layers are generated: the base layer, *enhancement layer* 1 and *enhancement layer* 2. Since enhancement layer 1 is a lower layer relative to the enhancement layer 2, decoding of enhancement layer 2 requires the availability of enhancement layer 1. Some examples of hybrid scalability follow.

7.3.5.1 Spatial and Temporal Hybrid Scalability.
This is perhaps the most common use of hybrid scalability. In this mode the three-layer bitstreams are formed by using spatial scalability between the base layer and enhancement layer 1, while temporal scalability is used between enhancement layer 2 and the combined base layer and enhancement layer 1, as shown in Figure 7.16.

In Figure 7.16, the input video is temporally partitioned into two lower temporal resolution image sequences, In-1 and In-2. The image sequence In-1 is fed to the spatial scalable encoder, where its reduced version, In-0, is the input to the base layer encoder. The spatial encoder then generates two bitstreams, for the base layer and enhancement layer-1. The In-2 image sequence is fed to the temporal enhancement encoder to generate the third bitstream, enhancement layer 2. The temporal enhancement encoder can use the locally decoded pictures of spatial scalable encoder as predictions, as explained in Section 7.3.4.

7.3.5.2 SNR and Spatial Hybrid Scalability.
Figure 7.17 shows a three-layer hybrid encoder employing SNR scalability and spatial scalability. In this coder the SNR scalability is used between the base layer and enhancement layer 1, and the spatial scalability is used between layer 2 and the combination of the base layer and enhancement layer 1. The input video is spatially down-sampled (reduced) to lower resolution as In-1 to be fed to the SNR scalable encoder. The

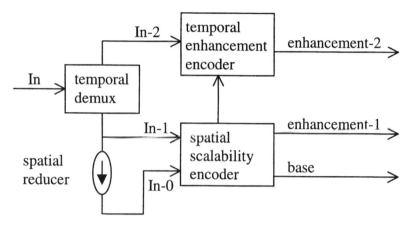

Figure 7.16   Spatial and temporal hybrid scalability encoder.

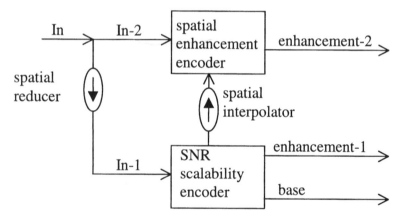

Figure 7.17   SNR and spatial hybrid scalability encoder.

output of this encoder forms the bitstreams of the base layer and enhancement layer 1. The locally decoded pictures from the SNR scalable coder are upsampled to the full resolution to form predictions for the spatial enhancement encoder.

7.3.5.3 SNR and Temporal Hybrid Scalability.   Figure 7.18 shows an example of an SNR–temporal hybrid scalability encoder. The SNR scalability is performed between the base layer and the first enhancement layer. The temporal scalability is used between the second enhancement layer and the locally de-

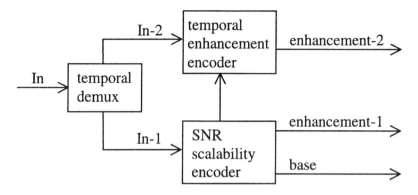

Figure 7.18   SNR and temporal hybrid scalability encoder.

coded picture of the SNR scalable coder. The input image sequence through a temporal demultiplexer is partitioned into two sets of image sequences, which are fed to each individual encoder.

7.3.5.4   SNR, Spatial and Temporal Hybrid Scalability Encoder.

Three scalable encoders might be combined to form a hybrid coder with a larger number of levels. Figure 7.19 shows an example of four levels of scalability, using all the three scalability tools mentioned.

The temporal demultiplexer partions the input video into image sequences In-1 and In-2. Image sequence In-2 is coded at the highest enhancement layer (enhancement-3), with prediction from the lower levels. The image sequence In-1 is first down-sampled to produce a lower resolution image sequence, In-0. This sequence is then SNR scalable coded, to provide the bitstreams for the base layer and the first enhancement layer. An upsampled and interpolated version of the SNR scalable decoded video forms the prediction for the spatial enhancement encoder. The output of this encoder results in the second enhancement layer bitstream (enhancement-2).

Figure 7.19 is just an example of how various scalablity tools can be combined to produce bitstreams of various degrees of importance. Of course depending on the application, the formation of the base and the level of the hierarchy of the higher enhancement layers might be defined in a different way to suit the application. For example, when the foregoing scalability methods are applied to each of the I, P, and B pictures, since these pictures have different levels of importance, their layered versions could increase the number of layers even further. Section 7.3.7 describes various applications of the basic scalability.

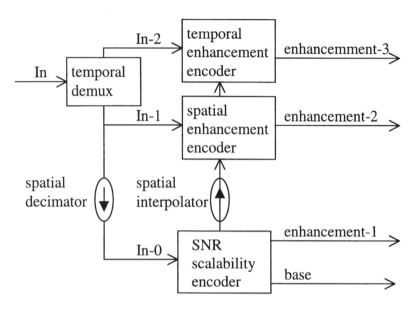

Figure 7.19   SNR, spatial, and temporal hybrid scalability encoder.

7.3.6   Scalability in the H.263+ Codec

H.263+ also supports temporal, SNR, and spatial scalability. This mode is normally used in conjunction with the error control scheme. The capability of this mode and the extent to which its features are supported is signaled by external means such as H.245 (22).

Details of the basic and multilayer scalabilities were given above. Owing to differences in the nature and application of H.263 and MPEG-2, however, there are some differences in the formation of scalability between the two standards.

The main difference between the MPEG-2 and H.263+ that might affect the scalability is the existence of a new type of picture, known as a composite PB-frames picture. This picture consists of a pair of P and B pictures, which are coded as *one* unit. The P part of the picture is predicted from the last decoded P picture and the B part is bidirectionally predicted from the last decoded P picture and the P picture currently being decoded. In an improved version of this optional PB-frames mode, a B macroblock in addition to the bidirectional prediction may have a separate forward or backward prediction (4).

There are three types of enhancement picture in the H.263+ codec, B, EI, and EP pictures (4). Each of these has an *enhancement layer number*, ELNUM, that indicates the layer to which it belongs, and a *reference layer number*, RLNUM, that indicates the layer used for its prediction. The encoder may use either its basic scalability of temporal, SNR, and spatial, or combinations of these in a multilayer scalability mode.

7.3.6.1 Temporal Scalability.
Temporal scalability is achieved by using bidirectionally predicted pictures or B pictures. As usual, B pictures use prediction from either a previous or a subsequent reconstructed picture, or both, in the reference layer. These B pictures differ from the B-picture part of PB or improved PB frames in that they are separate entities in the bitstream. They are not syntactically intermixed with a subsequent P or its enhancement part EP.

B pictures and the B part of PB or improved PB frames are not used as reference pictures for the prediction of any other pictures. This property allows for B pictures to be discarded if necessary without adversely affecting any subsequent pictures, thus providing temporal scalability. There is no limit to the number of B pictures that can be inserted between the pairs of reference pictures in the base layer. A maximum number of such pictures may be signaled by external means (e.g., H.245). However, since H.263 is normally used for low frame rate applications (low bit rates, e.g., mobile), the larger separation between the base layer I and P pictures, means that there is normally one B picture between them. Figure 7.20 shows the position of base layer I and P pictures and the B pictures of the enhancement layer for most applications.

7.3.6.2 SNR Scalability.
In SNR scalability, similar to MPEG-2, the difference between the input picture and the lower quality base layer picture is coded. The picture in the base layer that is used for the prediction of the enhancement layer pictures may be an I picture, a P picture, or the P part of PB or improved PB frames, but not be a B picture or the B part of a PB frame or its improved version.

In the enhancement layer, two types of picture are identified, EI and EP. If prediction is formed from the base layer only, the enhancement layer picture is referred to an EI picture. In this case the base layer picture can be an I or a P picture (or the P part of a PB frame). It is possible, however, to create a modified bidirec-

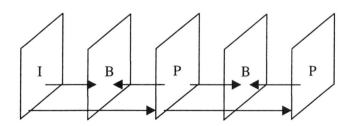

Figure 7.20   B-picture prediction dependency in temporal scalability.

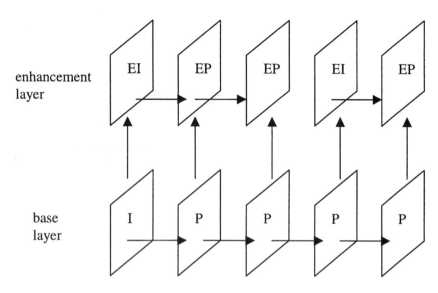

Figure 7.21   Prediction flow in SNR scalability.

tionally predicted picture by using both a prior enhancement layer picture and a temporally simultaneous base layer reference picture. This type of picture is referred to as an EP picture or "enhancement" P picture. Figure 7.21 shows the positions of the base and enhancement layer pictures in an SNR scalable coder. The figure also shows the prediction flow for the EI and EP enhancement pictures.

For both EI and EP pictures, the prediction from the reference layer uses no motion vectors. As with normal P pictures, however, EP pictures use motion vectors when predicting from their temporally prior reference picture in the same frame layer.

7.3.6.3   Spatial Scalability.   The arrangement of the enhancement layer pictures in the spatial scalability is similar to that of SNR scalability. The only difference is that before the picture in the reference layer is used to predict the picture in the spatial enhancement layer, it is downsampled by a factor of 2, either horizontally or vertically (1D spatial scalability), or both horizontally and vertically (2D spatial scalability). Figure 7.22 shows the flow of the prediction in the base and enhancement layer pictures of a spatial scalable encoder.

7.3.6.4   Multilayer Scalability.   Undoubtedly multilayer scalability will increase the robustness of H.263+ to channel errors. In the multilayer scable

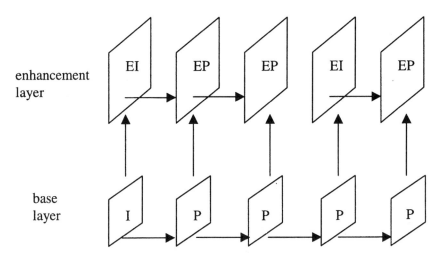

Figure 7.22 Prediction flow in spatial scalability.

mode, it is possible for B pictures to be temporally inserted not only between the base layer pictures of types I, P, PB, and improved PB, but also between enhancement pictures of types EI and EP, whether these consist of SNR or spatial enhancement pictures. It is also possible to have more than one SNR or spatial enhancement layer in conjunction with the base layer. Thus a multi-layer scalable bitstream can be a combination of SNR layers, spatial layers, and B pictures. With increasing of the layer number, the size of a picture cannot decrease. Figure 7.23 illustrates the prediction flow in a multilayer scalable encoder.

As with the two-layer case, B pictures may occur in any layer. However, any picture in an enhancement layer that is temporally simultaneous with a B picture in its reference layer must be a B picture or the B-picture part of a PB or improved PB frame. This is to preserve the disposable nature of B pictures. Note, however, that B pictures may occur in any layers that have no corresponding picture in lower layers. This allows an encoder to send enhancement video with a higher picture rate than the lower layers.

The enhancement layer number and the reference layer number of each enhancement picture (B, EI, or EP) are indicated in the ELNUM and RLNUM fields, respectively, of the picture header (when present). If a B picture appears in an enhancement layer in which temporally surrounding SNR or spatial pictures also appear, the RLNUM of the B picture is the same as the ELNUM. The

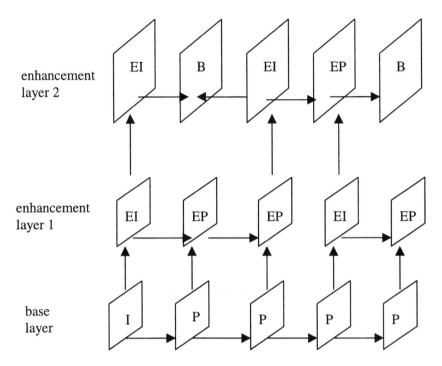

Figure 7.23   Positions of the base layer and enhancement layer pictures in a multilayer scalable bitstream.

picture height, the width, and the pixel aspect ratio of a B picture always equal those of its temporally subsequent reference layer picture.

7.3.6.5   Transmission Order of Pictures.   Pictures, which are dependent on other pictures, are located in the bitstream after the pictures on which they depend. The bitstream syntax order is specified such that for reference pictures (i.e., pictures having types I, P, EI, EP, or the P part of PB or improved PB), the following two rules apply:

1.   All reference pictures with the same temporal reference must appear in the bitstream in increasing enhancement layer order. This is because each lower layer reference picture is needed to decode the next higher layer reference picture.

2.   All temporally simultaneous reference pictures, as discussed in item 1 above, must appear in the bitstream prior to any B pictures for which any one of these reference pictures is the first temporally subsequent

reference picture in the reference layer of the B picture. This reduces the delay of decoding all reference pictures, which may be needed as references for B pictures.

Then, the B pictures with earlier temporal references follow (temporally ordered within each enhancement layer). For each B picture, the bitstream location must comply with the following rules:

1. It must come after that of its first temporally subsequent reference picture in the reference layer. This is because the decoding of a B picture generally depends on the prior decoding of that reference picture.
2. It must come after the bitstream location of all reference pictures that are temporally simultaneous with the first temporally subsequent reference picture in the reference layer. This is to reduce the delay of decoding all reference pictures, which may be needed as references for B pictures.
3. It must precede the location of any additional temporally subsequent pictures other than B pictures in its reference layer. Otherwise, the picture-storage memory requirement for the reference layer pictures would be increased.
4. It must come after the bitstream location of all EI and EP pictures that are temporally simultaneous with the first temporally subsequent reference picture.
5. It must precede the location of all temporally subsequent pictures within the same enhancement layer. Otherwise, needless delay and increased picture-storage memory requirements would be introduced for the enhancement layer.

Figure 7.24 shows two allowable picture transmission orders given by rules 1–5 for the layering structure. The numbers next to each picture indicate the bitstream order, separated by commas for the two alternatives.

7.3.7   Applications of Scalability

Considering the nature of the basic scalability of data-partitioning, SNR, spatial and temporal scalability, and their behavior with regard to picture drift, suitable applications for each method may be summarized in the following terms.

1. *Data partitioning*. This mode is the simplest of all, but since it has poor base layer quality and is sensitive to picture drift, it should be used only in environments that rarely experience any loss of enhancement data (e.g., loss rate $<10^{-5}$). Hence the best application would be video over ATM networks, where through admission control, the loss ratio can be maintained at low levels (23).

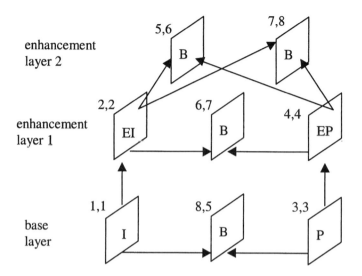

Figure 7.24   Example of picture transmission order.

2. *SNR scalability*. In this method two pictures of the same spatiotemporal resolution are generated, but one has lower picture quality than the
   other. This method has generally higher bit rate than a nonscalable encoder, but it can have good base picture quality and can be drift-free.
   Hence suitable applications include:
   a. Transmission of video at different qualities (e.g., multiquality
      video, video on demand, broadcasting of TV and enhanced TV)
   b. Video over networks with high error or packet loss rates, such as
      the Internet, or heavily congested ATM networks
3. *Spatial scalability*. This is the most complex form of scalability,
   where each layer requires a complete encoder/decoder. Such a loose
   dependency between the layers has the advantage that each layer is
   free to use any codec, with different spatiotemporal and quality resolutions. Hence there can be numerous applications for this mode,
   including:
   a. Interworking between two different standard video codecs (e.g.,
      H.263 and MPEG-2), or heterogeneous data networks
   b. Simulcasting of drift-free, good-quality video at two spatial resolu-
      tions, such as standard TV and HDTV.
   c. Distribution of video over computer networks
   d. Video browsing
   e. Reception of good-quality low spatial resolution pictures over mo-
      bile networks

  f. Similar to other scalable coders, transmission of error-resilient video over packet networks

4. *Temporal scalability.* This is a moderately complex encoder: either a single-layer coder encodes both layers, such as coding of B and the anchor I and P pictures in MPEG-1, MPEG-2, and H.263+, or two separate encoders operating at two different temporal rates. The major applications then can include:

  a. Migration to progressive HDTV from the current interlaced broadcast TV

  b. Internetworking between lower bit rate mobile and higher bit rate fixed networks

  c. Video over LANs, the Internet, and ATM networks for computer workstations

  d. Video over packet (Internet/ATM) networks for loss resilience

7.3.8 Coding Efficiency with Layered Coding

Layered coding schemes inevitably incur a coding penalty in the form of increased bit rate or decreased enhancement layer image quality in comparison to a single-layer coder of equivalent quality. Given comparable enhancement layer qualities, the "cost" in terms of increased total bit rate is the most important aspect of enhancement layer performance. Figure 7.25 illustrates this cost versus the percentage base layer bit rate measured as the percentage increase over the single-layer coder, for a typical video for data-partitioning and SNR scalable encoders. Note the difference in base layer bit-rate ranges, with SNR scalability able to operate between 20 and 70% of the total bit rate and data partitioning (DP) between 30 and 99%.

  Data partitioning incurs only a small increase in bit rate attributable to the duplication of slice header information, alone, resulting in our experiment in a constant 2.3% increase in bitrate over the single-layer coder. For the SNR scalable encoder, best performance is achieved with a 30% base layer bit-rate division, but as the base layer image quality is increased along with its share of the total bit rate, the total bit rate is seen to increase dramatically, culminating in as much as a 12–13% bit-rate increase. In ATM networks such an increase in bit rate can be critical. Under normal network conditions, simulations using two-layer video have shown that a 10% increase in bit rate can lead to a 50-fold increase in cell loss rate, essentially acting as the cause of the very cell losses a two-layer approach is meant to offer protection against (16).

  Similar behaviors from the other two scalable encoders (spatial and temporal) can also be expected. Owing to the duplication of the overhead information in coding of pictures, an increase in bit rate is similar to that found in SNR scalability expected. In temporal scalability, the larger temporal distances between the base layer pictures cause the encoding efficiency to drop, but this can be compensated by a

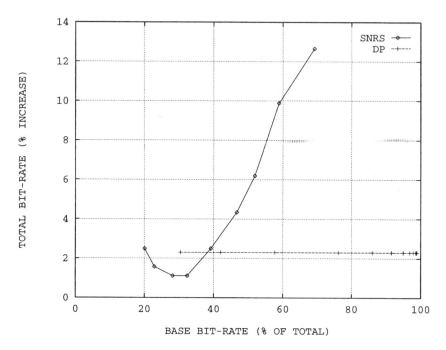

Figure 7.25   Percentage increase of total (base + enhancement) bit rate over equivalent single-layer versus percentage base layer of total bit rate for data-partitioning and SNR scalable coders.

better prediction of the enhancement layer. Overall, similar to the nature of P and B pictures in MPEG–1 and –2, the lower bit rate of the enhancement layer (like B pictures) can compensate for the increase in bit rate of the base layer, and the overall bit rate may not be very different from that of the single-layer encoder.

7.4   LAYERED CODING WITH WAVELETS

Since the introduction of an efficient method for coding of the wavelet transform coefficients by the *embedded zero-tree wavelet* (EZW) (7), there has been a great demand for coding of images with this method. One of the advantages of wavelet over DCT-based codecs is the absence of blocking artifacts. This method of coding has now been accepted for coding of still images in the future image codecs. Codecs such as MPEG-4 in still image mode and the future standard for still image coding (JPEG-2000) will be based on the wavelet transform (5,6).

From the layered coding point of view, the EZW method of coding makes spatial and SNR scalability an inherent part of the coding, as explained in the sections that follow. However, since with wavelet transforms one can generate several layers having various spatial and quality resolutions, the number of data layers can be much higher than what could be achieved with the DCT-based codecs, used in the current standard codecs. This advantage inevitably will increase the potential of wavelet coding for better delivery of images over networks with multipriority systems, such as, the IEEE 802.6 metropolitan area network, known as DQDB (24).

The coding principle is based of the discrete wavelet transform, which is a subclass of *subband coding*. The lowest subband after quantization is coded with a differential pulse code modulation (DPCM) and the higher bands with the *zero-tree* coding technique (7). The quantized DPCM and zero-tree data are then entropy-coded with an arithmetic encoder. Figure 7.26 shows a block diagram of the still image encoder. The sections that follow describe each part of the encoder is described.

7.4.1 Discrete Wavelet Transform

Subband coding/discrete wavelet transform, introduced by Crochiere et al. in 1976 (25), has proved to be a simple and powerful technique for speech and image compression. The basic principle is the partitioning of the signal spectrum into several frequency bands, which are then coded and transmitted separately. This format is particularly suited to image coding. First, natural images tend to have a nonuniform frequency spectrum, with most of the energy concentrated in the lower frequency band. Second, in the human visual system, the noise visibility tends to fall off at both high and low frequencies, and this characteristic enables the designer to adjust the compression distortion according to perceptual criteria. Third, since images are processed in their entirety, not in artificial blocks, there is no block structure distortion in the coded picture, as occurs in the transform-based image encoders.

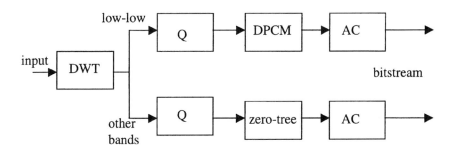

Figure 7.26 Block diagram of a wavelet-based still image encoder.

In subband/wavelet coding, the band splitting is done by passing the image data through a bank of band-pass *analysis filters*, as shown in Figure 7.27. To adapt the frequency response of the decomposed pictures to the characteristics of the human visual system, filters are arranged into octave bands.

Since the bandwidth of each filtered version of the image is reduced, the images can now in theory be downsampled at a lower rate, according to the Nyquist criteria, giving a series of reduced size subimages. The subimages are then quantized, coded, and transmitted. The subimages received are restored to their original sizes and passed through a bank of *synthesis filters*, where they are interpolated and added to reconstruct the image.

In the absence of quantization error, the reconstructed picture must be an exact replica of the input picture. This can be achieved only if the spatial frequency response of the analysis filters *tile* the spectrum without overlapping, which requires infinitely sharp transition regions and cannot be realized practically. Instead, the analysis filter responses have finite transition regions and do overlap, as shown in Figure 7.27, which means that the downsampling/upsampling processes introduce *aliasing* distortion into the reconstructed picture.

To eliminate aliasing distortion, the synthesis and analysis filters must have certain relationships such that the aliased components in the transition regions cancel each other out. To see how such a relation can make alias-free wavelet coding possible, consider a two-band wavelet transform, as shown in Figure 7.28.

The corresponding two-band wavelet transform encoder/decoder is shown in Figure 7.29, where filters $H_0(z)$ and $H_1(z)$ represent the z-transform transfer functions of the respective low-pass and high-pass analysis filters. Filters $G_0(z)$ and $G_1(z)$ are the corresponding synthesis filters. The downsampling factor is 2, and so is the upsampling factor.

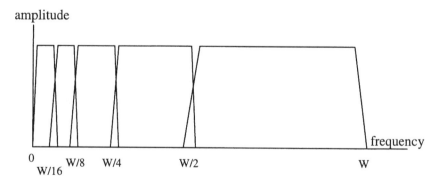

Figure 7.27   Bank of band-pass filters.

amplitude

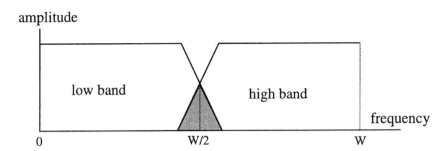

Figure 7.28   Two-band analysis filter.

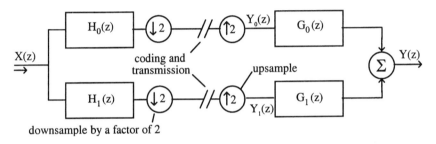

downsample by a factor of 2

Figure 7.29   Two-band wavelet transform encoder/decoder.

At the encoder downsampling by 2 is carried out by discarding alternate samples, the remainder being compressed into half the distance occupied by the original sequence. This is equivalent to compressing the source image by a factor of 2, which doubles all the frequency components present. The frequency domain effect of this downsampling/compression is thus to double the width of all components in the sampled spectrum.

At the decoder, the upsampling is a complementary procedure: it is achieved by inserting a zero-valued sample after each input sample and is equivalent to a spatial expansion of the input sequence. In the frequency domain, the effect is as usual the reverse, and all components are compressed toward zero frequency.

The problem with these operations is the impossibility of constructing ideal, sharp-cut analysis filters. This is illustrated in Figure 7.30a. Spectrum A shows the original sampled signal, which has been low-pass-filtered so that some energy remains above $F_s/4$, the cutoff of the ideal filter for the task. Downsampling compresses the signal and expands to give B, while C is the picture after expansion or upsampling. As well as those at multiples of F_s, this process generates additional spectrum components at odd multiples of $F_s/2$.

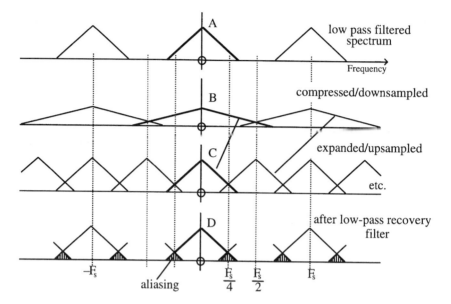

Figure 7.30a Low-pass subband generation and recovery.

These cause aliasing when the final subband recovery takes place, as at D. In the high-pass case (Figure 7.30b), the same phenomena occur, so that on recovery there is aliased energy in the region of $F_s/4$. The final output image is generated by adding the low-pass and high-pass subbands regenerated by the upsamplers and associated filters. The aliased energy would normally be expected to cause interference.

If the phases of the aliased components from the high-pass and low-pass subbands can be made to differ by π, however, cancellation occurs and the recovered signal is alias-free. How this can be arranged is best analyzed by reference to z transforms. Referring to Figure 7.29, after the synthesis filters, the reconstructed output in z-transform notation can be written as follows:

$$Y(z) = G_0(z) \cdot Y_0(z) + G_1(z) \cdot Y_1(z) \tag{13}$$

where $Y_0(z)$ and $Y_1(z)$ are inputs to the synthesis filters after upsampling. Assuming no quantization and transmission errors, the reconstructed samples are given by

$$Y_0(z) = \frac{1}{2}\left[H_0(z) \cdot X(z) + H_0(-z) \cdot X(-z)\right]$$

$$Y_1(z) = \frac{1}{2}\left[H_1(z) \cdot X(z) + H_1(-z) \cdot X(-z)\right] \tag{14}$$

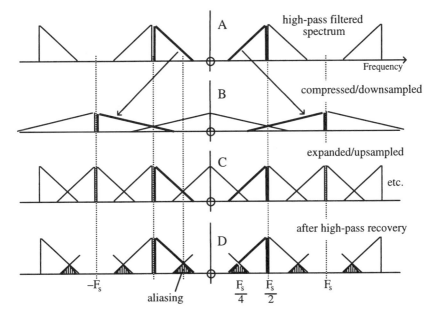

Figure 7.30b High-pass subband generation and recovery.

where the aliasing components from the downsampling of the lower and higher bands are given by $H_0(-z)X(-z)$ and $H_1(-z)X(-z)$, respectively. By substituting these two equations into Eq. (13), we get

$$Y(z) = \frac{1}{2}\left[H_0(z)\cdot G_0(z) + H_1(z)\cdot G_1(z)\right]X(z)$$
$$+\frac{1}{2}\left[H_0(-z)\cdot G_0(z) + H_1(-z)\cdot G_1(z)\right]X(-z)$$

(15)

The first term is the desired reconstructed signal, while the second term is aliased components. The aliased components can be eliminated regardless of the amount of overlap in the analysis filters by defining the synthesis filters as follows:

$$G_0(z) = H_1(-z) \qquad \text{and} \qquad G_1(z) = -H_0(-z)$$

(16)

With such a relation between the synthesis and analysis filters, the reconstructed signal now becomes:

$$Y(z) = \frac{1}{2}\left[H_0(z)\cdot H_1(-z) - H_0(-z)\cdot H_1(z)\right]X(z)$$

(17)

If we define the $P(z) = H_0(z).H_1(-z)$, then the reconstructed signal can be written as follows:

$$Y(z) = \frac{1}{2}[P(z) - P(-z)]X(z) \tag{18}$$

Now the reconstructed signal can be a perfect, but m-sample-delayed, replica of the input signal, if

$$P(z) - P(-z) = 2z^{-m} \tag{19}$$

Thus the z-transform input/output signals are given by

$$Y(z) = z^{-m}X(z) \tag{20}$$

This relation in the pixel domain implies that the reconstructed pixel sequence $\{y(n)\}$ is an exact replica of the delayed input sequence $\{x(n-m)\}$.

In these equations $P(z)$ is called the *product filter* and m is the delay introduced by the filter banks. The design of analysis/synthesis filters is based on factorization of the product filter $P(z)$ into linear phase components $H_0(z)$ and $H_1(-z)$. With the constraint that the difference between the product filter and its image be a simple delay, the product filter must have an odd number of coefficients. Le Gall and Tabatabai (26) have used a product filter $P(z)$ of the kind

$$P(z) = \frac{1}{16}\left(-1 + 9z^{-2} + 16z^{-3} + 9z^{-4} - z^{-6}\right) \tag{21}$$

and by factorizing have obtained several solutions for each pair of the analysis and synthesis filters:

$$H_0(z) = \frac{1}{4}\left(-1 + 3z^{-1} + 3z^{-2} - z^{-3}\right), H_1(-z) = \frac{1}{4}\left(1 + 3z^{-1} + 3z^{-2} + z^{-3}\right)$$

or

$$H_0(z) = \frac{1}{4}\left(1 + 3z^{-1} + 3z^{-2} + z^{-3}\right), H_1(-z) = \frac{1}{4}\left(-1 + 3z^{-1} + 3z^{-2} - z^{-3}\right)$$

or

$$H_0(z) = \frac{1}{8}\left(-1 + 2z^{-1} + 6z^{-2} + 2z^{-3} - z^{-4}\right), H_1(-z) = \frac{1}{2}\left(1 + 2z^{-1} + z^{-2}\right) \tag{22}$$

The synthesis filters $G_0(z)$ and $G_1(z)$ are then derived by using their relations with the analysis filters. Each of the equation pairs above gives the results $P(z) - P(-z) = 2z^{-3}$, which implies that the reconstruction is perfect, with a delay of three samples.

7.4.2 Higher Order Systems

Multidimensional and multiband wavelet coding can be developed from the two-band low-pass and high-pass analysis/synthesis filter structure of Figure 7.29. For example, wavelet coding of a two-dimensional image can be performed by carrying out a one-dimensional decomposition along the lines of the image and then down each column.

A seven-band wavelet transform coding of this type is illustrated in Figure 7.31, where band splitting is carried out alternately in the horizontal and vertical directions. In the figure, L and H represent the low-pass and high-pass filters with a 2:1 downsampling, respectively.

Figure 7.32 shows all seven subimages generated by the encoder of Figure 7.31 for a single frame of the FLOWER GARDEN test sequence, with 5-tap low and 3-tap high pass analysis filter pairs, (5,3), with the filter coefficients of $\{-1, 2, 6, 2, -1\}$ and $\{1,-2,1\}$, as given in Eq. (22).

The dimensions of the original image (not shown) were 352 pixels by 240 lines. Bands 1–4, at two levels of subdivision, are 88×60, while bands 5–7 are 176×120 pixels. In the figure, all bands but band -1 (LL) have been amplified by a factor of 4 and offset by $+128$ to enhance visibility of the low-level details they contain. The scope for bandwidth compression arises mainly from the low energy levels that appear in the high-pass subimages.

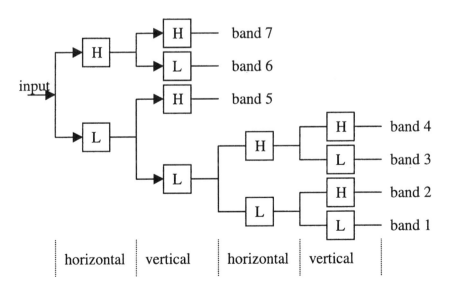

Figure 7.31 Multiband wavelet transform coding by means of repeated two-band splits.

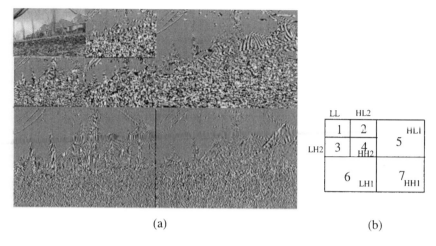

(a)   (b)

Figure 7.32   (a) The seven subimages generated by the encoder of Figure 7.31. (b) Layout of individual bands.

The number of decomposition levels of the luminance is defined by the encoder in the input bitstream. The chrominance components are decomposed to one level less than the luminance components. In MPEG-4 the wavelet decomposition is performed using a Daubechies (9,3) tap biorthogonal filter pair (27), which has been shown to have good compression efficiency. The Daubechies filter coefficients (rounded to three decimal points) are:

Low-pass $=\{0.033, -0.066, -0.177, 0.420, 0.994, 0.420, -0.177, -0.066, 0.033\}$

High-pass $=\{-0.354, 0.707, -0.354\}$ (23)

Since all the input pixels are not available at image borders, a symmetric extension of the input texture is performed before the wavelet transform is applied at each level (28). To satisfy the perfect reconstruction conditions with the Daubechies (9,3) tap analysis filter pairs, two types of symmetric extension are used.

Type –A is only used at the synthesis stage. It is used at the trailing edge of low-pass filtering and the leading edge of high-pass filtering stages. If the pixels at the boundary of the objects are represented by abcde, then the type–A extension becomes; edcba**abcde**, where the letters in bold type are the original pixels and the others are the extended pixels. Note that for a (9,3) analysis filter pairs of Eq. (23), the synthesis filter pairs will be (3,9) with:

$$G_0(z) = H_1(-z) \quad \text{and} \quad G_1(z) = -H_0(-z) \tag{24}$$

Type-B extension is used for both leading and trailing edges of the low- and high-pass analysis filters. For the synthesis filters, it is used at the leading edge of the low pass, but at the trailing edge of the high pass. With this type of extension, the extended pixels at the leading and trailing edges become edcb**labcde** and **abcde**ldcba, respectively.

7.4.3 Coding of the Lowest Band

In still image coding, the wavelet coefficients of the lowest band are coded independently from the other bands. These coefficients are DPCM-coded with a uniform quantizer. The prediction for coding a wavelet coefficient w_x is taken from its neighboring coefficients w_A or w_C, according to

$$w_{prd} = w_C, \quad \text{if } |w_A - w_B| < |w_A - w_C|; \quad \text{otherwise } w_{prd} = w_A. \tag{25}$$

The difference between the actual wavelet coefficient w_x and its predicted value w_{prd} is coded. The positions of the neighboring pixels are shown in Figure 7.33.

The coefficients after DPCM coding are encoded with an adaptive arithmetic coder. First the minimum value of the coefficient in the band is found. This value, known as *band_offset*, is subtracted from all the coefficients to limit their lower bound to zero. The maximum value of the coefficients as *band_max_value* is also calculated. These two values are included in the bitstream.

For adaptive arithmetic coding (29), the arithmetic coder model is initialized at the start of coding with a uniform distribution in the range of 0 to *band_max_value*. Each quantized and DPCM-coded coefficient after arithmetic coding is added to the distribution. Hence, as the encoding progresses, the distribution of the model adapts itself to the distribution of the coded coefficients (adaptive arithmetic coding).

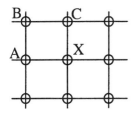

Figure 7.33 Prediction for coding the lowest band coefficients.

7.4.4   Zero-Tree Coding of Higher Bands

For efficient compression of higher bands as well as for a wide range of scalability, the higher order wavelet coefficients are coded with the *embedded zero-tree wavelet* (EZW) algorithm introduced by Shapiro (7). The method is based on the concept of quantization by *successive approximation*, and exploitation of the similarities of bands of the same orientation.

7.4.4.1   Quantization.

Quantization by successive approximation is the representation of a wavelet coefficient value in terms of progressively smaller quantization step sizes. The number of passes of the approximation depends on the desired quantization distortions. To see how successive approximation can lead to quantization, consider Figure 7.34, where a coefficient of length L is successively refined to its final quantized value of $\hat{L}$

The process begins by choosing an initial yardstick length l. The value of l is set to half the largest coefficient in the image. If the coefficient is larger than the yardstick, it is represented with the yardstick value; otherwise its value is set to zero. After each pass the yardstick length is halved and the error magnitude, which is the difference between the original value of the coefficient and its reconstructed value, is compared with the new yardstick. The process is continued, such that the final error is acceptable. Hence increasing the number of passes, the error in the representation of L by $\hat{L}$ can be made arbitrarily small.

With regard to Figure 7.34, the quantized length, $\hat{L}$, can be expressed as follows:

$$\hat{L} = 0 \times l + \left(1 \times \frac{l}{2}\right) + \left(0 \times \frac{l}{4}\right) + \left(0 \times \frac{l}{8}\right) + \left(1 \times \frac{l}{16}\right)\left(1 \times \frac{l}{32}\right) \times \cdots = \frac{l}{2} + \frac{l}{16} + \frac{l}{32} \quad (26)$$

where only yardstick lengths smaller than quantization error are considered. Therefore, given an initial yardstick l, a length L can be represented as a string of "1" and "0" symbols. As each symbol "1" or "0" is added, the precision in the representation of L increases, and thus the distortion level decreases. This process is in fact equivalent to the binary representation of real numbers, called bit-plane representation, where each number is represented by a string of "0s" and "1s." By increasing the number of digits, the error in the representation can be made arbitrarily small. It should be noted that the number of steps in this successive approximation can be made shorter, by approximating them in combined steps of $(\pm^1/_2$ and $(\pm 3^1/_2$. Hence making encoding more efficient. This method is used in the conventional successive approximation methods (see Section 7.4.4.3).

7.4.4.2   Similarities Among the Bands.

A two-stage wavelet transform (seven bands) of the FLOWER GARDEN image sequence, with the position of the bands, was shown in Figure 7.32. It can be seen that the vertical bands look like scaled versions of each other, as do the horizontal and diagonal bands. Of partic-

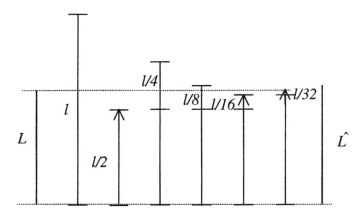

Figure 7.34 Principles of successive approximation.

ular interest in these subimages is the tendency of the nonsignificant coefficients from bands of the same orientation to be in the same corresponding locations. Also, the edges are approximately at the same corresponding positions. Considering that subimages of lower bands (higher stages of decomposition) have quarter-dimensions of their higher bands, one can make a quad-tree representation of the bands of the same orientation, as shown in Figure 7.35 for a 10-band (three-stage) wavelet transform.

In Figure 7.35, a coefficient in the lowest vertical band, LH_3, corresponds to 4 coefficients of its immediate higher band LH_2, of which relates to 16 coefficients in LH_1. Thus, if a coefficient in LH_3 is zero, it is more likely that its children in the higher bands of LH_2 and LH_1 will also be zero. The same is true for the other horizontal and diagonal bands. This tree of zeros, called a *zero tree*, is an efficient way of representing a large group of zeros of the wavelet coefficients. Here, the root of the zero tree is required to be identified, and then the descendant children in the higher bands can be ignored.

7.4.4.3 Embedded Zero-Tree Wavelet (EZW) Algorithm.

The combination of the zero-tree roots with successive approximation has opened up a very interesting coding tool for not only efficient compression of wavelet coefficients, but also as a means for spatial and SNR scalability (7,30). According to Shapiro (7), encoding algorithm, with slight modification on the successive approximation to ensure efficient coding, is described as follows:

1. The image mean is computed and extracted from the image. This depends on how the lowest band LL is coded. If it is coded independently of other bands, as with DPCM in MPEG-4, this stage can be ignored.

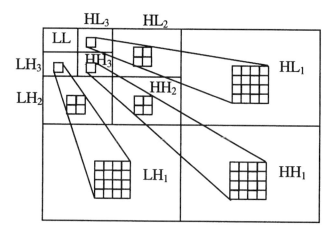

Figure 7.35   Quad-tree representation of bands of the same orientation.

2. An R stage ($3R + 1$ band) wavelet transform is applied to the (zero-mean) image.

3. The initial yardstick length l is set to half the maximum absolute value of the wavelet coefficients.

4. A list of the coordinates of the coefficients, called the *dominant list*, is generated. This list determines the order in which the coefficients are scanned. It must be such that coefficients from a lower frequency band (higher scale) are always scanned before the ones from higher frequency band. Two empty lists of coefficients coordinates, the *subordinate list* and the *temporary list*, are also created.

5. The wavelet transform of the image is scanned, and if, a wavelet coefficient is smaller than the current yardstick length l, it is reconstructed to zero. Otherwise, it is reconstructed as ($\pm 3^{l}/_{2}$, according to its sign.

6. Dominant pass. The reconstructed coefficients are scanned again, according to the order in the dominant list, generating a string of symbols as follows: if a reconstructed coefficient is positive or negative, a "+" or a "–" is added to the string, and the coordinates of this coefficient are appended to the subordinate list. If a reconstructed coefficient is zero, its coordinates are appended to the temporary list. In the case of a zero-valued reconstructed coefficient, two different symbols can be appended to the string; if all its corresponding coefficients in bands of the same orientation and higher frequencies are zero, a *zero-tree root* (ZT) is added to the string, and its corresponding coefficients are removed from the dominant list and added to the temporary list (since they are already known to be zero, they do not need to be scanned again). Otherwise, an *isolated*

zero (Z) is added to the string. The string generated from the four symbol alphabet of "+", "–", "ZT" and "Z" is encoded with an adaptive arithmetic encoder (29]) whose model is updated to four symbols at the beginning of this pass. However, during the scanning of the highest horizontal, vertical, and diagonal frequency bands (HL_1, LH_1, and HH_1 of Figure 7.35), no zero-tree roots can be generated. Therefore, just before, in the scanning of the first coefficient of these bands, the model of the arithmetic coder is updated to three symbols: "+", "–", and "Z."

7. The yardstick length l is halved.
8. Subordinate pass. The coefficients that have not yet been reconstructed as zero are scanned again to the order in the subordinate list, and each one has added either $+l/_2$ or $-l/_2$ to it to minimize the magnitude of its reconstruction error. If $l/_2$ is added, a "+" is appended to the string, and if $l/_2$ is subtracted, a "–" is appended. At the end of the subordinate pass the subordinate list is reordered so that the coefficients whose reconstructed values have higher magnitudes come first. The "+" and "–" symbols of this pass are encoded with the arithmetic coder, which had its model updated to two symbols ("+" and "–") at the beginning of this pass.
9. The dominant list is replaced by the temporary list, and the temporary list is emptied.
10. The whole process is repeated from step 5. It stops at any point at which the size of bitstream exceeds the desired bit rate budget.

In the dominant pass (step 6), only the reconstructed values of the coefficients that are still in the dominant list can be affected. Therefore, to increase the number of zero-tree roots, the coefficients not in the dominant list can be considered to be zero for the purpose of determining whether the zero-valued coefficient is a zero-tree root or an isolated zero.

The bitstream includes a header with extra information to the decoder. The header contains the number of wavelet transform stages, the image dimensions, the initial value of the yardstick length, and the image mean. Both the encoder and the decoder initially have identical dominant lists. As the bitstream is decoded, the decoder updates the reconstructed image, as well as its subordinate and temporary lists. In this way, it can exactly track the stages of the encoder and can therefore properly decode the bitstream. It is important to observe that the ordering of the subordinate list in step 8 is carried out based only on the reconstructed coefficient values, which are available to the decoder. If it was not so, the decoder would not be able to track the encoder, and thus the bitstream would not be properly decoded.

7.4.4.4 Analysis of the algorithm.
The algorithm above has many interesting features, which make it especially significant to note. Among them one can include the following points.

1. The use of zero trees, which exploit similarities among the bands of the same orientation, reduces the number of symbols to be coded.

2. The use of a very small alphabet to represent an image (maximum number of four symbols) makes adaptive arithmetic coding very efficient because such coding adapts itself very quickly to any changes in the statistics of the symbols.

3. Since the maximum distortion level of a coefficient at any stage is bounded by the current yardstick length, the average distortion level in each pass is also given by the current yardstick, being the same for all bands.

4. At any given pass, only the coefficients with magnitudes larger than the current yardstick length are encoded nonzero. Therefore, the coefficients with higher magnitudes tend to be encoded before the ones with smaller magnitudes. This implies that the EZW algorithm tends to give priority to the most important information in the encoding process, aided by the ordering of the subordinate in step 8. Thus for the given bit rate, the bits are spent where they are needed most.

5. Since the EZW algorithm employs a successive approximation process, the addition of a new symbol ("+," "–," "ZT" and "Z") to the string just further refines the reconstructed image. Furthermore, while each symbol is being added to the string, it is encoded into the bitstream; hence the encoding and decoding can stop at any point, and an image with a level of refinement corresponding to the symbols encoded/decoded so far can be recovered. Therefore, the encoding and decoding of an image can stop when the bit-rate budget is exhausted, which makes possible an extremely precise bit-rate control. In addition, owing to the prioritization of the more important information mentioned in item (4), no matter where in the bitstream the decoding is stopped, the best possible image quality for that bit rate is achieved.

6. *Spatial/SNR scalability.* To achieve both spatial and SNR scalability, two different scanning methods are employed. For spatial scalability, the wavelet coefficients are scanned in subband-by-subband fashion, from the lowest to the highest frequency subbands. For SNR scalability, the wavelet coefficients are scanned in each tree from the top to the bottom. The scanning method is defined in the bitstream.

7.4.5 Video Coding with the Wavelet Transform

The success of the zero-tree approach in the efficient coding of wavelet transform coefficients has encouraged researchers to use it for video coding. Although wavelet-based video coding is not part of the standard, here we show how the embedded zero-tree wavelet tool can be employed in video coding. The advantages are particularly significant if multiple spatio-SNR scalable video bitstreams are required.

Figure 7.36 shows a block diagram of a video codec based on wavelet transform. Each frame of the input video is transformed into n-band wavelet subbands. The lowest *LL* band is fed into a DCT-based video encoder, such as MPEG-1. The other bands undergo hierarchical motion compensation. First, the three high-frequency bands of the last stage are motion-compensated by means of the motion vectors from MPEG-1. The reconstructed picture from these four bands (*LL*, *LH*, *HL* and *HH*), which is the next-level *LL* band, requires only a ±1 pixel refinement (31). The other three bands at this stage are also motion-compensated by the same amount. This process is continued for all the bands. Hence, at the end, all the bands are motion-compensated. Now, these motion-compensated bands are coded with the EZW method.

For video networking in an environment supporting a multipriority system, the output of the MPEG-1 coded bitstream comprises the base layer data. That of the EZW is divided into layers of enhancement data of varying significance. For SNR scalability, the order of significance will be from earlier stages of successive quantization toward the finer step sizes. For spatial scalability, this will be from the root of the tree toward the children. As the network resources become more scarce, the less significant enhancement data will give their share of bandwidth to the more important ones.

It should be noted that since block-based motion compensation is used in Figure 7.36, the blocking artifacts may not be as well coded by wavelets as are natural images (32). For this type of codec, overlapped motion compensation, which smooths block edges, has proven to be much better (33).

7.4.5.1 Virtual Zero Tree (VZT).
Some problems are encountered when the EZW is used for video coding, with lowest band to be coded with an standard codec. First, the subband decomposition stops when the top-level *LL* band reaches a size of SIF/QSIF or sub-QSIF. At these levels there will be too many clustered zero-tree roots. This is very common for static parts of the pictures and

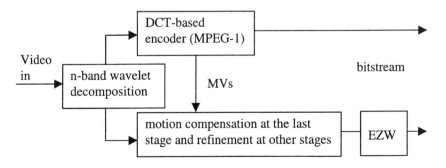

Figure 7.36 Hybrid MPEG/wavelet video coding scheme.

when motion compensation is very efficient. Even for still images or I pictures, a large part of the picture may contain only low spatial frequency information. As a result, at the early stages of quantization by successive approximation, when the yardstick is large, a vast majority of the wavelet coefficients fall below the yardstick. Second, even if the subband decomposition is taken to more stages, such that the top stage LL is a small picture of 16×16 pixels, it is unlikely that many zero trees can be generated. Hence the efficiency of EZW is greatly reduced.

To improve the efficiency of EZW, we have devised a version of it called *virtual zero tree* (VZT) (34). The idea is to build trees outside the image boundary, hence the word *virtual*, as an extension to the existing trees that have roots in the top stage, so that the significant map can be represented in a more efficient way. It can be imagined as replacing the top-level LL band with zero-value coefficients. These coefficients represent the roots of wavelet trees of several virtual subimages in normal EZW coding, although no decomposition and decimation actually takes place, as demonstrated in Figure 7.37.

In Figure 7.37, virtual trees, or a virtual map, are built in the virtual subbands on the high-frequency bands of the highest stage. Several wavelet coefficients of the highest stage form a virtual node at the bottom level of the virtual map. Then in the virtual map, four nodes of a lower level are represented by one node of a higher level, just as a zero tree is formed in EZW coding. The virtual map has only two symbols; *VZT root* and *non-VZT root*. If all four nodes of a 2×2 block on any level of a virtual tree are VZT roots, the corresponding node on the higher level will also be a VZT root. Otherwise this one node of the higher level will be a non-VZT node. This effectively constructs a long rooted tree of a clustered real zero trees. One node on the bottom level of the virtual map is a VZT root only when the four luminance coefficients of a 2×2 block and their two corresponding chrominance coefficients on the top-stage wavelet band are all zero tree roots. Chrominance pictures are also wavelet-decomposed, and for a 4:2:0 image format, four zero-tree roots of the luminance and one from each chrominance can be made a composite zerotree root (34).

It appears at first that by creating virtual nodes, we have increased the number of symbols to be coded, hence the bit rate will increase rather than decrease. However, these virtual roots will cluster the zero-tree roots into a bigger zero-tree root, such that instead of coding these roots one by one, at the expense of a large overhead by a simple EZW, we can code the whole cluster by a single VZT with only a few bits. VZT is more powerful at the early stages of encoding, where the vast majority of top-stage coefficients are zero-tree roots. This can be seen from Table 7.2, which gives a complete breakdown of the total bit rate required to code a P picture of the PARK SEQUENCE by both methods. The sequence

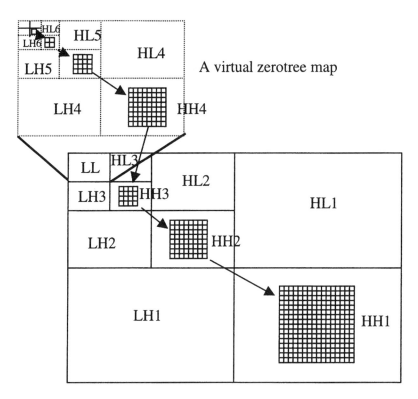

A virtual zerotree map

Figure 7.37 Virtual zero tree.

has a superhigh definition (SHD) quality [2048 × 2048 pixels at 60 Hz, courtesy of NHK Japan, (31)].

The SHD images after three-stage subband decomposition result in 10 bands. The *LL* band, with a picture resolution of 256 × 256 pixels, is MPEG-1 coded; the remaining nine bands are VZT- and EZW-coded in two separate experiments. The first row of the table shows that 171 kbit is used to code the *LL* band by MPEG-1. The second row shows that 15 kbit is used for the additional ±1 pixel refinement in all bands. For the higher bands, the image is scanned in five passes, where the bits used in the dominant and subordinate passes of VZT and EZW are shown. In VZT the dominant pass is made up of two parts: the one used in coding the virtual nodes and the other parts for real data in the actual nine bands. Note that although some bits are used to code the virtual nodes (i.e., nodes that do not exist in EZW), the total number of bits of the dominant pass in VZT is much lower than for EZW. The number of bits in the subordi-

Table 7.2   Comparison of VZT and EZW Coding Schemes

	VZT (kbit)					EZW (kbit)		
	Virtual pass	Real pass	Dominant pass	Subordinate pass	Sum	Dominant pass	Subordinate pass	Sum
MPEG	—	—	—	—	171	—	—	171
MV	—	—	—	—	15	—	—	15
Pass 1	1.5	3.2	4.4	0.16	4.9	25	0.16	25
Pass 2	7.7	31	39	1.7	41	153	1.7	156
Pass 3	18	146	164	11	175	465	11	476
Pass 4	29	371	400	41	441	835	41	896
Pass 5	42	880	992	128	1050	1397	128	1326
Grand total					1898			3265

nate passes, which code the real subordinate data, is the same for both methods. In Table 7.2, the grand total is the total bits used to code the P frame under the two coding schemes. It can be seen that VZT requires two-thirds the bit rate required by EZW.

We have also compared VZT against EZW in the coding of high-definition television pictures, using the test sequence GAYNOR courtesy of the British Broadcasting Corportation. For this image sequence, a two-stage (seven-band) wavelet transform is used and the LL band of the SIF size was MPEG-1 coded. Motion-compensated higher bands were coded with VZT and EZW. Our results show that while good-quality video at 18 Mbit/s can be achieved under EZW, the VZT only needs 11 Mbit/s (34).

7.4.6   Set Partitioning in Hierarchical Trees (SPIHT)

The compression efficiency of EZW as well as VZT is to some extent due to the use of arithmetic coding. Said and Pearlman have introduced a variant of coding of wavelet coefficients by successive approximation that even without arithmetic coding outperforms EZW (30). They call it set partitioning in hierarchical trees (SPIHT). The crucial parts of their coding process are the way the subsets of the wavelet coefficients are partitioned and the way the significant information is conveyed.

One of the main features of this scheme involves the way of transmitting the ordering data: it is based on the fact that the execution path of any algorithm is defined by the results of the comparisons of its branching points.

So, if the encoder and decoder have the same sorting algorithm, the decoder can duplicate the encoder's execution path if it receives the results of the magnitude comparisons, and the ordering information can be recovered from the execution path.

The sorting algorithm divides the set of wavelet coefficients $\{C_{i,j}\}$ into partitioning subsets T_m and performs the following magnitude test:

$$\max_{(i,j)_{(i,j)\in T_m}} \left\{ \left| C_{i,j} \right| \right\} \geq 2^n \, ? \tag{27}$$

If the decoder receives a "no" to that question (the subset is insignificant), it knows that all coefficients in T_m are insignificant. If the answer is "yes" (the subset is significant), then a certain rule shared by the encoder and decoder is used to partition T_m on new subset $T_{m,l}$, whereupon the significant test is applied to the new subsets. This set division process continues until the magnitude test has been done to all single-coordinate significant subsets to identify each significant coefficient.

To reduce the number of magnitude comparisons (message bits), a set-partitioning rule that uses an expected ordering in the hierarchy defined by the subband pyramid is defined (similar to Figure 7.35 used in zero-tree coding). In Section 7.4.4.2 we saw how the similarities among the subimages of the same orientation can be exploited to create an special orientation tree. The objective is to create new partitions such that subsets expected to be insignificant contain a huge number of elements and subsets expected to be significant contain only one element.

To make clear the relationship between magnitude comparisons and message bits, the following function is used:

$$S_n(T) = 1, \text{ if } \max_{(i,j)_{(i,j)\in T}} \left\{ \left| C_{(i,j)} \right| \right\} \geq 2^n$$
$$= 0, \text{ otherwise} \tag{28}$$

to indicate the significance of a set of coordinates T. To simplify the notation of single-pixel sets, $S_n(\{(i,j)\})$ is represented as $S_n(i,j)$.

To see how SPHIT can be implemented, let us assume $O(i, j)$ to represent a set of coordinates of all offspring of node (i, j). For instance, except for the highest and lowest pyramid levels, $O(i, j)$ is defined in terms of its offspring as follows:

$$O(i,j) = \{(2i, 2j), (2i, 2j+1), (2i+1, 2j), (2i+1, 2j+1)\} \tag{29}$$

We also define $D(i, j)$ as a set of coordinates of all descendants of the node (i, j), and H, a set of coordinates of all spatial orientation tree roots (nodes in the highest pyramid level). Finally, $L(i, j)$ is defined as follows:

$$L(\text{i}, j) = D(i, j) - O(i, j) \tag{30}$$

With the use of parts of the spatial orientation trees as the partitioning subsets in the sorting algorithm, the setpartitioning rules are defined as follows:

1. The initial partition is formed with the sets $\{(i, j)\}$ and $D(i, j)$, for all (i, j) "member of" $\in$ H.
2. If $D(i, j)$ is significant, it is partitioned into $L(i, j)$ plus the four single-element sets with $(k, l) \in O(i, j)$.
3. If $L(i, j)$ is significant, it is partitioned into the four sets $D(k, l)$, with $(k, l) \in O(i, j)$.
4. Each of the four sets now has the format of the original set, and the same partitioning can be used recursively.

7.4.6.1 Coding Algorithm.
Since the order in which the subsets are tested for significance is important, in a practical implementation the significance information is stored in three ordered lists: the *list of insignificant sets* (LIS), the *list of insignificant pixels* (LIP), and the *list of significant pixels* (LSP). In all lists each entry is identified by a coordinate (i, j), which in the LIP and LSP represents individual pixels, and in the LIS represents either the set $D(i, j)$ or $L(i, j)$. To differentiate between them, it is said that a LIS entry is of type A if it represents $D(i, j)$ and of type B if it represents $L(i, j)$ (30).

During the sorting pass, the pixels in the LIP, which were insignificant in the previous pass, are tested, and those that become significant are moved to the LSP. Similarly, sets are sequentially evaluated following the LIS order, and when a set is found to be significant, it is removed from the list and partitioned. The new subsets with more than one element are added back to the LIS, while the single-coordinate sets are added to the end of the LIP or the LSP depending whether they are insignificant or significant, respectively. The LSP contains the coordinates of the pixels that are visited in the refinement pass.

Thus the algorithm can be summarized as follows:

1. Initialization: Let the initial yardstick, n, be $n = \lfloor \log_2(\max_{(i,j)} \{ |C_{i,j}| \}) \rfloor$. Set the LSP as an empty set list, and add the coordinates $(i, j) \in H$ to the LIP, and only those with descendants also to the LIS, as the type A-entries.
2. Sorting pass
   2.1. For each entry (i, j) in the LIP do:
   2.1.1. output $S_n(i, j)$;

2.1.2. if $S_n(i, j) =1$ then move (i, j) to the LSP and output the sign of $C_{i,j}$;

2.2. For each entry (i, j) in the LIS do:

    2.2.1. if the entry is of type A then

        2.2.1.1. output $S_n(D(i, j))$;

        2.2.1.2. if $S_n(D(i, j)) = 1$ then

            2.2.1.2.1. for each $(k, l) \in O(i, j)$ do:

                2.2.1.2.1.1. output $S_n((k, l)$;

                2.2.1.2.1.2. if $S_n(k, l) =1$, then add (k, l) to the LSP and output the sign of $C_{k,l}$;

                2.2.1.2.1.3. if $S_n(k, l) = O$ then add (k, l) to the end of the LIP;

            2.2.1.2.2. if $L(i, j) \neq \emptyset$, then move (i, j) to the end of the LIS, as an entry of type B, and go to step 2.2.2; otherwise, remove entry (i, j) from the LIS;

    2.2.2. if the entry is of type B then

        2.2.2.1. output $S_n(L(i, j))$;

        2.2.2.2. if $S_n(L(i, j)) = 1$ then

            2.2.2.2.1. add each $(k, l) \in O((i, j)$ to the end of the LIS as an entry of type A;

            2.2.2.2.2. remove (i, j) from the LIS.

3. Refinement pass: for each entry (i, j) in the LSP, except those included in the last sorting pass (i.e., with same n), output the nth most significant bit of $|C_{i,j}|$.

4. Quantization-step update: Decrement n by 1 and go to Step 2.

One important characteristic of the algorithm is that the entries added to the end of the LIS in step 2.2 are evaluated before the same sorting pass ends. So, "for each entry in the LIS", means those that are being added to its end. Also similar to EZW, the rate can be precisely controlled because the transmitted information is formed of single bits. The encoder can estimate the progressive distortion reduction and stop at a desired distortion value.

Note that in this algorithm, all branching conditions based on the outcome of the wavelet coefficients are output by the encoder. Thus, to obtain the desired decoder's algorithm, which duplicates the encoder's execution path as it sorts the significant coefficients, we simply replace the word *output* with *input*. The ordering information is recovered when the coordinates of the significant coefficients are added to the end of the LSP. But note that whenever the decoder inputs data, its three control lists (LIS, LIP, and LSP) are identical to the ones used by the encoder at the moment it outputs the data, which means that the decoder indeed recovers the ordering from the execution path.

An additional task done by the decoder is to update the reconstructed image. For the value of n when a coordinate is moved to the LSP, it is known that $2^n \leq |C_{i,j}| < 2^{n+1}$. So, the decoder uses that information in the LSP, to set the reconstructed coefficients $\hat{C}_{i,j} = \pm 1.5 \times 2^n$. Similarly, during the refinement pass, the decoder adds or subtracts 2^{n-1} to/from $\hat{C}_{i,j}$ when it inputs the bits of the binary representation of $|\hat{C}_{i,j}|$. In this manner, the distortion gradually decreases during both the sorting and refinement passes.

In coding the LENA test image, Said and Pearlman showed that this method outperforms EZW in the entire bit-rate range by almost 0.4 dB. When this method is combined with arithmetic coding, the compression efficiency is further improved by almost another 0.4 dB (30).

7.5 SUMMARY

Transmission of video in a hostile environment of IP, ATM, and mobile networks, where there is always a danger of loss of information, demands protection of vital visual information against losses. Layered coding is a means of facilitating such protection by generating compressed image/video information at various importance levels.

This chapter introduced three general methods of layered coding techniques. In pyramidal coding, through recursive decimation and interpolation, an image is represented by successively condensed information. Denser images convey most important information about the image. Although this method has only historical importance, a variant of it, under the DCT pyramid, has proven to be very efficient in image condensation. Experimental results with static images show that with less than 10% of the compressed image, it is still possible to generate a meaningful image.

The second category of layered coding is used in the standard DCT-based codecs, under the scalability options. In terms of coding, only three methods of scalability (spatial, SNR, and temporal) have been recognized in the standard codecs. However, another method, known as data partitioning, is regarded as only the representation of the bitstream of the conventional codecs into two layers, rather than encoding them into two parts. Both MPEG-2 and H.263+ support these scalability functions. A hybrid combination of these scalabilities provides larger layers of bitstreams that facilitate internetworking operations.

The last category of layering is with the wavelet transform, currently recommended only for still images in JPEG-2000 and the still image coding option of MPEG-4. Owing to its ability to generate more layers than DCT-based codecs, this method is very attractive for video networking. However, work must be done to verify whether the method is capable of compressing video as efficiently as the most powerful DCT-based codecs such as H.263.

ACKNOWLEDGMENT

I acknowledge the work of numerous former and current students and research assistants, who have indirectly contributed to this work.

REFERENCES:

1. M Ghanbari. Two-layer coding of video signals for VBR networks. IEEE Selected Areas Commun. 8(5):771–781, June 1989.
2. ITU-T Recommendation I.363. B-ISDN ATM adaptation layer (AAL) specification. International Telecommunications Union, Geneva, June 1992.
3. MPEG-2. Generic coding of moving pictures and associated audio information. ISO/IEC 13818–2 Video. Draft International standard, November 1994.
4. Draft ITU-T Recommendation H.263+. Video coding for very low bit rates. International Telecommunications Union, Geneva, September 1997.
5. R Koenen, F Pereira, L Chiariglione. MPEG-4: Context and objectives. Image Commun 9:(4), 1997.
6. JPEG-2000. Coding of still pictures, requirements and profiles, version 4.0. ISO/IEC JTC1/SC29/WG1 (ITU-T SG8), N1105R, November 1998.
7. JM Shapiro. Embedded image coding using zerotrees of wavelet coefficients. IEEE Trans Signal Process 4(12):3445–3462, December 1993.
8. PJ Burt, EH Adelson. The Laplacian pyramid as an compact image code. IEEE Trans Commun 31(4):532–540, April 1983.
9. KH Tan, M Ghanbari. Layered image coding using the DCT pyramid. IEEE Trans Image Process 4(4):512–516, April 1995.
10. KN Ngan. Experiments on two-dimensional decision in time and orthogonal transform domains. Signal Process 11(3):249–263, October 1986.
11. L Vandendorpe. Hierarchical transform and subband coding of video signals. Signal Process Image Commun 4:245–262, June 1992.
12. H.261. ITU-T Recommendation H.261. Video codec for audiovisual services at p × 64 kbit/s, International Telecommunications Union, Geneva, 1990.
13. RE Crochiere, LR Rabiner. Interpolation and decimation of digital signals—A tutorial review. Proc IEEE, 69:300–331, 1981.
14. R Arvind, M Civanlar, A Reibman. Packet loss resilience of MPEG-2 scalable video coding algorithms. IEEE Trans Circuits Syst Video Technology, 6(5):426–435, October 1996.
15. M Ghanbari. An adapted H.261 two-layer video codec for ATM networks. IEEE Trans Commun 40(9):1481–1490, September 1992.
16. M Ghanbari, V Seferidis. Efficient H.261 based two-layer video codecs for ATM networks. IEEE Trans Circuits Syst Video Technology, 5(2):171–175, April 1995.

17. PAAA Assuncao, M Ghanbari. A frequency domain video transcoder for dynamic bit rate reduction of MPEG-2 bit streams. IEEE Trans Circuits Syst Video Technol 8(8):953–967, December 1998.

18. C Herpel. SNR scalability v.s data partitioning for high error rate channels. ISO/IEC JTC1/SC29/WG11 document. MPEG 93/658, July 1993.

19. G Morrison, IA Parke. Spatially layered hierarchical approach to video coding. Signal Process Image Commun. 5(5/6):445–462, December 1995.

20. M Ghanbari. Video Coding: An Introduction to Standard Codecs. London, Institution of Electrical Engineers, 1999.

21. MPEG-1. Coding of moving pictures and associated audio for digital storage media at up to about 1.5 Mbit/s. ISO/IEC 1117-2: video, November 1991.

22. ITU-T Recommendation H.245 Control protocol for multimedia communication. International Telecommunications Union, Geneva, September 1998.

23. ITU-T Draft Recommendation I.371, Traffic control and congestion control in B-ISDN. International Telecommunications Union, Geneva, 1992.

24. IEEE 802.6. Distributed-queue dual bus (DQDB) subnetwork of a metropolitan area network (MAN). Institute of Electrical and Electronics Engineers, Piscataway, NJ, July 1991.

25. RE Crochiere, SA Weber, JL Flanagan. Digital coding of speech in subbands. Bell Syst Tech J, 55:1069–1085, 1976.

26. D Le Gall, A Tabatabai. Subband coding of images using symmetric short kernel filters and arithmetic coding techniques. Proceedings of IEEE International Conference on Acoustics, Speech and Signal Processing, ICASSP'88 1988, pp 761–764.

27. I. Daubechies. Orthonormal bases of compactly supported wavelets. Commun Pure Appl Math XLI:909–996, 1988.

28. MPEG-4. Video verification model version-11. ISO/IEC JTC1/SC29/WG11, N2171, Tokyo, March 1998.

29. IH Witten, RM Neal, JG Cleary. Arithmetic coding for data compression. Commun ACM, 30(6):520–540, June 1987.

30. A Said, WA Pearlman. A new, fast and efficient image codec based on set partitioning in hierarchical trees. IEEE Trans Circuits Syst Video Technol 6(3):243–250, March 1996.

31. Q Wang, M Ghanbari. Motion-compensation for super high definition video. Proceedings of the IS&T/SPIE Symposium, Electronic Imaging, Science and Technology, very high resolution and quality imaging, San Jose, CA, January 27–February 2, 1996.

32. K Shen, E Delp. Wavelet based rate scalable video compression. IEEE Trans Circuits Syst Video Technol 9(1):109–122, 1999.

33. DG Sampson, EAB da Silva, M Ghanbari. Low bit-rate video coding using wavelet vector quantization. IEE Proc Vision, Image Signal Process 142(3):141–148, June 1995.

34. Q Wang, M Ghanbari. Scalable coding of very high resolution video using the virtual zerotree. IEEE Trans Circuits Syst Video Technol, Special Issue on Multimedia, 7(5):719–729, October 1997.

8
Error Resilience Coding

Guy Cote and Faouzi Kossentini
Department of Electrical Engineering, University of British Columbia,
Vancouver, British Columbia, Canada

Stephan Wenger
Technische Universitat Berlin,
Berlin, Germany

8.1 INTRODUCTION

The coding and transmission of compressed video information over existing and future communication networks with nonguaranteed quality of service (QoS) presents many challenges. Even though most networks provide some error control mechanism, media-based error recovery techniques are necessary in many scenarios, particularly in those that have real-time requirements and/or do not allow the use of feedback channel based mechanisms. These scenarios include a wide range of applications and environments: interactive video over the Internet, personal video communications over wireless networks, and video broadcasting over satellite, to name just a few. Thus, error resilience video coding has recently received a lot of attention from researchers in academia and industry alike.

In an error-prone environment, video-optimized error resilience techniques are necessary to accommodate the nature of compressed video bitstreams, which are very sensitive to bit errors and packet losses. Such errors may lead to the loss of synchronization at the receiver, which can, in turn, lead to the loss of many video blocks and (possibly) frames. For example, all current video coding standards typically employ variable-length codes (VLCs) to achieve high compression. However, a single bit error in a VLC can cause loss of synchronization, usually leading to the loss of many following VLCs. Moreover, the predictive coding process of motion compensation will cause errors to propagate in the spatial and temporal directions. In this chapter, we present error resilience coding methods that allow for more reli-

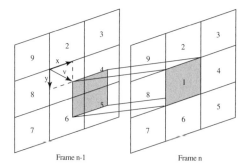

Figure 8.1 Temporal error propagation due to motion compensation.

able video communication in error-prone environments. We first describe the effects of errors on the compressed video bitstreams. Then, we discuss data recovery techniques applicable to video communication systems. Finally, we present the error resilience coding methods that have been developed to limit, or contain, the effects of error propagation.

8.2 ERROR PROPAGATION

The use of VLCs and predictive techniques in video coding leads to inevitable spatiotemporal error propagation. A single bit error can propagate to many bits, and error detection may not be able to locate the exact error location. Spatial predictive coding techniques such as motion vector prediction will cause errors to propagate spatially within a video frame. On the other hand, motion compensation, which is usually performed using one or more blocks* in a previous frame (see Figure 8.1), will cause spatiotemporal error propagation. If no action is taken to stop or limit the extent of spatiotemporal error propagation, the video reproduction quality can degrade substantially. In the remainder of this section, we discuss the effects of single bit errors and packet losses on spatiotemporal error propagation.

8.2.1 Effects of Bit Errors

In bit-oriented networks such as wireless networks (Chapter 5), bit errors can be detected at the transport level or at the source decoding level, depending on the adopted protocol environment and system design. At the transport level, error

---

* In this chapter, a block consists of a rectangular region of 16 pixels by 16 lines of luminance information and the corresponding chrominance information. This unit is also referred to as a macroblock in video coding standards (see Chapter 1 for a description of the frame structure, including group of blocks, slices, and macroblocks).

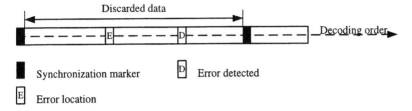

Figure 8.2 Error detection cannot locate a bit error when decoding VLCs: the data between two synchronization words is usually discarded.

detection techniques are normally applied to blocks of data. If a video decoder decides to drop a video segment that contains bit errors, the impact of errors is equivalent to that of the loss of the complete segment. If transport-level error detection is not available or if the system decides to process data known to be incorrect, bit errors will be present at the video decoder. Such errors can still be detected by using syntactic or semantic violations of the video bitstream (1). However, since the decoder almost always loses synchronization with the bitstream and fails to locate the bit errors while decoding corrupted VLCs, data between two synchronization (sync) words is usually discarded, as illustrated in Figure 8.2. Note, however, that it may be possible to recover additional information by means of alternative entropy coding methods that allow the decoder to stay synchronized with the bitstream. This is discussed later.

8.2.2 Effects of Packet Losses

Packet losses typically occur in packet networks, such as the Internet (Chapter 3) and ATM networks (Chapter 4). Other networks that use some form of blocking structure for channel coding or multiplexing may also experience packet losses.* Packet sizes, spatiotemporal location of packets within the video sequence, and the extent of predictive coding will determine the impact of packet losses on error propagation. Depending on the size of packets, a packet loss may affect only a small spatial location of a video frame, or it can lead to the loss of complete coded video frame(s). If the packet loss occurs in a limited spatial location within a video frame, error concealment may be applied to the missing video data. If complete frames are lost, the decoder can choose to repeat the last correctly received frame, or it can perform temporal frame interpolation to maintain an adequate frame rate. Nevertheless, when any type of error occurs in a predictive coding system, proper action is necessary at the encoder to limit the effects of spatiotemporal error propagation.

---

* This is particularly true in many practical applications (e.g., H.324 or MPEG-2 transport over satellites).

8.2.3   Error Handling

Once errors have been detected at either the transport or the video layer, proper action must be taken by the video decoder. The video encoder can provide tools and/or additional information to ensure better system performance in case of erroneous transmission. Such *error resilience* video coding methods are described in this chapter. Even with effective error resilience coding methods, residual errors may be present, and the video decoder must be able to perform error concealment operations, as discussed in Chapter 6.

8.3   VIDEO-OPTIMIZED CHANNEL CODING TECHNIQUES

In this section, we describe the forward error correction (FEC) and automatic repeat request (ARQ) channel coding techniques that have been applied to video coding for transmission over error-prone networks.

8.3.1   Forward Error Correction

FEC techniques, widely employed in data communication systems (2), can be used effectively in a video communication system for the detection and correction of bit errors. In this open-loop method, the recovery from errors is the responsibility of the decoder. The transmitter adds redundant parity bits, which can be used, to a certain extent, to detect and (possibly) recover lost information. FEC methods add some amount of delay, since the information is grouped into blocks of bits before parity information is added. Using FEC techniques, recovery from single-bit errors is possible, but protection from long bursts of errors would require the addition of an excessive amount of parity bits and, consequently, a substantial increase in bandwidth and delay. On the other hand, the performance of FEC codes on channels with bursty errors can be enhanced by interleaving (3), with an increase in complexity and delay.

To be more effective, FEC techniques can take into account the importance of the different parts of a video bitstream, thereby applying unequal error protection (UEP) (4,5). The video bitstream is first partitioned into classes of different sensitivities. Important information such as frame size, temporal location of a frame, spatial location indication, coding mode, and quantization information must be protected to ensure a minimum level of video reproduction quality. Errors in these header bits will not only affect the video reproduction quality, but also can cause the decoder to reset in response to resource allocation problems. For example, if the encoder changes picture size from QCIF to CIF and this information is not correctly received, the decoder may have to reset to accommodate higher than expected number of blocks and display resolution. FEC coding can be applied in a cascade manner, where the same FEC code is first applied to all header information, and then reapplied to the more important part of the same information. Since header information is usually a relatively small part of the bitstream, FEC overhead can be minimal.

FEC techniques can also be employed in a packet-based network (6). In this case, one or more packets with parity information are calculated for a group of packets. A missing packet can be reconstructed by using the information of the correctly received packets and the parity packet. Interleaving schemes can be employed to achieve resilience against burst packet losses. The main drawbacks of packet-based FEC techniques are similar to those of bit-oriented techniques: the need of similar data packet sizes, and the added complexity, bandwidth requirements, and delay. Note that when the locations of the missing packets are known, the decoding complexity can be significantly reduced. FEC techniques for packet-based video transmission have been proposed for ATM networks (7–9) and more recently for the Internet (10,11).

8.3.2 Automatic Repeat Request

ARQ techniques are used extensively for channel error recovery in data communication (12). ARQ is effective against burst errors and packet losses. In this closed-loop error recovery method, a feedback channel is maintained from the receiver to the transmitter. This feedback channel conveys the status of received packets, providing the encoder with the possibility of either retransmitting erroneously received packets or containing the effect of their losses.

Different ARQ techniques have already been proposed for video communication in (13,14). An ARQ buffer is present at the transmitting side, which contains the video data frames that have been transmitted but not yet acknowledged, as well as the frames not yet transmitted. The decoder sends an acknowledgment (ACK) or a negative acknowledgment (NACK) back to the transmitter to inform it of the status of the received data frames. The transmitter will determine whether the lost data frames should be retransmitted, based on the delay requirements of the system. It is important to avoid losing complete video frames. This can be done, for example, with a layered coder, which ensures that the base layer is received through retransmission, and the enhancement layer is transmitted only when the ARQ buffer fullness is below a certain threshold based on the delay requirements and/or the network condition.

While ARQ techniques are usually more effective than the FEC ones, they cannot be used in many video communication applications such as TV broadcasting, which do not support a feedback channel. Even when a feedback channel is available, real-time constraints require that ARQ delays be kept within an application-specific limit. Therefore, ARQ techniques are generally not suited for real-time video communication over error-prone networks.

8.4   SPATIAL ERROR RESILIENCE CODING TECHNIQUES

An important aspect of error resilience video coding is to contain the effects of errors. As mentioned earlier, locating the exact position of bit errors in a compressed video bitstream is often not possible, and, depending on the extent of the predictive coding and the entropy coding methods employed, a large amount of possibly correct information must be discarded. In this section, we first describe techniques that contain the effects of such errors to small spatial regions without an excessive overhead rate increase. These techniques include the placement of synchronization markers, data partitioning, and network-aware video packetization.

It is also possible to use error resilience entropy coding methods to recover information within a corrupted video segment. Example methods discussed here are reversible variable-length coding, the error-resilient entropy code, fixed-length coding, and semi-fixed-length coding.

Error resilience entropy coding methods are useful for bit-error-prone networks. However, they provide limited error resilience performance in a packet lossy environment. Multiple-description (MD) coding techniques, which allow for the recovery of data in a packet lossy network, are discussed in Section 8.4.8.

8.4.1   Synchronization Markers

Sync markers are codewords that are uniquely identifiable in the bitstream. Therefore, the entropy decoder can resynchronize once such a codeword has been detected. A VLC, a combination of VLCs, or any other codeword combination in the bitstream cannot reproduce the sync word. Moreover, while shorter sync words introduce less overhead, they also increase the probability of emulating sync words in the bitstream in bit-error-phone environments. These restrictions put a limit on the minimum length of the sync word. In H.263, for example, a 17-bit sync word equal to 00000000000000001 is employed. Another desirable feature of a sync word is its detection properties in error-prone environments. Such sync words have been proposed (15). Although it may be possible to design self-synchronizing VLCs (16,17), all video coding standards employ sync markers. This is because sync markers not only provide for bitstream synchronization, they also ensure spatial synchronization at the decoder. This is achieved by inserting additional fields after the sync word for critical information, such as the block address and quantizer value. Moreover, to contain the errors within a slice, data dependencies across slice boundaries within the video frame are usually forbidden by video coding standards. To remove such dependencies, the encoder modifies the coding strategy at the beginning of a new slice. For example, the motion vector of the first block of a new slice is not predicted.

To contain the errors to a small spatial region, sync words may be inserted at various locations, either at a uniform spatial interval in the coded frame, or at a uniform bit interval in the bitstream. In H.263 or MPEG-4, for example, sync words can be inserted at the beginning of every row of blocks (uniform spatial interval), thus forming groups of blocks (GOBs). Using the slice structure makes it possible to insert sync markers before any coded block, regardless of the block's spatial position. It is then possible to insert a sync marker after a target number of bits and thus start new slices at uniform bit intervals.* When sync words are inserted between uniform bit intervals, they will be closer (spatially) in high-activity regions, since more bits are necessary to represent these parts of a picture.

While the placement of sync markers according to a uniform pattern often performs quite well, a significant improvement in performance can be obtained when more sophisticated algorithms are used. In fact, we next briefly describe a rate distortion (RD) optimized algorithm for the insertion of synchronization markers for video transmission in a bit-error-prone environment (18). A summary of research work on RD-optimized video coding using the Lagrangian multiplier method (19) for an error-free environment can be found elsewhere (20). Ortega and Ramachandran (21) have given an overview of RD methods, with insight on RD optimization in error-prone environments.

Next, we present an RD-optimized mode decision algorithm that takes into account the network condition and the error concealment method used by the decoder. Let us assume that the video is packetized by means of slices, and that a sync marker can be placed at the start of the slice. Let us also assume that a bit error occurring within a slice will result in the whole slice being discarded. Using the size of the slice $L(s)$ and the channel average bit error rate (BER) P_e, the slice error rate (SER) is first evaluated. The probability of error of a video block, p, is then set to the value of the SER. The SER will depend on the video coding mode, since a different coding mode will produce a different bit rate. The SER is computed for two scenarios: (a) a slice header is inserted at the beginning of the current block, and (b) no slice header is inserted. In the first case, $L(s)$ is the number of bits of the slice header plus the number of bits of the current block, and in the second case, $L(s)$ is the number of bits since the location of the last slice header plus the number of bits of the current block. Given $L(s)$, we obtain

$$\text{SER} = 1 - (1 - p_e)^{L(s)} \tag{1}$$

for both cases a and b.

---

* VLC codewords should not be divided by a sync marker. Therefore, sync markers are inserted at the next possible location after the target number of bits in the slice has been reached.

The rate of the synchronization marker R(sync) is taken into consideration in the Lagrangian minimization. For a small increase in bit rate from inserting a sync marker, a large improvement in video reproduction quality at the decoder can be achieved. The Lagrangian cost function for the slice header localization J_{sync} is then given by

$$J_{snyc} = (1 - p)D_q(\text{mod } e) + pD_c + \lambda_{sync}R_{sync} \tag{2}$$

where sync $\in \{0, 1\}$, with 0 meaning no sync marker is inserted and 1 meaning a sync marker is inserted; D_q is the distortion due to quantization if the block is received with probability $(1 - p)$, and D_c is the distortion due to error concealment if the same block is lost and concealed with probability p.

To obtain the value of the Lagrangian parameter λ_{sync} for different average BERs, we find the average slice length that yields the minimum Lagrangian J_{sync} for different values of λ_{sync}. Values of slice length (in units of coded blocks) versus λ_{sync} are presented for the sequence FOREMAN in Figure 8.3. coded at 48 kbit/s, QCIF resolution, and 10 frames/s. The Lagrangian parameter λ_{sync} is employed to control the trade-offs between coding efficiency and error resilience. It can be chosen according to system parameters to yield a desired average slice length.

To illustrate the advantage of the RD sync insertion algorithm, we com-

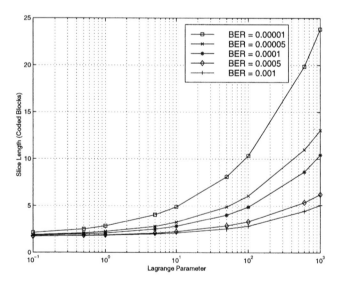

Figure 8.3   Average slice length (in units of coded blocks) versus the Lagrangian parameter λ_{sync} for different average BERs for the sequence FOREMAN.

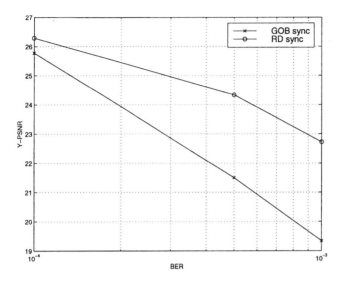

Figure 8.4 Performance of the RD sync marker insertion algorithm versus GOB sync for the sequence FOREMAN.

pare its performance to that of inserting a sync marker at the start of every GOB. Results are presented in Figure 8.4 for the sequence FOREMAN coded at 48 kbit/s with λ_{sync} = 100 and sent over the binary symmetric channel (BSC). For a given average BER, the BSC model is actually the worst channel model, yielding the highest probability of error in a slice, compared to a channel with correlated errors (burst errors). As much as 3 dB improvement in reproduction quality is achieved at a BER of 10^{-3}.

8.4.2 Data Partitioning

Without the use of data partitioning, the motion vectors and discrete cosine transform coefficient information in a DCT-based video coder usually are coded together for every block. This eliminates the overhead for addressing a block when both classes of information are skipped. When data partitioning is used, the motion vector and DCT coefficient information within a slice are, respectively, grouped together and separated by a boundary marker. The boundary marker is a uniquely decodable codeword that signals the end of the motion vector information and the beginning of the DCT coefficient information. This arrangement yields several advantages. First, errors can be localized to data of a certain type, and the unaffected information can be employed for video reconstruction at the decoder. For example, when an error occurs in the DCT data but the motion vector data are not affected, the motion vector information can still be used to assist in error concealment. Second, if undetected errors occur in the video packet, the received data can be considered invalid if the boundary marker is not detected. However, if the boundary marker is detected but the block address is incorrect after the sync word at the start of the next slice has been detected, the decoder can assume that the motion vector information was correct and discard the DCT coefficients information.

Data partitioning provides improved video quality under different error conditions, as reported for MPEG-4 (22) and for H.263 (23). We present some results for MPEG-4 data partitioning in Figure 8.5, where PSNR plots are shown for the sequence CONTAINER coded at QCIF resolution and 24 kbit/s with and without data partitioning. Video packets having a pseudoconstant length of 480 bits, delimited by sync words, are employed. It is clear that a substantial performance improvement can be achieved with data partitioning when motion vector information is employed to assist error concealment (22). Over a wide range of error conditions, bit rates, and test sequences, data partitioning improves the quality of the reproduced video by over 2 dB, assuming that missing blocks in the nonpartitioning case are concealed by simply repeating the blocks in the previous frame at the same spatial location.

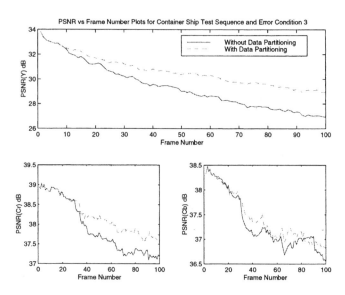

Figure 8.5 Performance of data partitioning for the test sequence CONTAINER for burst errors, BER 10-2, burst length 10 ms. (Reproduced from Ref. 22.)

8.4.3   Network-Aware Video Packetization

In packet lossy environments, the use of appropriate packetization techniques can improve error resilience substantially. Whenever it is possible, a video communication system will attempt to start a packet with a synchronization point of the video bitstream, allowing the independent decoding of the packet. The size of a packet is either fixed (e.g., ATM networks) or chosen subject to network constraints such as those dictated by the maximum transfer unit (MTU) size and packetization payload/overhead trade-off considerations (e.g., the Internet). The size of a coded video segment can be adapted to a target packet size by using slices, as discussed earlier.

Every coded frame carries, in the picture header, information relevant to all slices of a frame. If the first packet of a picture is lost, it will then be impossible to decode any of the slices of that picture, even if the packets containing such slices are available. One possible solution to this problem is to add a redundant representation of the picture header to each packet. Many current video systems and standards allow for such a redundant representation (24). The visual part of MPEG-4, for example, provides a tool called *header extension code* (HEC) that allows for important header information to be duplicated at the slice level.

8.4.4   Reversible Variable-Length Codes

Reversible variable-length codes (RVLCs) (25) are VLCs that have the prefix property in the forward and reverse directions, and they can therefore be uniquely decoded in both directions. When the decoder detects an error while decoding in the forward direction, it can look for the next sync marker and start decoding in the reverse direction until an error is encountered. Based on the position of the detected errors in the forward and reverse directions, the decoder is able to locate the error within a smaller region in the bitstream and recover additional data, as illustrated in Figure 8.6.

One simple method of constructing RVLCs is to add a fixed-length prefix

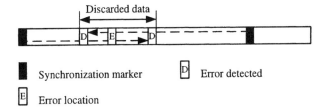

Figure 8.6   Reversible variable-length codes enable the recovery of data by allowing decoding in the forward and reverse directions.

and suffix to a constant Hamming weight VLC code set. The decoder is able to decode in the forward and reverse directions by counting the number of 1s in the code to detect the end of the code. More complete RVLCs can be generated by increasing the length of the prefix. RVLCs can also be designed by modifying the Golomb–Rice code, usually providing better compression efficiency (26).

RVLCs can be constructed to be symmetric (25). However, since asymmetrical RVLCs allow a more flexible bit assignment, they provide better compression efficiency than symmetrical RVLCs. To construct an asymmetrical RVLC, we start with an optimal nonreversible VLC, such as a Huffman code, which satisfies the prefix condition. The suffix of each codeword can be extended by adding bits, as illustrated in Figure 8.7 and described below:

1. A reverse binary tree is set up in such a way that the ends of the codewords are placed on the root of the reverse tree from the shorter codewords to the longer codewords (see Figure 8.7b and c).
2. When a suffix, which is also a prefix in the reverse tree, coincides with a shorter codeword, another codeword with the same bit length is assigned in the reverse tree instead. In Figure 8.7d, D is assigned in the reverse tree instead of C, since the suffix of C coincides with A.
3. When there is no other codeword with the same bit length whose suffix does not coincide with one of the shorter codewords, the minimum number of bits needed to satisfy the suffix condition are added to the end of the codeword. In Figure 8.7e, one bit "1" is added to the end of C.
4. When bit length assignment has been completed, new codewords are sorted by bit length, and codewords are reassigned to the symbols according to their occurrence probabilities (Figure 8.7f).

Other methods of generating RVLCs have been proposed (25–27). In general, the disadvantage of two-way decodable RVLCs is a reduction in compression efficiency. RVLCs can be designed to match the probability distribution of the coded video data, being motion vector information or run-length coded DCT coefficients, such that the compression efficiency is maximized. Also, to take full advantage of the RVLCs' properties, codewords representing data of the same type should be grouped together. Thus, RVLCs are usually employed with data partitioning.

8.4.5   The Error-Resilient Entropy Coding (EREC) Method

The EREC method, originally proposed in (1996) (28), is used to convert VLCs to fixed-length blocks of data. This allows the decoder to be synchronized with the bit-stream at the start of each EREC frame with minimal additional redundancy.

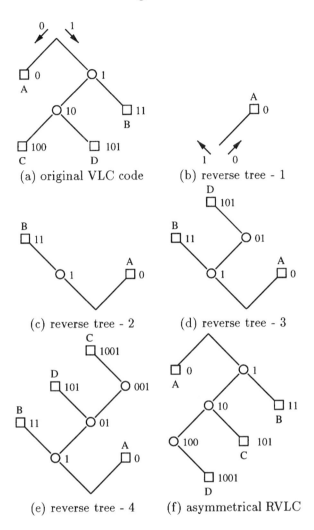

(a) original VLC code   (b) reverse tree - 1

(c) reverse tree - 2   (d) reverse tree - 3

(e) reverse tree - 4   (f) asymmetrical RVLC

Figure 8.7 Conversion from a VLC set into an asymmetrical RVLC one.

The EREC frame structure is composed of N slots, each of length s_i bits, for a total length of $T = \sum_{i=1}^{N} s_i$ bits per EREC frame. It is assumed that the values of s_i, T, and N are known by the decoder. The slot lengths s_i can be predefined as a function of T. The number of EREC slots N can usually be fixed in advance, and thus, only T needs to be transmitted to the decoder.

The VLC blocks of data of length b_i are placed into an EREC frame by means of a bit reorganization structure that relies on the ability to determine the end of each variable-length block. Figure 8.8 shows an example of the reorganization algorithm. The first stage is to allocate each block of variable-length data to a corresponding EREC slot. Blocks with an equal number of bits to those available in the slot are coded completely, leaving the slot full. Blocks with $b_i <$ s_i are coded completely, leaving the slot with $s_i - b_i$ bits unused. Blocks with b_i $> s_i$ have s_i bits coded to fill the slot, and $b_i - s_i$ bits are left to be allocated. In the subsequent stages, each block of data still to be coded is allocated to a partially filled slot. At stage n, the remaining bits of the VLC code at slot i are allocated to the slot $i + \phi_n$ mod N, if space is available. Provided the bits can fit in the set of N slots, all the bits are placed within N stages of the algorithm. The remaining spaces in the EREC slots are filled with redundant bits. In the absence of channel errors, the decoder follows this algorithm by decoding the variable-length data until it detects the end of each VLC block, at which point the remaining bits of the slot are declared parts of other VLC blocks placed later in the algorithm.

The parameter ϕ_n is a predefined offset sequence, and it is set to 1 in the example illustrated in Figure 8.8. A pseudorandom offset sequence ϕ_n was shown to provide better error resilience properties (28) because of its uncorrelated nature (i.e., $\phi_{n+k} - \phi_n$ is independent of n). Thus, two VLC blocks k slots apart will not be searched in the same order.

It was shown (28) that the EREC method provides a relatively large improvement in reproduction quality when applied to DCT-based still image and video coding compared to using VLCs with GOB sync markers. In 1998 (29) a joint source channel coder using H.263 video coding and the EREC method was developed, yielding a significant improvement over the use of VLCs. It is impor-

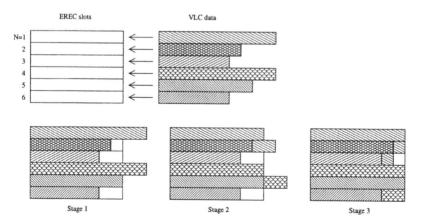

Figure 8.8   Example of the EREC bit reorganizing procedure.

tant to note that the EREC method requires that some information be transmitted on highly protected channels and that it does not guarantee image/video frame spatial synchronization. Therefore, sync markers should still be employed.

8.4.6 Fixed-Length Codes

Fixed-length codes (FLCs), also known as block codes, are less sensitive to error propagation than VLCs. As opposed to the VLC case, where the input symbols are of fixed length and the output codewords are of variable length, the FLC process converts variable-length input codewords to fixed-length block codes. An algorithm to construct optimal FLCs, in terms of minimum output bit rate, was proposed in 1968 by Tunstall (30).

The lower bound on the average length of an FLC is the same as that of a VLC, which is the entropy of the source U, $H(U)$, for a discrete memoryless source. However, the lower bound of an FLC is limited by the probability of the less likely symbol, p_{min}. As a result, the coding efficiency decreases as the alphabet size increases. Modified Tunstall codes to address this particular drawback were first presented in 1992 (31), and more recent work is available (32).

The upper bound of the average length of an FLC is different from that of a VLC. In a VLC, the upper bound is $H(U) + 1$. In an FLC, the upper bound decreases as the length of the output codewords, N, increases. This puts a limit on the minimum output codeword length possible to achieve a certain level of compression efficiency.

As for RVLCs, data partitioning should be used with FLCs to improve their coding efficiency, since different data types may use different fixed block sizes. Even though FLCs allow codeword synchronization, they do not guarantee spatial synchronization, and sync codewords are therefore still necessary.

8.4.7 Semi-Fixed-Length Codes

Video information in a bitstream has different levels of error sensitivity. This property can be exploited by using semi-fixed-length codes, where unequal error protection techniques are used to ensure that the critical part of the code highly protected and the less important part moderately protected. In this section, we present an example of the application of semi-fixed-length codes to the coding of motion vectors (33). By protecting the important part of the motion vector bits, we can minimize the probability that the decoder will lose synchronization with the motion vector part of the bitstream, at the expense of only a small increase in the total bit rate.

Experimental results indicate that a large percentage of the motion vector differences resulting from predictive motion estimation belong to either region 0 or region 1 in Figure 8.9. Based on the statistical behavior of the motion vector

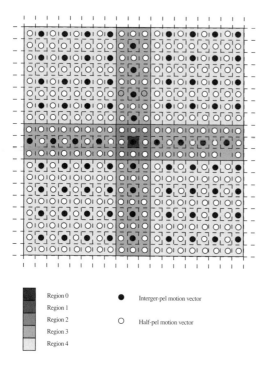

Region 0
Region 1
Region 2   ●   Interger-pel motion vector
Region 3
Region 4   ○   Half-pel motion vector

Figure 8.9   The semi-fixed-length coding method: motion vector coding regions.

differences, the search area centered at the predicted motion vector is divided
into *five* regions. Figure 8.9 depicts the difference motion vector regions, and
Table 8.1 represents the associated codewords and their probabilities, for an
H.263 encoder and QCIF video sequences. A tree representation of the header
part is shown in Figure 8.10. The popular *gray* encoding method was employed
to generate the specific codes for the difference motion vectors. Region 0 corresponds to the (0, 0) difference motion vector and is represented by *one* bit, as this
vector is the most probable one. Region 1 represents the half-pel vectors around
the (0, 0) integer–pel difference vector. Region 2 represents the (1, 0), (0, 1), (-1,
0), and (0, -1) integer–pel difference motion vectors, and their corresponding
half-pel vectors. The remaining difference vectors are represented by regions 3
and 4, both extending to the (≈16.5, ≈16.5) rectangular boundaries. In regions 1,
2, and 3, *three* additional bits are necessary to represent the half-pel vectors.
However, only *two* bits are necessary to represent the same half-pel vectors in
region 4.

  In terms of encoding efficiency, semi-fixed-length coding is very close to
VLC. When a set of 11 QCIF video sequences is used, semi-fixed-length coding

Table 8.1 Semi-Fixed-Length Codes for the Difference Motion Vectors

	Integer-pel code			
Region	Variable-length header	Fixed-length portion	Half-pel code	Probability
0	0		N/A	0.4387
1	1 00		XXX	0.3683
2	1 01	XX	XXX	0.1295
3	1 10	XX XXXX	XXX	0.0242
4	1 11	XXXXX XXXXX	XX	0.0473

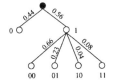

Figure 8.10 Tree representation of the headers of the semi-fixed-length codes (with their respective probabilities).

yields an average difference motion vector code length of 4.64, compared to an average of 4.21 for the VLC coding. The advantage of semi-fixed-length coding, however, is that a small portion of the motion vector code (header shown in Figure 8.10) can be protected at a higher rate by using UEP techniques. To enable UEP, data partitioning is applied. The motion vector codes are further separated into two fields by a synchronization marker. The header information is blocked first, followed by the remaining data, and ending with another synchronization marker.

To illustrate its higher channel error resilience, the foregoing semi-fixed-length coding method was compared to the VLC one, within an H.263 framework and using a rate-compatible punctured convolutional (RCPC) channel coder (34). The two methods were compared by simulating transmission over a BSC. Table 8.2 lists the source coding and channel coding rates for the semi-fixed-length motion vector codes and H.263's VLCs. The video sequence MISS AMERICA is coded at 10 frames/s and at an overall code rate of 9.6 kbit/s, which includes both the source coding and the channel coding bits in both the semi-fixed-length coding and the VLC cases. The simulation results are shown in Figure 8.11. The source channel coding simulation for each BER is repeated more than 50 times, and the average PSNR value is recorded.

As expected, when no protection is applied, both the VLC and the semi-fixed-length coding methods lead to significantly lower PSNR and subjective

Table 8.2 Source Coding and Channel Coding Rates
for BSC

BSC		Semi-Fixed Length Code	
error pattern	VLC	Header	Fixed part
RCPC rate	8:11	8:16	8:10
Source coding	73%	50%	80%
Channel coding	27%	50%	20%

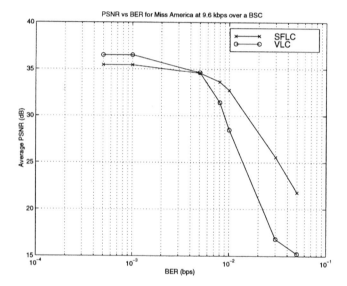

Figure 8.11 PSNR performance comparison between the semi-fixed-length-based coder (SFLC) and the VLC-based coder for a binary symmetric noisy channel model as a function of BER for the sequence MISS AMERICA.

quality levels. Employing equal error protection (EEP) for the VLC-based coder improves the performance at the lower BERs. However, the performance degrades significantly at the higher BERs. Clearly, UEP applied to the semi-fixed-length codes provides a substantial subjective and objective performance advantage, by as much as 6 dB at a 5% BER.

8.4.8 Multiple-Description Coding

Multiple-description (MD) coding allows a video decoder to extract meaningful information from a subset of the bitstream. For example, an SNR scalable bit-

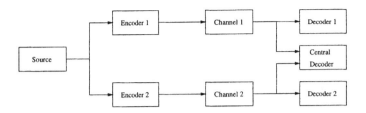

Figure 8.12 Multiple-description coder.

stream allows meaningful information to be retrieved when only the base layer is received. However, to make use of the enhancement layers, the base layer must be received correctly. This can be assured only if priority classes are supported by the network (e.g., ATM). MD coders also have the ability to produce descriptions that may be equally important (balanced descriptions) and are also mutually refinable, that is, are receiving two descriptions together (and combining them is better than receiving the descriptions separately).

Figure 8.12 shows a block diagram of a typical MD coder. An encoder produces two descriptions that are transmitted over two channels. The encoder has no knowledge of the status of the channels. The two-channel model is usually employed to represent two different network packets transmitted on the same network. At the receiving end, we have three decoders: a channel 1 decoder, a channel 2 decoder, and a combined channel 1 and 2 decoder. If information from channel 1 or channel 2 only is received, the corresponding decoder is able to reconstruct a video sequence with distortion level D_1 or D_2, respectively. If information from both channels is received correctly, the central decoder is able to reconstruct a video sequence with distortion level D_0. The achievable rates for given distortion levels D_0, D_1, and D_2 were derived in 1982 (35) for a Gaussian source.

8.4.8.1 Multiple-Description Scalar Quantizers.
Different methods have been proposed for the design of MD coders. One method is the design of multiple-description scalar quantizers (36). The input signal x is quantized to yield an integer index $l = q(x)$, where $q(\cdot)$ represents the mapping of a uniform threshold quantizer with central bin index l. Information about l is mapped to a pair of indexes $(i, j) = a(l)$. The index i is transmitted on channel 1, while the index j is transmitted on channel 2. If information for channel 1 or 2 only is received, the distortion level D_1 or D_2 will be incurred, respectively. If information from both channels is received, the index pair (i, j) is mapped back to the central index l through $a(l)$ to reconstruct x with distortion level D_0. Figure 8.13 presents an example of an MD quantizer mapping. If only one index is received, it is possible to estimate the index l by choosing the central index in the row/column of

i →

j	1	3					
↓	2	4	5				
		6	7	9			
			8	10	11		
				12	13	15	
					14	16	17
						18	19	21
							20	22

Figure 8.13 Example of a multiple-description quantizer assignment for a 22-level quantizer.

the received index i or j, respectively. Details of index assignments can be found elsewhere (36). The technique has been applied to intra coding of blocks in a DCT-based image/video coding framework. Significant gains in video production quality were reported in a packet lossy environment (36).

8.4.8.2 Multiple-Description Transforms. Another method of obtaining multiple descriptions is to use transforms that introduce a controlled level of correlation between the two descriptions (37,38). This is realized by forcing dependencies between pairs of transformed coefficients, allowing either coefficient to be estimated from the other when one is lost. A transform-based MD method codes a pair of input variables A and B by forming and coding a pair of transformed variables C and D, where

$$\begin{bmatrix} C \\ D \end{bmatrix} = T \begin{bmatrix} A \\ B \end{bmatrix} \tag{3}$$

Redundancy is added by controlling the correlation in the pair (C, D) of transformed coefficients through **T**. The one-channel distortion is reduced because the correlation between C and D allows the information from the unreliable channel to be estimated from information received on the reliable channel.

A transform MD method can be applied to blocks of transform coefficients in a DCT-based video coder as follows. Quantized DCT coefficients of the same frequency belonging to spatially neighboring blocks are paired as input variables (A, B). Blocks are paired spatially far apart to minimize correlation between paired coefficients. A correlating transform T is designed for each group of paired frequencies, depending on their visual importance. These correlating transforms are applied to each quantized transform coefficient pair, then entropy coding is applied to the correlated variables. DC coefficient pairs, being the most important, would be coded with high redundancy (correlation).

8.5 TEMPORAL ERROR RESILIENCE CODING TECHNIQUES

As seen earlier, motion compensation can cause errors to propagate over a large frame area and over many frames. This section describes methods to contain the effects of errors due to temporal prediction.

Temporal error resilience can be achieved when it is possible to use an earlier picture than the last transmitted one for temporal prediction. This reference picture is chosen to minimize error propagation. This can be done with or without a feedback channel, by means of reference picture selection or video redundancy coding, respectively. These two techniques are discussed next. On the other hand, temporal error resilience can also be achieved by random intra coding of blocks, intra coding of blocks based on feedback information, or RD-optimized intra coding of blocks. Such intra coding methods are discussed in Sections 8.5.3 and 8.5.4.

8.5.1 Reference Picture Selection

Reference picture selection (RPS) dynamically replaces reference pictures in the encoder in response to an acknowledgment signal from the decoder sent through a feedback channel (39,40). Two modes of operation are defined depending on the acknowledgment message. In the ACK mode of operation, the decoder sends a positive acknowledgment message to the encoder every time a picture is received correctly. The encoder replaces the reference picture according to the returned ACK. If an error occurs, no ACK is sent back and the reference picture remains the last known to be correct frame. In the NACK mode of operation, the decoder send a negative acknowledgment message to the encoder only when a picture has not been received correctly, and the encoder adjusts the reference picture accordingly. Once a NACK message has been sent by the decoder, the decoding process may proceed or temporarily stop, resulting in some degradation or a frame-freeze, respectively, that is, until a frame employing an error-free picture for prediction is received. RPS can be employed not only on complete video frames, but also on video segments (GOBs or slices).

Both the ACK and NACK methods have their advantages and disadvantages. If the round-trip delay is longer than the video frame interval, using the ACK method will lead to a loss in coding efficiency, since the temporal distance of the reference picture will be further than necessary. However, temporal error propagation will not occur, since a reference picture that is not available at the decoder will not be used for prediction at the encoder. In the NACK method, feedback delay will not lead to a loss in coding efficiency. However, incorrect frames are displayed, or a temporary freezing of the decoder will occur, for the duration of a round-trip delay.

Both methods are sensitive to errors in the feedback channel. In the ACK case, if an error in the feedback channel occurs, the reference picture is not replaced, leading to a decrease in coding efficiency, but no serious picture quality degradation at the decoder. In the NACK case, if an error occurs in the feedback channel, the encoder will not use the correct reference picture until a NACK has been correctly received, leading to significant picture degradation at the decoder. It has been confirmed that the NACK method is effective for low error rates, while the ACK method is effective for high error rates (39).

8.5.2 Video Redundancy Coding

Video redundancy-coding (VRC) improves temporal error resilience by means of multiple prediction options without the use of a feedback channel (41). The principle of VRC is to divide the sequence of pictures into two or more threads in such a way that all pictures are assigned to one of the threads in a round-robin fashion. Each thread is coded independently. Obviously, the frame rate within one thread is much lower than the overall frame rate: half in case of two threads, a third in case of three threads, and so on. This leads to a substantial coding efficiency penalty because of the generally larger changes and the longer motion vectors, typically required to represent accurately the motion-related changes between two P/pictures a thread. In regular intervals, all threads converge into a so-called sync frame. From this sync frame, a new thread series is started.

Figure 8.14 illustrates VRC with two threads, five pictures per thread, and three threads, three pictures per thread. If one of these threads is damaged because of a packet loss* the remaining threads stay intact and can be used to predict the next syncframe. VRC is a good example of multiple-description coding in the time domain, where each thread corresponds to one description. Experimental results (41) show that VRC with three threads and three pictures per thread provides good video quality for a picture loss rate of 20%.

8.5.3 Random Intra Coding

A simple technique to avoid error propagation in the temporal direction is to increase the frequency of intra-coded frames. However, intra-coded frames require a substantially larger number of bits than inter-coded frames, resulting in high latency and error sensitivity in a constant bit rate, error-prone environment. Instead of intra coding a complete video frame, it is often preferable to intra-code only some blocks within a frame. One simple technique is to intra-code blocks in a random pattern. Random intra coding of blocks has been sug-

---

* It is here assumed that every coded picture is transmitted as a packet.

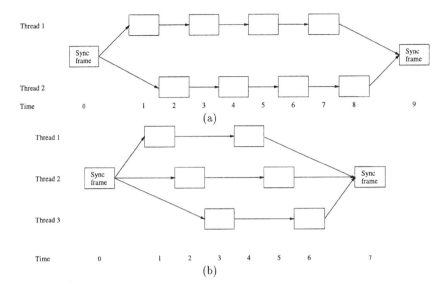

Figure 8.14 VRC example: (a) two threads, five pictures per thread and (b) three threads, three pictures per thread.

gested (42,43). Haskell and Messerschmitt (42) propose that the portion of blocks to be intra-updated in a coded frame be chosen based on the life expectancy of the errors. They state that this life expectancy depends on the intra block refresh rate but is fairly independent of the probability p that a block is in error. In another proposed content adaptive method (44), only blocks with high activity are intra-coded.

A simple relationship between the probability that a block is corrupted by errors, p, and the intra updating frequency, I_{freq}, can be obtained based on experimental results (45). To obtain this relationship, different video sequences are encoded with a fixed bit rate, and the intra refresh rate is varied over four different block loss rates $p = 0, 5, 10,$ and 20%. Decoder Y-PSNR results are presented for the sequence PARIS encoded at 64 kbit/s wit H.263 in Figure 8.15. From a large set of video sequences, it can be observed that the frequency of the intra updating can be roughly approximated by

$$I_{freq} = \frac{1}{p} \tag{4}$$

For example, for a probability of block loss p of 20%, each candidate block should be coded in the intra mode once for every five times it is coded in the inter mode. A detailed analysis of random updating was presented in 1999 (46).

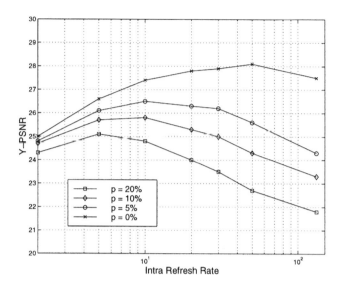

Figure 8.15   Performance of intra block refresh with picture loss rate for the sequence
PARIS.

8.5.4   Intra Coding Based on Feedback Information

The coding strategy of video blocks is modified by means of feedback information to minimize the reproduction quality degradation given the motion compensation error propagation and the error concealment method employed (47).
Because the exact locations of the errors are known by the encoder, the coding
strategy can be modified to prevent prediction from erroneously received blocks.
Each time an error is detected during decoding, the video receiver reacts in the
following manner. Damaged blocks are specified, based on the packetization
structure. For example, all blocks between two sync words may be considered to
be lost if any part of the bitstream between those sync words is corrupted by errors. Information about the lost blocks and their addresses is then sent back to
the transmitter. Finally, the damaged blocks are concealed.

After receiving the feedback information, the video encoder responds by
adapting its coding strategy in one of the following two methods. In method A,
the affected picture area in the encoder reference frame is evaluated, and a tree is
built to track the temporal propagation of errors resulting from the damaged
blocks. The error propagation tree is constructed by keeping a table entry for
each block, which includes spatiotemporal addresses of blocks used for its prediction. More sophisticated encoder error tracking methods have been developed
(48). More specifically, the affected blocks at the encoder are weighted to reflect

the number of pixels used for motion compensation. Encoding is then resumed without using the affected picture area (e.g., by intra coding the affected blocks). In method B, the decoder error concealment is also applied to the damaged blocks at the encoder. The encoder's decoding loop is then updated.

Method A is less complex than method B, in as much as only the propagation tree used to determine the affected picture area needs to be stored and updated at the encoder. However, method A also decreases coding efficiency. For a short round-trip delay method B is clearly more efficient.

8.5.4.1 Rate Distortion Optimized Intra Coding. In this section, we discuss an RD-optimized intra coding algorithm that takes into account the network condition and the error concealment method used by the decoder (18). Three coding modes are considered: skip, inter, and intra. In the case of an RD mode decision in an error-free environment, independently for every block at the spatial location (x, y) and in frame n, we choose the mode that minimizes the Lagrangian given by

$$J_{mode}(n, (x, y)) = D(n, (x, y), mode) + \lambda_{mode} R(n, (x, y), mode) \qquad (5)$$

That is, we choose the coding mode that yields the best RD trade-offs for the block. The distortion D is the sum of squared differences (SSD) between the original block and the coded block, and R is the incurred rate of coding the block. The use of

$$\lambda_{mode} = 0.45(Q/2)^2 \qquad (6)$$

has been shown to provide good RD trade-offs for the coding mode considered here (18), where Q is the quantization step size of the block.

For error-prone environments, the distortion at the decoder is first divided between two sources: distortion D_1 (attributed to a block being received, but possibly predicted from an already concealed block) and distortion D_2 (attributed to a block being lost and concealed). Assuming a block error probability of p, the following Lagrangian:

$$J_{mode}(n,(x,y)) = \left[1 - p(n,(x,y))\right]D_1(n,(x,y),\text{mode}) +$$
$$p(n,(x,y))D_2(n,(x,y)) + \qquad (7)$$
$$\lambda_{mode}R(n,(x,y),\text{mode})$$

is minimized. Then, D_1 is weighted by the probability $(1 - p)$ that this block is received, and D_2 is weighted by the probability p that the same block is lost and concealed at the decoder. D_2 is the distortion incurred by using a particular concealment method to conceal the block. It is constant for all coding modes considered, but its contribution to the overall distortion will depend on p, which may vary depending on the coding mode considered. For each coded block, D_2 is stored and used for the computation of D_I in subsequent frames. D_I is the coding distortion and includes the incurred distortion from predicting from already concealed blocks. D_I depends on the coding mode considered. For the intra mode, the distortion D_I is the same as the error-free coding distortion. For the inter mode, D_I is the quantization distortion plus the concealment distortion of the block(s) from which it is predicted. More precisely, for the considered block in frame n at position (x, y), we obtain

$$D_1(n,(x,y),\mathrm{mod}\, e) = D_q(n,(x,y),\mathrm{mode}) +$$
$$\sum_{k=1}^{N} p\big[n - k,(x + v_x, y + v_y)\big] D_2\big[n - k,(x + v_x, 6 + v_y)\big] \tag{8}$$

where D_q represents the quantization distortion. The distortion $D_2[n - k, (x + v_x, y + v_y)]$ represents the concealment distortion of the block in the previous frame $(n - k)$, k time intervals before the current frame, at the current spatial location (x, y) displaced by the motion vector $v = (v_x, v_y)$. The motion vector v is set to the motion vector of the considered block in the inter mode. The maximum number of frames considered, N, is set to the number of coded frames since the last intra-coded block at the current spatial location. The actual coding distortion perceived at the decoder will be higher, since Eq. (8) is based on the assumption that the intra-coded block will be received error free, and that only single loss patterns within the last N frames are considered.

To obtain $p[n - k, (x + v_x, y + v_y)]$ and $D_2[n - k, (x + v_x, y + v_y)]$, we use the stored values of $p[n - k, (x, y)]$ and $D_2[n - k, (x, y)]$ computed in the mode decision process. The $D_2[n - k, (x, y)]$ values are the constant (with respect to the mode) concealment distortion values at $(v_x, v_y) = (0,0)$. We assume a maximum motion vector range of $(\pm16, \pm16)$, and a block size of 16×16. We compute $D_2[n - k, (x + v_x, y + v_y)]$ by weighting the distortions of the surrounding blocks in the previous frame(s) that overlap with the motion compensated block, as illustrated in Figure 8.1. For each of the surrounding blocks numbered 1 to 9, a weight w_n, $n = 1, \dots, 9$, which is proportional to the overlap area, is computed. These weights are presented in Table 8.3. We then obtain

$$p\big[n - k,(x + v_x, y + v_y)\big] D_2\big[n - k,(x + v_x, y + v_y)\big]$$
$$= \sum_{l=1}^{9} w(l) p\big[n - k,(x,y)_l\big] D_2\big[n - k,(x,y)_l\big] \tag{9}$$

where $(x, y)_l$ represents the block l overlapping the considered block at position (x, y) as shown in Figure 8.1. The values of $w(l)$ are set to *zero* if the conditions in Table 8.3 are not met: that is, if the block used for prediction does not overlap with the block represented by the weight $w(l)$.

Table 8.3   Weight Values for the Computation of Distortion $D_2(n - k, v)$

Weights		Conditions			
		$v_x \geq 0$		$v_x < 0$	
$w(l)$	Value	$v_y \geq 0$	$v_y < 0$	$v_y \geq 0$	$v_y < 0$
$w(1)$	$[(16 - \lfloor v_x \rfloor) \times (16 - \lfloor v_y \rfloor)]/256$	X	X	X	X
$w(2)$	$[(16 - \lfloor v_x \rfloor) \times \lfloor v_y \rfloor]/256$		X		X
$w(3)$	$[v_x \times \lfloor v_y \rfloor]/256$			X	
$w(4)$	$[v_x \times (16 - \lfloor v_y \rfloor)]/256$	X	X		
$w(5)$	$[v_x \times v_y]/256$	X			
$w(6)$	$[(16 - \lfloor v_x \rfloor) \times v_y]/256$	X		X	
$w(7)$	$[\lfloor v_x \rfloor \times v_y]/256$		X		
$w(8)$	$[\lfloor v_x \rfloor \times (16 - v_y)]/256$		X	X	
$w(9)$	$[\lfloor v_x \rfloor \times \lfloor v_y \rfloor]/256$			X	

To demonstrate the advantages of this method, we present some results for different bit rates and block loss rates. Results are presented for the video sequence FOREMAN in Figure 8.16 for a block probability of error p of 20%. Results of the RD-optimized intra coding method are compared to those of the random intra update method, with an update frequency of once every five coded frames. The same error concealment used by the decoder is assumed at the encoder. The same decoder is employed for the comparison. The RD intra coding improves significantly the video reproduction quality, especially in poor network conditions. An improvement in quality of over 3 dB is achieved at a block loss rate of 10% and a bit rate of 256 kbit/s for the video sequence considered.

8.6   ERROR RESILIENCE TOOLS IN CURRENT STANDARDS

Version 2 of H.263, also known as H.263+, includes error resilience tools that are defined in the baseline syntax and in four of its normative annexes (49,50). The visual part of the MPEG-4 standard also provides support for error resilience (1,51). We here discuss briefly the error resilience tools included in these video coding standards as listed in Table 8.4.

8.6.1   Forward Error Correction

The FEC mode, the oldest of the error resilience oriented optional modes, is available in H.261 and H.263. If this mode is enabled, the video bitstream is

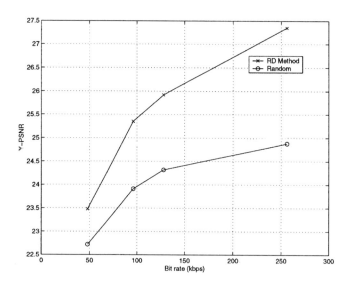

Figure 8.16 Performance of RD-optimized intra coding for the sequence FOREMAN and a block loss rate *p* of 20%.

Table 8.4 Error Resilience Tools Supported in H.263 Version 2 and MPEG-4

Standard	FEC	Sync words	RVLCs	Data partitioning	Independent segment decoding	Reference picture selection	HEC
H.263	Yes	Yes	Yes	No[a]	Yes	Yes	No[b]
MPEG-4	No	Yes	Yes	Yes	No	No[c]	Yes

[a] Data partitioning will be included in Version 3 of H.263.
[b] Although H.263 does not support this mode, the transport protocol for H.263 may support it, for example, in RFC-2429.
[c] Reference picture selection will likely be included in Version 2 of MPEG-4.

divided into FEC frames of 493 bits each. A (511,493) BCH forward error correction checksum is calculated for all the bits of each frame, including one bit that is necessary for the synchronization to the frame structure. This code adds 18 parity bits to a source block of 493 bits and allows correction of 2-bit random errors. This code is typically employed for error correction for ISDN and may be used for error detection in highly error-prone environments such as mobile networks.

8.6.2 Synchronization Words

For both packet lossy and bit-error-prone channels, the intelligent use of synchronization markers is necessary to ensure fast resynchronization during decoding. Even in the baseline mode of operation, synchronization markers can be inserted by using the optional GOB headers. Unfortunately, the size of coded GOBs cannot be chosen according to a fixed packet size, or adapted freely to a bit interval chosen according to the error rate. More freedom in placing synchronization markers is allowed when slices are employed, which are optionally supported in H.263 and MPEG-4. As seen earlier, slices permit the insertion of synchronization markers after each coded block, thus allowing for a more judicious placement of the synchronization markers within a coded picture. In addition to providing bitstream resynchronization, sync words allow for spatial resynchronization within a coded video frame.

8.6.3 Reversible Variable-Length Codes

When Annex D of H.263 is used within H.263 Version 2, the coding of motion vector information is performed by means of RVLCs. In MPEG-4, when the data-partitioning mode is employed, DCT coefficient information is coded by means of RVLCs. RVLCs are discussed in Section 8.4.4.

8.6.4 Data Partitioning

The forthcoming third version of H.263 will likely include data partitioning, already supported by MPEG-4. Data partitioning was presented in Section 8.4.2.

8.6.5 Independent Segment Decoding

As already described, slices are self-contained insofar as all prediction mechanisms within a coded picture are interrupted. This, however, does not prevent error propagation due to motion compensation. Error propagation can be prevented by using the independent segment decoding (ISD) mode, supported in H.263, which enforces the treatment of segment boundaries as if they were picture boundaries. A segment is defined as a slice, a GOB, or a number of consecutive GOBs with empty GOB headers. In such a case, error propagation outside the segment boundaries (due to motion compensation) can be avoided. Note that by using video objects, similar error resilience gains can be achieve in MPEG-4 (1).

8.6.6 Reference Picture Selection

The reference picture selection mode, defined in Annex N of H.263, supports reference picture selection and video redundancy coding. The methods can be applied either to pictures or to individual rectangular (GOB or slice) picture segments. If feedback messages are employed, they can be either multiplexed into the H.263 datastream of the opposite direction (video multiplex backchannel submode), or conveyed out of band (separate logical channel submode) (49).

8.6.7 Header Extension Code

The header extension code allows the introduction of duplicate copies of important picture header information in the video packets. The HEC includes information such as spatial dimension of the frame, temporal location, and the coding mode of the frame. This technique reduces significantly the number of discarded video frames in error-prone environments. This mode is supported in the visual part of MPEG-4, and a similar tool is included in the RTP payload specification for H.263 Version 2, defined in Request for Comments 2429 (24).

8.7 CONCLUSIONS

Existing and future communication networks do not always guarantee error-free transmission; thus transmission of compressed video in such environments presents many challenges. In this chapter we discussed error resilience coding methods that allow reliable video communication in error-prone environments. We first described the effects of errors on the compressed video bitstreams. Then, we discussed data recovery techniques that have been applied to video communication systems. Finally, we presented the error resilience coding methods, which have been developed to limit, or contain, the effects of spatiotemporal error propagation. Many of these error resilience methods are now supported by video standards such as H.263 and MPEG-4. The effects of random and often time-varying errors on compressed video bitstreams are still not well understood, and the design of error-resilient coding methods for both bit-oriented and packet-based networks is often empirical. Error-resilient video coding is a relatively new area of research, and many more error resilience coding methods are yet to be developed.

REFERENCES

1. R Talluri. Error resilient video coding in the MPEG-4 standard. IEEE Commun Mag 26(6): 112–119, June 1998.
2. SB Wicker. Error Control Systems for Digital Communication and Storage. Toronto: Prentice Hall Canada, 1995.
3. JG Proakis. Digital Communication. 3rd ed. McGraw-Hill, New York, 1995.
4. A Andreadis, G Benelli, A Garzelli, S Susini, FEC coding for H.263 compatible video transmission. Proceedings of International Conference on Image Processing, Santa Barbara, CA, October 1997, pp 579–581.

5. W Rabiner Heinzelman, M Budagavi, R Talluri. Unequal error protection of MPEG-4 compressed video. Proceedings of International Conference on Image Processing, Kobe, Japan, October 1999.
6. J Rosenberg, H. Schulzrinn. An RTP payload format for generic forward error correction. Internet draft, February 1999, Available from http://info.internet.isi.edu:80/in-drafts/files/draft-ietf-avt-fec-05.txt.
7. SH Lee, PJ Lee, R Ansari. Cell loss detection and recovery in variable rate video. Proceedings of the Third International Workshop on Packet Video, Morristown, NJ, March 1990.
8. EW Biersack. Performance evaluation of forward error correction in an ATM environment. IEEE Selected Areas Commun 11(4):631–640, May 1993.
9. E Ayanoglu, R Pancha, AR Reibman, S Talwar, Forward error control for MPEG-2 video transport in a wireless ATM LAN. ACM/Baltzer Mobile Networks Appl 1(3): 245–258, December 1996.
10. U Horn, KW Stuhlmueller, M Link, B Girod. Robust Internet video transmission based on scalable coding and unequal error protection. EURASIP Image Commun. Special issue on real-time video over the Internet 15:77–94, September 1999.
11. W Tan, A Zakhor. Error control for video multicasting using hierarchical FEC. International Conference on Image Processing, Kobe, Japan, October 1999.
12. S Lin, D Costello, M Miller. Automatic-repeat-request error-control schemes. IEEE Commun Mag 22(12):5–17, December 1984.
13. M Khansari, A Jalali, E Dubois, P Mermelstein. Low bit-rate video transmission over fading channels for wireless microcellular system. IEEE Trans Circuits Syst Video Technol. 6:1–11, February 1996.
14. H Lui, M El Zarki. Performance of H.263 video transmission over wireless channels using hybrid ARQ. IEEE J Selected Areas Commun 15(9):1775–1786, December 1997.
15. WS Lee, MR Pickering, MR Frater, JF Arnold. Error resilience in video and multiplexing layers for very low bit-rate video coding systems. IEEE J Selected Areas Commun 15(9):1764–1774, December 1997.
16. TJ Ferguson, JH Rabinowitz. Self-synchronizing Huffman codes. IEEE Trans Info Theory IT-30(4):687–693, July 1984.
17. JC Maxted, JP Robinson. Error recovery for variable length codes. IEEE Trans Inf Theory IT-31:794–801, 1985.
18. GCôté, S Shirani, F Kossentini. Optimal mode selection and synchronization for robust video communications over error prone networks. IEEE J Selected Areas Commun (accepted for publication).
19. H Everett. Generalized Lagrange multiplier method for solving problems of optimum allocation of resources. Oper Res 1:399–417, 1963.
20. GJ Sullivan, T Wiegand. Rate-distortion optimization for video compression. IEEE Signal Process Mag 15(6):74–90, November 1998.
21. A Ortega, K Ramchandran. Rate-distortion methods for image and video compression. IEEE Signal Process Mag 15(6):23–50, November 1998.
22. R Talluri, I Moccagatta, Y Nag, G Cheung. Error concealment by data partitioning Signal Process: Image Commun Mag 14:505–518, May 1999.

23. DS Park, JH Park, JD Kim, YS Kim. Error-resilient video coding in H.263+ against error-prone mobile channels. SPIE Proceedings on Visual Communications and Image Processing, San Jose, CA, January 1999, vol 3653, pp 200–207.

24. C Bormann, L Cline, G Deisher, T Gardos, C Maciocco. D Newell, J Ott, G Sullivan, S Wenger, C Zhu. RTP payload format for the 1998 version of ITU-T Recommendation H.263 video (H.263+). Request for Comments 2429, May 1998. Available from ftp://ftp.isi.edu/in-notes/rfc2429.txt.

25. Y Takishima, M Wada, H Murakami. Reversible variable length codes. IEEE Trans Commun 43(2):158–162, February 1995.

26. J Wen, JD Villasenor. A class of reversible variable length codes for robust image and video coding. Proceedings of International Conference on Image Processing, Santa Barbara, CA, October 1997, vol 2, pp 65–68.

27. B Girod. Bidirectionally decodable streams of prefix code words IEEE Commun Lett 3(8), August 1999.

28. DW Redmill, NG Kingsbury. The EREC: An error resilient technique for coding variable-length blocks of data. IEEE Trans Image Process 5:565–574, April 1996.

29. KN Ngan, CW Yap. Combined source-channel video coding. Signal Recovery Techniques for Image and Video Compression and Transmission. Kluwer Academic Publishers, Boston, 1998.

30. BP Tunstall. Synthesis of noiseless compression codes, Ph.D. dissertation, Georgia Institute of Technology, 1968.

31. T Algra. Fast and efficient variable-to-fixed-length coding algorithm. Electron Lett 1399–1401, July 1992.

32. R Llados-Bernaus, RL Stevenson. Fixed-length entropy coding for robust video compression. IEEE Trans Circuits Syst Video Technol 8(6):745–755, October 1998.

33. G Côté, M Gallant, F Kossentini. Semi-fixed length motion vector coding for H.263-based low bit rate video compression. IEEE Trans. Image Process 8(10):1451–1455, October 1999.

34. J Hagenauer. Rate-compatible punctured convolutional codes and their applications. IEEE Trans Commun 36(4):389–400, April 1988.

35. A El Gamal, T Cover. Achievable rates for multiple descriptions. IEEE Trans Inf Theory IT-28(6):851–857, November 1982.

36. V Vaishampayan. Design of multiple description scalar quantizers. IEEE Trans Inf Theory 39(3):821–834, May 1993.

37. J-C Batallo and V Vaishampayan. Asymptotic performance of multiple description transform codes. IEEE Trans Inf Theory 43:703–707, March 1997.

38. Y Wang, M Orchard, A Reibman, V Vaishampayan. Redundancy rate distortion analysis of multiple description image coding using pairwise correlating transforms. Proceedings of International Conference on Image Processing, Santa Barbara, CA, October 1997, pp 608–611.

39. S Fukunaga, T Nakai, H Inoue. Error resilient video coding by dynamic replacing of reference pictures. Proceedings of IEEE Global Telecommunications Conference, New York, November 1996, vol 3, pp 1503–1508.

40. M Khansari. Performance of predictive coders over noisy channels with feedback.

Proceedings of IEEE International Conference on Acoustics, Speech, and Signal Processing, Seattle, WA, May 1998, vol 6, pp 3473–3476.

41. S Wenger. Video redundancy coding in H.263+. Proceedings of AVSPN, Aberdeen, Scotland, September 1997.

42. P Haskell, D Messerschmitt. Resynchronization of motion compensated video affected by ATM cell loss. Proceedings of the IEEE International Conference on Acoustics Speech and Signal Processing, San Francisco, March, 1992, vol 3, pp 545–548.

43. N Naka, S Adachi, M Saigusa, T Ohya. Improved error resilience in mobile audio-visual communications. Proceedings of IEEE International Conference on Universal Personal Communications, Tokyo, November 1995, vol 1, pp 702–706.

44. JY Liao and JD Villasenor. Adaptive intra update for video coding over noisy channels. Proceedings of International Conference on Image Processing, Lausanne, Switzerland, September 1996, vol 3, pp 763–766.

45. G Côté, F Kossentini. Optimal intra coding of blocks for robust video communication over the Internet. Signal Process: Image Commun. special issue on real-time video over the Internet 15:25–34, September 1999.

46. N Fäerber, KW Stuhlmueller, B Girod. Analysis of error propagation in hybrid video coding with application to error resilience. Proceedings International Conference on Image Processing. Kobe, Japan, October 1999.

47. M Wada. Selective recovery of video packet loss using error concealment. IEEE J Selected Areas Commun 7(5):807–814, June 1989.

48. E Steinbach, N Fäerber, B. Girod. Standard compatible extension of H.263 for robust video transmission in mobile environment. IEEE Trans Circuits Syst Video Technol 7(6):872–881, December 1997.

49. ITU-T Recommendation H.263, Version 2. Video coding for low bitrate communication. International Telecommunications Union, Geneva, January 1998.

50. S Wenger, G Knorr, J Ott, F Kossentini. Error resilience support in H.263+. IEEE Trans Circuits Syst Video Technol 8(6):867–877, November 1998.

51. ISO/IEC 14496-2. Coding of audio-visual objects: Visual Final draft international standard. ISO/IEC JTC1/SC29/WG11 N2502, October 1998.

9
Variable Bit Rate Video Coding

Antonio Ortega
Department of Electrical Engineering–Systems,
University of Southern California, Los Angeles, California

9.1 INTRODUCTION

The goal of this chapter is to establish the importance of variable bit rate (VBR) coding of video as a means of providing good decoded video quality, and to show how VBR video can be best incorporated within a networking infrastructure, and in particular within a network environment that supports VBR transport. Throughout this chapter we use the terms VBR and CBR (constant bit rate) to refer to both coding modes (where the rate refers to the number of bits used per frame) and transport modes (where rate refers to the number of bits that can be transmitted during certain periods of time). Whether coding or transmission is at issue should be clear from the context or is stated explicitly.

We start by showing how video compressed at constant quality will result in a variable number of bits per frame. Thus, if the bitstream generated by a video encoder must be kept very close to a constant rate (e.g., for transmission over a CBR channel), there will be a penalty in terms of quality. If a particular scene requires too many bits for the available channel bandwidth, for example, the quality will have to be lowered.

Emerging networks provide a great deal more flexibility than traditional point-to-point dedicated links or circuit-switching networking techniques when it comes to bandwidth utilization. For example, new network environments based on packet switching, such as the Internet, lend themselves very naturally to VBR transmission and thus seem to be better suited to transmit video streams, which tend to be VBR in nature. Therefore the variable rate produced by the encoder can potentially be matched to a variable transport rate, whereas in a CBR transmission environment the video encoder would have to adjust its rate to match the constant channel rate constraint. Still, while VBR transport is appealing, even if the network supports variable rate transmission it is not necessarily true that it can transport without loss any arbitrary video bitstream, in particular if transmission is subject to strict delay constraints. In this chapter we concentrate on the problem of matching VBR video coding to VBR transport modes of various kinds. Details on these various modes can be found in other chapters in this book, as well as in papers dealing with VBR transport of video (1–3).

In Section 9.2 we begin by providing concrete examples of the variable rate nature of video sequences by examining bit-rate traces for a video sequence coded with a single quantization step size. Obviously a variable rate compression can be achieved in many different ways, and this section briefly highlights some popular techniques that lead to different coding rates for the same input sequence.

In Section 9.3, we devote our attention to the delay constraints that arise in typical video applications. These delay constraints are the most general constraints imposed on a video communications system, since they depend solely on the specific video application being considered, rather than on the channel characteristics or the type of transport mode (VBR or CBR) that is selected. Networked video applications can be categorized into three main classes: (a) live interactive video (LIV; e.g., video conferencing), (b) live noninteractive video (LNIV; e.g., broadcasting), and (c) playback of preencoded video (PEV). For each of these scenarios we discuss the specific form of the delay constraints. While all three application classes are likely to be encountered in practice, in this chapter we discuss mainly live applications (LIV or LNIV), which are more challenging in general.

Typically the video encoder must select the coding parameters, and thus the coding rate, to avoid violating the delay constraints. Clearly, the degree of difficulty in meeting these constraints will depend on the bandwidth and delay characteristics of the transmission channel. Thus, in a network with unlimited bandwidth and low delay, one could transmit very high quality video without risk of violating the delay constraints. In Section 9.4 we discuss several possible transmission modes that are often encountered in existing systems. These modes differ in the variability of the channel rate (e.g., CBR vs. VBR) as well as in the amount of information the encoder has about the channel conditions.

Given these transmission classes, in Section 9.5 we define three general problems, each of which leads to a different set of rate constraints for the encoder. These cases are the CBR channel, the VBR channel with deterministic rates, and the VBR channel with randomly varying rates. For each of these scenarios we provide rate constraints the decoder must meet to avoid data loss due to excessive delay.

Section 9.6 presents a summary of the work that has been done in recent years to enable rate control at the encoder to meet the aforementioned constraints. A complete survey of rate control techniques falls outside the scope of this chapter, and thus we emphasize approaches that attempt to optimize the selection of rates. While in real-world applications simpler techniques may be selected, focusing on the optimized approaches allows us to discuss some of the desirable features that all rate control algorithms (whether emphasizing optimality or simplicity) should seek to achieve. Finally, Section 9.7 summarizes the key ideas in the chapter and points to some of the transmission environments in which VBR transmission of video is likely to remain a challenging area of research in the short term.

9.2   VARIABLE RATE COMPRESSION OF VIDEO

It is easy to define VBR video encoding: a video encoder is VBR if it produces a variable number of bits per frame. Of course this is not a very useful definition in that, as described in the video coding standards chapters, practically all video encoders of interest are VBR. Thus in this section we discuss in more detail how VBR video is produced and what its quality implications are. In particular we emphasize that for practical video coding schemes there are many ways of producing a VBR stream, and these must be compared in terms of quality or distortion. (How the quality or the distortion is measured will be discussed next, in Section 9.2.1.)

Three factors explain the variable rate nature of compressed video, namely, the coding frame type, the input video characteristics, and the coding parameters. First, in most practical coders there exist various frame coding modes, which result in different rates for the same input frame. For example, MPEG-2 coders include I, P, and B frames, and since P and B frames utilize motion-compensated prediction, while I frames do not, P and B frames result in lower overall coding rate (refer to the chapters on video coding standards in Part 1 for further details).

Second, even if one considers a single type of frame (e.g., all frames are coded in intra mode), and the remaining coding parameters are fixed, there will be rate variations due to the changes in the scene contents. These variations, as will be seen in Section 9.2.2, can be very significant. For example, a difference of a factor of 2 in bit rate between frames in a given sequence is fairly common.

Finally, the output rate depends on the selection of coding parameters. For the sake of flexibility, and to incorporate the maximum number of features into the encoder, most standard video compression systems incorporate many different coding parameters (from quantizers to coding modes to motion compensation modes) that can be used to modulate the output rate. Section 9.2.3 provides a brief overview of these, and we once again refer to the video coding standards chapters for detailed descriptions of these algorithms.

9.2.1 Rate Distortion Trade-offs for VBR Video

Video compression algorithms aim to achieve the best possible quality *delivered to the end user.* Thus, the video quality provided to the end user will depend not only on decisions made at the encoder, but also on how the video data is transported over the network (e.g., if the encoder produces too much data for the channel bandwidth, some data may be lost). Thus, an important theme in this chapter is that end-to-end video quality depends on both source and network, and for this reason knowledge of the channel characteristics (e.g., bandwidth, loss, or delay characteristics) should be incorporated into the way the video encoder operates. With this knowledge, through intelligent rate control, the video encoder will be able to get the most end-to-end video quality out of the available channel.

For most applications of interest, video is compressed in a lossy manner; that is, the decoded sequence is not an exact copy of the original video sequence. Perhaps a lossless compression is needed in only two situations: scientific applications, where all the available information is likely to be needed for later processing and analysis, and entertainment applications, where lossy compression could lead to artifacts during production and thus is likely to be introduced only when the final version of the video is ready.

Thus, we consider here lossy compression only. To meet our stated goal of providing the best video quality to the end user, we first need to determine ways of measuring this lossy video quality. Knowledg e of perceptual issues is more developed for image coding (4) than for video, although in the latter case some basic facts are known (5). The quality of individual frames in a video sequence can be assessed in much the same way as for still images. Video quality may change over time, however and this possibility must be taken into account. A typical assumption is that overall perceptual quality for a complete sequence will depend on the quality of its worst quality scene, given that the worst scene is sufficiently long (5).

While some general guidelines may apply, the quality assessment will also depend on the type of application being considered. Thus, quality expectations for a videoconferencing application are likely to be much lower than for the delivery of a movie over a network. Note also that we do not consider here the effect of packet losses on perceptual quality (these are considered in Chapter 6, on error concealment).

A popular approach for perceptually based compression is to introduce in the encoding process some constraints that are perceptually meaningful and then let the encoder optimize an objective metric, such as mean-squared error (MSE) or weighted MSE. One example of this approach is the design of quantization matrices for coding based on discrete cosine transforms DCT (see Chapter 2, on video coding standards), where frequencies are given different weights according to their relative perceptual importance. Another example comes in the bit allocation among frames, where a generally accepted rule of thumb is that quality should be kept more or less constant from frame to frame, and therefore a good bit allocation should try to penalize large changes in quantization step size within a set of frames.

For applications that involve real-time encoding and transmission (i.e., applications that need low overall delay) these so-called objective distortion metrics will be sufficient. As will be seen, for offline encoding applications more sophisticated techniques are required to supplement MSE-based approaches as it becomes possible, for example, to determine which scenes in a given video sequence require more rate to achieve similar perceptual quality.

9.2.2 Achieving Constant Quality Requires Variable Rate

Compression is achieved by exploiting the existing redundancies in the source (e.g., spatial, temporal, and statistical redundancy). Since the level of redundancy varies from frame to frame, it comes as no surprise that the number of bits per frame must be variable, even if the same quantization parameters are used for all frames.

Consider, for example, the spatial allocation of bits in a frame. As described in earlier chapters, the number of bits required to encode an image block, with a given quantization step size, will depend on the frequency contents of the block. Therefore, images containing high-frequency information will require more bits than frames having predominantly low-frequency content. Similarly, scenes with significant motion will require more bits than scenes exhibiting little or no motion.

Thus, a fundamental result in video coding is that maintaining a constant (perceptual or objective) quality throughout a sequence requires a variable rate allocation. This large variability has been observed in video trace analysis work such as that of Garrett (6), or Rose (7). For example, the trace shown in Figure 9.1 corresponds to the movie *Mission Impossible,* where the sequence has been coded with a constant quantization parameter in a Motion JPEG framework*. As can be seen, changes of over a factor of 2 are common, and for longer sequences even larger variations are likely. Figure 9.2 also shows how the MSE varies substantially from frame to frame. Note that if an MPEG coder (9) were used instead, the average rate per group of pictures (GOP) would show similar

---

* Each frame is coded using JPEG (8), and the same JPEG coding parameters are used for every frame. We use the measured total number of bits per frame and the average distortion (MSE) in our traces.

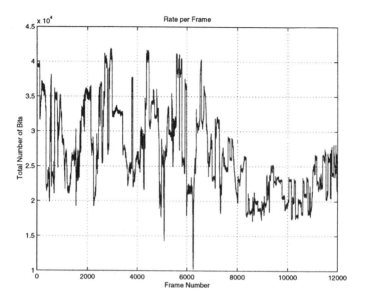

Figure 9.1 *Mission Impossible* trace: rate.

variability, but variations in rate within a GOP would depend mostly on the frame type (e.g., I frames vs. B frames).

These traces illustrate how the problem of achieving constant perceptual quality for a whole sequence takes different forms depending on whether live or preencoded video is considered. On the one hand, it is not possible to guess what the contents of future frames of live video will be, and therefore, at a given time, the encoder will have to make coding decisions to target the quality of the current frames.

On the other hand, let us consider authoring of compressed movies for DVD storage as an example of preencoded video. In this particular scenario the only constraint is the overall storage capacity in the DVD (since data can be read into the player at a rate much higher than the typical video coding rates), and therefore the number of bits assigned to different scenes can show significant variations. Moreover, given that these movies are compressed once but decoded many times, a relatively complex encoding process is acceptable as long as the achievable quality gains are significant.

Thus, a two-pass approach is typically used, where the first pass aims at locating scenes that have higher "complexity" (i.e., will require a larger amount of bits to achieve the desired quality). This can be accomplished by coding the whole sequence with a single quantizer scale and then determining which parts of the sequence have required more bits (see, e.g., Refs. 10, 11). This information is then used in the second pass of the algorithm, where the encoder is al-

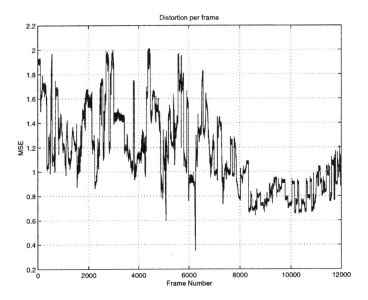

Figure 9.2 *Mission Impossible* trace: distortion.

lowed to adapt the quantization step size, based on the results of the first pass. For example, for "easy" scenes it may possible to decrease the rate, with respect to the first pass, without affecting the perceptual quality.

The concept of scene complexity is illustrated by the plots of Figure 9.3. The top two plots are normalized versions of Figures 9.1 and 9.2, where we have normalized by dividing all rate or MSE values by the maximum rate or MSE in the sequence [e.g., $R'_i = R_i/\max_i(R_i)$, where R_i and R'_i are, respectively, the rate and the normalized rate for frame i]. The bottom plot shows the normalized value per frame of the product of rate and MSE (i.e., $D \cdot R$) for each of the selected quantizers. Note that since typical rate distortion characteristics can be roughly modeled as having the form $D = K/R$, for a given constant K, then $D \cdot R$ does provide an approximation to the complexity of a particular frame. Under the $D = K/R$ modeling assumption, a large K means that many bits are required to achieve low distortion, and thus a frame with large $D \cdot R$ can be deemed to have high complexity. Conversely, a small K would indicate low complexity, since a small number of bits can significantly reduce distortion. In the particular example of the bottom curve of Figure 9.3, the final section of the sequence (say, after frame 8000) seems to be less complex than the beginning, and thus a two-pass algorithm would tend to allocate more bits to the beginning of the sequence than to the end.

Interestingly, two-pass algorithms are not enough for professional DVD applications, and there is usually a third stage before the final compressed ver-

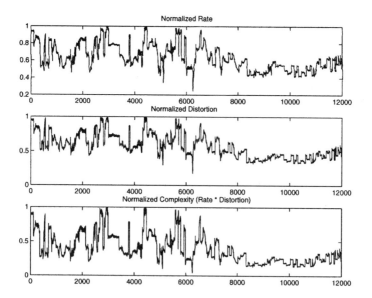

Figure 9.3 *Mission Impossible* trace: normalized rate, distortion, and complexity per frame. Note that variations from scene to scene are very significant.

sion is produced. In this final stage a person actually views the decoded sequence and applies selected modifications to the coding parameters to ensure that any remaining visible artifacts are removed. The role of this person (sometimes called the "compressionist"!) clearly demonstrates not only that MSE has its limitations but also that reliable, automatized, perceptual quality metrics remain difficult to define. Therefore achieving near-perfect perceptual quality (under rate constraints) remains almost an art.

In summary, we can assume, as in Reference 11, that through frame complexity estimation or other techniques it will be possible to determine the "ideal rate" for each segment of a sequence. Here ideal rate is defined as the minimum number of bits that produces transparent quality (i.e., such that the original segment and the decoded one are indistinguishable). Such an ideal rate, or an alternative rate allocation aiming at constant perceptual quality, will be different for each segment in the sequence, and therefore coding at constant quality will necessarily require variable rate per frame.

9.2.3 Mechanisms Available to Produce Variable Rate Video

In the example of Figures 9.1 and 9.2 we kept a fixed quantization step size for all frames and employed intra-only coding (i.e., all frames were coded by using

JPEG, with the same coding parameters for all frames). Obviously, as indicated in the video coding standards chapters, a state-of-the-art coder incorporates many other coding options. Examples of how these coding options can be judiciously chosen to optimize performance are given elsewhere (12). Here we provide just a rapid overview of available mechanisms. We refer to the chapters in Part 1 for further details about the various parameters that can be chosen for each frame, and to Reference 12 for a detailed description of techniques that can enable efficient selection of parameters.

9.2.3.1 Quantizer Selection.

The most immediate approach to the production of a variable rate is to change the quantization step size. All video compression algorithms used in practice, including those based on standards, allow flexibility in the selection of quantizer (see the chapters in Part 1). Typically, each individual block or macroblock within a frame can be assigned a different quantization step size. These features are included in video compression algorithms primarily to allow the systems to operate at several channel rates and to provide the benefits of a good bit allocation within a given image. For example, one can allocate a finer quantizer to parts of the image that may be more sensitive to quantization errors. Well-known techniques such as Lagrangian optimization can be used to achieve an efficient allocation in the rate distortion (RD) sense among the blocks (12–14).

For video coding, quantizer selection is further complicated by the practice of using motion-compensated prediction. Because motion-compensated prediction is based on transmitting the difference between a previously quantized frame and the current frame, quantizer selection for one frame affects the RD performance for future frames (15).

9.2.3.2 Coding Mode Selection.

In addition to the quantization step size, other coding parameters (or coding modes) can be chosen for use for each macroblock. In particular, for inter frames each macroblock can be predicted, skipped, or coded in intra mode. Typically, this decision can be made by considering which of the modes provides the least energy residue in the motion-compensated predicted frame. However, alternative approaches can be used, where the trade-off between rate and distortion is considered. More generally, other modes of operation might be selected, including, for example, the type of motion compensation used (e.g., overlapped vs. nonoverlapped, motion vector block size, etc.) (12).

9.2.3.3 Frame-Type Selection.

Consider as an example MPEG-2 (see Chapter 2). The three frame types (I, P, B) can be chosen according to several criteria. For example, a specific application such as stored video may require that I frames be placed at fixed intervals (e.g., one every 0.5 second) to enable random access and features such as fast forward and rewind. In a real-time application, frame selection can be used to modulate the encoding rate. For example, the spacing between I frames can increase if lower rate is desired. As before, the frame-type selection can be optimized based on the RD trade-off (16).

9.2.3.4 Frame Skipping. Finally, certain video coding standards allow frame skipping, leading to a variable frame rate and therefore variable rate video. Frame skipping means reducing the number of frames per second that are transmitted (e.g., from the original rate of 30 frames/s to, say, 10 frames/s) so that if a lower source rate is required, one can transmit fewer frames but use more bits per frame. This option is obviously more suitable for interactive video and in general low-quality applications, where it is not crucial to maintain a constant number of frames per second. In particular, for computer-based applications, as opposed to systems in which specialized hardware is used, it may be easy to support the display of a variable number of frames per second and even to introduce techniques for interpolation at the receiver.

9.3   DELAY CONSTRAINTS FOR REAL-TIME DECODING
AND DISPLAY OF VIDEO

The two main ideas presented in Section 9.2 are that constant quality video tends to require a variable bit rate and that there are many ways in which a variable rate bitstream can be generated. The encoder has the ability to select parameters for each of these modes and as in Reference 12, methods such as Lagrangian optimization and dynamic programming (14) can be used to search the space of all possible operating points to find the one that is better in a rate distortion sense. Section 9.6 discusses issues of rate control, that is, how to allocate bits among different frames in a sequence. Obviously these problems arise only when there are constraints (as there surely will be) on the total rate that can be used. The goal of this section is to describe the possible delay constraints that will make transmission at the ideal rate unfeasible in practice. More detailed discussions of the various delay constraints can be found elsewhere (17–19).

9.3.1   Delay Constraints: Preventing Decoder Buffer
Underflow

Let us assume that a video sequence with a total of M frames is transmitted at a fixed number of frames per second.* Let R_i be the number of bits assigned to the ith frame.[†] Let $t_d = 0$ be the time at which the first bit of the video sequence is received by the decoder. Time is measured in units of number of frames at the decoder. Thus, $t_d = i$ corresponds to i frame intervals having passed, where one

---

* Our formulation could be easily adapted to having a variable number of frames per second, but we make this assumption for simplicity.
[†] It would be possible to consider smaller basic units (e.g., a set of blocks within a frame), but for simplicity we consider frames as our basic unit.

frame interval lasts δ_f seconds. For example, assuming that 30 frames/s are being displayed at the decoder, $\delta_f = 1/30$ second. Let C_i be the number of bits received by the decoder buffer during the ith frame interval. Note that C_i does not correspond necessarily to compressed data for the ith frame. This is because data for a particular frame could be transmitted over several frame intervals, depending on bandwidth conditions and the number of bits used to code the frame.

We will assume that the decoder actually begins decoding and displaying frames after ΔN_d frame intervals, or $\Delta T_d = \Delta N_d \cdot \delta_f$ seconds, have passed. Thus, the first frame (frame 1) will be decoded and displayed at time $t_d = \Delta N_d$. Although a more detailed analysis of the delays involved—for example, computation delay, is possible (see, e.g., Ref. 20), here we assume that frames are instantaneously decoded and displayed.

Under this framework, the system will function normally as long as the decoder buffer is "fed" frames fast enough that after time $t_d = \Delta N_d$, the decoder can play δ_f^{-1} frames per second. Note that so far we have made no assumption about how the frames are generated at the transmitter or when they are transmitted. Since we assume that frames are played back at a constant rate, it follows that if the first frame is decoded at time ΔN_d, then the ith frame must be available at time $i - 1 + \Delta N_d$: that is, $(i - 1 + \Delta N_d) \cdot \delta_f$ seconds after the first bit was received at the decoder. In the most general case, the goal of the transmitter will be to avoid decoder buffer underflow (see also Figure 9.4). Obviously decoder buffer overflow as well as encoder buffer overflow and underflow also must be addressed. However overflow at either buffer can be addressed by providing sufficient buffer memory. Given the continued decrease in memory costs, the assumption that sufficient memory is available seems to be reasonable for many applications. Encoder buffer underflow can be easily avoided by not transmitting data. Thus from now on we focus on decoder buffer underflow prevention, and this is the main objective of the rate control algorithms of Section 9.6.

In our system, the compressed video data is placed in a transmission buffer, then drained and transmitted. We assume that the video encoder and the transmitter are combined so that the video encoder can control when data is transmitted.

Formulation 1 Decoder buffer underflow prevention *To prevent the decoder from losing frames the transmitter must ensure that all the information corresponding to frame i has arrived to the decoder before $t_d = i - 1 + \Delta N_d$. This is equivalent to the channel rates having been sufficient to transmit all the necessary data:*

$$\sum_{k=1}^{i-1+\Delta N_d} C_k \geq \sum_{k=1}^{i} R_k, \forall_i \tag{1}$$

that is, the total channel rate used up to time $i - 1 + \Delta N_d$ has been enough to transport the first i frames.

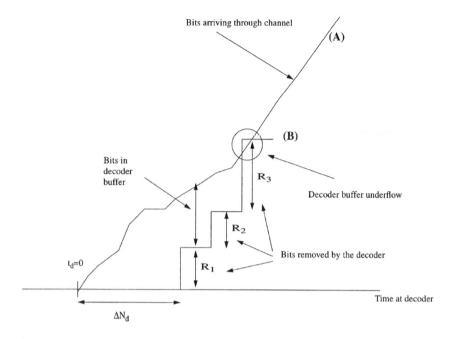

Figure 9.4   Data received at the decoder and data that must be available for decoding to proceed. Clearly, if the decoder demand (B) exceeds the channel supplied data (A) at any time, the decoder will be unable to operate correctly. This is what is called decoder buffer underflow.

Note that we are assuming that no frames are skipped at the encoder. Clearly, if the encoder was allowed to skip frames, some of the time and delay constraints might be less stringent than if all frames had to be encoded and delivered. However, even when the encoder generates a variable number of frames per second, constraints similar to those above would hold, except that the frame intervals would have variable size.

We continue to assume that the encoding and decoding delays are constant and thus are not taken into account in what follows. Thus, the two delay components that can result in a violation of the constraint of Eq. (1) are transmitter buffer delay and transmission channel delay.

Transmitter buffer delay, δ_{tb}: the delay due to the time needed to drain video data corresponding to a particular frame, after it has been placed in the transmit buffer by the encoder. This delay exists only if the channel bandwidth is limited and does not match the data produced for all frames; otherwise, data could be drained into the channel as soon as it is produced. Clearly, given the video data, the lower the channel rate, the longer this delay will be.

Transmission channel delay, δ_{ch}: the delay suffered by packets of video data being transmitted through the network (i.e., from the time they have been extracted from the transmit buffer to the time when they are available at the receiver buffer). This delay may be variable in numerous scenarios, such as transmission over a shared network or transmission over a lossy link (here delay is assumed to include the time needed for retransmission of lost data if applicable).

Clearly, then, for a given coded sequence the channel resources must be selected such that the total delay $\delta_{tb} + \delta_{ch}$ incurred by each video frame does not result in a violation of the decoder buffer underflow constraint.

As an example of the delay variability, consider Figure 9.5, which depicts the number of frame intervals required to transmit 100 frames at a constant rate

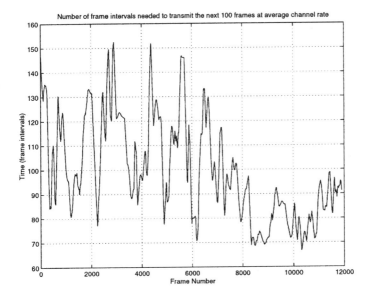

Figure 9.5 Total delay in transmitting 100 frames. For each frame, we plot the number of frame intervals that would be needed to transmit the next 100 frames under the assumption that the average rate per frame for the whole sequence is used as the constant channel rate. Note that the delay oscillates around 100 frames and that some scenes require more than 100 frames for transmission.

equal to the average rate of the sequence. This was generated by taking the rate trace of Figure 9.1, computing the overall average rate, and dividing the total rate for each group of 100 frames by the average frame rate. As can be seen, when most of the frames are below the average rate, transmission can be completed in less than 100 frame intervals, while when the rate is greater, a longer delay is incurred. In other words, if a delay constraint of 100 frame intervals ($\Delta N_d = 100$) were to be enforced, lower average rate would be required for many frames in the initial part of the sequence

9.3.2 Real-Time Versus Pre-encoded Video

The delay constraint comes into play because the decoder cannot "wait" for late frames. Thus, to know whether the delay $\delta_{tb} + \delta_{ch}$ exceeds this maximum delay we must first know *when* the encoded frames first become available. To make this determination, we differentiate between live and preencoded video.

9.3.2.1 Preencoded Video.
Let us consider first offline playback of a preencoded source. In this case the whole video sequence has already been encoded and is ready to be transmitted. Thus, in this scenario we can assume that the transmission buffer is very large and contains the whole video sequence at the beginning of transmission. Even if, as is the case for disk-based video servers, there are two separate levels of storage (e.g., disk and transmission buffer), it is still likely that the bottleneck will be in transmission, rather than in moving data from the storage device into the transmission buffer. Thus, since all the frames are available at the transmitter from the beginning, and the deadline depends only on the decoder, the maximum delay that a frame can experience will be variable. For example, as illustrated by Figure 9.6, for a given channel rate, if the number of frames per second transmitted is large (e.g., > 30 frames/s), subsequent frames may be transmitted over a longer interval of time without being lost at the decoder. Thus, in the PEV case, ignoring the channel delay, we have ΔN_d frame intervals to transmit the first frame and in general $\Delta N_d + i$ intervals to transmit the ith frame, since all the frames are available at the transmitter at the start of the video transmission. In summary, as seen in Figure 9.6, the maximum delay per frame is different for each frame, and there is more flexibility in transmission than in the live video case, which we consider next.

9.3.2.2 Live Video.
Consider the scenario of video captured in real time, then compressed and transmitted. Assume that the first frame experiences delays δ^1_{tb} and δ^1_{ch} after the time the frame has been captured and compressed. Normally δ^1_{tb} will tend to be very small or zero, since there are no other frames waiting to be transmitted. A delay may exist, however, because time is needed to set up the transmission or because the encoder decides to store a few frames in the

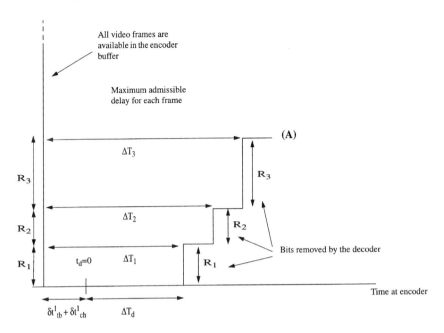

Figure 9.6 Delay constraints in the preencoded video case.

encoder buffer before transmission actually starts (e.g., to avoid encoder buffer underflow).

Thus, the first frame will experience, from capture to display, an overall end-to-end delay ΔT, which can be written as follows:

$$\Delta T = \delta_{tb}^1 + \delta_{ch}^1 + \Delta T_\lambda \qquad (2)$$

where ΔT_d is the time the decoder waits before starting the decoding process, measured from the time the first bits of video data were received. That is, the time between the capture and encoding of frame i and its decoding and display will be ΔT for any i. It is important to note that even though all the delay components will vary over time, so that frame i will experience delays δ_{tb}^i and δ_{ch}^i, the overall delay ΔT must remain constant. This is illustrated by Figure 9.7.

Thus, in this real-time encoding case, frames arrive at the encoder at a constant rate (δ_f^{-1} frames per second), are encoded, and are put in the encoder buffer. The first frame is decoded after $\Delta N_d = \Delta T_d/\delta_f$ frame intervals and, unless frames are dropped, the ith frame also must be available at the decoder by time $i + \Delta N_d$. In this case each frame spends exactly ΔT seconds in the system, and there are always exactly $\Delta N = \Delta T/\delta_f$ frames in the system.

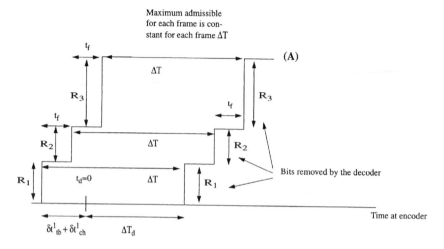

The interval between video frame arrival at the encoder is constant and equal to t_f

The interval between video frame decoding and display is also constant and equal to t_f

Maximum admissible for each frame is constant for each frame ΔT

t_f (A)

ΔT

R_3 R_3

t_f

t_f

R_2 ΔT R_2

R_1 $t_d=0$ ΔT R_1

Bits removed by the decoder

Time at encoder

$\delta t^l_{tb} + \delta t^l_{ch}$ ΔT_d

Figure 9.7   Delay constraints in the live video case.

Clearly, given that ΔT determines the maximum delay a frame experiences, having a large ΔT chosen will tend to reduce the chance of violating the delay constraint. As Section 9.6 reveals, this can alternatively be seen as meaning that the rate control algorithm will have more degrees of freedom and thus the overall video quality will be better.

9.3.3   Interactive Versus Noninteractive Video

The tightness of the constraint will also depend on how much overall delay the specific application can withstand, that is, how large can ΔT be for a specific application.

In a noninteractive application, this delay ΔT has the effect of an initial latency in the playback. Anyone who has used video or audio feeds from the Internet may have observed how data is initially buffered before playback begins. One question that comes to mind is, What benefit, if any, can be derived from having a large ΔT? In the case of unreliable environments such as the Internet, the answer is immediate. Since the end-to-end delay determines the delay constraint for any given frame, longer ΔT means that larger variations in the delay components can be tolerated. This means that the system will be more robust to losses and jitter (more time for retransmission) but also that the individual transmission delays of each frame (source rate for the frame divided by allocated channel rate) can vary significantly. This enables more flexibility in allocating bits per frame and allows us to approach "ideal" VBR coding rates. Thus, in general, larger ΔT tends to result in higher quality.

The live interactive video scenario differs from the case above only in that the overall delay must be lower (i.e., ΔT must be small). A typical assumption in this case is that of a 150 ms round-trip delay (from the time one of the users of the system says something, until the time this user receives an answer). This constraint severely limits the potential for improving performance through rate control. Under these delay constraints, only a few frames are in the system at any given time, and the encoder and decoder buffers must be small.

9.4 THE IMPACT OF TRANSMISSION MODES ON END-TO-END VIDEO QUALITY

To this point we have described the delay constraints as observed by the encoder and decoder but have not considered how the achievable end-to-end performance is affected by the selection of transmission mode.

As an example, consider the extreme case of negligible channel delay δ_{ch}, with each frame at the transmitter buffer transmitted completely within a single frame interval, that is, $C_i = R_i$. In this case, an example of VBR transmission, the system would be able to operate with practically no delay. However, given rate traces such as those presented earlier, it is unlikely that such a network service will be available unless capacity is significantly overdimensioned with respect to the expected number of users.

VBR transmission of video encoded at variable rate seems to be a desirable objective, since it would match the variable rate output of a coder to a variable transmission rate over the channel. Substantial activity in exploring VBR transmission of video dates back to the mid- to late 1980s (e.g., Refs. 21–23) and is ongoing (24). However, researchers have used the term VBR to describe transmission modes of different types, ranging from modes that guarantee quality of service (QoS) in the data delivery to approaches with "best-effort" performance, as is the case with transmission over the Internet. Each of these VBR modes presents different challenges to the video application to ensure transmission under the constraints of Formulation 1 above.

Numerous transmission modes can be used to transport video data. Our objective here is not to provide an exhaustive enumeration, and we refer the reader to Chapters 4 and 10, on ATM and feedback of rate and loss information, respectively, where some of these transmission modes are presented. Instead, we provide an overview of the properties of these transmission modes. We present these at a high level, emphasizing the clarification of how selecting one mode or another will affect the video transmission. Our motivation is to provide a simple classification of transmission characteristics, and in particular as they are relevant to the video encoder.

9.4.1   CBR Versus VBR Transmission

VBR transmission has been deemed attractive for both source quality and network utilization. Thus, some of the promised advantages of VBR video combining VBR coding and transport are as follows.

1. *Better video quality* for the same average bit rate, by avoiding the need to adjust the quantization as in CBR. That is, we may be able to operate close to the "ideal rate" for the source.
2. *Shorter delay,* since the encoder buffer size can be reduced without encountering an equivalent delay in the network. In the simplest case, if we can use for each frame as many bits as needed to transmit it within a single frame interval, the delay will be low indeed.
3. *Increased call-carrying capacity* because the bandwidth per call for VBR video may be lower than for CBR for equivalent quality. This is also described as statistical multiplexing gain: the basic idea is that if a number of VBR sources are grouped together, they are unlikely to all make use of their maximum rate at the same time, so that lower-than-peak-rate bandwidth allocation is possible.

While these potential advantages were heavily emphasized in early packet video papers, further research has shown that no design can maximize them simultaneously. In this chapter we concentrate on video coding aspects, but it is clear that, as argued elsewhere (24), a VBR transport design can have advantages for both video and network sharing and thus it would have to be evaluated based on both types of metric.

9.4.2   Quality-of-Service Guarantees Versus Best Effort

Much of the early work on packet video assumed the availability of transmission under some sort of quality-of-service (QoS) guarantees. These QoS guarantees are generally assumed to be probabilistic. For example, for a particular service there may be a guarantee that the delay will not exceed a given value more than a certain percentage of the time. While there has been extensive research on QoS guarantees in small-scale ATM environments (e.g., a local network, or a switch) there is as yet no deployment of services with end-to-end QoS over the Internet. For this reason, video over the Internet operates under completely best-effort conditions. From the perspective of the video encoder/transmitter, operating in a best-effort environment may require that a transmission scheme be designed with features to ensure robustness to packet losses as well as potentially significant variations in delay.

9.4.3 Constrained Versus Unconstrained Transmission Rate

Normally, if QoS guarantees exist, there are also some constraints on the number of bits that can be transmitted through the channel. Obviously, this is true in the CBR transmission case, where rate is guaranteed to be constant but a strict limit on the channel rate exist. More interestingly, constraints will also be applied in the VBR transmission case. That is, even though a variable number of bits can be transmitted, the transmission rate is subject to some conditions. For example, the long-term sustainable rate may have to be below some maximum value, and the short-term or "peak" rate may likewise be limited.

These constraints are typically defined in terms of some operational measurements (typically simple counters are used) by which the network determines whether specific sources are complying with the constraints. These are called policing functions, and examples include the leaky bucket, the sliding window, and the jumping window (25,26). Note that in some cases the constraints are explicit (e.g., when policing functions such as the leaky bucket are used). This is particularly likely when QoS is provided, since the transmitter agrees to abide by certain rules to receive the promised guarantees from the service provider. In other cases, especially if only best-effort transmission is available, the constraints will be implicit and will be observed only indirectly. With transmission using TCP/IP, for example, there will be no explicit conditions on the rate to be transmitted; as congestion arises, however, the transmission rate will have to be lowered.

9.4.4 Feedback Versus No Feedback

Feedback to the video encoder is one of the key characteristics of video (as opposed to data) transmission over packet networks (24). In data transmission, feedback can be used only to adapt the way the information is sent (e.g., reducing the transmission rate if congestion occurs as in TCP/IP), but the information itself cannot be changed. Thus, in a TCP/IP transmission, rate reduction means that the overall transfer time will be longer, since the data to be transmitted remains the same but the channel rate is lower. Instead, video encoders can modulate the data they produce by adjusting a number of parameters, including quality, frame rate, and resolution. This property is particularly useful when there are time variations in the channel characteristics (e.g., due to network congestion).

An example of the role of feedback can be seen by considering a generic system, where the video encoder sends encoded data to a buffer and encoded data, or video traffic, is then drained at a variable rate, which is monitored at the user–network interface (UNI) (27). This system would be typical of an ATM-based interface, but similar methods might be applied under other transport mechanisms. The UNI monitors the transmitted rate and compares the connection parameters to those negotiated between the user and the network at the time of connection setup. The network policing functions, if used, can be considered to be implemented at the UNI. Finally, traffic transmitted through the network experiences a certain QoS level. Information about the currently available QoS, as determined, for example, by the existence of congestion, might be also transmitted back to the UNI and thence to the source [as, e.g., in an available bit rate (ABR) scheme (28)].

Under this generic system setup we can define the following modes of operation (24):

1. Unconstrained VBR (U-VBR), where the video encoder operates independently of the UNI. For example, the encoder operates with a constant quantization scale throughout transmission. Most video rate modeling efforts have been based on U-VBR traces.

2. Shaped VBR (S-VBR), where the buffer is linked to the UNI but is not connected to the encoder. In this case, the encoder produces a bitstream that is identical to that in U-VBR. However, now a shaping algorithm can determine the actual transmission rates C_i. While the content of the bitstream is unaffected, the traffic patterns may be smoothed out at the cost of some additional delay.

3. Constrained VBR (C-VBR),* where the encoder has knowledge not only of the buffer state but also the networking constraints at the UNI. Thus the video encoder can modulate its output to maximize the video quality, given all the applicable constraints, including those related to delay and transmitted rate. Here, the bitstream content *is* affected, but the changes are made by the video encoder, which can change the rate in a manner that has the least impact on perceptual quality.

4. Feedback VBR (F-VBR), which adds information about the network state to what is made available to the encoder. This allows the same trade-offs as in C-VBR to be considered, with the additional advantage that the encoder can adjust to changes in the state of the network (e.g., congestion periods).

In this chapter we concentrate on the C-VBR and F-VBR scenarios, which are the only two modes of operation that entail some sort of feedback to the video encoder. These are the most likely to provide the best performance. The rate constraints presented in Section 9.5 make explicit how the encoder has to operate under the delay constraints of Formulation 1 for each channel transmis-

---

* This was referred to as shaped bit-rate (SBR) by Hamdi et al. (29,30), but here we use the naming convention we proposed recently (24).

sion scenario. Section 9.6 provides an overview of algorithms that can be used to meet these constraints.

It is worth emphasizing that in much of the early work (e.g., Refs. 21–23), feedback was disregarded. For example, the experimental performance analysis work employed bit traces that were generated by video encoders operating "open loop," that is, without any kind of feedback. On the other hand, most practical systems will incorporate some sort of feedback, and therefore feedback should be incorporated into the analysis.

9.5 ENCODER RATE CONSTRAINTS

In the preceding sections we described the delay constraints and the various transmission modes available. We now derive the rate constraints that the encoder/transmitter must meet to avoid violating the delay constraints for a given channel configuration. For the purposes of our discussion, we divide the channels into three classes, namely, CBR, VBR with predictable, but constrained, channel rates, and VBR with unpredictable channel rates.

Note that in designing a complete video transmission system, several parameters, other than transmission rate, must be taken into account. For example, one can think of end-to-end delay as a resource, since for the same rate the coded quality increases when ΔT_d increases. While this improvement comes at the cost of increased initial latency, it may be a worthwhile trade-off for LNIV or PEV applications. Likewise, memory may be a limited resource even if delay is not, so that the overall buffer space in the decoder will have to restricted (e.g., a handheld device or a set-top box).

In Figure 9.8, which provides an illustration of the relevant rate constraints, A represents the total accumulated bits in the transmitter buffer (each step represents the bits corresponding to one frame), and B represents the bits corresponding to frames that have been removed from the decoder buffer (each step corresponds to removing one frame so that it can be decoded). Note that A and B are simply shifted versions of each other, since the frames that are put in the transmitter buffer are eventually removed from the decoder buffer to be decoded. Also note that in this example the delay, the difference in the time axis between the A and B, is made up of two components, a delay in starting the transmission and a delay in starting the decoding.

In Figure 9.8 C represents the rate at which bits are transported from encoder to decoder. In this case we are representing a CBR transmission mode, since C is shown as a straight line. Thus A - C corresponds to the bits remaining in the encoder buffer and C - B to those present in the decoder buffer.

From Figure 9.8 we can also visualize the four possible constraints that one may have to take into account in the coding process, namely, the overflow

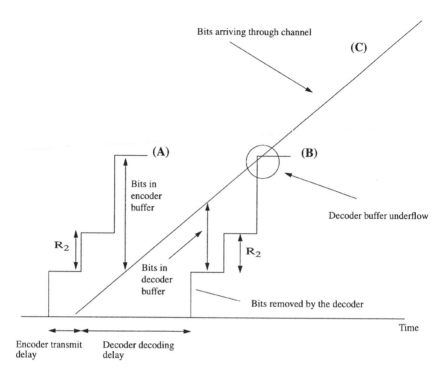

Figure 9.8   Rate constraints.

and underflow conditions at encoder and decoder buffers. Encoder buffer overflow occurs when the buffer memory at the encoder is exceeded, that is, if the difference A – C becomes greater than the maximum memory. Conversely, if the difference A – C becomes zero (it cannot be negative), what we observe is encoder buffer underflow, and in this situation no transmission takes place, or "filler bits" are sent. At the decoder, if C – B is too large, the decoder buffer may overflow. On the other hand, if C – B becomes negative (as in the example of Figure 9.8), that means that the decoder demand exceeds the bits supplied by the channel and therefore decoder buffer underflow occurs.

In this chapter we concentrate on the problem of decoder buffer underflow (frames arriving too late at the receiver). As mentioned before, encoder/decoder buffer overflow problems can be solved easily if sufficient memory is available and decoder buffer underflow is avoided. Moreover, we will assume that encoder buffer underflow can be handled without penalty through the introduction of filler bits.

9.5.1 CBR

Clearly, a constant bit rate (CBR) transmission mode, because of its predictable traffic patterns, makes the task of network management easier (in that all decisions can be based on deterministic traffic characteristics), although it also precludes gain via statistical multiplexing. Further, the CBR mode is not well matched to the inherently VBR characteristics of coded video. However, it is difficult to support good-quality video by using VBR transport unless the network provides feedback to the source, or provides end-to-end delay and loss guarantees with VBR transmission constraints that are known to the source.*

In a CBR environment we have, as in Figure 9.8, a fixed number of bits transmitted through the channel. Let us consider now the state of the encoder and decoder buffers, under the condition that, as in Formulation 1, frames put in the encoder are removed from the decoder buffer after a fixed number of frame intervals ΔN_d has passed. To simplify the notation, we assume that the channel delay is negligible and that data is sent from the transmitter as soon as it is available (i.e., $\delta^1_{tb} + \delta^1_{ch} = 0$, and in general $\delta^i_{ch} = 0$). Thus the only delay in the system corresponds to the ΔN_d frame intervals that the decoder waits before removing the first frame from the buffer. Under these conditions, the encoder and decoder buffer states at the i frame interval are respectively,

$$B^e(i) = \sum_{j=1}^{i} R_j - \sum_{j=1}^{i} C \tag{3}$$

$$B^d(i) = \begin{cases} \displaystyle\sum_{j=1}^{i} C - \sum_{j=1}^{i-\Delta N_d} R_j & \text{when } i \ge \Delta N_d \\ \displaystyle\sum_{j=1}^{i} C & \text{when } i < \Delta N_d \end{cases} \tag{4}$$

Thus the encoder contains simply all the bits produced up to that time, minus those that have been transmitted, at the constant channel rate C. The decoder buffer at time i, on the other hand, contains all the bits received from the channel up to that time; minus the frames that have been decoded. Note that consistent with our delayed decoding assumption, at time i the $(i - \Delta N_d)$th frame is being decoded. Note also that we assume that there is no encoder buffer underflow;

---

* Transmission of video over channels without such feedback is possible, as demonstrated by live video multicasts over the Internet. However, the resulting video quality cannot be as high as in a guaranteed transmission environment, since the video encoding algorithm must be made robust to almost certain channel losses (and thus both video quality and compression factors suffer).

that is, ΣR_j is always greater than ΣC, to preserve the linearity of the constraints. This is an easy constraint to meet in practice, since the encoding rate can be increased to avoid underflow.

If we now combine the encoder buffer occupancy from Eq. (3) at time i and decoder buffer occupancy from Eq. (4) at time $i + \Delta N$, we have

$$B^d(i + \Delta N_d) = \sum_{j-1}^{i+\Delta N_d} C - \sum_{j=1}^{i} R_j = \sum_{j=i+1}^{i+\Delta N_d} C - \left(\sum_{j=1}^{i} R_j - \sum_{j=1}^{i} C \right)$$
$$= \sum_{j=i+1}^{i+\Delta_d} C - B^e(i) \tag{5}$$

Thus, to prevent the decoder buffer from underflowing, we have to keep the right-hand side of Eq. (5) always greater than zero. We can introduce the concept of *effective buffer size*, $B_{eff}(i)$, which we define as the maximum level of buffer occupancy the encoder can reach at time i such that the channel rates are adequate to transport all the bits without violating the end-to-end delay constraint (i.e., without producing decoder underflow). From Eq. (5) the maximum level of encoder buffer occupancy is $\sum_{j=i+1}^{i+\Delta N} C$, thus we have

$$B_{eff}(i) = \sum_{j=i+1}^{i+\Delta N_d} C \tag{6}$$

and thus we have that the effective buffer size

$$B_{eff}(i) = \Delta N \cdot C \tag{7}$$

should be constant.

We summarize this result in Formulation 2.

Formulation 2 Rate Constraints for CBR   *In a CBR channel operating under end-to-end delay ΔN_d at a rate C, to prevent decoder buffer underflow, the encoder must avoid the encoder buffer size exceeding $B_{eff} = \Delta N_d \cdot C$. It can be shown that if the encoder buffer does not exceed the maximum occupancy B_{eff} then the decoder buffer will not exceed that maximum buffer occupancy either (17).*

Note that we refer to *effective* buffer size because, given that there is sufficient memory available at encoder and decoder, this effective memory is determined by the delay, rather than by memory considerations. As an example, assume that large amounts of memory are available at encoder and decoder; then the same system could operate with different end-to-end delays ΔN_d and for each chosen value there would be a different B_{eff}.

9.5.2 VBR with Known Channel Rates

Consider now the VBR transmission case in which the channel rates are known. This would be the case in a VBR transmission under leaky-bucket constraints, where the encoder will be able to decide on the channel rate during the frame interval i, C_i, as long as it complies with the leaky-bucket constraints. We can then revisit Formulation 2 and replace the constant rate C by a variable one, C_i. The encoder and decoder buffer occupancies are now

$$B^e(i) = \sum_{j=1}^{i} R_j - \sum_{j=1}^{i} C_j \tag{8}$$

$$B^d(i) = \begin{cases} \displaystyle\sum_{j=1}^{i} C - \sum_{j=1}^{i-\Delta N_d} R & - \text{ when } i \geq \Delta N_d \\[4mm] \displaystyle\sum_{j=1}^{i} C & \text{ when } i < \Delta N_d \end{cases} \tag{9}$$

where as before the decoder waits ΔN_d frame intervals before starting to decode the video frames available in its buffer. Again, we can combine the encoder buffer occupancy from Eq. (8) at time i and decoder buffer occupancy from Eq. (9) at time $i + \Delta N$, giving

$$B^d(i + \Delta N) = \sum_{j=1}^{i+\Delta N} C_j - \sum_{j=1}^{i} R_j = \sum_{j=i+1}^{i+\Delta N} C_j - \left(\sum_{j=1}^{i} R_j - \sum_{j=1}^{i} C_j \right)$$

$$= \sum_{j=i+1}^{i+\Delta N} C_j - B^e(i) \tag{10}$$

so that decoder buffer underflow is prevented if the right-hand side of Eq. (10) is always greater than zero. And from Eq. (10) the maximum level of encoder buffer occupancy is $\sum_{j=i+1}^{i+\Delta N} C_j$ so that the effective buffer size is now

$$B_{eff}(i) = \sum_{j=i+1}^{i+\Delta N} C_j \tag{11}$$

The main difference between this and the CBR case is that now the effective buffer size depends on the frame interval, i, and is equal to the sum of the future ΔN_d channel rates. We can guarantee that if the encoder buffer fullness $B^e(i)$ is always smaller than $B_{eff}(i)$, the decoder buffer will not underflow.

Thus in the VBR transmission case we can have the following constraints.

Formulation 3 Rate Constraints for VBR   *In a VBR channel operating under end-to-end delay* Δ_d *at a known rate* C_i*, to prevent decoder buffer underflow, the encoder must prevent the encoder buffer size exceeding* $B_{eff}(i) = \sum_{j=i+1}^{i+\Delta N} C_j$*.*

Note that in a "controlled" VBR channel environment the transmitter may be able to decide the number of bits to use for both source and channel. As shown elsewhere (19), this can be done in practice, and the channel rate selection can be performed so that the rates comply with some of the constraints (e.g., leaky bucket) mentioned above.

9.5.3 VBR with Unpredictable Channel Rates

The most important characteristic of Formulation 3 becomes apparent when one considers the case of rates that are not deterministically known. There are, of course, numerous instances of this scenario, such as a reliable channel with variable delay (where the effective throughput thus varies over time), an unreliable channel with retransmission (20), or a congestion-controlled channel.

The key difficulty in dealing with these scenarios is that the encoder must make decisions on the source coding, which are based on deterministic knowledge of the source, but must somehow take into account the random behavior of the channel. The channel behavior is such that the data may arrive reliably to the receiver but owing to random delay or to the need for retransmission, *it may arrive at the decoder too late* to be decoded in time for display. Thus, while the encoder cannot control the channel behavior, it can use whatever knowledge of the channel is available to avoid decoder buffer underflow.

Formulation 3 provides a simple way to formulate the desired behavior of the system. To ensure that the decoder buffer will not underflow, it is sufficient to guarantee that

$$B_e(i) \leq B_{eff}(i) = \sum_{j=i+1}^{i+\Delta N_d} C_j \tag{12}$$

The future channel rates C_{i+1} through $C_{i+\Delta N_d}$ are not known at time i. However, the deterministic part of the system (the selection of source rates at the encoder) in Eq. (12) is clearly separated from the random components (the channel behavior).

If there is no knowledge about the channel, very little can be done, other perhaps than to assume worst-case behavior. On the other hand, if we have an a priori model of the channel and/or some online observation of its current state, it is possible to attach a likelihood of achieving a certain channel rate.

Let us call $P_i(c) = P_i(c \neq$ model observation), the probability (given applicable observations and prior channel model) of the available channel rate being c at time i. Note that this model could be discrete or continuous, and will depend on specific channel characteristics. An example of such a model can be found in Reference 20, where a point-to-point wireless link based on the CDMA IS-95 standard is used. Note also that such a formulation can also be extended to the case in which a random delay, rather than a random rate, must be considered. Finally, it should be clear that the overall performance of a system under such random channel behavior will depend both on the rate control algorithms to be discussed in the next section and on the accuracy of the channel models.

Given the model $P_i(c)$, we can define two different formulations as follows.

Formulation 4 Expected Rate Constraints   *Let the system operate with delay* ΔN_d *and random channel rate characterized by* $P_i(c)$. *Then the goal is to select the encoding rate to meet the expected rate constraints. That is, for each frame i choose the rates such that:*

$$B_e(i) \le E\left[\sum_{j=i+1}^{i+\Delta N} C_j\right] \tag{13}$$

where $E[\cdot\cdot]$ *indicates the expectation with respect to the probabilities* $P_i(c)$.

It is obvious that Formulation 4 does not guarantee that the data will be transmitted correctly, but it is simple and it can be easily incorporated into a rate control algorithm in the form of a table that provides expected values for each possible observed channel state.

Formulation 4 lead us to a more general formulation, where we take into account the likelihood of losses due to decoder buffer underflow.

Formulation 5 Minimizing Loss Probability   *With the system again operating with delay* ΔN_d *and random channel rate characterized by* $P_i(c)$, *the goal is to select the encoding rate to meet a certain threshold in the loss probability. That is, select the* $B_e(i)$ *such that*

$$P\left[B_e(i) > \sum_{j=i+1}^{i+\Delta N} C_j\right] \le \text{threshold} \tag{14}$$

where the probability obviously depends on $P_i(c)$.

Examples of these two approaches can be found in Reference 20.

9.5.4   Special Cases

We now consider two special cases in which transmission may fall in one of the categories considered above (say CBR or VBR) but additional constraints may have to be taken into account. Without going into details, we point out that the formulations provided before may have to be modified to address these scenarios.

9.5.4.1   VBR for Stored Video.   For preencoded video, we can consider two different scenarios, namely, local playback (e.g., from a DVD player) and networked playback (e.g., video-on-demand service to a home). The former case, as discussed earlier, involves a global allocation among the different scenes in the movie, while the channel constraints do not play much of a role (the "channel," i.e., the connection between storage device and decoder, is supposed to have sufficient bandwidth to accommodate even the highest rate scenes).

In the second, and more interesting, scenario, the video sequence must be encoded in such a way that meets any applicable channel constraints. This will result in different encoding results depending on whether a CBR or a VBR transmission mode is selected. In addition to these transmission-related issues, designers must take into account the impact of the storage medium on performance. As an example, consider the case of data to be stored on a disk. Typically a disk is organized into segments that constitute the basic storage unit. Thus disk reading hardware is designed to be able to read one complete disk segment into a buffer and then move on to another segment. There will be a latency involved in moving from one disk segment to another, and since the disk is rotating, the latency will depend on the relative position of the two segments. Thus the disk placement policies will have an impact on performance. For example, if the system incurs excessive latency in some of its read operations the output buffer may empty and a decoder buffer underflow may occur.

Examples of studies of data placement on a disk for later playback can be found in the literature (31–34). An example of work that incorporates the disk placement constraints into the rate control algorithm is also available (35).

9.5.4.2   Video Caching.   Proxy caching is playing an increasing role in evolving network infrastructure. However, while proxy caching of web objects is commonplace (36) and there are several commercially available proxy caching products, the same is not true of video objects. A few examples of recent work in this area are cited (37–41).

We consider two potential benefits of proxy caching. First, it provides more efficient sharing of network resources, since several users can have access to data stored locally, without needing to access it directly from the server. In particular, given that the data is available from a network node close to the user, it is possible to greatly reduce, or even remove, the initial latency in the video display. Since our system requires the decoder to wait to receive ΔN_d frames before starting to decode, we are normally constrained by the time it takes to transport these frames, and this creates an initial latency (users of audio or video over the Internet will have experienced this). Instead if all these initial frames are available from the proxy, the delay will be less than ΔN_d frame intervals. Second, even if users do not share data, it can be shown (see Ref. 39) that caching allows a more robust delivery of data, since it is less likely that losses (or excessive delay) will occur in transmitting data from the cache to the decoder, whereas transfer from the more "distant" (in terms of network topology) server would be less reliable.

We can roughly divide the approaches uses for video caching into four classes. First it is possible to store complete video sequences only, thus replicating parts of the content of a server in the cache. This approach is attractive in its simplicity, and indeed is the one most widely used nowadays. For example, this is achieved by replicating video sequences close to the end users, so that in effect mirror sites are built that store the relevant video sequences and from which end users can directly stream sequences of interest. This mirroring has the disadvantage of not being very scalable, given the relatively large sizes of the video data.

Second, it is possible to store only a prefix of the video data, that is, all the frames the decoder will need to start decoding and for which it would normally wait ΔT_d seconds. If this prefix is cached as proposed by Wang et al. (38), all the initial latency will be absorbed without requiring that the whole sequence be stored. A third approach (37,39) would allow both the prefix and a set of intermediate frames to be stored. This approach provides the same benefits of prefix caching but adds the attractive feature of more robust delivery. The intuition is simple: if intermediate samples are stored, and these can be delivered reliably to the decoder, then the probability that the decoder buffer will "starve" is clearly reduced. Finally, it is possible to define caching strategies that rely on a scalable format for the video stream (41). In this scenario, the cache will store some of the layers of the video stream so that the server needs to provide only the higher resolution layers if the cache already contains the coarse layers. This approach is similar to the "soft caching" approach used for images (42,43) and preserves the video delivery at lower quality in cases of low network bandwidth.

It is not necessary in general to perform the encoding in a special manner because the data is going to be cached. In fact it may be preferable for the encoder to make no assumptions about whether the data will be cached. However, the problem of deciding which frames to cache (or at what resolution) is very similar to the rate control problems we will consider next, and similar techniques can be used to solve them.

9.6 RATE CONTROL ALGORITHMS

We have just seen how guaranteeing that the decoder always has data to decode requires the transmitted bitstream to comply with a series of rate constraints. These constraints depend on the type of transmission environment considered, including the variability, or lack of it, in the transmitted rate, and the end-to-end delay. Thus, after a transmission environment has been chosen, the video encoder will be responsible for producing a bitstream that meets the relevant delay constraints. To accomplish this, we need a rate control algorithm at the video encoder: that is, an algorithm to assign a quantizer to each frame or coding unit, such that the constraints are met and the video quality is good. Note that such a rate control algorithm is needed regardless of the scenario considered (LIV, LNIV, or PEV). However in the PEV case the rate selection must be done based solely on a priori assumptions on the channel behavior, while in the other two cases it is possible to take into account current channel conditions to determine the rate to use at the encoder.

In this section we provide an overview of rate control techniques that have been proposed in recent years. It is worth noting that while much of the research in video coding has been driven by the definition of widely accepted standards (H.263, MPEG-2, etc.), these standards do not define the operation of the encoder (in fact this probably has a lot to do with their success, since this approach allows companies to offer optimized encoders that provide a differentiated product while maintaining standard compatibility). Thus, rate control, which is performed at the encoder, is not part of the standard, so that many different rate control techniques can be applied while standard compatibility at the decoder is preserved.

In Section 9.2 we outlined techniques to estimate rates at which sequences or segments within a sequence may be encoded such that degradation is practically imperceptible. While the discussion focused on offline encoding (e.g., using a two-pass algorithm), it is conceivable that approximate online techniques could be derived from these approaches. The next step in analyzing the performance of a system for video delivery over a network is to determine what resources are required to deliver this perceptually lossless video. We are interested in the channel characteristics, including its rate and delay performances, the delay experienced by the user before video data playback starts, and the memory required at the decoder. It is because these other resources (e.g., the network bandwidth) are not abundant or free that delivering the sequence at its ideal rate may not be feasible.

9.6.1 Basic Problem Formulation

In each of the formulations discussed in the preceding section, we derived a set of constraints on the rates produced by the video encoder. Note that all these constraints had the form of restrictions on the average rate, or the total rate for particular sets of frames. In other words, these constraints did not specify the number of bits to be used for individual frames but rather indicated the overall rate for *a set of frames.*

Assume that we consider one such constraint: that the total number of bits for a set of frames must be less than some prescribed amount. Then we must decide how to allocate bits among the frames: the goal should be to provide the maximum overall quality. The issue of quality is, as mentioned early in the chapter, a difficult one for video. In many cases the selected quality criterion is to minimize the average distortion over the set of frames, although other approaches are also used in practice, such as the lexicographic optimization (44) or the min-max criterion (45). These two techniques seek, in different ways, to minimize the distortion of the worst frame in the set, and thus are somewhat closer to the known characteristics of the human visual system. Still, owing to its relative simplicity, average distortion continues to be widely used, and many of the algorithms described below seek to minimize this metric.

Given that the goal of rate control is to maximize a quality measure while complying with some rate constraints, a natural way of tackle these problems is to formulate them as rate distortion (RD) optimization problems. Thus a typical formulation poses a problem of the following sort: find the bit allocation to the frames such that the overall distortion is minimized and the applicable rate constraints are met.

The overview we provide next is not exhaustive. Rather, our goal is to provide examples of rate control algorithms that have been proposed in recent years. Our emphasis is on algorithms based on rate distortion optimization. This class of algorithms is useful even though their complexity tends to be high. RD algorithms can be used to provide benchmarks for other approaches. Moreover, one can also use them to derive approximate algorithms, where, for example, the "true" RD values are replaced by values obtained from models.

We refer the reader to our earlier work (14) for an overview of rate distortion optimization techniques and their application to resource allocation problems in image and video compression. More detailed examples of the benefits of these techniques in image and video compression can be found elsewhere (12).

9.6.2 CBR Algorithms

For many applications of interest constant bit rate transmission is used. When one is transmitting over a CBR channel, buffers at the encoder and decoder are required to smooth out the variations in the encoding rates. Buffering data requires extra memory at both encoder and decoder and introduces additional delay to data transmission. As the encoder is allowed to produce a more variable rate (more bits for difficult frames, fewer bits for easy frames, e.g.) the overall quality will be better. Thus larger buffers, or equivalently, increased end-to-end delay, will tend to result in higher video quality (17,18). Traditionally, rate control has been studied from the point of view of memory. That is, rate control was required to avoid overflowing the available buffers at encoder and decoder. However, as in earlier work (17,19) we have assumed that sufficient physical memory is available and have formulated the problem from the point of view of end-to-end delay.

Algorithms for rate control under CBR channel conditions have been studied for years. The initial emphasis was to derive approaches that would prevent encoder buffer overflow, and in the beginning these algorithms were targeted at live video and were required to be relatively simple. In early examples (46,47), the emphasis was on simplicity. Another example is the test model 5 (48) algorithm in MPEG-2. In this simple algorithm the rate controller defines bit-rate targets for each of the frame types and then attempts to keep the rate within the target by varying the quantization step size. Other examples of rate control include work by Keesman et al. (49), as well as algorithms targeted for more recent standards, such as MPEG-4 (50,51).

Rate distortion based optimization techniques start with the assumption that each coding unit (e.g., each frame) can be coded with one among a finite number of coding parameters, and that each of these coding parameters will correspond to a rate and distortion pair. A typical approach consists then in measuring those RD parameters and then searching the space of all admissible solutions for the one that provides the lowest distortion without violating the rate constraints. Early examples of RD optimization algorithms (18,52) deal with frame level optimization.

One issue that must be taken into account in typical video coding algorithms is dependency, the fact that quantizer selections for some frames affect the rate distortion performance for other frames. This problem was first studied by Ramchandran et al. (15). Algorithms that take into account these dependencies have been published (16,53).

Blockwise allocation algorithms are then needed to determine how to distribute the bits among the blocks in a frame. Approaches based on RD optimization include those described in References 54–56, while simple techniques such as the test model 5 quantization selection scheme are also useful if complexity is a concern.

Complexity in RD-optimized rate control algorithms is due to two factors: first the rate distortion values at each of the operating points would have to be computed; then the best among all the available operating points would have to be found. The first complexity term is by far the most expensive, since obtaining the RD data entails compressing and then decompressing the data, possibly for a large number of operating points. Thus, several authors have proposed applying the RD optimization after models of the RD characteristics have been derived. Examples of this approach include work reported in References 57–59.

As new standards for compression are defined, there are frequently new modes of operation that were not possible with earlier standards and must be taken into account by the rate control algorithm.

As an example, the H.263 standard allows the use of a variable number of frames per second. Song and coworkers have published an example of rate control using a variable number of frames (60,61). There are two main difficulties in making a decision about the "ideal" frame rate for a given scene. First consider rate. For a given rate target, lowering the frame rate to lower the coding rate (fewer frames to be coded) may become counterproductive because the energy in the residue frames increases as the frame rate decreases (since frames are further apart, there is less temporal redundancy). Thus there is likely to be, for a given coding rate, an optimal frame rate, in the sense of the quality of the reconstructed sequence, including error that is possibly the effect of frame interpolation. Second, consider the issue of perceptual quality. Even if the sequence being considered does not have a very high level of motion, reducing the frame rate will come at a cost of significant perceptual quality degradation, since the decoded sequence may appear to have "jerky" motion. Jerkiness can be removed to some extent by using frame interpolation techniques, in particular motion-compensated frame interpolation techniques such as those described by Kuo and Kuo (62).

The new MPEG-4 standard raises other interesting questions, such as methods to optimize the coding of contour information in video objects (63), where again nonstandard distortion measures need to be used. Once the objects have been defined, it is necessary to decide how to allocate bits among the various objects (64). These new areas present significant challenges and are still the object of very active research.

9.6.3 VBR Algorithms

We will consider two different VBR transmission environments. First, in this section, we consider situations in which the encoder has the freedom to choose the transmission rate, and it is assumed that the network will permit transmission at this rate, perhaps under the restriction that some channel rate constraints be met. In Section 9.6.4, we analyze the case of random channel rates and consider the benefits of performing rate control to increase robustness.

While VBR transmission has been said to produce better quality than CBR, it is often difficult to quantify the gains because there are many parameters involved in the comparison (e.g., rate, delay, etc.). While the benefits of VBR transmission have often been touted, comparisons have sometimes ignored some of the factors. For example, as discussed elsewhere (24), while VBR transmission has been said to provide benefits in lower delay, higher video quality, and increased network utilization (statistical multiplexing gain), it is unclear that all these benefits can be achieved simultaneously. There is evidence of the potential benefits of VBR video transmission terms of perceptual quality (65), although it is difficult to quantify the exact increase in performance.

One particularly interesting and realistic scenario is that of the variable channel rates being subject to constraints—for example, as in the leaky bucket (25,26). In this scenario, the encoder, while able to select the channel rates, will have to ensure that these are within the prespecified constraints. As shown by Reibman and Haskell (17), and derived in an earlier section, each selection of channel rates leads to different constraints for the encoder. Recent work (19,66) has derived algorithms to optimally select the source and channel rates. For algorithms such as the leaky bucket, which tends to monitor the long-term average transmission rate and keep it close to a given value, it can be shown (19) that the main benefit of VBR transmission is to achieve the same quality as a CBR scheme with the same long-term average rate, but with a reduced end-to-end delay. Intuitively, in CBR transmission quality increases as the end-to-end delay increases, while in VBR transmission it is possible to reap the same benefit by having the rate of several frames averaged in the network, rather than in the encoder/decoder buffers.

It is worth pointing out that once rate control has been performed, as in Reference 19, there will be many choices of channel rate that will (a) meet the desired channel rate constraints, and (b) accommodate the optimal video quality. Thus there interesting arise opportunities to explore channel rate selections that have good properties in terms of smoothness or other network-based criteria. One can assume, as Rexford and Towsley (67) did, that the source has been coded and then find the transmission rate that accommodates transmission within the delay constraints while meeting applicable rate smoothness constraints.

9.6.4   Real-Time Adaptation to Channel Conditions

In the second VBR scenario of interest, the rate is random. As shown earlier (20) and outlined above, it is possible to use available channel information (assuming that there is a back channel) to modify the encoder's behavior. The main intuition is that the encoder should lower the rate per frame once it becomes clear that the channel bandwidth is lower. While we have provided RD-optimized solutions to Formulations 4 and 5 (20), it is also possible to derive simpler solutions.

Clearly the success of these approaches will depend on the existence of a feedback channel, as will be seen in Section 9.7, but also on the application and the type of channel considered. Rate control at the encoder will be effective only if it is possible for the encoder to react to the channel changes. Thus, these techniques will be effective if (a) the channel memory is sufficiently long (e.g., when the channel remains in a given state for times that are of the order of magnitude of a few frame intervals), (b) the end-to-end delay is longer or of the same order of magnitude as the channel memory, and (c) the channel feedback delay is not too long.

9.6.5   Layered/Scalable Video

The foregoing discussions have assumed that rate control involves selecting coding parameters at the video encoder on a frame-by-frame or block-by-block basis. However it is worth mentioning that in one situation rate control is particularly easy, namely, the bitstream that has already been organized in layers by means of a scalable or multiresolution encoding algorithm. This solution is attractive in its simplicity, since it allows the transmitter, or an intermediate node in the network, to decide the number of layers to send, given the current channel conditions. The basic idea is that the video encoder produces a base layer, which gives a coarse (relatively low quality) approximation to input sequence, and then a series of enhancement layers that successively can be used to improve the quality.

While scalable video coding has been proposed by numerous authors, and was incoporated in the MPEG-2 standard, its widespread application has been hampered by a real or perceived reduction in performance compared to nonscalable algorithms. This lower performance can be measured in terms of higher complexity and lower quality at the same rate compared to a single-layer algorithm. In the MPEG-2 context there are three modes of scalability: temporal, spatial, and SNR. Temporal and spatial scalability provide low-resolution coded streams that represent the input data with an approximation comprising fewer frames or smaller size frames, respectively. For the purpose of rate control as discussed in this chapter, the SNR scalability mode (each layer represents a coarse version of the input) seems to be better suited. It is worth mentioning that a coarse of multiresolutions coding, the so-called data-partitioning approach (68), can be used for rate control.

For all its simplicity, few real applications of scalable video in a communications context have been reported. One of the few examples of application of these techniques to Internet video is the proposed layered multicast approach (69), where the end clients can subscribe the number of layers (and thus overall resolution) that their bandwidth can support.

9.7   CONCLUSIONS: TRANSMISSION ISSUES FOR VBR VIDEO

To conclude this chapter we summarize the key ideas and comment on some of the issues that remain to be addressed before true VBR video networking becomes reality. We have shown that VBR coding is the natural form of representation for video, and thus it would be desirable to transmit video end-to-end in a way that allows the "ideal" VBR representation of the data. We have shown that the real-time nature of video decoding and display constrains transmission to follow certain rules, to guarantee that transmitted data will arrive in time to be decoded (i.e., without producing decoder buffer underflow). We also made the case that the actual constraints in fact depend on the channel conditions.

There are already numerous systems in operation that allow transmission of video over constant rate channels. These require that the video coding parameters be adjusted so that the long-term average transmitted rate remains constant, thus resulting in some quality degradation with respect to a purely VBR coding and transmission mode. Other environments, such as the Internet, can support variable rate transmission but provide no QoS guarantees on the rate provided.

It is likely that near-term efforts in networked video transmission, and in related video compression issues, will focus on the two extreme cases of VBR transmission, namely, VBR transmission over channels with QoS guarantees, and transmission over lossy channels. Both environments present significant challenges for compression and transmission alike.

In the case of VBR transmission with QoS guarantees, establishing conditions that will assure these guarantees is still a subject of research. Even the notion of QoS is itself somewhat misleading in that the end user of a video transmission will really care about the decoded video quality, rather than about the parameters (losses, delay jitter, etc.) that usually are taken to measure the transmission quality. One question of interest that has been addressed only partially to date includes the definition of algorithms to map levels of desired decoded video quality into combinations of networking parameters. For example, the video application may have to determine the combination of network services needed to provide, say, broadcast quality at the receiver. As shown in this chapter, the video encoder is best placed to make decision about what coding information is most important, and so it is the video encoder that can best handle the trade-offs, given any applicable network constraints. Thus, a promising direction will be in the definition of simple interfaces between the video server and the network that abstract the details of the operation of one from the other. The example we discussed with a video coder optimizing its quality to match a given leaky-bucket constraint constitutes a simple instance of this approach.

The second area that needs significant progress is accessing video over a wireless link. The potential benefits, however, are substantial. In this case the video encoder will have to be robust enough to handle potential data losses, as well as able to accommodate changes in bit rate. Here again, one of the possible solutions is to introduce feedback about the state of the channel, so that the encoder can adjust its behavior depending on channel conditions.

ACKNOWLEDGMENT

The author was supported in part by the National Science Foundation under grant MIP-9804959 and by the Integrated Media Systems Center, a National Science Foundation Engineering Research Center, with additional support from the Annenberg Center for Communication at the University of Southern California, and the California Trade and Commerce Agency.

REFERENCES

1. I Dalgic, F Tobagi. Performance evaluation of ATM networks carrying constant and variable bit-rate video traffic. IEEE J Selected Areas Commun, 15:1115–1131, August 1997.
2. S Gringeri, K Shuaib, R Egorov, A Lewis, B Khasnabish, B Basch. Traffic shaping, bandwidth allocation, and quality assessment for MPEG video distribution over broadband networks. IEEE Network Mag November/December 1998, pp 94–107.
3. M Krunz, S Tripathi. Bandwidth allocation strategies for transporting variable-bit-rate video traffic. IEEE Commun Mag January 1999, pp 40–46.
4. N Jayant, J Johnston, R Safranek. Signal compression based on models of human perception. Proc. IEEE, October 1993.
5. B Girod. Psychovisual aspects of image communications. Signal Process 28:239–251, 1992.
6. M W Garrett. Contributions toward real-time services on packet switched networks. PhD dissertation, Department of Electrical Engineering Columbia University, New York, 1993.
7. O Rose. Statistical properties of MPEG video traffic and their impact on traffic modeling in ATM systems. Technical Report 101. University of Wuerzburg, Institute of Computer Science Research Series, February 1995.
8. W Pennebaker, J Mitchell. JPEG Still Imaqe Data Compression Standard. New York: Van Nostrand Reinhold, 1994.
9. J Mitchell, W Pennebaker, CE Fogg, DJ Le Gall. MPEG Video Compression Standard. New York: Chapman & Hall, 1997.
10. I Koo, P Nasiopoulos, R Ward. Joint MPEG-2 coding for multi-program broadcasting of pre-recorded video. Proceedings of International Conference on Acoustics, Speech and Signal Processing, ICASS'99, Phoenix, AZ, March 1999.
11. N Duffield, K Ramakrishnan, AR Reibman. SAVE: An algorithm for smoothed adaptive video over explicit rate network. IEEE/ACM Trans Networking 6:717–728, December 1998.
12. G Sullivan, T Wiegand. Rate-distortion optimization for video compression. IEEE Signal Process Mag November 1998, pp 74–90.
13. Y Shoham, A Gersho. Efficient bit allocation for an arbitrary set of quantizers. IEEE Trans Acoust Speech Signal Process 36:1445–1453, September 1988.
14. A Ortega, K Ramchandran. Rate-distortion techniques in image and video compression. IEEE Signal Process Mag 15:23–50, November 1998.
15. K Ramchandran, A Ortega, M Vetterli. Bit allocation for dependent quantization with applications to multiresolution and MPEG video coders. IEEE Trans Image Process 3:533–545, September 1994.
16. J Lee, BW Dickinson. Rate distortion optimized frame-type selection for MPEG coding. IEEE Trans Circuits Syst Video Technol 7:501–510, June 1997.

17. AR Reibman, BG Haskell. Constraints on variable bit-rate video for ATM networks. IEEE Trans Circuits Syst Video Technol 2:361–372, December 1992.
18. A Ortega, K Ramchandran, M Vetterli. Optimal trellis-based buffered compression and fast approximation. IEEE Trans Image Process 3:26–40, January 1994.
19. C-Y Hsu, A Ortega, A Reibman. Joint selection of source and channel rate for VBR video transmission under ATM policing constraints. IEEE J Selected Areas Commun 15:1016–1028, August 1997.
20. C-Y Hsu, A Ortega, M Khansari. Rate control for robust video transmission over wireless channels. IEEE J Selected Areas Commun 17:756–773, May 1999.
21. W Verbiest, L Pinnoo, B Voeten. The impact of the ATM concept on video coding. IEEE J Selected Areas Commun 6:1623–1632, December 1988.
22. B Maglaris, D Anastassiou, P Sen, G Karlsson, J Robbins. Performance models of statistical multiplexing in packet video communications. IEEE Trans Commun 36:834–843, July 1988.
23. P Sen, B Maglaris, N Rikli, D Anastassiou. Models for packet switching of variable-bit-rate video sources. IEEE J Selected Areas Commun 7:865–869, June 1989.
24. TV Lakhsman, A Ortega, AR Reibman. VBR video: Trade-offs and potentials. Proc IEEE, 86:952–973, May 1998.
25. EP Rathgeb. Modeling and performance comparison of policing mechanisms for ATM networks. IEEE J Selected Areas Commun 9:325–334, April 1991.
26. L Dittmann, SB Jacobsen, K Moth. Flow enforcement algorithms for ATM networks. IEEE J Selected Areas Commun 9:343–350, April 1991.
27. ATM Forum. ATM User-Network Interface Specification, Version 3.0. Englewood Cliffs, NJ: Prentice-Hall, 1993.
28. R Jain, S Kalyanaraman, S Fahmy, R Goyal, S-C Kim. Source behavior for ATM ABR traffic management: An explanation. IEEE Commun Mag 34:50–57, November 1996.
29. M Hamdi, JW Roberts. QoS guaranty for shaped bit rate video connections in broadband networks. Proceedings of International Conference on Multimedia Networking, MmNet'95, Aizu-Wakamatsu, Japan, October 1995.
30. M Hamdi, JW Roberts, P Rolin. Rate control for VBR video coders in broadband networks. IEEE J Selected Areas Commun 15:1040–1051, August 1997.
31. E Chang, A Zakhor. Disk-based storage for scalable video. IEEE Trans Circuits Syst Video Technol 7:758–770, October 1997.
32. E Chang, H. Garcia-Molina. Reducing initial latency in media servers. IEEE Multimedia, Fall 1997, pp 50–61.
33. DW Brubeck, LA Rowe. Hierarchical storage management in a distributed VOD system. IEEE Multimedia, Fall 1996, pp 37–47.
34. S Ghandeharizaheh, SH Kim, C Shahabi. On configuring a single disk continuous media server. Proceedings of the ACM SIGMETRICS/PERFORMANCE, May 1995.
35. Z Miao, A Ortega. Rate control algorithms for video storage on disk based video servers. Proceedings of 32nd Asilomar Conference on Signals, Systems, and Computers, Pacific Grove, CA, November 1998.
36. A Chankhunthod, PB Danzig, C Neerdals, MF Schwartz, KJ Worrell. A Proceedings of hierarchical Internet object cache. USENIX Technical Conference, 1996.

37. Y Wang, Z-L Zhang, D Du, D Su. A network conscious approach to end-to-end video delivery over wide area networks using proxy servers. Proceedings of IEEE Infocom, San Francisco, April 1998.

38. S Sen, J Rexford, D Towsley. Proxy prefix caching for multimedia streams. Proceeding of IEEE Infocom, New York, March 1999.

39. Z Miao, A Ortega. Proxy caching for efficient video services over the Internet. Proceedings of Packet Video Workshop, PVW'99, New York, April 1999.

40. S Acharya. Techniques for improving multimedia communication over wide area networks. PhD dissertation, Cornell University, Ithaca, NY, 1999.

41. R Rejaie, M Handley, H Yu, D Estrin. Proxy caching mechanism for multimedia playback streams in the Internet. Proceedings of WWW Caching Workshop, San Diego, CA, June 1999.

42. A Ortega, F Carignano, S Ayer, M Vetterli. Soft caching: Web cache management techniques for images. Proceedings of the First IEEE Signal Processing Society Workshop on Multimedia Signal Processing, Princeton, NJ, June 1997.

43. J Kangasharju, Y Kwon, A Ortega. Design and implementation of a soft caching proxy. Proceedings of the Third WWW Cachinq Workshop, Manchester, England, June 1998. Will also appear in a special issue of Computer Networks and ISDN Systems, Elsevier, North-Holland.

44. DT Hoang, EL Linzer, JS Vitter. Lexicographic bit allocation for MPEG video. Visual Commun Image Represent, vol 8, December 1997.

45. GM Schuster, G Melnikov, AK Katsaggelos. A review of the minimum maximum criterion for optimal bit allocation among dependent quantizers. IEEE Trans Multimedia, 1:3–17, March 1999.

46. J Zdepsky, D Raychaudhuri, K Joseph. Statistically based buffer control policies for constant rate transmission of compressed digital video. IEEE Trans. Commun 39:947–957, June 1991.

47. C-T Chen, A Wong. A self-governing rate buffer control strategy for pseudo-constant bit rate video coding. IEEE Trans Image Process 2:50–59, January 1993.

48. MPEG-2. Test Model 5 (TM5) Doc. ISO/IEC JTC1/SC29/WG11/93-225b. Test Model Editing Committee, April 1993.

49. G Keesman, I Shah, R Klein-Gunnewiek. Bit-rate control for MPEG encoders. Signal Process: Image Commun, Vol. 6, pp. 545-560, Feb. 1995.

50. T Chiang, Y-Q Zhang. A new rate control scheme using quadratic rate distortion model. IEEE Trans Circuits Syst Video Technol 7:246–250, September 1997.

51. J Ribas-Cordera, S Lei. Rate control in DCT video coding for low-delay communications. IEEE Trans Circuits Syst Video Technol 9:172–185, February 1999.

52. J Choi, D Park. A stable feedback control of the buffer state using the controlled Lagrange multiplier method. IEEE Trans Image Process 3:546–558, September 1994.

53. GM Schuster, AK Katsaggelos. A video compression scheme with optimal bit allocation among segmentation, displacement vector field and displaced frame difference. IEEE Trans Image Process 6:1487–1502, November 1997.

54. A Ortega, K Ramchandran. Forward-adaptive quantization with optimal overhead cost for image and video coding with applications to MPEG video coders. Proceed-

ings of SPIE, Digital Video Compression: Algorithms & Technologies '95, San Jose, CA, February 1995.

55. T Wiegand, M Lightstone, D Mukherjee, T Campbell, SK Mitra. Rate-distortion optimized mode selection for very low bit-rate video coding and the emerging H.263 standard. IEEE Trans Circuits Syst Video Technol 6:182–190, April 1996.

56. GM Schuster, AK Katsaggelos. A video compression scheme with optimal bit allocation between displacement vector field and displaced frame difference. IEEE J Selected Areas Commun 15:1739–1751, December 1997.

57. L-J Lin, A Ortega. Bit-rate control using piecewise approximated rate-distortion characteristic. IEEE Trans Circuits Syst Video Technol 8:446–459, August 1998.

58. H-M Hang, J-J Chen. Source model for transform video coder and its application. IEEE Trans Circuits Syst Video Technol 7:287–311, April 1997.

59. W Ding, B Liu. Rate control of MPEG video coding and recording by rate-quantization modeling. IEEE Trans Circuits Syst Video Technol 6:12–20, February 1996.

60. H Song, J Kim, C-C J Kuo. Real-time encoding frame rate control for H.263+ video over the Internet. Signal Process: Image Commun, Vol 15, Nos. 1–2, Sept. 1999.

61. H Song. Rate control algorithms for low variable bit rate video. PhD dissertation, University of Southern California, Los Angeles, May 1999.

62. T-Y Kuo, C-C J Kuo. Motion compensated frame interpolation for low-bit-rate video quality enhancement. Proceedings of Visual Communications and Signal Processing, VCIP'99, San Jose, CA, January 1999.

63. GM Schuster, AK Katsaggelos. An optimal boundary encoding scheme in the rate-distortion sense. IEEE Trans Image Process 7:13–26, January 1998.

64. A Vetro, H Sun, Y Wang. MPEG-4 rate control for multiple video objects. IEEE Trans Circuits Syst Video Technol 9:186–199, February 1999.

65. MR Pickering, JF Arnold. A perceptually efficient VBR rate control algorithm. IEEE Trans Image Process 3:527–532, September 1994.

66. J-J Chen, DW Lin. Optimal bit allocation for coding of video signals over ATM networks. IEEE J Selected Areas Commun 15:1002–1015, August 1997.

67. J Rexford, D Towsley. Smoothing variable-bit-rate video in an internetwork. IEEE/ACM Trans Networking 7:202–215, April 1999.

68. A Eleftheriadis, D Anastassiou. Constrained and general dynamic rate shaping of compression digital video. Proceedings of ICIP'95, Washington, DC, vol III, 1995, pp 396–399.

69. S McCanne, M Vetterli, V Jacobson. Low-complexity video coding for receiver-driven layered multicast. IEEE J Selected Areas Commun 15:983–1001, August 1997.

10
Feedback of Rate and Loss Information for Networked Video

N. G. Duffield and K. K. Ramakrishnan
AT&T Labs–Research, Florham Park, New Jersey

10.1 MOTIVATION FOR FEEDBACK AND ADAPTATION

As the availability of high-bandwidth networks increases, the desire and ability to transport video are expected to grow correspondingly. Users will expect to be able to use interactive video as an integral part of the overall communication experience. Stored video is increasingly transported over the Internet by means of video streaming applications; however, maintaining good quality remains a challenge. This is because video is a demanding application, requiring a significant and consistent amount of bandwidth from the network. Furthermore, to support good-quality video, packet loss should be rare. Interactive video is even more demanding, requiring not only consistent bandwidth but also reasonably good latency. Just as with interactive voice, having a round-trip latency considerably greater than about 300 ms impacts interactive communication in undesirable ways. Unlike voice, overcoming delay jitter for video requires substantial buffering at the receiver, impacting cost.

Congestion in the network impacts video transport in all three dimensions: inconsistent bandwidth availability for the video stream, increased latency and jitter, and packet loss. Even when video streams have priority for transport over the network, potential sources of congestion in the network may be other video streams competing for capacity, or other even higher priority flows, such as network control traffic. Because of the high variability of the bandwidth requirements even for a single video source (see, e.g., Ref. 1), congestion due to competing video sources is likely to pose a major challenge to maintaining quality. The first defense against congestion is to utilize buffers in the network to overcome short-term mismatches between the available capacity in the network and the rate required for transporting the video stream. However, when the rate mismatch lasts a sufficiently long period (maybe a few milliseconds, or sometimes even less, depending on the amount of buffering available), packet loss results. Since video is typically transported over the network using an unreliable transport protocol such as UDP, packet losses typically result in the loss of video frames. Depending on the encoding, video has varying amounts of tolerance to frame loss. Typically, no more than a very small probability of frame loss is acceptable. Frame loss arises from the loss of one or more packets, depending on the encoding. The requirement for video on the network transport is to have a very small packet loss probability, in the range of 0.1–5%, depending on use. This is quite difficult to achieve, unless the network is considerably overprovisioned.

Compressed video exhibits burstiness over multiple time scales (see, e.g., Ref. 1). Over the short time scale, burstiness occurs because of the compression algorithm (e.g., with MPEG, because of the I-, B-, and P-frame structure). Over the longer term, burstiness is due to varying scene complexity, because of motion or extra detail in the scene. This can occur for fairly long periods—several tens of seconds or even minutes—depending on the content. Thus, there can be fairly long periods when the data rate of the video source is high, much higher than its average rate.

There are several avenues available to deal with the burstiness of compressed video. The first is to buffer the bursts. Buffers could be provided in the network, the destination, or the source. The motivation for providing network buffering is to ride over brief transient mismatches in the input rate relative to the network capacity, either from an individual video stream when per-flow buffering is employed in the network, or from the aggregate of all input flows when the buffer is shared. Destination buffering accommodates the jitter perceived by the receiver in receiving frames from the network and enables the video stream to be played out smoothly, without degradation in quality. Source buffering is primarily used as a smoothing buffer, when the source attempts to overcome a mismatch between the required rate and the permissible transmission rate over short intervals.

There are two somewhat simple ways of supporting video in an open-loop manner. (By "open-loop," we mean that the source transmits at a rate of its choosing, without reacting to any feedback from the network about its state of congestion.) The first is to use a constant bit rate (CBR) service, where the video source transmits at a constant rate that is negotiated a priori with the network. Use of a constant bit rate service will likely result in variable video quality. Ensuring that quality is not degraded severely, by ensuring that there is no loss of packets, requires the allocation of an adequately large CBR rate. This can lead to underutilization of the network resources, because resources may be committed to this video flow, and other sources are not allowed to use these network resources. Later in the chapter, we discuss the potential trade-offs between using a constant bit rate service and other service alternatives.

A second option is to use a variable bit rate (VBR) service, which still uses the network in an open-loop fashion. The VBR service uses a small number of descriptors, as described in Chapter 4 of this volume: a peak rate, a token bucket size (which controls the number of packets that may be sent at the peak rate), and a token fill rate (which determines the average rate). The average rate at which the network serves the video stream is based on the token fill rate. During the sustained peaks typically found in video, it will be quite difficult to avoid losses unless the buffers provided in the network to deal with such peaks are extremely large. Without adequate buffering in the network, packet loss would be excessive, impacting quality severely. On the other hand, packets can encounter excessive queueing delays in large buffers, impacting quality for real-time use.

Approaches supporting video in an open-loop fashion are also unable to react to changing conditions in the network. A video source that is not capable of adapting to changes in network capacity due to congestion can suffer packet losses, leading to frame loss and the impairment of quality. There is little that a source can do to control which frames are lost under these circumstances. To ensure that there is negligible loss requires the network to be very conservative in admission control when capacity for a video stream is allocated.

We have seen that open-loop transport of video can suffer from three drawbacks: the requirement for conservative admission control; large buffers, impacting delay; and the potential for packet loss, impacting quality. Requiring the source to adapt its transmission rate to network conditions represents a different approach. The source may negotiate a rate of transmission with the network as and when necessary, so that there is minimal loss and delivered video quality is acceptable. Further, the source may adapt itself to minimize the mismatch between the desired rate inherent for the video stream and the available network capacity. We believe that adaption at the video source is feasible and desirable. We describe broadly the possible approaches for adaptation available to the source.

The desired quality of the video to be delivered to the receiver varies widely, depending on the application, the potential cost to the user, and the network infrastructure that is available for transporting the video. There is a relatively large class of applications that can tolerate some variability in the perceived quality of the video, including video teleconferencing, interactive training, low-cost information distribution such as news, and even some entertainment video.

There are several possible approaches to adapting the video source. The method of adaptation is likely to vary depending on the content, what it is used for, and so on. For example, with a video teleconference among users having limited expectation of quality, it may be acceptable to modify the frame rate. Thus the frame grabbing rate might be reduced, while the same resolution is retained (by keeping the video encoding parameters the same). This would reduce the number of frames transmitted by the source. Alternatively, the source could reduce the number of samples in the frame. Finally, the more frequently examined approach for adaptation of the video source is to modify the source rate dynamically by adjusting the video encoding parameters. One parameter particularly suitable for adaptation is the quantization parameter, which determines the level of detail of the encoded frame. However, it is important that the quality of the video not be impacted substantially in the process. Later in the chapter we describe criteria for evaluating the quality of video being transported in the network, including the impact of the source adaptation.

Among the promising approaches for adapting to the short-term fluctuations in the rate required for video are renegotiated CBR (RCBR) (2) and feedback-based congestion control (3b–6). The approach described in Reference 5 attempts to achieve the goals of increasing the multiplexing gain by frequently negotiating bandwidth between the source and the network, with the desire to be responsive to the needs of the video source, while at the same time relying on the adaptation of source rates to match available bandwidth.

The type of adaptation that is feasible depends on the information that is available from the network regarding the current state of the network, including the available capacity to carry the particular video stream. Using the Internet's current suite of protocols (TCP, UDP, and IP), the primary feedback that is received about congestion in the network is indication of lost packets. Several research and experimental efforts have been undertaken to adapt the source rate of the video stream in reaction to this indication of loss (7,8). We discuss these in greater detail in Section 10.2.

We now describe in more detail the framework for source adaptation and the role of network feedback; Figure 10.1 illustrates the set of possible elements discussed. The uncompressed video from the source is fed to an encoder, which is capable of encoding in one or more frames that conform to sizes determined in part by the network feedback. We refer to Chapters 7 and 9 for detailed surveys of video coding schemes. In single-layer coding schemes, such as JPEG and MPEG, the frame size can be specified not to exceed a given byte size by selection of the appropriate value of the quantization parameter. The output of the encoder is fed to a rate adaptation buffer at the source that is used to accommodate the variability in the demand from the encoder. It also accommodates the difference between the rate coming into the buffer and the output rate from the source into the network. In addition to adjusting the size of the frame being encoded, the drain rate of the buffer into the network may be adjusted according to the feedback information. Depending on the application requirements, some shortfall in available capacity relative to the desired rate may be acceptable over shorter

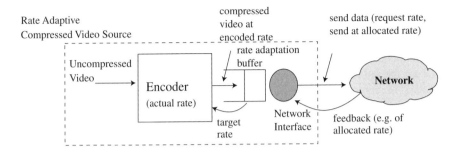

Figure 10.1 Framework for rate-adaptive video in an explicit-rate environment.

times scales. The advantage of network feedback is that it enables the adaptation to the rate shortfall to be performed gracefully at the source (e.g., by buffering, or by adaptation of the encoder to reduce frame size) rather than in an uncontrolled manner in the network (through packet loss or delay). This feedback may be explicit in the rate, or it may only indicate the presence of congestion. The source itself may request a transmission rate of the network. In responding to such requests, it is the function of network connection admission control to ensure that the available capacity meets the required capacity over long time scales.

Another approach is to use a layered coding scheme. The layers can be *independent,* where each layer completely describes the video information at a given resolution, or the layering can be *cumulative* in that each layer builds on the lower layers. Adaptation may be performed in a variety of ways. In one example of adaptation with a layered coding scheme, the different frequency components are transmitted separately, and the rate adaptation is accomplished by choosing not to carry the high-frequency components.

A specific example for a source using feedback for adaptation is found when the source uses the *available bit rate* (ABR) service defined by the ATM Forum (9), using the explicit rate option. The source is allowed to request a rate from the network, and the network responds with an allocated rate based on the contention for resources in the network, with the assurance that the rate allocated will not go below a minimum rate negotiated at connection setup time. The minimum rate the source requests may be selected so that the quality for the video does not go below a minimum acceptable level. It is possible to keep the queueing delays seen by connections using the ABR service fairly small, since the explicit-rate schemes can ensure that the aggregate rate of all sources sharing a link remains below the link bandwidth. To ensure that the delays experienced by video flows are reasonably small, it may be necessary to separate flows that are admission-controlled and require low delay (e.g., video) from others that may not be admission-controlled (e.g., bursty data). There may be a concomitant service discipline at the switches to serve the separate classes in proportion to the rates allocated to each of the classes (e.g., as in Ref. 10).

An integral part of source rate adaptation for video is the smoothing of the video either at a source or at a gateway, when the original encoding of the stream cannot be controlled. Smoothing involves the use of a buffer at the source or gateway. This enables the source to smooth the rate it requests from the network for transmission of the video, a feature having the potential to achieve higher multiplexing gains in the network. The smoothing buffer enables us to smooth out the bursts in the rate required for the video. We cover smoothing in more detail later in this chapter.

In the next section, we discuss the proposals that have been discussed in the literature to transport real-time video over a best-effort Internet. Most of these proposals depend on loss as an indication of congestion and use feedback of received rates from the destination. The source uses this information to estimate the available bandwidth and adapts to it. We briefly address the work on feedback-based transport of video over the Internet for multicast in Section 10.3. A significant amount of work remains to be done in the area of feedback-based multicast transport of real-time video. One of the more promising approaches for unicast feedback-based transport of real-time video is the use of explicit-rate feedback. We discuss this method in detail in Section 10.4. In Section 10.5, we discuss in more detail the issues related to smoothing and to the characterization of the rate required for a video stream. A particular example of a smoothing and rate adaptation algorithm is SAVE (smoothed adaptive video over explicit rate networks), which we have worked on (11,12). We describe the SAVE algorithm in detail in Section 10.6. The traditional means for evaluation of video transport focuses on minimizing loss (frame, packet, or cell loss). SAVE modifies the quantization parameter as the primary means of rate adaptation. We believe that it is necessary to evolve the metrics for evaluation of such rate adaptation algorithms. Section 10.7 describes the criteria we used for evaluating SAVE. The next two sections present evaluation results of SAVE obtained through simulation. Finally, in Section 10.10 we present a summary.

10.2 TRANSPORT OF VIDEO OVER THE BEST-EFFORT INTERNET

The current Internet provides a best-effort service, without providing guarantees with respect to bandwidth, delay, or loss. Transporting video over such networks, especially when capacity is not in plenty, is a significant challenge. We refer the reader to Chapters 3 and 4 of this volume for the fundamental issue related to congestion control in IP and ATM networks.

Without the predictability offered by the network, applications must adapt in response to packet loss indication. Bolot and Turletti (7) describe their experience with a rate control mechanism for transport of video over the Internet. The mechanism was incorporated in their software videoconferencing system IVS. (13). The experimental work examined ways of adapting the source coder's output rate within the existing network and transport layer protocols in the Internet (RTP, RTCP, UDP, and IP). The feedback information provided in RTCP packets in receiver reports (RR) is used to derive loss rates at the sender. A somewhat coarse approximation of the block loss rate is made based on the packet loss rate. The source then uses a control algorithm to adjust λ, the maximum rate of the coder. The adjustment algorithm uses the principles of linear increase and multiplicative decrease of λ to ensure that reasonable efficiency and fairness are maintained (14,15). Congestion in the network is deduced from the RRs. When the loss rate reported by RTCP exceeds a high-loss threshold (e.g., 5%), the source declares that the network is *Congested* and that λ needs to be reduced. When the loss rate drops below a low-loss threshold (e.g., 2%, although we believe this low threshold should be smaller), the source declares that the network is *UnCongested*.

Bolot and Turletti (7) also briefly outlined a way of declaring congestion in the case of multicast and a way of accommodating heterogeneity. When a reasonable percentage of receivers (say, 10% or more) indicate that they are experiencing excessive loss in the RRs, the source infers that the environment is congested and that it needs to reduce λ. Similarly, when more than 10% of the receivers indicate that they are experiencing low loss, the source increases λ.

The paper (7) defined two variables: a reduction factor, $\alpha \leq 1$, and an increase factor, β. The source periodically adjusts the rate λ, using the following rules:

if(Congested)
   $\lambda = \max\{\lambda * \alpha, \text{minimum\_rate}\}$;
if(UnCongested)
   $\lambda = \min\{\lambda + \beta, \text{maximum\_rate}\}$;

The algorithm ensures that the source coder's rate neither goes below a *minimum_rate* nor exceeds a *maximum_rate*.

Bolot et al. primarily examined the approach of adapting the frame rate at the source (adjusting the frame grabbing rate). Experiments were performed on the Internet between three sites, and the rate control mechanism described above was observed to improve performance by dramatically reducing the loss rate experienced. However, there is considerable variation in λ, frequently reaching the *minimum_rate*. When there is considerable delay to get the notification of losses to the source (e.g., in a video teleconference between France and California), λ tends to rapidly oscillate between the *maximum_rate* and the *minimum_rate*. Because the frame rate is modified (rather than the quantizer value), the impact on quality from such a wide variation is possibly acceptable for use in videoconferencing only. However, better guarantees on the bandwidth and finer control would be required if the quality requirements for the content were higher (e.g., entertainment video).

More recently, a further refinement to support streaming video from a server over the Internet has been explored (8). This protocol, called RAP, involves a rate-adaptive source at a server and a corresponding rate-adaptive receiver at every client, with the receiver acknowledging every packet. These acknowledgments provide timely feedback to the source of packet losses (more precisely, the lack of packet loss). Because the application is primarily streaming video, the source adaptation is of the packet transmission rate, rather than the encoder's rate. Unlike a window flow control mechanism, where the window size is adjusted, the interpacket gap (IPG) is adjusted in RAP in response to congestion. The IPG is adjusted according to the additive increase, multiplicative decrease policy. By taking advantage of the acknowledgments generated for every packet by a RAP receiver, the source maintains a smoothed round-trip time (SRTT) estimate. Knowledge of the SRTT allows the source to update the source rate approximately once every round-trip time. When the congestion indication is a coarse one, such as packet loss (14) or a binary explicit congestion notification (16), it is important that the source not react to such indications more than once in a round-trip time. A change made at the source needs to take effect in the network, and a subsequent indication needs to arrive before the source reacts again. With explicit rate based feedback mechanisms, on the other hand, there exists the potential for sources to react more frequently within a round-trip time, as we explore later in this chapter. The availability of the SRTT enables a RAP source to adjust the interval between updates to the packet transmission rate, just as TCP implicitly does with a window-based protocol. Thus, unlike the periodic updates used in the work by Bolot and Turletti (7), RAP updates the source packet rate approximately once every round-trip time. A small further enhancement in RAP is to include a finer grained control of the transmission rate by updating the IPG on every acknowledgment. This is similar to TCP's modification of the window size upon receiving each acknowledgment during its congestion avoidance phase.

The design of rate adjustment protocols in the Internet for real-time streams such as video also needs to take into account the existence of other data streams that use TCP, especially the congestion control mechanisms used by TCP. Unfairness may result when a real-time stream generates a load on the network causing the bottleneck router buffer occupancy to build up. This eventually leads to packet loss, and TCP sources may react to the loss and reduce their transmission rate. Real-time streams that do not use TCP (e.g., they may use UDP) may not react to the packet loss, thus gaining an unfair advantage. This has been a real concern in the Internet, and several rate control protocols proposed for real-time streams have included the notion of being "TCP-friendly". Additional details in RAP include the determination of a source packet transmission rate that is suitably friendly to the other TCP sources.

Simulation results published in 1999 (8) primarily focus on the TCP friendliness of the proposed protocol. However, some results on RAP indicates that the source packet transmission rate with RAP is smoother than the transmission rate of a source using TCP. The encoder runs independently, without taking into account the source transmission rate. We believe that the variation in transmission rate and the lack of explicit modification of the encoder behavior are still likely to impact perceived video quality. We explore the modifications to the encoder behavior in the subsequent sections of this chapter.

Many of the studies on adaptive rate control of a video source attempt to ensure that the output rate does not go below a minimum rate, so that the quality is not severely degraded (i.e., below an acceptable level). We will see this in the approaches taken for supporting rate-adaptive video over a network that provides bandwidth guarantees, such as asynchronous transfer mode (ATM) networks, in subsequent sections of this chapter.

10.3 SUPPORTING VIDEO IN A MULTICAST ENVIRONMENT

It is likely that multicast will be used increasingly in the future for carrying real-time multimedia. The heterogeneity that we are likely to see in the network, due to both receiver characteristics and variability in link bandwidths, poses a challenge to techniques of adaptation. McCanne et al. published a seminal paper (17) on moving the rate adaptation to the receivers by means of what they called receiver-driven layered multicast (RLM). The paper combines layered video compression with a layered transmission scheme. The assumption is that the compression algorithm encodes the video into a number of layers that incrementally provide enhanced video quality. The network is used to transport each video layer as a different multicast group. End points receive the different layers by explicitly joining a multicast group. The quality as seen at a receiver is a function of the groups (from the lowest up to the highest group) that the receiver has joined. Congestion at an intermediate point in the network results in packet loss. This acts as an indication to receivers to leave a multicast group and to be able to adapt to the capacity available in the end-to-end path.

A critical assumption made in RLM is that packet loss occurs uniformly across all layers. McCanne et al. go further to suggest that uniform dropping has the potential to discourage greedy users who request rates well above the bottleneck rate.

A simple scheme in which a receiver drops a layer when congestion is encountered needs to be enhanced to do the reverse action to add a layer. RLM receivers actively experiment to add layers at "well-chosen" times. If a join experiment results in congestion, the receiver drops the new, offending layer. Join experiments involve overhead and need to be carefully managed. RLM uses a *join timer* with an exponential back-off procedure to ensure that join experiments that are likely to fail are done with sufficient infrequency. To scale RLM to a large number of receivers, the scheme uses a notion of "shared learning." Before a receiver conducts a join experiment, it notifies the entire group by multicasting a message identifying the experimental layer. Because all receivers can learn from the failed join experiments of other receivers for a layer, they can scale back their join timer for that layer. This technique of shared information relies on the network's way of signaling congestion, namely, by dropping packets across all layers.

RLM has been studied in the context of smooth, constant bit rate sources for each layer. A typical compressed video source may in fact be bursty at each layer, and it may be useful to look at smoothing the source by adaptive quantization even for layered video sources. Simulation experiments suggest that as the number of receivers grows with RLM, the time to converge to the optimal point is aided by allowing the receivers to share information on failed join experiments. Long-term loss rates were under 1%, while medium-term loss rates stayed in the range of a few percent (>10% when averaged over periods of 1 second). Further understanding of the impact of RLM on actual video quality with traces appears to be needed.

McCanne et al. assumed that packet loss occurs uniformly across all the layers. In subsequent work, Bajaj et al. compared the consequence of uniform versus priority dropping for layered video (18a). They examined whether there would be a sufficient disincentive for greedy users if the network were to uniformly drop packets across all the layers. Alternatively, if the network were to use priority dropping, where packets belonging to the base layer are marked with high priority, while the lower layers are marked with successively lower priority, there might be a benefit for transmission of layered video (18). While their results are inconclusive, Bajaj et al. conjecture that there is an upper bound of about 36% improvement that may be obtained with priority dropping over uniform dropping. They also observe uniform dropping with FIFO service does not offer very good incentive properties. Incentive properties are useful to examine because they show whether a greedy user can derive an unfair benefit over other users by transmitting more layers. Bajaj et al. point out that a user may in fact obtain a benefit by transmitting more layers than the social optimal (which is the level at which all the other users are transmitting to match the capacity available in the network). One way to overcome the problems associated with FIFO service and uniform dropping is to use fair queueing (10) in the network. Priority dropping helps with FIFO service by constraining usage somewhat more easily.

10.4 SOURCE ADAPTATION USING RATE-BASED FEEDBACK CONTROL

Video transmitted in real time inherently expects to be able to transmit the data at a rate that is commensurate with the needs of the video content. Compressed video is inherently bursty, with rate fluctuations happening over multiple time scales, and a source that uses constant bit rate transport requires a local buffer for smoothing. Buffer overflow or underflow is prevented by continually adjusting the quantizer step size, resulting in *variable quality*. The advantage of CBR transport is that it makes admission control simple. On the other hand, using a variable bit rate transport allows the maintenance of a more constant quality by accommodating the rate fluctuations of compressed video. Transmitting video at a variable bit rate is especially attractive when the source and network cooperate in matching the source transmission rate to the network's available capacity. This is facilitated by mechanisms that allow the source to request varying amounts of bandwidth over time from the network to transmit the video stream. The network then notifies the source of the available rate through feedback. Sections 10.4.1 and 10.4.2 describe the constraints under which these rates are characterized and computed and discuss specific mechanisms for rate renegotiation between the source and the network.

10.4.1 Constraints on Rate Required for Transporting Real-Time Video

Selection of a specific transmission rate for the video source depends on the balance of three elements: application constraints (e.g., on delay and quality), the rate required by the source to satisfy those constraints, and the capacity available from the network. Balancing the required source rate and the available network rate requires that the source be able to characterize both.

10.4.1.1 Buffering and Delay Constraints. A rate adaptation buffer at the source smooths the source rate but introduces delay when the instantaneous source rate is greater than the buffer drain rate. Delay variation due to buffering at the source and in the interior of the network can be accommodated in a receiver playout buffer at the expense of increasing mean delay. Thus end-to-end delay constraints imposed by the application (e.g., teleconferencing) limit the degree of rate smoothing attainable. At the destination, complete frames are removed from the decoder buffer to be rendered at the frame frequency; the condition at the receiver when a frame is not present when it should be rendered is termed *underflow*.

At the encoder, overflow occurs when its buffer capacity is exceeded. In real-time video, frames are deposited in the source buffer every interframe time, so the encoder buffer may potentially empty during an interframe period, since the next frame may not be available on demand. Although underflow may signify the inefficient use of network resources, its avoidance is not viewed as a hard constraint.

10.4.1.2 Source Adaptation Constraints. For real-time video, encoders may adapt to a given network rate by adjusting the coarseness of the encoding, a lower rate entailing lower quality. If the original encoding of the real-time stream cannot be controlled (e.g., with recorded video, or at a network gateway), the same adaptation mechanism can be employed at a transcoder. The main constraint to this approach is its impact on perceived quality at the destination and the potential for delays (especially at the network gateway).

10.4.1.3 Lookahead Constraints. If future source rates are known (e.g., for recorded video), the network rates required to satisfy buffer and delay constraints can be calculated precisely; we review specific schemes later. This approach generalizes when source rates are not known in advance, but some latency can be tolerated. The latency period is equivalent to a lookahead window in which source rates are known.

10.4.1.4 Implicit Versus Explicit Feedback. Feedback is not necessarily given to the source in the form of an explicit rate; instead, notification may just be of the presence or absence of congestion within the network. In explicit congestion notification (ECN) (16) for IP networks, network elements may set the ECN bit in packets according to a policy that may penalize packets that encounter congestion. The source may then reduce its transmission rate, although now the reduced rate is not supplied by the network and must be determined at the source. The transmission rate may be reduced by reducing the window size in TCP. Without explicit congestion notification, congestion would have to be inferred from packet losses. The time to recover from packet losses, especially when they occur in a burst, can be high, impacting the real-time requirements of video transport.

10.4.1.5 Signaling Frequency and Latency Constraints. When the source employs some prediction of its future demands to characterize its future rate requirements, increasing the time between renegotiations will typically entail higher rate requirements. This is because prediction is more uncertain over longer intervals, and so a higher network rate is required to accommodate variability in the source demands. Renegotiation latency can impact source buffering requirements, hence source delay, since source traffic after an upward change in desired source rate may have to be buffered until the upward renegotiation is complete.

Explicit rate renegotiation can be performed in hardware, as an integral part of the datalink layer and in switch implementations. Alternatively, it may be performed with additional messaging at the network layer. In the former case, we may be able to renegotiate with higher frequency and lower latency. In the available bit rate (ABR) transport in ATM (9), resource management (RM) cells are issued from the source periodically (e.g., every 32 cells), and the source sets a rate request in the RM cell. This rate may be adjusted downward by network elements on the path to the destination (18b); the final rate is then returned back, and the source transmission rate must not exceed this rate returned in the RM cell. The RM cells are frequent (roughly once every 14 ms for a 1Mbit stream) and have the latency of a round-trip time to communicate available bandwidth. There is no network-imposed constraint on changing the requested rate as frequently as every RM cell. (However, the network resource allocation algorithms attempting to achieve max-min fairness [3], typically take a small number of round-trip times to stabilize after a change.) By contrast, when rates are renegotiated by means of explicit additional messages—for example, through Resource Reservation Protocol (RSVP) 19—the per-renegotiation processing cost at network elements is expected to bound the time between renegotiations to time scales of seconds or even minutes.

10.4.1.6 Rate Prediction Errors. The greater the information on source demands and network rate availability, the more accurately the two can be matched. Uncertainty in either leads to inefficiency if increased safety margins are applied to rate estimates. Factors leading to uncertainty in network rate include higher renegotiation latency, lower renegotiation frequency, and a simple notification of congestion in place of explicit rate feedback. The primary factor leading to uncertainty in source rate is the degree to which rate prediction is required. If the lookahead window exceeds the time between rate renegotiations, this factor will be absent.

10.4.2 Rate Renegotiation Mechanisms and Adaptation

We now look at specific mechanisms for rate renegotiation with the network and approaches for adaptation at the video source. One proposal for rate renegotiation by a video source is the renegotiated constant bit rate (RCBR) scheme proposed in (2). RCBR overcomes the medium-term variations in compressed video. It uses renegotiation of the traffic parameters of a constant bit rate connection by means of ATM signaling messages. This potentially limits the variation in quality while also avoiding overflow of buffers in the network.

For compressed video, the rate fluctuations over the medium to long time scale are due to scene changes. These can typically last tens of seconds or even minutes. With RCBR, the video application uses network layer signaling over the connection, requesting the desired bandwidth for the video flow. If there is enough bandwidth in the network and if the request is satisfied, the long-term fluctuations for the video flow can be accommodated. Since bandwidth is shared between several users, a renegotiation failure is always possible. There are several options at this point. The application may adapt to the bandwidth currently allocated to the connection until the next renegotiation, as described in this chapter, and attempt to maintain an acceptable level of perceptual quality. Alternatively, with measurement-based admission control, it may be possible to maintain a sufficiently low probability of blocking of the renegotiation request (2).

In the case of on line compressed video, the evolution of the compressed video flow is not known in advance (e.g., for videoconferencing) Therefore, RCBR uses a prediction of the flow to generate the sequence of renegotiation. Grossglauser et al. (2) studied algorithm based on a very simple AR(1) model to show that reasonable performance can be achieved. A similar prediction mechanism was used by Lakshman et al. (5).

Signaling is often performed by software in the end systems and typically, although not necessarily, involves considerable processing, including the invocation of connection admission control (CAC) functions in switches. This processing load may be a limitation for the RCBR approach, in that it may result in limiting the frequency with which renegotiations may be performed. The primary emphasis on the work with RCBR has been to examine the probability of renegotiation failure.

To overcome the constraints that may be present in using a CBR transport or in using RCBR and infrequent renegotiation, we may also exploit feedback of the available capacity from the network to adapt the rate of transmission at a video source. Network feedback enables a source to adjust its transmission rate based on the bandwidth currently available to the source. Moreover, when the video source's bandwidth demand cannot be met, the network feedback of the currently available bandwidth can be used to match the video source rate. Several papers (3–5,11,20) have described ways of using the feedback of rate and buffer occupancy at the bottleneck link/switch in the network. Even with a scheme like RCBR, renegotiation failures may be handled gracefully by adapting the quantization parameter of the encoder. Rate-based congestion management has been examined in considerable detail in proposals for end-to-end, feedback-based congestion control of ATM networks (21), in particular for the available bit rate service.

One of the early efforts to use rate-based congestion control approaches for adapting real-time compressed video was described by Kanakia et al. (3b). The video encoder and decoder mechanisms are essentially the same as those used for a CBR encoder. However, the actual bitstream produced by the encoder has a variable bit rate, and there is a buffer at the encoder and decoder (just as with a CBR encoder and decoder). The encoder uses its buffer occupancy levels to modulate its generation of video data to be transmitted. Most of these rate-based adaptation schemes make the fundamental assumption that the video encoder has a rate control mechanism that can be used to match the target rate computed at the source as a result of feedback from the network. The feedback information sent from the network is used to reduce the input rate from video sources, with a conscious attempt to gracefully degrade the quality of the image. Because the feedback information sent from the network switches arrives at the encoder after a substantial delay (based on the propagation delays and the size of the network), a carefully constructed control mechanism is needed at the source. The goal is to ensure that the rate of transmission of video into the network does not exceed the capacity available for the video flow, while at the same time not overflowing both the encoder buffer and the buffers at the routers in the network.

The control mechanism proposed by Kanakia et al (3b) is based on predicting the evolution of the system over time and using that prediction to compute a target sending rate for each frame of video data. The feedback information assumed in this work is generally a little more elaborate than is available on the current Internet or with the currently proposed ATM service classes. However, it serves as a model of what may be achieved if more information (such as both available rate and queue occupancy) is made available. The network routers feed back both the service rate, μ_n and the queue occupancy χ_n at the bottleneck router for a particular flow, along with timestamp information for the packet generated at the router. The feedback information is reported multiple times per frame interval. Because of feedback delay, the information available at a source may be k frames old. For both μ_n and χ_n, estimates $\hat{\mu}_n$ and $\hat{\chi}_n$ are maintained at the source, based on a prediction of the evolution of the bottleneck state. The target sending rate, λ_n, for a frame, n, is calculated as follows:

$$\lambda_n = \begin{cases} \lambda_{n-1} + \delta & \text{if } x_{n-k} = 0 \\ \hat{\mu}_n + \dfrac{x^* - \hat{x}_n}{\text{gain} \cdot F} & \text{otherwise} \end{cases} \qquad (1)$$

Here, χ^* is the target value of the buffer occupancy at the bottleneck for this video flow, and $1/F$ is the frame rate for this video. When the reported buffer occupancy at the bottleneck is zero, the sending rate is increased linearly until the reported occupancy is nonzero. The value δ controls the increase rate, and *gain* is a gain factor controlling the influence of the extent to which the current buffer occupancy differs from the target value χ^*. When the occupancy is nonzero, the control mechanism attempts to maintain the bottleneck buffer occupancy close to the target value, χ^*.

Knowing the last known buffer occupancy level at the start of the $(n - k)$th frame, the source estimates the buffer occupancy x_n. The information used in this estimate is the amount of data sent by the source since the last time the buffer occupancy was estimated (at the time of the start of the previous frame), and the estimate of the amount of data drained from the bottleneck queue in the same interval of time. Since the actual service rate at the bottleneck for this flow is also known only on a delayed basis, the source also maintains an exponentially weighted moving average estimate of the bottleneck service rate. Thus there are two predictors, the current buffer occupancy at the bottleneck and the current service rate at the bottleneck. These predictors were described in detail by Kanakia et al. (3b). The effectiveness of the scheme depends somewhat on the robustness of these predictors.

The service rate at the bottleneck is likely to depend on the frame size. Given that the size of the frames generated by the encoder for an encoding criterion such as the MPEG standard depends on the type of the frame (I, B, or P frame), Kanakia et al. suggest maintaining three separate estimators for the service rates. Thus, the source keeps track of the value of the group of pictures (GOP) parameter and the frames being transmitted. Correlating the feedback received from the bottleneck, the source then maintains the estimate of the service rate for each type of frame.

Kanakia et al. (3b) limited their view of congestion, in the network to the case of a single bottlenecked node/router. However, they examined through simulations the case of multiple congested routers that have a significant buffer occupancy because of cross-traffic.

The evaluation metrics used are the per-frame signal-to-noise ratio (SNR) as well as the average SNR over a sequence of frames. The authors suggest that this is an initial, crude indication of the perceptual quality of video that users are likely to observe. In addition, the authors reconstructed the video sequence received at the decoder based on trace-driven simulations and conducted subjective evaluations of the quality of the video. This served as a basis for comparing the evaluation metric of SNR versus the subjective, perceived quality. The authors also studied the benefit of a *priority loss* scheme, where packets from B frames are assigned a low priority while packets from P and I frames are assigned a high priority. The priority assignment is based on the observation that the loss of P and I frames adversely affects the signal quality not only of those frames but also that of other frames.

Experiments were conducted with trace-driven simulations. The highlight of the observations was that the average SNR value is an imperfect measure of the perceptual quality. Even though the SNR value for the priority loss scheme and for the feedback-based scheme were similar, the actual difference in perceptual quality was high. With feedback control, there appeared to be barely noticeable flicker (due to packet losses), in contrast to highly visible flashing and blurring of picture quality with the priority loss scheme for video sequences examined in their earlier paper (3b).

The results of this work suggest that there is good promise for feedback-based control of compressed video. The work we describe in the following sections builds on the concepts presented earlier (3b). The motivation for the subsequent work was to limit the dependence on the extent of elaborate information being fed back from the network. In addition, the motivation was to simplify the estimation and prediction needed at the source of the precise state of the network.

10.5 RATE CHARACTERIZATION AND SMOOTHING

Smoothing the source rate entails selecting a transmission schedule of frames across the network that is feasible in the sense that it is compatible with delay and buffering constraints at the source and destination. When the sequence of frame sizes is known exactly, as in the the case of stored video, conditions for feasibility can be formulated exactly. This has been achieved for various combinations of constraints at the source and destination in a number of different works; see References 20, 22–28.

We elaborate on the case of constraints at the destination buffer, following the notation from Salehi et al. (26). Let l_i, $i = 1, 2, \ldots, N$ denote the sizes of frame in a stream of N video frames stored at a server which are to be transmitted across a network to a decoder buffer of capacity B. For convenience, time will be measured in units of the fixed interframe time; let s_i denote the amount of data transmitted during the ith interframe time, so that $S(t) = \sum_{i=1}^{t} s_i$ is the cumulative amount of data sent up to time t. Complete frames are to be removed from the decoder buffer at the frame frequency (i.e., frame i at time i), hence avoidance of underflow requires that

$$L(t) \leq S(t) \tag{2}$$

where $L(t) = \sum_{i}^{t}=l_i$ is the cumulative size of the first t frames. Avoidance of overflow of the decoder buffer requires that the amount of data it receives be bounded above as follows:

$$S(t) \leq U(t) := \min \{L(t-1) + B, L(N)\} \tag{3}$$

Salehi et al. (26) call a transmission schedule S feasible if both the constraints represented by Eqs. (2) and (3) are satisfied. (Here we use the term feasible schedule more generally to describe a transmission schedule that is compatible with any given set of constraints under consideration). Several extensions of this basic framework are possible. First, identical constraints at an encoder buffer can be incorporated, namely, that a finite source buffer should not overflow or underflow (20,25,26). Second, a playback delay can be added to smooth out transmissions at the start of the video (27). Third, delay jitter can be bounded by making the constraints of Eqs. (2) and (3) more conservative (26).

For a given set of constraints, feasible schedules are not generally unique. This raises the question of which representative schedule among the set of feasible schedules should be used for transmission. Once equipped with a quantitative notion of the optimality of a schedule, one naturally tends to identify and use the optimal schedule. Examples of optimal properties of the transmission schedule include minimization of either the peak rate, the rate variance, or the number of rate changes. Algorithms that minimize the peak rate have been proposed (29, 30), but these did not simultaneously minimize variability. Elsewhere (20) it was proposed to use the feasible schedule with the shortest length (of the two-dimensional trajectory of cumulative rate vs. time). Using techniques from the theory of majorization, it was proved (26) that this trajectory minimizes a number of quantities, including peak rate, variance, and the empirical effective bandwidth for a bufferless resource. Moreover, it is the unique such trajectory.

Unlike the case of smoothing of stored video, in online smoothing the sequence of frame sizes is not known in advance. The prime example of this is live video. Another case is streaming video, which may be live or recorded; however, additional smoothing may take place at gateways in the network interior. These gateways will generally be unaware of future frame sizes, even for recorded video. For one-way video transmission, such as for entertainment, a substantial playback delay (say a small number of seconds) may be tolerable. Thus it is possible to smooth over a substantial window of frames. The optimal smoothing algorithm of Reibman and Berger (20) was adapted in 1998 (27) to operate on such finite windows.

However, in interactive applications such as teleconferencing, delay requirements are far more stringent, requiring as little as a few hundred milliseconds round-trip delay. This limits smoothing, which now must occur over smaller windows, and consequently the required bandwidth will be larger on average and also more variable. Prediction can be used to alleviate this stringency, and several different forms have been proposed. They share the premise that at time scales shorter than the scene time scale, patterns of frame rates should be approximately constant. One method is to make use of the GOP structure in MPEG-encoded video, with the working approximation that the sizes of frames at the same position of successive groups will be unchanged (see [24]). In practice, these corresponding frame sizes differ from group to group, so such prediction will be imperfect. A modification that ameliorates the inaccuracy is to supplement with statistical prediction; autoregressive models for frame sizes have been proposed (23,31,32). In this approach the parameters of the model are determined from the video source in question; since these vary between different video sources, they must be either precalculated (possible only in the case of stored video) or calculated progressively (in the case of online video). Additional robustness to departures in the actual frame sizes from prediction can be achieved by systematic overestimation of the bandwidth required (e.g., by applying a multiplier to the predicted bandwidth).

Additional mechanisms can be supplied to provide robustness to prediction errors. This is particularly important at scene boundaries, where both the deterministic and statistical predictors may take some time to respond to the frame rates of the new scene. In these circumstances, unexpectedly large frames and a shortfall in bandwidth from the network can result in violation of the delay constraint. In the SAVE algorithm (11), robustness is provided by characterizing the largest frame of the current scene and choosing the buffer drain rate such that a frame of this size could always be drained within the delay constraint, were it to arrive. Others have proposed (23) to monitor the level of the source adaptation buffer and switch the drain rate to a larger value if this level is exceeded, irrespective of current predictions.

Prediction can play a further role when the transmission rate is to be negotiated between the source and the network. Typically there is some latency between the issuance of the request and its granting. Hence the source should request the rate it expects to require when the request is granted, rather than when it is made.

10.6   THE SAVE ALGORITHM

As an example of a smoothing and rate adaptation algorithm, we have worked on the algorithm called SAVE (smoothed adaptive video over explicit rate networks) (11,12). SAVE is a source algorithm used for transporting compressed video in conjunction with explicit rate based feedback control in the network. In this chapter, we describe SAVE and the evaluation of the algorithm as an example of how network feedfack can be used to achieve (a) compressed video sources that are rate adaptive, good quality simultaneously with (b) good multiplexing gains, and (c) assurance that the delay at the source buffer does not exceed a bound.

The SAVE algorithm adapts to the demands of the video source, but imposes controls just when the uncontrolled demand of the sources would lead to excessive delay. The algorithm comprises two parts. The *rate request algorithm* specifies how the source requests bandwidth from the system. The *frame quantization algorithm* specifies how the frame sizes are controlled to avoid excessive delay. We now motivate these two parts by examining the characteristics of the source video. The material in this section is based on the work reported earlier (11,12).

10.6.1   Heuristics for the Requested Rate

We estimate the rate required of the network as the maximum of two components: one reflecting the short-term average rate requirements and the other based on the typical large frame at the scene time scale. The work is based on compressed video that uses compression algorithms such as MPEG. In this case there may be a number of relatively large frames that have been intra-frame-coded and occur periodically. These may be interspersed with inter-frame-coded frames that are typically smaller; these carry motion information and temporal changes from the previous frame. With MPEG, the I frames are typically large frames. A group of pictures (GOP) typically consists of one I frame followed by a series of other (not-I) frames, although this need not necessarily be the case.

It is desirable to have a network rate that is smoothed over the GOP period to avoid systematic fluctuations within it; otherwise poor performance can result. Without smoothing, the allocation of rate could systematically lag demand, and the mismatch of a large allocation with a small demand leads to wastage of network resources. So one determinant of the required rate will be the smoothed rate $r_{sm} = f_{sm}/\tau$, where τ is the interframe time, and f_{sm} is the ideal frame size—that required by the encoder to encode the frame at ideal perceptual lossless quality—smoothed over some window of w_{sm} frames. For encodings without a periodic structure, we could in principle take w_{sm} as small as 1.

While r_{sm} gives the average requirement over a small number w_{sm} of frames, the larger frames in the smoothed set will suffer increased delay. These large frames are potentially the I frames in MPEG-2, the initial frames of a new scene, or the frames generated when there is considerable activity in the scene. We aim to allocate a rate to ensure that the frame delay does not exceed some target τ_{max}. So we keep track of the maximum frame size f_{max} at the time scale of scenes of a few seconds (i.e., over some window w_{max}, which may be substantially larger than the smoothing window w_{sm}). There are evidently correlations in the frame sequences, especially over intervals of a few seconds (e.g., at the scene time scale). By keeping track of the peak sizes over this time scale and ensuring that the rate is adequate to meet their requirements, we can be responsive to the requirements of the scene. Also, we can be responsive to the needs of any periodic, relatively larger I frames in an I-B-P frame structure for MPEG compression.

However, just as correlations decay over larger time scales, the use of the finite window w_{max} means that the changes in activity at the scene level are reflected in f_{max}. Nonetheless, we do find it useful to keep a historical estimate of f_{max} through autoregression. The rate we associate with the estimate f_{max} of the maximum frame size is $r_{max} = f_{max}/\tau_{max}$, that is, the rate required to drain the frame of size f_{max} from an empty buffer within the delay target τ_{max}. The requested rate in SAVE is at least the maximum of (r_{sm}, r_{max}). In practice we find that the ratio f_{max}/f_{sm} is usually larger than τ_{max}/τ. Because the large frames are comparatively isolated, the source buffer will usually be relatively empty immediately before the large frame enters it, if the requested rate is allocated.

The requested rate has a built-in safety factor. To allow us to drain the buffer, especially when it has been built up, we ask for a *small* overallocation of the rate, over and above the rate that was computed above. This is in keeping with the intuition that the mean rate requested is likely to be slightly higher than the mean of the source's ideal rate, just so that we can ride out peaks in the source's ideal rate. We also assume that there is an initial rate allocated to the source, to drain the first few frames, until the feedback arrives from the network in response to the request generated when the first frame is being encoded and transmitted.

10.6.2 Heuristics for Frame Quantization

In parallel with the rates above, we also keep track of available size f_{avail} for a frame to be drained within the delay target τ_{max}, given the current rate allocation and buffer occupancy. This size is supplied to the encoder. If the ideal frame size exceeds the available size f_{avail}, the quantization level in the encoder is adjusted to permit the encoded frame size to be reduced to meet f_{avail} if possible, but never by more than some fixed factor. Clearly it is desirable that the frequency and amount of cropping not be excessive. One of the consequences of tracking the maximum frame size on a scene time scale is that typically, only the first frame of a new scene is vulnerable to cropping. We now specify the two parts of the SAVE algorithm precisely.

10.6.3 The Rate Request Algorithm

The requested rate is (essentially) the maximum of two rates: r_{sm}, the average rate per frame (over some short smoothing window of w_{sm}), and r_{max}, the maximum rate (over a medium-term window w_{max}) required to drain a frame from an empty buffer within the delay constraint. Let $f(n)$ be the size of frame n, τ the interframe time, and τ_{max} the buffer delay constraint. Then for the nth frame

$$r_{sm}(n) = (\tau w_{sm})^{-1} \sum_{i=0}^{w_{sm}-1} f(n-i) \tag{4}$$

$$r_{max}(n) = (\tau_{max})^{-1} \quad \max_{i=0,1,\ldots,w_{max}-1} f(n-i) \tag{5}$$

The heuristic for this choice is as follows. We clearly want to request a rate that is commensurate with at least the average rate of the source. By choosing w_{sm} quite small, we will make this responsive to rate changes within the medium term. (But if there is a GOP structure of period p present in the encoding, we want $w_{sm} \geq p$ to avoid systematic variations in the requested rate.) However, if the allocated rate were just r_{sm}, when the short-term peak-to-mean ratio exceeds τ_{max}/τ (typically only 2 to 3), large frames will suffer delay beyond τ. So with allocation of the maximum of r_{sm} and r_{max}, the large frames typically find the buffer empty, and so drain within time τ_{max}. By taking w_{max} sufficiently large we aim to anticipate the large frame typical of a scene. (Actually there is a little more detail

in the earlier work (11): we take the maximum also with an autoregressive estimate r_{ar} of the maximum frame size divided by τ_{max}). Finally, we systematically
over request by a factor $\beta > 1$; the requested rate at frame n is then

$$r_{req}(n) = \beta \max\{r_{sm}(n), r_{max}(n), r_{ar}(n)\} \tag{6}$$

10.6.4 THE FRAME QUANTIZATION ALGORITHM

Given a buffer occupancy $b(n)$ and allocated rate $r_{all}(n)$ at frame n, the estimated
size of a frame that will empty within the delay bound is $f_{avail}(n) = \tau_{max}r_{all}(n-1)-$
$\max\{0, b(n)-\tau r_{all}(n-1)\}$. We stipulate that no frame can be encoded in a size less
than some proportion γ of its ideal size. The encoded size of frame n will be

$$f_{enc}(n) = \min\{f(n), \max\{f_{avail}(n-1), \gamma f(n)\}\} \tag{7}$$

Choosing $\gamma > 0$ risks that a frame will be delayed more than τ, the interframe
time. However, since the network component of the delay is a variable quantity,
it may be better to risk that a frame will be delayed slightly more (but within the
maximum buffer delay constraint τ_{max}) than to encode only very coarsely.

10.7 EVALUATION CRITERIA

In this section, we describe the criteria for evaluating the performance of the
overall system: delay, quality, and networking performance. While the criteria
for video quality are somewhat heuristic, they are based on known characteristics of how people subjectively rate the quality of video (33).

10.7.1 Source Delay

The source buffer should not introduce delay so large that it eats into the delay budget of the network; this would make the network less attractive for real-time services. We assume that there is a sufficiently large playout buffer at the receiver to
overcome delay jitter. Hence the primary concern for the work is the aggregate delay introduced in the source buffer and the network. We assume that an overall (one-
way) delay budget around 200–300 ms is acceptable, and that, of this, a delay target
of about 100 ms for the source buffer is reasonable for interactive applications. We
assume that the source buffer is large enough to accommodate any backlog arising
because of a shortfall of the allocated rate from the encoded rate; at the operating
point, such differences will last only a short time if the delay target is reached.

10.7.2 Quality and Adaptation

We assume that it is desirable to keep the quality of the video transmitted by the
source as close to the ideal quality as possible. The premise is that sources are

adaptive enough that even if the encoded rate falls below the ideal rate, the video quality at the receiver will not suffer significant perceptual impairment. We think this is true provided the shortfalls are sufficiently small, rare, and short-lived. We shall use the term *cropping* to describe the reduction from the ideal rate to the encoded rate. In particular, cropping entails a reduction in encoding detail rather than a truncation of the size of the image. Cropping can occur either because of delay in the network to respond to changes in the short-term average rate or because congestion forces the network to allocate less than the requested rate. In the latter case, the network is unable to know either the actual video quality aimed for or the effect the reduction of allocated rate will have on quality; rate allocation among sources is done entirely on the basis of the requested rates. The rate allocated by the network itself may be based on a weighted max-min fair allocation (32, 5), where the weights are proportional to the requested rate. This enables the network to favor a video source that has a higher requested rate (possibly because of a higher ideal rate) than another, even though they share the same bottleneck.

In evaluating the operation of SAVE with a given video source, we look at the pattern of cropping over the entire sequence of frames. We strive to keep the proportion of cropping below 20%, exceeding this level at most for 0.1% of all the frames. At the rates in question, this amount of reduction of the encoded rate will degrade video quality as measured by the peak signal-to-noise ratio (PSNR) by about 1–2 dB. We believe that greater than this amount of degradation is generally perceivable by moderately experienced viewers.

We also look at the dynamics of cropping. In addition to meeting the foregoing criteria for cropping amount and frequency over the whole trace, we want to avoid long sequences of consecutively cropped frames. So we looked at the distribution of the length of bursts of successive frames cropped above (or below) the 20% threshold (other thresholds could also be considered). We expect that viewers will perceive the quality of video to be equivalent to the quality of the worst segment, provided this segment is long enough (33). Thus we will be particularly interested in the maximum burst length of cropping greater than the threshold of 20%. Conversely, during periods when cropping is below the threshold (including the case of no cropping) we expect there to be little impact on perceivable quality, even for experienced viewers.

We aim to keep the maximum burst length of cropping not much greater than any GOP period present in the encoding. Otherwise cropping of the large frame in successive GOPs could lead to noticeable quality reduction over timescales of up to 1 second. An example of this would be the cropping of consecutive I frames in a 12-frame GOP encoded at 24 frames/s. Cropping of an I frame can impair quality for subsequent frames. In addition, the periodic nature of the impairments will make them more noticeable (33). For this reason, when there is a GOP structure present, if two frames cropped more than 20% are separated by less than the GOP length, then for statistical purposes we treat all the intermediate frames as though they have been cropped more than 20%.

10.7.3   Robustness to Network Feedback Delay

The rate allocation mechanism of the explicit rate network is not expected to instantaneously allocate a rate in response to requests. To include the time needed for the stabilization of the rate allocation algorithms (34), we need to verify that quality measures are preserved even for a relatively large feedback delay (considered in the number of frame times). Even in the absence of network congestion, frame cropping is likely to occur when the short-term average demand suddenly changes. Therefore, some frames are likely to suffer cropping until the network allocates an increased rate.

10.7.4   Channel Capacity and Multiplexing Gain

We look at the number of sources that may be multiplexed within a link of a given capacity when the delay constraints and cropping criteria are met. This is eventually the criterion that will guide us to choose one algorithm over another. For statistical multiplexing gain, we want to be able to assign capacity to an aggregate of sources at less than the peak of their aggregate requested rate. During transient periods in which the aggregate requested rate exceeds the capacity, the explicit rate mechanism of the network will proportionately reduce the allocation to each source so as to avoid congestion. We use the term *rate reduction* when the allocated rate is less than the requested rate. We determine the sufficiency of such an allocation by establishing the extent to which such rate reduction is compatible with the delay and quality targets described above.

10.7.5   Sensitivity to Algorithm Parameters

Finally, SAVE has a number of tunable parameters. We shall investigate the sensitivity of the quality metrics to variations in w_{sm} and w_{max}.

10.8   FRAMEWORK FOR SIMULATION-BASED EVALUATION

The effectiveness of rate adaptation algorithms is evaluated by means of trace-driven simulations. Currently, the ability of analytical or synthetic models to represent a range of video sequences with reasonable accuracy is still limited. Even with trace-driven simulations, we have found that it is important to study the algorithms across a wide range of video sequences and coding algorithms of different types.

In our study of feedback-based rate adaptation and source smoothing, we used 28 different traces, ranging from video teleconference traces to entertainment video and advertisements. It is also important to evaluate the algorithms with traces of sufficient length, because that allows us to capture the effect of scene changes, where significant burstiness may exist. We have also looked at the behavior of the algorithm with different coding types, such as H.261, MPEG-1, and MPEG-2, because their effect may also be different.

We use frame-level simulation to understand the behavior of the algorithm from the point of view of the source. This allows us to abstract out the details of network behavior at the packet level on the very short time scale and to study a large number of alternatives rapidly. However, it is also important to understand the detailed, network-level effects such as those from packet loss, queueing delay in the network, and short time scale variation of available bandwidth. We therefore use both approaches. We depend on the detailed network-level simulation to validate and refine our understanding derived from the frame-level simulations.

We assume that the rate allocation mechanisms in the network act by allocating a rate to each source in proportion to its requested rate, so that the total allocated rate over all sources is no greater than the link capacity (5). We can investigate the frequency, duration, and magnitude of such events through simulations of the aggregate requested rate, and in particular its crossing of the link capacity. Figure 10.2 is typical; rare excursions above a level may be bursty. For this reason, for simulations, we model the dependence of the allocated rate on the requested rate in two stages. We first model the impact of contention by proportionately reducing the allocated rate in accordance with a rate reduction process, accounting for the network feedback delay. We then model the evolution of the source adaptation buffer behavior. This is described in more detail in the next section.

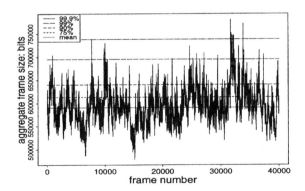

Figure 10.2 Aggregated requested rate: nineteen 40,000-frame traces in set E. The vertical range is about half the lowest value.

10.8.1   The Experimental Traces

We used five sets of traces to represent sequences of ideal frame sizes. Table 10.1 describes the individual traces in more detail. The experiments reported below use trace sets A and E; results on sets B, C, D are reported elsewhere (11). The sets of traces were as follows:

A. An MPEG-2 encoding of a 40,680-frame portion of *The Blues Brothers*, with M=1. There is no periodic structure, and no B frames. The frame rate was 24 frames/s.

Table 10.1   Trace Properties: Trace Sets B and E Are MPEG1; Trace Set A Is MPEG 2; Trace Sets C and D Are H.261

Set	Name	Type[a]	Length (frames)	Rate (frames/s)	Mean Bits per frame	Peak Bits per frame
A	*Blues Brothers*	ent	40,680	24	54,823	339,304
B	*Star Wars*	ent	174,138	24	15,598	185,267
C	C1	vtc	9,000	30	10,495	99,250
	C2	vtc	9,000	30	28,330	112,549
	C3	vtc	9,000	30	10,736	78,464
	C4	vtc	9,000	30	11,704	78,004
	C5	vtc	7,500	30	7,214	88,141
D	D1	vtc	45,000	25	66,202	322,048
	D2	vtc	38,137	25	168,720	539,616
E	mrbean	ent	40,000	24	17,647	229,072
	asterix	ent	40,000	24	22,349	147,376
	atp	ent	40,000	24	21,890	190,856
	bond	ent	40,000	24	24,308	244,592
	dino	ent	40,000	24	13,078	119,632
	fuss	ent	40,000	24	27,129	187,176
	lambs	ent	40,000	24	7,312	134,224
	movie2	ent	40,000	24	14,288	172,672
	mtv	ent	40,000	24	24,604	229,200
	mtv2	ent	40,000	24	19,780	251,408
	news2	ent	40,000	24	15,358	189,888
	race	ent	40,000	24	30,749	202,416
	sbowl	ent	40,000	24	23,506	140,840
	simpsons	ent	40,000	24	18,576	240,376
	soccer	ent	40,000	24	25,110	190,296
	star2	ent	40,000	24	9,313	124,816
	talk2	ent	40,000	24	17,915	132,752
	talk	ent	40,000	24	14,537	106,768
	term	ent	40,000	24	10,905	79,560

[a] vtc, video teleconference; ent, entertainment (movie or television).

B. A 174,138-frame MPEG-1 trace of *Star wars* (1). The GOP is 12 frames, with an IBBPBBPBBPBB pattern. The frame rate was 24 frames/s.

C. H.261 encodings of five video teleconferences, of either 7500 or 9000 frames. Each has an initial I frame, followed by P frames only. The frame rate was 30 frames/s.

D. H.261 encodings of two video teleconferences. No periodic structure. The frame rate was 25 frames/s.

E. Nineteen MPEG-1 traces, each with 40,000 frames, compiled by Rose and originating from cable transmissions of films and television; see Rose's report (35) for further details. The GOP is 12 frames with an IBBPBBPBBPBB pattern. For the experiments we assumed a uniform rate of 24 frames/s.

10.8.2 Modeling Network Characteristics with Frame-Level Simulations

When we use a frame-level simulation, we use a synthetic model of the characteristics of the network, such as available bandwidth and feedback delay. Included in the synthetic model are the dynamics that result from bursty traffic that acts as cross-traffic and reduces the amount of available bandwidth.

10.8.2.1 Model for Network Contention and Feedback Delay.
The feedback delay for the network to allocate requests was assumed to be fixed in the frame-level simulation as follows:

$$r_{all}(n) = \begin{cases} r_{req}(n-\delta) & n > \delta \\ r_0 & n \leq \delta \end{cases} \tag{8}$$

Here r_0 is an initial rate given to the source until the network responds to the first rate request after the feedback delay of δ. We used the mean ideal rate as r_0.

Consider a channel carrying the aggregated traffic from these sources. If the capacity C of a channel is less than the maximum aggregate requested rate, then periods of congestion will occur from frames n (of the aggregate stream) for which the aggregate requested rate $R(n)$ exceeds the capacity C. The ABR rate allocation algorithm responds to instances of the demand exceeding the available bandwidth by allocating bandwidth to individual sources in proportion to their requests, the proportion being such that the total allocation equals the available bandwidth. We achieve this by using a weighted max-min fair allocation algorithm in the network (5). Thus when $R(n) > C$ the rate allocated to each source will be a proportion $C/R(n)$ of its request. This models the characteristic when all the sources share a common bottleneck.

We can gauge the effect of attempting to use a network link that has less capacity than the peak aggregate rate as follows. For a given set of traces. we run the SAVE algorithm to construct the requested rate for each trace as before, then sum to yield the aggregate requested rate $R(n)$. For a capacity C, we construct the proportional rate reduction process

$$p(n) = \max\{1, C/R(n)\} \tag{9}$$

To assess the impact of contention on an individual source, we rerun the SAVE algorithm, but now proportionately reduce the allocated rate, subject to the network roundtrip delay δ. Hence (8) is replaced by

$$r_{all}(n) = \begin{cases} p(n-\delta)r_{req}(n-\delta) & n > \delta \\ r_0 & n \le \delta \end{cases} \tag{10}$$

The buffer evolution is

$$b(n) = f_{enc}(n) + \max\{0, b(n-1) - r_{all}(n-1)\tau\} \tag{11}$$

Note that this scheme ignores some second-order effects: reduction of the allocated rate for a given frame may increase buffer occupancy at the end of that frame time; hence the rate request on the next frame may be increased to remain within the delay target. Or, cropping might be increased. In addition, the feedback delay has the potential to vary because of queueing at the switches, although we try to keep this small.

We overcome the approximations in the frame-level simulation using a cell-level network simulation, where we obtain an accurate characterization of the effects of a reduced rate being returned by the network and the dynamics of contention at the links in the network. The cell-level network simulation described below also models the more general case of sources sharing multiple bottlenecks.

10.8.3 Network-Level Simulation

We also developed a network simulation at the cell level that was driven with the same traces. The explicit-rate feedback control mechanism was used at the ATM layer to control the rate of transmission from each source. The switches in the network use a rate allocation scheme that achieves weighted max-min fairness (5).

In the explicit-rate ABR scheme, *in-band* resource management (RM) cells are periodically (in terms of cells sent by the source) transmitted by each source. A source specifies a "demand" or desired transmit rate in each transmit-

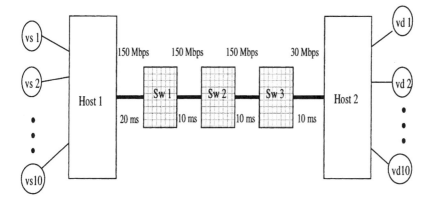

Figure 10.3   Network configuration for cell-level simulation.

ted RM cell in an *ER field*. Also specified in the RM cell is the currently allowed rate. Switches compute the rate they may allocate to each VC and overwrite this rate in the RM cell's ER field if the computed rate is lower than what was in the received RM cell. As the RM cell progresses from the source to destination, the ER-field value reflects the minimum rate allocated by any of the switches in the path for the VC. On reaching its destination, the RM cell is returned to the source, which now sets its allocated rate, ACR, based on the ER-field value in the returned RM cell. The information returned in the RM cells may be used to adapt the bit rate of the video encoder appropriately.

Sources transmit an RM cell once every 32 cells in the simulations. Because the rate returned from the network has the potential to vary considerably, reflecting the changes in the network, we perform an averaging of the ACR over a period of time. In the cell-level network simulation reported, we use an averaging interval of one frame time (41.67 ms for trace sets A and E).

We used a relatively simple configuration (shown in Figure 10.3) for examining the performance of the SAVE algorithm. Several video sources ("vs" in the figure), ranging from 10 sources in the case of trace A to 19 sources for trace set E, "fan in" to the first switch. The bottleneck is the link between the third switch and the destination host. The destination host is the sink ("vd" in the figure) for all the video sources. The capacity of the bottleneck is varied. The initial one-way delay is 50 ms. We also varied the link delays by doubling the propagation delay of each of the individual links, to understand the impact of feedback delay. The simulation was run for approximately 20,000 frames from each source.

10.9 SIMULATION RESULTS

10.9.1 Impact of Network Congestion and Feedback Delay on Attained Quality

If contention between sources causes congestion on a link, the allocated rate is reduced below the requested rate; this can give rise to cropping. In this section, we present results from trace-driven simulations. We use a relatively simple approach of frame-level analysis and corroborate its accuracy with the corresponding results for the full cell-level network simulation of the multiplexed system.

10.9.1.1 Pathwise Comparison of Cropping and Rate Reduction. A segment of trace set A was subjected to contention from the aggregate requested rate of 10 traces from set E, as modeled by Eqs. (9) and (10). The effects are shown in Figure 10.4. The points show the ratio of encoded to ideal rate (i. e., one minus the cropping proportion). The base behavior without contention, for a

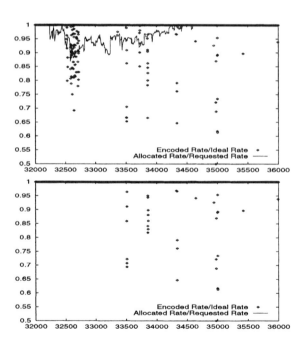

Figure 10.4 Pathwise comparison of cropping and rate reduction. Top: Segment of trace of set A, impacted by contention with 10 traces from set E, the total allocated at the 90th percentile of the peak requested rate. The encoded/ideal rate (= 1 - cropping proportion) drops below 1, partially in response to contention. Bottom: The encoded/ideal rate for the same trace without contention. The horizontal axis is the frame number.

single trace, is shown at the bottom. At the top is shown the modified ratio in the presence of contention. Also shown is the extent of contention experienced, as reflected by the ratio of allocated to requested rate. Note the additional cropping that now occurs between frames 32,500 and 33,000. Most of the cropping is less than 20% (i.e., encoded/ideal rate > 0.8) even when the allocated rate is only about 90% of the requested rate.

10.9.1.2 Effects of Rate Reduction and Feedback Delay on Cropping.
The distribution of the proportion of cropped frames, for various link bandwidths, is shown for the multiplex of 19 sources from trace set E in Figure 10.5, for network feedback delays of 100 ms (top) and 200 ms (bottom). For 100 ms delay, the target cropping (no more than 1 in 1000 frames suffer more than 20% cropping) is attained at a link capacity of about 25 Mbit/s; only twice as many frames suffer this much cropping when the delay is doubled. In both cases, attained quality is insensitive to an increase of capacity beyond this point, indicating that contention for resources is statistically negligible thereafter. If higher quality were required, the window w_{max} could be increased. These results were insensitive to long-term relative shifts of the traces; this indicates that although long time scale fluctuations in the frame sizes are to be expected (see e.g., Ref. 1), these are smoothed over by means of multiplexing many sources. The results were similar with simulations using trace A: the probability of frames being cropped more than 20% was as follows: no more than 3 in 1000 frames are cropped at 100 ms feedback delay; slightly more at 200 ms delay.

10.9.2 Behavior of the Frame Delay

We use a cell-level network simulation to investigate the delay experienced by 10 simultaneously active sources. Each copy was offset by 3999 frames relative to the previous one so that the long-term behaviors of the individual sources would be out of phase to some extent. The bottleneck link rate (of the link between switch 3 and the destination host 2 in Figure 10.3) is 30 Mbit/s. The total one-way network propagation delay was 50 ms.

In Figure 10.6 we show the requested rate and the allocated rate (the ACR smoothed over a 1-frame time) for a 2000-frame segment. We show the one-way, end-to-end delay, including both the smoothing buffer delay and the network delay (propagation time and queueing delay), in Figure 10.7. We chose a target of 90 ms for the smoothing buffer delay.

The delay behavior follows the pattern of the rates: larger delays occur not only for isolated large frames, but also at transitions from lower to higher frame rates (e.g., around frame 34,250). This happens because the requested rate initially tracks the lower rate, leading to a buildup in buffer occupancy due to the

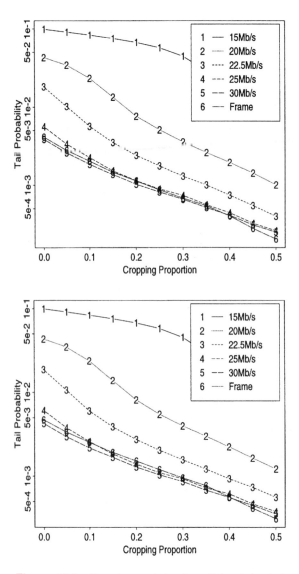

Figure 10.5 Cropping statistics for cell-level simulation: Data for network feedback delays of 100 ms (top) and 200 ms (bottom). Trace set E, tail distribution proportion of frames cropped, averaged over 19 multiplexed sources, as a function of link bandwidth. Cropping is acceptable for bandwidth more than 25 Mbit/s; statistics are similar to those obtained for single-source frame-level simulation, shown for comparison. Quality is insensitive to further increase in link bandwidth.

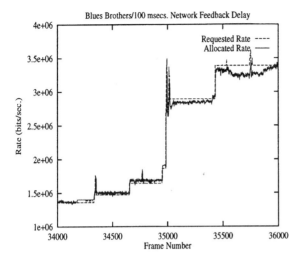

Figure 10.6 Network simulation rates: Trace A, 1 trace within a multiplexed set. For short periods, the allocated rate is lower than requested as a result of network contention.

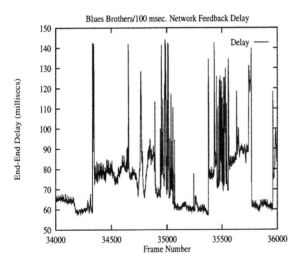

Figure 10.7 End-to-end network delay: Trace A, 1 trace within a multiplexed set.

larger frames within a period of duration in the order of the smoothing window, w_{sm}, after the rate jumps. After this time, the requested rate, and finally the allocated rate, increase in response to the increased frame size; this brings the buffer occupancy back down. We observe that the buffer occupancy, reflected by the delay, is kept low in periods of lower activity, so that when a new large frame shows up, or when there is a scene change, there is adequate free buffer to accommodate the large frames.

Even though we have multiplexed 10 sources over the network (with mean ideal rate for each source of 1.3 Mbit/s), the amount of queueing delay experienced in the network is not significant. This supports our expectation that the explicit rate based congestion management mechanism maintains small queues at the network's switches. Indeed, comparisons with frame-level simulations using the same traces show that the variability of frame delay is due almost entirely to source buffer delay.

10.9.3 Multiplexing Gain and Impact on Quality

We now examine the multiplexing gains achieved by using the smoothing algorithm at the source. We assess the impact of statistical multiplexing on the delay and cropping of single sources by subjecting SAVE to the simulated rate reduction process $p(n)$ from Eq. (9). Table 10.2 summarizes experiments with fivefold aggregates of traces from set E; for aggregations of 5, 20, and 35 sources, see Figure 10.8. In each case the capacity is expressed as a quantile of the aggregate requested rate.

Table 10.2 and Figure 10.8 show that mean and maximum of the delay are quite insensitive to both aggregation size and the degree to which capacity is set below the peak aggregated requested rate. This shows that one of the design criteria of SAVE (cropping to avoid delay) operates well, over a wide range of conditions. However, both frequency and duration of cropping increase as the capacity decreases. Our criterion that the *maximum* burst of cropping that exceeds 20% should not exceed a GOP (12 for the traces of set E) is met when capacity is a little less than the 90th percentile of the peak aggregate requested rate. The overall cropping criterion (no more than 1 in 1000 frames to be cropped more than 20%) is already satisfied at this capacity.

Figure 10.8 shows that as the size of the aggregate increases, performance measures improve for capacity at a given quantile of the aggregate requested rate. The smoothing by SAVE of individual sources reduced the variability of the requested rate compared with the ideal rate. This smoothing within sources in turn makes smoothing across sources in an aggregate more effective. We demonstrate this by displaying in Figure 10.9 the tail distribution of the aggregate rate per source for the ideal and requested rates, for aggregations of 1, 5, and 38 sources from set E. Although quantiles below about the 90th percentile (and also

Table 10.2   Impact of Statistical Reductions in Allocated Rate[a]

| Capacity | Delay | | Fraction cropped | |
(quantile)	Mean	Max	> 0%	> 20%
1.0	20.4	99.0	0.003	0.0006
0.9	20.5	99.9	0.004	0.0006
0.8	20.8	102.2	0.006	0.0008
0.7	21.1	103.8	0.008	0.0010
0.6	21.5	104.9	0.011	0.0017
0.5	21.8	106.2	0.013	0.0022

| Capacity | Burst crop > 20% | | Burst crop ≤ 20% | |
(quantile)	Mean	Max	Mean	Min
1.0	2.2	7.3	2900.	108.
0.9	2.2	8.9	2600.	106.
0.8	2.7	13.8	2297.	79.
0.7	3.3	20.2	1869.	28.
0.6	7.2	75.6	1405.	25.
0.5	9.0	96.9	1235.	20.

[a] Averaged impact on single traces within five-fold aggregation in set E. Capacity is expressed as a quantile of the aggregated requested rate. As capacity decreases, insensitivity of delay and mean burst length of cropping over 20% are observed.

the mean) are higher for the requested rate than the ideal rate, the higher quantiles are very much lower for the requested rate. Even for large aggregates, the high quantiles of the ideal rate (curve 3) remain far higher than for the aggregate requested rate (curve 6).

An important feature to observe from Figure 10.9 is that for larger aggregations, the curve becomes nearly vertical, indicating that the various quantiles become very close; see particularly curves 5 and 6 for the aggregate requested rate. This has an important potential benefit for measurement-based admission control. We think of an effective bandwidth for a source as a rate required to accommodate its extremes of variability. The narrowness of the distribution of the requested rate means that measurements of the effective bandwidth will be less influenced by statistical errors than for the ideal rate and will, in any case, be relatively insensitive to how it is specified.

10.9.3.1   Single-Source Behavior and Comparative Multiplexing Gain.
When SAVE is employed for transport of a single source's video stream, we shift the focus away from the statistical properties of aggregations and instead seek to determine the *constant rate* required for a given source in order for SAVE to achieve the quality targets. We refer to this mode as "buffered CBR." In this

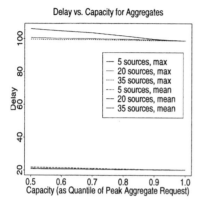

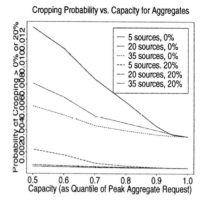

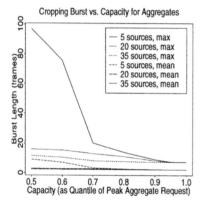

Figure 10.8 Dependence of delay and cropping on reduced capacity. For aggregations of 5, 20, and 35 sources, averaged impact on single traces within aggregate; capacity expressed as quantile of peak aggregate requested rate. Top left: mean and maximum delay. Top right: proportion of cropping > 0% and > 20%. Bottom: mean and maximum burst length of cropping > 20%.

mode, the parameter γ (the minimum proportion of the frame to be encoded) is set to zero: since the rate given to the source is constant, we are unable to adaptively increase the allocated rate. When this occurs over lengthy periods of high activity, it leads to either excessive delays or buffer overflow.

Over the 19 traces of set E, the required CBR rate was found to exceed the mean ideal rate by a factor of between about 2.4 and 6.0, with an average of about 3.6. For the trace A, it is about 2.2 times the mean ideal rate. To examine

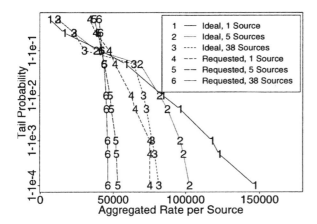

Figure 10.9 Rate smoothing and aggregation: tail distribution for ideal and requested rates per source, for aggregations of 1, 5, and 38 sources of set E. High quantiles of requested rate are lower than those of ideal rate.

the multiplexing performance of the SAVE algorithm working in conjunction with an explicit rate feedback based network, we compare these buffered CBR bandwidth requirements to the bandwidth required when SAVE is used in a network with explicit-rate feedback. For buffered CBR, we use the sum of the CBR rates of the constituents of the aggregate. For SAVE, we use the 90th percentile of the peak aggregated requested rate. These are displayed for 1- to 38-fold aggregations from set E in Figure 10.10 including protocol overhead. The CBR, SAVE, and mean ideal rates (neglecting any protocol overhead) are in the approximate proportions 3.6:2.3:1.

The bandwidth requirements of SAVE from the network-level simulation are displayed as points in Figure 10.10. The other traces in the figure have been adjusted for protocol overhead. All include a factor for the ATM cell header (about 10%); the SAVE frame simulation also contains a factor to account for the overhead of resource management cells (about another 3%). We see that the full network simulation and the frame-level simulation of individual traces are in close agreement. The difference between them was at most 10%.

The higher rate allocation for the buffered CBR reflects the necessity to allocate a sufficient rate to accommodate long-lived trends found in the video sources. If bandwidth allocated by the network is slightly lower than needed, degradation of quality will occur, often over a long burst. Since this is an inherent property of the video source, we expect that similar allocations will be required for other algorithms that adapt and transport real-time video at a constant rate and at similarly high quality. We compared the buffered CBR rates with the

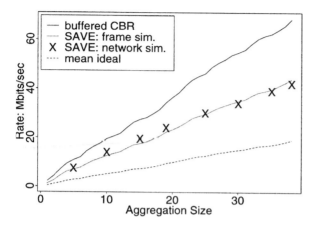

Figure 10.10   Utility of explicit rate for multiplexing gain: bandwidth requirements, normalized by the mean ideal rate, for 1-to 38-fold aggregates of set E. Middle Curve: SAVE, 90th percentile of aggregate requested rate. Upper Curve, CBR rate for 100 ms source buffer. Bottom Curve, mean ideal rate capacity estimate based on full network simulation described in text.

peak smoothed rate of the algorithm in Reference 24 under the same delay constraint; the rates were similar.

We quantified the relative sensitivities of SAVE and buffered CBR to systematic rate reduction (for SAVE) or underallocation (for buffered CBR). One motivation for this is to try to understand the effect of errors in traffic characterization at admission control time. We compared the sensitivity of the quality metrics (frequency of cropping > 20%, and maximum burst length of such cropping). For SAVE we reduced the time-varying allocated rate by a fixed proportion; for buffered CBR we reduced the constant rate by the same proportion. The results for trace A are summarized in Figure 10.11 for proportions from 0.6 to 1. Burstiness of cropping is not very sensitive for SAVE for rate reductions down to at least 0.75, but then increases rapidly. Buffered CBR, on the other hand, is quite sensitive to underallocation, for reasons outlined above. Cropping frequency for SAVE is more sensitive, in this case degrading to 1 in 1000 for a systematic rate reduction of about 0.9.

10.9.4   Sensitivity to Smoothing Parameters

The SAVE smoothing algorithm has two components of smoothing, as described in Section 10.6: the short-term smoothing window w_{sm} and the medium-term maximum window w_{max}. We nominally choose w_{sm} to be 12 frames, the GOP length of the traces in set E. The maximum window w_{max}, which aims to

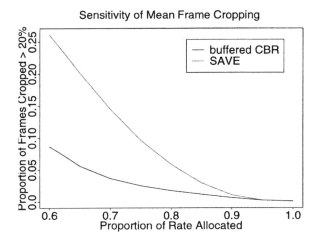

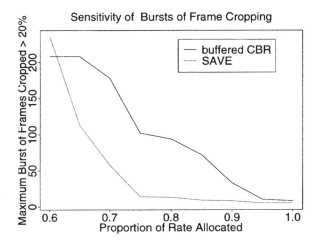

Figure 10.11 Comparative sensitivity of frame cropping in SAVE and buffered CBR to systematic rate reduction or underallocation of bandwidth. Top: average cropping is more sensitive for SAVE. Bottom: burst cropping is more sensitive for buffered CBR.

capture the characteristic of the large frames of a scene, was nominally set to 1000 frames. In this section, we use the frame-level simulation to study the sensitivity of SAVE, specifically its quality and bandwidth usage, to these two smoothing parameters.

Figure 10.12 shows the variation of the mean requested rate with w_{max} and w_{sm}. There is little sensitivity to the value of w_{sm}. There is a small reduction in the mean requested rate only when w_{sm} falls below 8 frames. However, there is considerable sensitivity to the value of w_{max}. We isolate this in Figure 10.13 by plotting the mean requested rate, averaged over w_{sm}, as a function of w_{max}. Note the logarithmic horizontal scale. The mean requested rate increases with w_{max}, re-

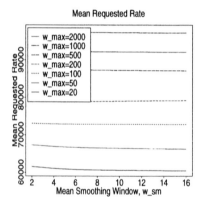

Figure 10.12   Mean requested rate versus w_{sm}; trace set A, for varying w_{max}.

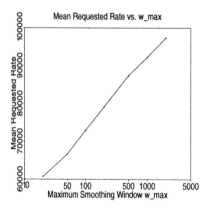

Figure 10.13   Mean requested rate versus w_{max}, averaged over w_{sm}.

flecting the tendency of one large frame to raise the requested rate for a longer duration. The mean requested rate increases only slowly with w_{max}, approximately logarithmically.

The maximum requested rate is insensitive to w_{max}, as shown in Figure 10.14: the curves of the maximum requested rate as a function of w_{sm} coincide for values of w_{max} in a range from 20 to 2000. However, the maximum requested rate is a decreasing function of the smoothing window w_{sm}. It reduces rapidly as w_{sm} increases up to 8. Beyond that, we begin to reach a point of diminishing returns, and the maximum requested rate reduces slowly as w_{sm} goes beyond the GOP value of 12. The form of dependence on w_{max} and w_{sm} indicates that the largest requested rate is governed by the short-term average over a few large frames, and the mean requested rate is governed by the large frames observed over a longer, scene-level, time scale.

We turn to the impact on quality as w_{sm} and w_{max} are varied. Figure 10.15 shows how the proportion of frames cropped by more than 20% varies. For values of w_{max} greater than 100, the proportion of frames cropped over 20% remains below 0.5% for the entire range of w_{sm} that we examined. For smaller values of w_{max} (< 100), the proportion of cropped frames shows a small amount of sensitivity to w_{sm}. Thus, the primary sensitivity is once again to w_{max}; this property is isolated in Figure 10.16. Note the log–log scale: the proportion of frames cropped more than 20% decays slowly, as a power law, in w_{max} (in fact $\approx$ const $\cdot w_{max}^{-0.85}$). For the acceptability criterion that we selected (no more than 0.1% of frames cropped > 20%), w_{max} needs to be reasonably large, of the order of 500 frames or more. This supports our initial intuition that w_{max} needs to capture the scene-level be-

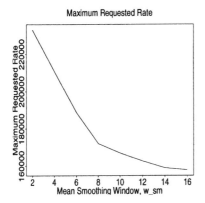

Figure 10.14 Maximum requested rate versus w_{sm}: trace set A. Curves coincide for w_{max} from 20 to 2000.

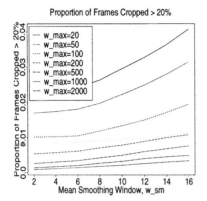

Figure 10.15   Proportion of frames cropped > 20% versus w_{sm}: trace set A for varying w_{max}.

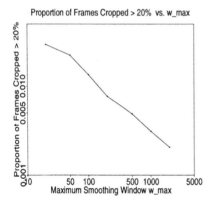

Figure 10.16   Proportion of frames cropped > 20% versus w_{max}; trace set A, averaged over w_{sm}.

havior, which is likely to be of the order of a few seconds. We also observed the statistics of the burst length of cropping with varying w_{sm} and w_{max}; generally, the mean burst length ranged from 1.5 to 3.5, increasing with w_{sm}. The maximum burst length was a decreasing function of w_{max}, in a range from 25 to 2, and generally increasing with w_{sm}. Finally, Figure 10.17 shows that maximum source buffer delay is reasonably insensitive to w_{sm} once w_{max} is greater than about 50 frames; it is within the 100 ms target for

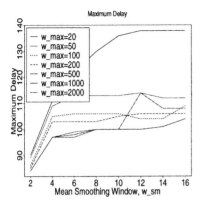

Figure 10.17   Maximum delay versus w_{sm}; trace set A for varying w_{max}.

$w_{max} \geq 1000$. In summary, w_{max} is the main tunable parameter determining quality.

10.10 CONCLUSIONS

This chapter discussed the use in the transport of video of feedback information over a communication network. The feedback information could be in the form of an available rate or of loss in the network.

Depending on the encoding, video has varying amounts of tolerance to frame loss. Typically, no more than a very small probability of frame loss is acceptable. Loss of one or several packets can lead to frame loss, the sensitivity depending on the packetization. The requirement for video on the network transport is to have a very small packet loss probability (in the range 0.1–5%). This is quite difficult to achieve.

Congestion in the network impacts video transport in three dimensions: inconsistent bandwidth availability for the video stream, increased latency and jitter, and packet loss. The first defense against congestion is to utilize buffers in the network to overcome short-term mismatches between the available capacity in the network and the rate required for transporting the video stream. Burstiness also may be overcome by having the source negotiate a rate of transmission with the network as and when necessary, so that there is minimal loss, and delivered video quality is acceptable. Finally, the source may adapt itself, to minimize the mismatch between the ideal rate for the video stream and the available network capacity.

There are several possible approaches to adaptation at the video source. The method of adaptation is likely to vary depending on the content, use, and so on. The approach for adaptation of the video source more frequently examined, and studied in detail in this chapter, is to modify the source rate dynamically by adjusting the video encoding parameters.

We initially examined ways in which the video source may be able to adapt to indication of loss in the network (as with the current Internet). We then explored the use of an explicit rate based feedback mechanism, similar to that used for ATM's ABR service class, for transporting compressed video traffic. The adaptation of compressed video is based on negotiation of the bandwidth with the network by means of feedback-based congestion control and adapting the quantization parameter when necessary. The rate allocation mechanism in the network is based on a weighted max-min fairness criterion. This allows the network to treat flows unequally (in proportion to their weights), so that higher rate sources whose quality is more likely to be affected are treated preferentially (instead of all sources experiencing the same rate reduction).

In the adaptation mechanisms we discuss, the video source rate is matched to the available bandwidth returned in the feedback from the network by modifying the quantization level used during compression. We believe that the overall perceptual quality of the video is likely to be higher with this form of source adaptation to congestion, where the source modifies the quantizer, than when the network drops cells or packets under congestion (thus losing frames).

Smoothing and aggregation of flows helps reduce variability in the rate requested of the network. We studied SAVE, our source smoothing and rate adaptation algorithm, which has the following components:

1. A source smoothing algorithm that finds a rate that is the maximum of:
   a. A smoothed rate over a small moving window that is intended to capture the short-term average behavior, smoothing over the periodic structure introduced by the compression algorithm. The smoothed rate would drain the average frame over an interframe time.
   b. An estimate of the maximum frame size over a sufficiently long term, to capture the characteristics of the peak rate required for a *scene*. This maximum frame must be drained within the delay bound for the source buffer.
2. A rate adaptation mechanism at the source that determines a target frame size so that a bound on the delay contributed at the source smoothing buffer is not exceeded.
3. Finally, a rate is requested from the network, as a demand in the ex-

plicit-rate congestion control mechanism used by the network to allocate a rate to this flow.

For this form of adaptation, it appears necessary to evolve the quality metrics typically used to evaluate the efficacy of mechanisms to transport video. The metrics relate to how frequently we have to adapt the video and by how much. We are quite stringent in setting quality targets for SAVE, suggesting that no more 1 in 1000 frames should suffer more than a 20% cropping. Further, we examined the burstiness of the impairment, because we believe that having a long string of consecutive frames that are cropped results in noticeable degradation in quality. We showed some of the results of trace-driven simulations of SAVE that demonstrate its effectiveness in meeting our quality targets. We also looked at the "traditional" measures of effectiveness in the context of SAVE: the multiplexing gain, the source buffer delay, and the behavior of the rate requested from the network.

We believe adaptation algorithms need to be robust to variations in the feedback delay and to network congestion, failing which we would see buffer occupancy at the source increase. We find that SAVE's adaptation based on smoothing the short-term variations in ideal frame rate (over a GOP interval) and tracking the maximum ideal frame size over a scene time scale allows us to be relatively insensitive to feedback delay.

Finally, we showed that the most significant parameter in SAVE is the maximum smoothing window w_{max}. The proportion of frames cropped decreases as a power law with w_{max}, and the mean requested rate goes up logarithmically with w_{max}. Thus w_{max} serves as a dial that we may use to manage a trade-off between quality and the average of the rate we request from the network. The short-term smoothing window w_{sm} helps us in reducing the peak requested rate from the network, without much impact on the quality. The maximum requested rate goes down as w_{sm} goes up to about a GOP, beyond which we see diminishing benefits. Thus, the combination of w_{max} and w_{sm} can be used to manage the resources we use from the network, while managing quality to be within acceptable limits. We believe that SAVE demonstrates considerable promise as a method of online rate adaptation for compressed video.

REFERENCES

1. M W Garrett, W Willinger. Analysis, modeling and generation of self-similar VBR traffic. *Proceedings of the ACM SIGCOMM'94* Conference, London, August 1994, pp 269–280.
2. M Grossglauser, S Keshav, D Tse. RCBR: A simple and efficient service for multiple time-scale traffic. Proceedings of the ACM SIGCOMM'95 Conference, September 1995.

3a. D Bertsekas, R Gallagher. Data Networks. Englewood Cliffs, NJ, Prentice Hall, 1992.

3b. H Kanakia, PP Mishra, A R Reibman. An adaptive congestion control scheme for real-time packet video transport. Proceedings of the ACM SIGCOMM'93 Conference, September 1993.

4.   H Kanakia, P P Mishra, A Reibman. Packet video transport in ATM networks with single-bit feedback. *Proceedings of the Sixth International Workshop on Packet Video,* Portland, OR, September 1994.

5.   T V Lakshman, P P Mishra, K K Ramakrishnan. Transporting compressed video over ATM networks with explicit rate feedback control. Proceedings of IEEE Infocom '97, Kobe, Japan, April 1997.

6.   P P Mishra. Fair bandwidth sharing for video traffic sources using distributed feedback control. *Proceedings of IEEE GLOBECOM,* Singapore City, Singapore, November 1995.

7.   J-C Bolot, T Turletti. Experience with control mechanisms for packet video in the Internet. Comput Commun Rev 28(1): 4–15, January 1998.

8.   R Rejaie, M Handley, D Estrin. An end-to-end rate-based congestion control mechanism for realtime streams in the Internet. Proceedings of IEEE Infocom '99, New York, March 1999.

9.   ATM Forum. ATM Forum Traffic Management Specification Version 4.0. af-tm-0056.00, April 1996. Available as: ftp://ftp.atmforum.com/pub/approved-specs/af-tm-0056.000.pdf

10. A Demers, S Keshav, S Shenker. Analysis and simulation of a fair queueing algorithm. Proceedings of the ACM SIGCOMM'89 Conference, September 1989.

11. N G Duffield, K K Ramakrishnan, A R Reibman. SAVE: An algorithm for smoothed adaptive video over explicit rate networks. IEEE/ACM Trans Networking 6(6):717–728, December 1998.

12. N G Duffield, K K Ramakrishnan, A R Reibman. Issues of quality and multiplexing when smoothing rate adaptive video. Proceedings of the Eighth International Workshop on Network and Operating Systems Support for Digital Audio and Video (NOSSDAV'98), Cambridge, July 1998.

13. T Turletti, C Huitema. IVS videoconferencing in the Internet. *IEEE/ACM Trans Networking* 4(3): 340–351, June 1996.

14. V Jacobson. Congestion avoidance and control. Proceedings of the *ACM SIG-COMM'88* Conference, Stanford, CA, August 1988, pp. 314–329.

15. K K Ramakrishnan, R Jain. A binary feedback scheme for congestion avoidance in computer networks. *ACM Trans. Comput Syst* 8(2): 158–181, May 1990.

16. K K Ramakrishnan, S Floyd. A proposal to add explicit congestion notification (ECN) to IP. *RFC 2481,* January 1999. Available from: *ftp://ftp.isi.edu/in-notes/rfc2481.txt*

17. S McCanne, V Jacobson, M Vetterli. Receiver-driven layered multicast. Proceedings of the ACM SIGCOMM'96 Conference, Stanford, CA, September 1996, pp 117–130.

18a. S Bajaj, L Breslau, S Shenker. Uniform versus priority dropping for layered video. Proceedings of the ACM SIGCOMM'98, Conference, Vancouver, British Columbia, Canada, August 1998, pp 131–143.

18b. L Kalampoukas, A Varma, K K Ramakrishnan. An efficient rate allocation algorithm for ATM networks providing max-min fairness. Proceedings of Sixth IFIP International Conference on High Performance Networking, HPN'95, Spain, September 11–15, 1995.

19. R Braden, L Zhang, S Berson, S Herzog, S Jamin. Resource reservation protocol (RSVP)—version 1 functional specification. Internet Engineering Task Force Request for Comments 2205, September 1997.

20. A R Reibman, AW Berger. On VBR video teleconferencing over ATM networks. Proceedings of IEEE Global Telecommunications Conference (GLOBECOM), December 1992.

21. F Bonomi, K W Fendick. The rate-based flow control framework for the available bit rate ATM service. IEEE Network. 9(2); March/April 1995.

22. S Lam, S Chow, D K Y Yau. An algorithm for lossless smoothing of MPEG video. Proceedings of the ACM SIGCOMM'94, Conference, London, August 1994.

23. TJ Ott, Lakshman T V Lakshman, A Tabatabai. A scheme for smoothing delay sensitive traffic offered to ATM networks. Proceedings of IEEE Infocom '92, May 1992, pp 776–785.

24. AR Reibman, AW Berger. Traffic descriptors for VBR video teleconferencing over ATM networks. *IEEE/ACM Trans Networking* 3(3): 329–339, June 1995.

25. AR Reibman, B Haskell. Constraints on variable bit-rate video for ATM networks. IEEE Trans Circuits Syst Video Technol 2:361–372, 1992.

26. J D Salehi, Z-L Zhang, J F Kurose, D Towsley. Supporting stored video: Reducing rate variability and end-to-end resource requirements through optimal smoothing. Proceedings of the ACM Sigmetrics Conference on Measurement and Modeling of Computer Systems, May 1996, pp 222–231.

27. S Sen, J Rexford, J Dey, J Kurose, D Towsley. Online smoothing of variable bit-rate streaming video. University of Massachussetts Technical Report 98–75, 1998.

28. N Shroff, M Schwartz. Video smoothing within networks using deterministic smoothing at the source. Proceedings of IEEE Infocom'94, 1994, pp 342–349.

29. W Feng, F Jahanian, S Sechrest. An optimal bandwidth allocation strategy for the delivery of compressed pre-recorded video. ACM Multimedia Syst J 5:297–309, 1997.

30. J Zhang, J Hui. Traffic characteristics and smoothness criteria in VBR video transmission. Proceedings of IEEE Conference on Multimedia Computing and Systems, Ottawa, Canada, June 1997.

31. A Elwalid, D Heyman, TV Lakshman, D Mitra, A Weiss. Fundamental bounds and approximations for ATM multiplexers applications to video teleconferencing. *IEEE J Selected Areas Commun.* 13(6): pp 1004–1016, August 1995.

32. D Heyman, A Tabatabai, TV Lakshman. Statistical analysis and simulation study of VBR video teleconference traffic in ATM networks. *IEEE Trans Circuits Syst Video Technol* March 1992, pp 49–59.

33. B Girod. Psychovisual aspects of image communications. *Signal Processing* 28:239–251, 1992.

34. A Charny, K K Ramakrishnan, A Lauck. Time scale analysis and scalability issues for explicit rate allocation in ATM networks. *IEEE/ACM Trans Networking,* 4(4), August 1996.
35. O Rose. Statistical properties of MPEG video traffic and their impact on traffic modeling in ATM systems. University of Wuerzburg. Institute of Computer Science Research Report Series. Report 101, February 1995.

Part 4
Transport of
Compressed Video

11
Internet Video

M. Reha Civanlar
AT&T Labs–Research, Red Bank, New Jersey

11.1 INTRODUCTION

By now, almost everyone who has "surfed" the World Wide Web has received some form of video over the Internet. Considering that packet video was classified among the advanced research topics just a decade ago, it is not hard to believe that the Internet may become the main video distribution network of the near future. Achieving this state at a reasonable cost, however, is not effort free.

As discussed in Chapter 3 on IP networks, the Internet is a heterogeneous collection of networks. Currently, it does not provide any quality-of-service guarantees[*] (1), and QoS transmission for all video streams in their entirety may stay infeasible for a long time owing to economical constraints. Unavoidable packet losses and delay jitter caused by congestion make effective streaming of video over the Internet a challenging task.

In the near future, many problems with video delivery over the Internet will be alleviated as a result of the following factors:

availability of higher access bandwidth through cable and digital subscriber loop modems
server load and network traffic reduction through the large-scale deployment of IP multicast
the increasing backbone bandwidth

---

[*]QoS guarantees may give upper bounds for several network performance parameters, such as packet loss rates, delay, and delay jitter. Clearly, offering such guarantees requires infrastructure support, which is not free. Moreover, sharing limited resources makes the establishment of a price structure unavoidable.

However, they will not be completely eliminated. The demand for better quality has no limits. When broadcast quality TV becomes available over the Internet, the users will ask for high-definition TV (HDTV). And, when that becomes available, probably, three-dimensional or holographic TV will be requested! It is reasonable to expect that the resources needed for video applications will continue to increase hand in hand with the improving network conditions.

A successful real-time Internet video delivery system should not only survive in the presence of extremely adverse network conditions, but also minimize the effects of common network problems on the delivered video quality. Several techniques described in this book, particularly layered coding and error resilient coding techniques, are promising steps in achieving this target. Further developments in these fields, theoretical as well as implementation-related, will help with the wide-scale deployment and use of Internet video applications.

The heterogeneity of the Internet will continue to require that video delivery applications operate over wide range of bandwidths. Additionally, video applications must be adaptive to avoid congesting the network (i.e., they must act in a network-friendly manner). With adaptation, wide-scale deployment of video applications will not deteriorate the performance of other Internet applications.

The Internet with its comprehensive protocol stacks offers many tools for building the video network of the future. As discussed in Chapter 3, a complete video communications system based on the Internet depends on many protocols for handling various tasks such as call control, session control, directory assistance, and channel reservations. This chapter focuses on the time-related media delivery issues that are handled by the Real-Time Transport Protocol (RTP) (2) developed by the Internet Engineering Task Force (IETF). Over the Internet, compressed media of any kind (e.g., H.26x, MPEG, G.728), along with other data types, can be transported, multiplexed, and synchronized by using the services provided by the RTP/UDP/IP (3) stack. This approach has a high potential in providing the path for the unified information infrastructure of the future.

RTP has a hierarchical architecture in which the main protocol provides the common re-usable functionalities that are needed by all real-time delivery applications. The specific support required by various coding types is provided through the definition of RTP payload formats. Defining a specific RTP payload format requires a thorough understanding of the underlying coding technique as well as the details of the transport protocol.

In this chapter, we present a brief review of the video delivery impairments and possible remedies, followed by a discussion of the factors that make a video stream easy to transport over the Internet. We discuss the current techniques for video transport over the Internet through a detailed investigation of selected video payload formats for RTP. The chapter closes with a discussion of future directions.

11.2   DELIVERY IMPAIRMENTS AND REMEDIES

Delivery of video packets in real-time differs fundamentally from delivery of data packets in that video packets are time sensitive, and there is usually not enough time for redelivering lost video packets. Additionally, most video coding algorithms employ interframe and/or intraframe prediction, where decoding a picture may require availability of the previous pictures or previously transmitted parts of the current picture. Although prediction is a very effective tool for video compression, it may cause propagation of the effects of packet losses. On the other hand, in many cases, the effects of lost packets can be concealed with little effort (e.g., by displaying the parts from a previously received picture corresponding to the lost packets). Actually, among all the real-time media types, video may have the highest tolerance to packet losses. The challenge of video delivery over the Internet is to make the best use of this loss tolerance in dealing with the delivery impairments.

Logically, only two bad things may happen to a packet delivered over the Internet: it may be lost, or it may be delayed. In reality, a delay longer than a certain length is considered to be a loss because video packets received after a long delay may become useless. Other anomalies such as out-of-order delivery of packets and packet replication (4) can be detected by means of the timestamps and the sequence numbers provided by RTP, and handling of these is quite straightforward. As for bit errors, owing to the checksum operation at the transport layer, the number of the corrupt packets that reaches the video decoder at the application layer is negligible.*

11.2.1   Packet Loss

The result of several studies on the packet losses on the Internet is that *"in a large conference, it is inevitable that some receivers will experience packet loss (5)"* (6). Consequently, we cannot expect a loss-intolerant system to be useful for the Internet video delivery. Several techniques for designing loss-resilient codecs were discussed in Part 3 on systems for video networking of this book. In this chapter, we focus on transporting the output of such codecs over the Internet in a manner consistent with the overall architecture of the Internet.

A well-established principle for loss-resilient transmission of video over the Internet is *application layer framing* (ALF) (7). According to the ALF principle, the packets must be constructed consistent with the structure of the underly-

---

*Although the transport layer may be adjusted to pass packets containing bit errors to an application, the author is not aware of any application that uses this mechanism to deal with such packets. Under normal configurations of common TCP/IP stacks, corrupt packets are dropped at the transport layer (e.g., UDP, before an application receives them).

ing coding algorithm. For example, in MPEG-2 based video delivery, if each packet carries an integer number of complete MPEG-2 video slices, recovery and resynchronization after a packet loss become much easier than in a blind, chop-and-ship packetization system. Fortunately, recent international video coding standards, such as ITU's H.263+ and ISO's MPEG-4, which are described in Chapters 1 and 2, respectively, include the necessary provisions for *ALF*-based packetization. Even older standards can be adapted to use *ALF* packetization, as can be seen from the payload formats for H.261 and MPEG discussed in the later sections.

Scalable or *layered* coding is another established approach for efficient Internet video delivery. As discussed in Chapter 7 on layered coding, this approach allows a base layer for video and one or more enhancement layers. The base layer can be protected better and is expected to be delivered even in the poorest network conditions with sufficiently high reliability. The enhancement layers, on the other hand, are delivered only if the network conditions are favorable (i.e., using best-effort delivery) to enhance the spatial resolution, temporal resolution, or signal-to-noise ratio level of the video. Clearly, layered coding is also useful for addressing the heterogeneity issues. In recognition of the power of these tools, some classic (MPEG-2) and most of the newer video coding standards (H.263+, MPEG-4) include scalable video coding tools in addition to the error-resilient delivery techniques. The latest RTP specification defines generic mechanisms for transporting layered video bitstreams (8).

An extension of the use of layered coding for loss resilience to general codecs is based on improved delivery of *high priority segments* (9). It is well known that not all bits in a compressed video bitstream are of equal importance. Some bits belong to segments defining vital information such as picture types, quantization values, parameter ranges, and average intensity values for image blocks. In the transport of compressed video bitstreams over packet networks, packet losses from such segments cause a much longer lasting and severe degradation on the output of a decoder than that caused by packet losses from other segments. We call the segments that carry vital information *high priority* (HP) segments. The rest of the bitstream consists of *low priority* (LP) segments. Clearly, the video outputs resulting from transport techniques that protect the *HP* segments against packet losses are more resilient to packet losses in general.

The higher reliability needed to transmit the base layer of a layered codec or the HP segments of any codec can be obtained over the current Internet by using reliable multicast protocols that are being standardized in the IETF (10). These protocols are based on proper use of the two well-established error recovery techniques: automatic repeat request (ARQ) and forward error correction (FEC) (11). Increased reliability obtained this way over the existing infrastructure requires increased delay due to *ARQ* and/or increased bandwidth due to

FEC. In the near future, there will be network support for prioritized delivery over the Internet through differentiated services (12).

It is quite likely that even with the use of intelligent delivery techniques, some packet losses will remain. As discussed in earlier chapters, the effects of these losses may be eliminated or, at least, reduced by using error-resilient video coding, which aims to minimize the damage due to packet losses. Error-resilient coding includes data recovery tools (e.g., reversible variable-length coding) and error concealment tools (e.g., postprocessing), which may be used to hide the visual effects of any lost data on the displayed pictures.

11.2.2 Delay Jitter

Two components of the Internet packet delivery delay are the propagation delay on the wires and the queuing delay on the routers. The propagation delay depends on the distance and is constant. The queuing delay, on the other hand, depends on the network congestion and may vary significantly during a session creating *delay jitter.*

Handling the delay jitter by intelligent use of *play out buffers* is fundamental to a successful Internet video delivery system. The basis for designing common Internet "streaming" media applications is the intelligent use of receiver-side buffering. The target of the receiver-side buffering is to reduce the packet losses due to delay, using the minimum possible buffer size (or overall delay.) Using large play out buffers decreases the effects of delay jitter but results in long start-up delays. For example, in delivering stored video, if the entire material is buffered at the receiver before the playback is started, effectively converting a *streaming* application into a *download-and-play* application, the amount of delay jitter will be irrelevant! Clearly, interactive applications put much stricter constraints on the play out buffer size, hence, their tolerance to delay jitter is much lower. This is one of the main reasons why the video-on-demand applications are much more advanced and popular than video conferencing applications over the Internet.

Play out buffer size management has two components. The first one is to determine the initial minimum buffer size (i.e., the initial waiting time). If the initial buffer is too small, the playback will have to pause; if it is too large, we will have an unnecessarily long initial wait. Since the delay jitter is variable, the buffer size should adapt to its variations also. The second component of the buffer management is implementing a mechanism to change the buffer size in real time with minimal effect on the quality of the playback. Fortunately, video is a particularly suitable medium for this purpose because occasional frame repeating and frame dropping are usually acceptable.

Effective sampling rate modification based on frame repeat/drop is also useful in adjusting the mismatch between the transmitter and the receiver clocks.

Theoretically, these clocks can be adjusted quite accurately by running the Network Time Protocol (NTP) (13) at both ends. However, this may be unrealistic, mainly owing to hardware codec implementations with fixed clock rates. In the current practice, the buffer overflows and underflows due to clock mismatches are handled the same way as the buffer adjustment for delay jitter, repeating or dropping frames as needed.

Systems that are designed mainly for synchronous delivery channels with low loss rates, such as the system layer of the MPEG standard, use transmitter-based control of the receiver buffers. On the transmitter side, the rate control algorithms usually manage the quantization scale parameters to avoid receiver buffer overflow and underflow based on a specified receiver buffer size and fixed end-to-end delay. The clock synchronization is accomplished by transmitting special clock reference signals. However, this approach is not suitable in multicast scenarios, where a large number of heterogeneous receivers located at the different network segments try to receive video from the same source.

11.2.3 Congestion Control

A vital parameter for effective video streaming over the Internet is the *bottleneck bandwidth*, which gives the upper limit to the speed of a network in delivering data from one end point to the other. If a codec tries to send data over this limit, all extra packets will be lost. On the other hand, sending under this limit will clearly result in suboptimal video quality. Although accurate estimation of this time-varying limit is difficult, techniques that adapt their rates to a measured bottleneck bandwidth are reported in the literature (14,15). The bursty nature of the Internet traffic is the main obstacle in estimating the bottleneck bandwidth. Another problem associated with rate adjustment at the transmitter side is that for a multicast application, each receiver may experience a different bottleneck bandwidth. A rate adjustment algorithm based on a combination of the RTCP reports from all receivers is presented elsewhere (16). Another solution for rate control in a multicast scenario may be obtained through sending different layers of the output of a layered codec to different multicast groups. This way, each receiver can adjust its own reception bandwidth by selecting the multicast groups to which it subscribes (17).

Rate control poses a problem with the stored media also. Changing the rate of a stored, compressed video stream requires real-time transcoding, which increases the computational load on the server. Storing the output of a layered coder may provide a solution for this problem. Currently, a simple approach based on storing the same video material encoded at several rates is preferred for many commercial products.

It may be possible to design delivery techniques that give some performance improvements at the expense of creating unnecessary traffic. Congesting the Internet may not be considered to be a delivery impairment for video per se, but use of uncontrolled video sources may end up clogging the network. This may result in installation of new Internet mechanisms to prevent the use of such applications (18). Therefore, appropriate rate control mechanisms must be a part of all video delivery applications that will be used on the Internet. The definition of such mechanisms is currently an active research area (16,19,20), and there is no globally accepted solution.

11.3 VIDEO STREAM PROPERTIES FOR NETWORK USE

Although it is possible to improve the real-time delivery performance of video encoded in any form over the Internet, real-time video streams with certain properties are more convenient for networked applications. Some of these properties are described in Sections 11.3.1–11.3.8.

11.3.1 Natural Breakpoints for Packetization

Applying the ALF principle to packetizing a stream that has natural breakpoints can be easier and more efficient. For example, if a picture is JPEG-coded and presented to a packetizer, the resulting packets will contain arbitrary sections of the encoded data. If one of these packets is lost, it will be practically impossible to decode the remaining packets even if they are received. However, if the same JPEG-coded picture contains special *"restart markers"* indicating starting of independently decodable blocks, a lost packet will not cause such a severe problem.

11.3.2 Adjustable Packet Sizes

As discussed in Chapter 3 on IP networks, different technologies used as parts of the Internet have different frame (largest data unit) sizes. A packet whose size is larger than the smallest frame size allowed on its path, a maximum transmission unit (MTU) (21), must be fragmented and reassembled before it can be carried. Fragmentation increases the effects of packet losses[*] while imposing extra work on the network elements. If the size of a packet can be changed based on the MTU while staying consistent with ALF, fragmentation can be avoided. To reduce the packet header and packet processing overheads, it is desirable to have packet sizes as close to the MTU as possible (22). However, particularly for low bit rate applications, the acceptable delay may limit

---

[*]Usually, loss of a fragment causes loss of the entire packet.

the largest packet size to a value much smaller than the MTU. In such cases, header compression (23) may be used to reduce the overhead. In applications that use more than one medium, multiplexing these may provide another solution.

11.3.3 No Bit Level Shifts During Packetization

If the packets can be constructed without performing bit level shifts on the encoded stream, a significant number of unnecessary operations can be avoided at the decoder and the encoder.

11.3.4 Well Defined High-Priority Information

If certain parts of a data stream are vital for decoding the rest of it, it is preferable to have them in easily identifiable and separable sections for more reliable parsing and transmission.

11.3.5 Flexible Rate Control

An encoding scheme whose rate can easily be changed in a predictable way is useful in adapting its output to network conditions for preventing congestion. Usually, the actions to be taken for changing the rate of an encoder are well known (e.g., dropping the frame rate or resolution, increasing the quantization step size). The main problem is predetermination of the rate and the quality after such actions are taken.

11.3.6 Ease of Transcoding

The heterogeneity of bandwidths used for the Internet connections requires the use of different rates for the same multimedia material. Data streams that can easily be transcoded to change their bandwidth are definitely preferable.

11.3.7 Layered Coding

As discussed in Section 11.2, layered coding is beneficial for two purposes. The first is to remove the need for transcoding by providing representations of the same multimedia source at different bit rates without noticeably increasing the overall bandwidth. The second benefit is to provide for a price/performance compromise by sending only a selected portion of a video stream through channels with special QoS provisions, such as guaranteed delivery, while sending the rest over cheaper, best-effort connections.

11.3.8   Resilience to Error Propagation

Given that packet losses will be unavoidable in the foreseeable future, techniques that prevent or reduce the propagation of data loss effects are preferable.

11.4   RTP PAYLOAD FORMATS

Now we analyze selected payload formats for RTP, to demonstrate the use of several packetization techniques for effective video transport over the Internet.

11.4.1   H.261

An IETF Request For Comment, RFC 2032 (24), defines one of the earliest RTP payload formats for packet video transport over the Internet. It is still being successfully used in several Mbone tools such as Vic (25) as well as several commercial products (26,27). This payload format demonstrates a successful approach to packetizing a video payload that was not originally designed for packet networks. Since H.261 is designed for operation over synchronous links, this payload format does not use the companion framing and multiplexing standards.

As explained in Chapter 1 on H series video coding standards, in the H.261 hierarchy, the elements are pictures, groups of blocks (GOBs) and macroblocks (MBs). Each layer in this hierarchy contains information needed to decode lower layers. For example, the picture level specifies information such as the delay from the previous frame and the image format. The GOB number and the default quantizer that will be used for the MBs are specified at the GOB level. The blocks, which are present, and optionally, a quantizer and motion vectors, are specified at the MB level. Therefore, the natural data unit is a picture. However, a picture and even a GOB may be larger than the *path MTU*. Under these circumstances, to apply ALF, this payload format uses macroblocks as its basic data unit. The implementation of this approach is not straightforward, however, for the following reasons:

Since the macroblock start and end points are not marked in an H.261-encoded stream, their identification requires Huffman decoding of the bitstream.

The encoded streams are not byte-aligned. To prevent bit-level shifts during packetization that may be caused by this nonalignment, the payload format uses bit counts in its payload-specific header.

Each packet contains the payload specific header shown in Figure 11.1. The functions of the fields in this header are as follows:

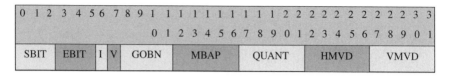

Figure 11.1   H.261 payload specific header.

Start bit position (SBIT) and *end bit position (EBIT)*: number of most and
least significant bits that should be ignored in the first and last payload
bytes, respectively. These fields are needed to prevent bit shifts as mentioned above.

Intra-frame-encoded data (I), motion vector flag (V): *"hint"* *flags*. That is,
their values can be derived from the bitstream. They are included to allow decoders to make optimizations before the bitstream is decoded.
Their values must be the same during an entire RTP session. If I is 1,
this bitstream contains only intra frames (no predictive coding). If V is
0, motion vectors are not used for this stream. An H.261-conformant implementation sets V=1 and I=0. The proper use of such hint flags can be
quite effective in simplifying the decoder design for packetized video
transmission.

In addition, the following fields are used to repeat the vital information that may
be lost because of previous packet losses. This is a specific example for a technique to protect the HP information, as discussed in the preceding section.

GOB number (GOBN): the GOB number for the data at the start of the
packet.

Macroblock address predictor (MBAP): the last MB address encoded in
the previous packet.

Quantizer (QUANT): the quantizer value (MQUANT or GQUANT) in effect prior to the start of this packet. Set to 0 if the packet begins with a
GOB header.

Horizontal motion vector data (HMVD) and *vertical motion vector data
(VMVD)*: references for the horizontal and the vertical motion vector
data.

11.4.1.1   Enhancing the Packet Loss Resilience.

Because of the predic-
tive coding, after a packet loss, parts of the displayed image may remain corrupt
until all MBs involved have been encoded in Intra-frame mode (i.e., encoded independently of past frames). This payload format has provisions to use one of
the following approaches to mitigate error propagation:

1. Use only intra-frame encoding and MB-level conditional replenishment. That is, only MBs that change (beyond some threshold) are transmitted with no predictive coding. Clearly, this approach has less bandwidth efficiency than a compliant application. In addition, the time variations of the camera noise cause a visible difference between the transmitted and not-transmitted MBs that may be annoying.

2. Adjust the Intra-frame encoding refreshment rate according to the packet loss observed by the receivers. The H.261 recommendation specifies that an MB is intra-frame-encoded at least every 132 times it is transmitted. When the measured loss rate is significant, however, the intra-frame refreshment rate can be raised to speed the recovery. Again, using frequent intra-frames reduces the compression efficiency.

3. Repair a corrupted image by requesting an intra-frame-coded image refreshment after detection of a packet loss. Based on such a request, the coder may send the following frame in full intra-frame-encoded mode. Alternatively, if the decoder sends to the coder a list of lost packets, the encoder can save bandwidth by sending only MBs that are lost in intra-frame mode. This mode is particularly efficient in point-to-point connections or when the number of participating decoders is low.

Approach 1 is implemented in the Vic videoconferencing software (25). Approaches 2 and 3 are implemented in the IVS videoconferencing software (28).

11.4.1.2 Use of Optional H.261-Specific Control Packets.

As discussed earlier, RTP's companion control protocol RTCP is extendable. This payload format defines two H.261-specific RTCP control packets, full Intra-frame request" and negative acknowledgment (NACK). Their purpose is to speed up refreshment of the video when their use is feasible (option 3 above). Support of these H.261-specific control packets by the H.261 sender is optional. Some reported experimental results show that use of this feature could have very negative effects when the number of sites is very large (24). Thus, it is recommended these control packets should be used with caution.

The H.261-specific control packets differ from normal RTCP packets in that they are not transmitted to the normal RTCP destination transport address for the RTP session (which is often a multicast address). Instead, these control packets are sent directly via unicast from the decoder to the coder. The destination port for these control packets is the same port that the coder uses as source port for transmitting RTP (data) packets. Therefore, these packets may be considered "reverse" control packets.

Consequently, these control packets may be used only when no RTP mixers or translators intervene in the path from the coder to the decoder. If such intermediate systems do intervene, the address of the coder would no longer be present as the source address in the IP packets received by the decoder. In fact, it might not be possible for the decoder to send packets directly to the coder.

Some reliable multicast protocols use similar NACK control packets transmitted over the normal multicast distribution channel, but they typically use random delays to prevent a NACK implosion problem (29). The goal of such protocols is to provide reliable multicast packet delivery at the expense of delay, which is appropriate for applications such as a shared whiteboard.

On the other hand, interactive video transmission is more sensitive to delay and does not require full reliability. For video applications, it is more effective to send the NACK control packets as soon as possible (i.e., as soon as a loss is detected), without adding any random delays. In this case, multicasting the NACK control packets would generate useless traffic between receivers, since only the coder will use them. However, this method is effective only when the number of receivers is small. In IVS (28), for example, the H.261-specific control packets are used only in point-to-point connections or in point-to-multipoint connections when there are fewer than 10 participants in the conference.

11.4.2 Motion-JPEG

The JPEG still image compression standard can be used for video coding by compressing each frame of video as an independent still image. Video coded in this fashion is often called motion-JPEG or MJPEG. As discussed in the preceding section, under heavy packet losses, error propagation may render the use of predictive coding inefficient, and a solution based on intra-only coding may be preferable. In such cases, the existence and costs of hardware- or software-based JPEG codecs may make MJPEG an attractive alternative, especially for applications that need higher resolution frames and nonstandard interframe times.

The viewgraph transmission system discussed elsewhere (30) is a good example of the use of MJPEG. In this system, effective transmission of the viewgraphs and the pointer used in a presentation is accomplished by using MJPEG to encode the viewgraphs. A straightforward approach to transmitting the viewgraphs and the pointer by means of regular video of a presenter's display is problematic because, while the viewgraphs require a high spatial resolution, the pointer movements need to be sampled and transmitted at a high temporal resolution so that the presenter's pointing actions can be displayed synchronously with the corresponding audio and video signals. To satisfy both these requirements, at least S-VHS quality video needs to be used. Codecs that can compress S-VHS video effectively in real time are expensive, and transmitting it uncompressed requires very high bandwidths. Considering that a viewgraph usually stays displayed for a couple of minutes, its transmission need not be at video frame rates. This makes it possible to use MJPEG, which can be implemented in software running on inexpensive computers, even for compressing and decompressing high-resolution ($\geq 640 \times 480$), full-color viewgraphs.

The RTP payload format for MJPEG (31) is optimized for such video streams where the JPEG codec parameters change rarely from frame to frame. This payload format assumes JPEG's sequential discrete cosine transform (DCT) operating mode (32, Annex F) and single-scan, interleaved images. While these conditions are more restrictive than even baseline JPEG, many hardware implementations can be used with this setting.

In practice, it is rare for most of the table specification data related to a JPEG picture to change from frame to frame within a single video stream. Therefore, RTP/JPEG data is represented in abbreviated format, with all the tables omitted from the bitstream where possible. Each frame begins immediately with the entropy-coded scan. The information that would otherwise be in both the frame and scan headers is represented entirely within an RTP/JPEG header (defined below).

While parameters like Huffman tables and color space are likely to remain fixed for the lifetime of the video stream, other parameters should be allowed to vary, notably the quantization tables and image size (e.g., to implement rate-adaptive transmission or to allow a user to adjust the "quality level" or resolution manually for flexible rate control). Thus, explicit fields in the RTP/JPEG header are allocated to represent this information. Since only a small set of quantization tables is typically used, the entire set of quantization tables is encoded in a small integer field. Customized quantization tables are accommodated by using a special range of values in this field, and then placing the table before the beginning of the JPEG payload. The image width and height are encoded explicitly.

Because JPEG frames are typically larger than the underlying network's path MTU, frames must often be fragmented into several packets. One approach is to allow the IP layer to perform the fragmentation. However, this precludes rate-controlling the resulting packet stream or partial delivery in the presence of loss, and frames may be larger than the maximum network layer reassembly length (see Ref. 33 for more information). To avoid these limitations, RTP/JPEG defines a simple fragmentation and reassembly scheme at the RTP level.

RTP's MJPEG payload format uses a payload specific header. The first 8 bytes of the payload specific header, called the *main JPEG header*, are as shown in Figure 11.2. All fields in this header except for the Fragment Offset field are

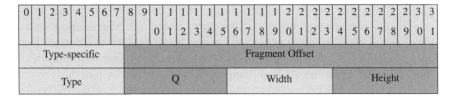

Figure 11.2 Main JPEG header.

the same in all packets from the same JPEG frame. A Restart Marker header and/or Quantization Table Header may follow this header, depending on the values of the Type and Q fields. The usage for the fields in the main JPEG header is as follows:

> *Type-specific*. Interpretation of this field depends on the value of the Type field.
>
> *Fragment offset*. This is the offset in bytes of the current packet in the JPEG frame data. It is useful for handling out-of-order and lost packets if the JPEG frames do not have restart markers.
>
> *Type*. This field specifies the information that would otherwise be present in a JPEG abbreviated table specification as well as the additional JPEG file interchange format (JFIF) style (34) parameters not defined by JPEG. Such parameters that include the color space definitions that are necessary for accurate interpretation and display of the decoded images but not for the decoding process.
>
> *Q*. This field is used in defining the quantization tables for the current frame. The Q value determines whether the quantization tables are computed by means of an algorithm determined by the Type field or explicitly specified through a Quantization Table header. If the second alternative is chosen, the Quantization Table header is added after the main JPEG header in the first packet of the frame, providing for an "*in-band*" specification.
>
> *Width, height*. The width and the height of the image are given in 8-pixel multiples. The largest image resolution is 2040 × 2040 pixels.

11.4.2.1 Restart Markers. Restart markers in the JPEG data denote a point at which the decoder should reset its state. It is possible to start a partial decoding of a JPEG stream from a restart marker. These are the only types of marker that may appear embedded in the entropy-coded segment, and they may appear only on a minimum coded units (MCU) boundary. An MCU is the smallest group of image data coded in a JPEG bitstream. Each MCU defines the image data for a small rectangular block of the output image. A "restart interval" is defined to be a block of data containing a restart marker followed by some fixed number of MCUs. When these markers are used, each frame is composed of some fixed number of back-to-back restart intervals.

The original JPEG specification provides a sequence number field in the restart markers to identify the location of this partially decoded frame segment in the original frame. Unfortunately, this field is not large enough to properly cope with the loss of an entire packet's worth of data at a typical network MTU size. The restart marker header contains the additional information needed to accomplish this.

The *restart interval* field specifies the number of MCUs that appear between restart markers. The size of restart intervals always should be chosen to allow an integral number of restart intervals to fit within a single packet. This will guarantee that packets can be decoded independently from one another. If a restart interval ends up being larger than a packet, the F and L bits in the restart marker header can be used to fragment it, but for that restart interval to be decoded properly, the resulting set of packets must be received in its entirety by a decoder.

Once a decoder has received either a single packet with both the F and the L bit set on, or a contiguous sequence of packets (based on the RTP sequence number) that begins with an F bit and ends with an L bit, it can begin decoding. The position of the MCU at the beginning of the data can be determined by multiplying the restart count value by the restart interval value. A packet (or group of packets as identified by the F and L bits) may contain any number of consecutive restart intervals.

11.4.3 MPEG-1 and MPEG-2

As discussed in Chapter 2, the MPEG-1 and MPEG-2 standards define efficient and popular techniques for encoding video. However, as in H.261, these standards were developed in complete independence of the Internet architec-

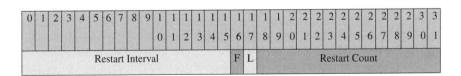

Figure 11.3   Restart marker header.

ture. The RTP MPEG payload format (35) is an excellent example for demonstrating how to adapt an independently designed payload type for effective Internet transport.

The MPEG-1 system specification defines an encapsulation of the elementary streams (ES) that contains presentation time stamps (PTS), decoding time stamps (DTS), and system clock references, and performs multiplexing of MPEG-1 compressed video and audio ESs with user data. The MPEG-2 standard defines two system stream formats: the MPEG-2 transport stream (TS) and the MPEG-2 program stream (PS). The TS is tailored for communicating or storing one or more programs of MPEG-2 compressed data and also other data in relatively error-prone environments. The PS is tailored for relatively error-free environments.

The RTP MPEG payload format (35) seeks to achieve interoperability among end points based on both MPEG systems (MPEG-1 systems and MPEG-2 TS and PS) and MPEG ES. In this way, existing hardware codecs and stored multimedia material on servers that employ one of these formats can be used without any change, using RTP as the base transport protocol.

When operating only among ES-based systems, a payload format that provides greater compatibility with the Internet architecture is defined as a part of this payload format. In this approach, consistent with the overall Internet architecture, solutions of some of the system issues are left to other protocols defined in the Internet community.

In many instances of transporting MPEG-2 video, an associated audio channel is always present. A separate, experimental payload format defined to handle this important case is described in RFC 2343 (36) and discussed in Section 11.4.3.3.

11.4.3.1 Encapsulation of MPEG System Streams.
For this payload format, each RTP packet contains a timestamp derived from the sender's 90 kHz clock reference. This clock is synchronized to the system stream program clock reference (PCR) or system clock reference (SCR) and represents the *target transmission time* of the first byte of the packet payload. The target transmission time is not necessarily the time the packet is put on the network. It is the time at which data in the packet must be transmitted as implied by the coding algorithm. This timestamp will not be passed to the MPEG decoder because the necessary timestamps for the decoder are carried within the payload. In this format, the primary purposes of the RTP timestamp are to estimate and reduce any network-induced jitter and to synchronize relative time drift between the transmitter and receiver.

For MPEG-2 transport streams, the RTP payload will contain an integral number of MPEG transport packets. To avoid end-system inefficiencies, data from multiple small packets (normally fixed in size at 188 bytes) can be aggregated into a single RTP packet.

For MPEG-2 program streams and MPEG-1 system streams there are no packetization restrictions; these streams are treated as a packetized stream of bytes. That is, the ALF principle cannot be used.

The M bit of the RTP header is used for a special purpose in this payload format. It is set to 1 whenever the timestamp is discontinuous (such as might happen when a sender switches from one data source to another). This allows the receiver and any intervening RTP mixers or translators that are synchronizing to the flow to ignore the difference between this timestamp and any previous timestamp in their clock phase detectors.

11.4.3.2   Encapsulation of MPEG Elementary Streams.   A distinct RTP payload type is assigned to MPEG-1 and MPEG-2 video ESs. Further indication of whether the data is MPEG-1 or MPEG-2 is not provided in the RTP- or MPEG-specific headers of this encapsulation, because this information is available in the ES headers. MPEG-1 video can be distinguished from MPEG-2 video at the video sequence header; that is, for MPEG-2 video a *sequence_header()* is followed by *sequence_extension()*. The particular profile and level of MPEG-2 video (*MAIN_Profile@MAIN_Level*, *HIGH_Profile@HIGH_Level*, etc.) are determined by the *profile_and_level_indicator* field of the *sequence_extension* header of MPEG-2 video.

The MPEG bitstream semantics were designed for relatively error-free environments, and there is a significant amount of dependency (both temporal and spatial) in the stream, such that loss of some data makes other uncorrupted data useless. The format as defined in this encapsulation uses the ALF information plus additional information in the RTP-stream-specific header to allow recovery mechanisms, as discussed below.

11.4.3.2.1   Fragmentation.   Since MPEG pictures can be large, they will normally be fragmented into packets of size less than a typical path MTU. The following fragmentation rules apply:

1.   The MPEG Video_Sequence_Header, when present, will always be at the beginning of an RTP payload.
2.   An MPEG GOP_header, when present, will always be at the beginning of the RTP payload, or will follow a Video_Sequence_Header.
3.   An MPEG Picture_Header, when present, will always be at the beginning of an RTP payload, or will follow a GOP_header.

Each ES header must be completely contained within the packet. Consequently, a minimum RTP payload size of 261 bytes must be supported to contain the largest single header defined in the ES (i.e., the *extension_data()* header containing the *quant_matrix_extension()*). Otherwise, there are no restrictions on where headers may appear within packet payloads.

11.4.3.2.2 Slice Indicators. In MPEG, each picture is made up of one or more "slices," and a slice is intended to be the unit of recovery from data loss or corruption. An MPEG-compliant decoder will normally advance to the beginning of the next slice whenever an error is encountered in the stream. To facilitate this, MPEG *slice begin* and *end* bits are provided in the encapsulation header. The beginning of a slice either must be the first data in a packet (after any MPEG ES headers) or must follow some integral number of slices in a packet. This requirement ensures that the beginning of the next slice after one with a missing packet can be found without requiring the receiver to scan the packet contents. Slices may be fragmented across packets as long as all the foregoing rules are observed.

11.4.3.2.3 Periodical Repetition of the Sequence Headers. An implementation based on this encapsulation assumes that the Video_Sequence_Header is repeated periodically in the MPEG bitstream. In practice (though not required by MPEG standard), this repetition is used to allow channel switching and to receive and start decoding a continuously relayed MPEG bitstream at arbitrary points in the media stream. It is suggested that during play back of an MPEG stream from a file format (where the Video_Sequence_Header may be represented at the beginning of the stream only), the first Video_Sequence_Header (preceded by an *end-of-stream* indicator) be saved by the packetizer for periodic injection into the network stream.

11.4.3.2.4 Header Information. The timestamp field of the RTP header reflects the presentation time for the picture whose data is contained in the current packet measured with a 90 kHz clock. It is the same for all packets that make up a picture, and it may not be monotonically increasing if B pictures are present. For packets that contain only a video sequence and/or GOP header, the timestamp is that of the subsequent picture.

The M bit is set to 1 on packets containing MPEG frame end code.

A payload-specific header (Figure 11.4) is attached to each RTP packet after the RTP header. It has the following fields:

MBZ: unused; must be set to zero.

T: MPEG-2-specific header extension present; set to 1 when the MPEG-2 video-specific header extension follows this header.

TR: temporal reference: the temporal reference of the current picture within the current GOP. This value ranges from 0 to 1023 and is constant for all RTP packets of a given picture.

AN: active N bit for error resilience. Set to 1 when the following bit (N) is used to signal changes in the picture header information for MPEG-2 payloads. It must be set to 0 for MPEG-1 payloads or when the N bit is not used.

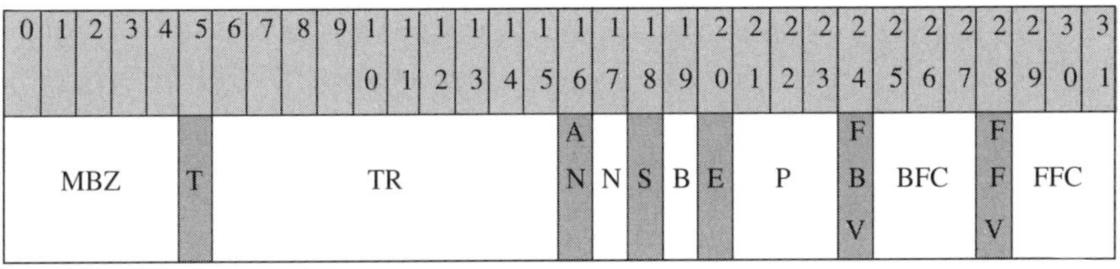

0	1	2	3	4	5	6	7	8	9	1 0	1 1	1 2	1 3	1 4	1 5	1 6	1 7	1 8	1 9	2 0	2 1	2 2	2 3	2 4	2 5	2 6	2 7	2 8	2 9	3 0	3 1
MBZ					T		TR									AN	N	S	B	E		P			FBV		BFC			FFV	FFC

Figure 11.4 Payload-specific header for MPEG-1 and MPEG-2.

N: New picture header: used for MPEG-2 payloads when the previous bit (AN) is set to 1; otherwise, it must be set to zero. It is set to 1 when the information contained in the previously transmitted picture headers cannot be used to reconstruct a header for the current picture. This happens when a set of parameters different from those for the previous pictures of the same type is used to encode the current picture. The N bit must be constant for all RTP packets that belong to the same picture so that receipt of any packet from a picture allows the detection of whether information necessary for reconstruction was contained in that picture (N=1) or a previous one (N=0).

S: sequence header present. normally 0 and set to 1 at the occurrence of each MPEG sequence header. Used to detect the presence of a sequence header in an RTP packet.

B: beginning-of-slice: set when the start of the packet payload is a slice start code, or when a slice start code is preceded by only the following: Video_Sequence_Header, GOP_header, and/or Picture_Header.

E: end-of-slice (ES) (1 bit). Set when the last byte of the payload is the end of an MPEG slice.

P: picture type (3 bits): I (1), P (2), B (3), or D (4). This value is constant for each RTP packet of a given picture. Value 000B is forbidden and 101B–111B are reserved to support future extensions to the MPEG ES specification.

FBV, BFC, FFV, FFC: obtained from the most recent picture header; constant for each RTP packet of a given picture. For I frames none of these values are present in the picture header, and they must be set to zero in the RTP header. For P frames only the last two values are present, and FBV and BFC must be set to zero in the RTP header. For B frames all four values are present.

11.4.3.2.5 MPEG-2 Video-Specific Header Extension.   In this header extension (Figure 11.5), the X bit is unused and must be set to zero. The E bit is for extensions present. If set to 1, this header extension, including the com-

0	1	2	3	4	5	6	7	8	9	1	1	1	1	1	1	1	1	1	1	2	2	2	2	2	2	2	2	2	2	3	3
										0	1	2	3	4	5	6	7	8	9	0	1	2	3	4	5	6	7	8	9	0	1
X	E	f_[0, 0]			f_[0, 1]				f_[1, 0]				f_[1, 1]				Dc		PS			T	P	C	Q	V	A	R	H	G	D

Figure 11.5 MPEG-2 video-specific header extension.

posite display extension when D=1, will be followed by one or more of the following extensions: quant matrix extension, picture display extension, picture temporal scalable extension, picture spatial scalable extension, and copyright extension.

Since they may not be vital in decoding of a picture, the inclusion of any one of these extensions in an RTP packet is optional even when the MPEG-2 video-specific header extension is included in the packet (T=1). If present, they should be copied from the corresponding extensions following the most recent MPEG-2 picture coding extension, and they remain constant for each RTP packet of a given picture.

The following values are copied from the most recent picture coding extension and are constant for each RTP packet of a given picture; their meanings are as explained in connection with the MPEG-2 standard:

$$f\_[0,0], f\_[0,1], f\_[1,0], f\_[1,1], DC, PS, T, P, C, Q, V, A, R, H, G, D$$

11.4.3.3 Audio/Video Bundled Payload Format (BMPEG).

The bundled packetization scheme (36) is needed because it has several advantages over other schemes for some important applications including videoondemand (VoD), where audio and video are always used together. Its advantages over independent packetization of audio and video are as follows:

1. Uses a single port per "program" (i.e. bundled A/V). This may increase the number of streams that can be served (e.g., from a VoD server). In addition, it eliminates the performance hit when two ports are used for the separate audio and video streams on the client side.

2. Provides implicit synchronization of audio and video. This is particularly convenient when the A/V data is stored in an interleaved format at the server.

3. Reduces the header overhead. Since using large packets increases the effects of losses and delay, audio-only packets need to be smaller, increasing the overhead. An A/V bundled format can provide about 1% overall overhead reduction. Considering the high bit rates used for MPEG-encoded material (e.g., 4 Mbit/s), the number of bits saved (e.g., 40 kbit/s,) may provide a noticeable improvement in audio or video quality.

4. May reduce overall receiver buffer size. Audio and video streams may

experience different delays when transmitted separately. The receiver buffers need to be designed for the longest of these delays. For example, let us assume that using two buffers, each with a size B, is sufficient with probability P when each stream is transmitted individually. The probability that the same buffer size will be sufficient when both streams need to be received is P times the conditional probability of B being sufficient for the second stream, given that it was sufficient for the first one. This conditional probability is, generally, less than one, requiring use of a larger buffer size to achieve the same probability level.

5. May help with the control of the overall bandwidth used by an audiovisual program.

Moreover, there are two main advantages over packetization of the transport layer streams:

1. *Reduced overhead.* This scheme does not contain systems layer information, which is redundant for the RTP (essentially, they address similar issues).
2. *Easier error recovery.* Because of the structured packetization consistent with the ALF principle, loss concealment and error recovery can be made simpler and more effective.

In addition to the encapsulation rules used for MPEG ESs, the BMPEG format requires that each packet contain an integral number of video slices. It is the application's responsibility to adjust the slice sizes and the number of slices put in each RTP packet so that lower level fragmentation does not occur. This approach simplifies the receivers, while somewhat increasing the complexity of the transmitter's packetizer. Considering that a slice can be as small as a single macroblock, it is possible to prevent fragmentation for most cases. If a packet size exceeds the path maximum transmission unit (path MTU), this payload type depends on the lower protocol layers for fragmentation, although this may cause problems with packet classification for other services.

The video data is followed by a sufficient number of integral audio frames to cover the duration of the video segment included in a packet. For example, if the first packet contains three slices of video each 1/900 second long, and layer 1 audio coding is used at a 44.1 kHz sampling rate, only one audio frame covering 384/44100 second of audio need be included in this packet. Since the length of this audio frame (8.71 ms) is longer than that of the video segment contained in this packet (3.33 ms), the next few packets may not contain any audio frames until the packet in which the covered video time extends outside the length of the previously transmitted audio frames. Alternatively, it is possible, in this proposal, to repeat the latest audio frame in "no-audio" packets for packet loss resilience. Again, it is the application's responsibility to adjust the bundled packet size according to the minimum MTU size to prevent fragmentation.

11.4.3.3.1 RTP Fixed Header for BMPEG Encapsulation. The RTP header fields are used as follows:

M: set to 1 for packets containing the end of a picture.

Timestamp: 32-bit, 90 kHz timestamp representing the sampling time of the MPEG picture; may not be monotonically increasing if B pictures are present. The timestamp is the same for all packets belonging to the same picture. For packets that contain only a sequence, extension, and/or GOP header, the timestamp is that of the subsequent picture.

11.4.3.3.2 BMPEG Specific Header. In this case (Figure 11.5), the header fields are as follows:

P: picture type. I (0), P (1), B (2).

N: header data changed. Set if any part of the video sequence extension, GOP, and picture header data is different from that of the previously sent headers. It is reset when all the header data is repeated.

MBZ: reserved for future use.

Audio length: length of the audio data in this packet in bytes. Start of the audio data is found by subtracting "Audio Length" from the total length of the received packet.

Audio offset: the offset between the start of the audio frame and the RTP timestamp for this packet in number of audio samples (for multichannel sources, a set of samples covering all channels is counted as one sample for this purpose).

Audio offset is a signed integer in two's-complement form. It allows an offset of approximately ± 750 ms at a 44.1 kHz audio sampling rate. For a very low video frame rate (e.g., a frame per second), this offset may not be sufficient and this payload format may not be usable.

If B frames are present, audio frames are not reordered along with video. Instead, they are packetized along with video frames in their transmission order (e.g., an audio segment packetized with a video segment corresponding to a P

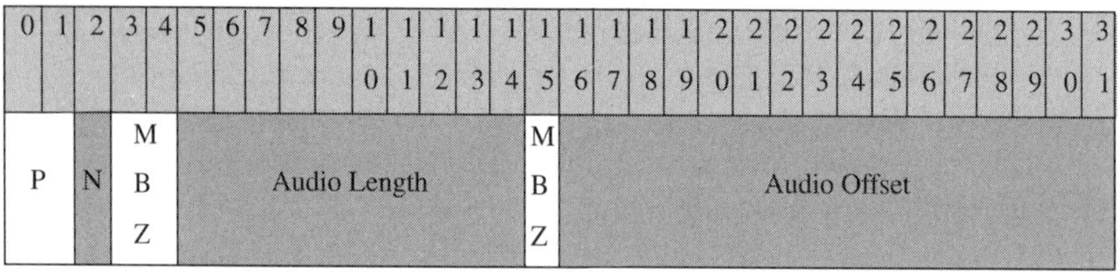

0	1	2	3	4	5	6	7	8	9	1 0	1 1	1 2	1 3	1 4	1 5	1 6	1 7	1 8	1 9	2 0	2 1	2 2	2 3	2 4	2 5	2 6	2 7	2 8	2 9	3 0	3 1
P	N	MBZ			Audio Length									MBZ				Audio Offset													

Figure 11.6 BMPEG-specific header.

picture may belong to a B picture, which will be transmitted later and should be rendered at the same time with this audio segment). Even though the video segments are reordered, the audio offset for a particular audio segment is still relative to the RTP timestamp in the packet containing that audio segment.

11.4.3.4 Error Recovery and Resynchronization Strategies. During the initial decoding of an RTP-encapsulated MPEG elementary stream, the receiver may discard all packets until the sequence-header-present bit is set to 1. At this point, sufficient state information is contained in the stream to allow processing by an MPEG decoder.

According to the IETF (35), loss of packets containing the GOP_header and/or Picture_Header is detected by an unexpected change in the temporal-reference and picture-type values. If desired, a GOP header can be reconstructed by using a "null" time_code, repeating the closed_gop flag from previous GOP headers, and setting the broken_link flag to 1. Since RFC 2343 (36) does not provide a special picture counter, such as the "temporal reference (TR)" field of RFC 2250 (35), lost GOP headers may not be detected by this payload format. However, the only effect of this may be incorrect decoding of the B pictures immediately following the lost GOP header for some edited video material.

The loss of a Picture_Header can also be detected by a mismatch in the temporal reference contained in the RTP packet from the appropriate counters at the receiver.

For MPEG-1 payloads, after scanning to the next Beginning-of-slice, the Picture_Header is reconstructed from the P, TR, FBV, BFC, FFV, and FFC contained in that packet, and from stream-dependent default values.

For MPEG-2, additional information is needed for the reconstruction. This information is provided by the MPEG-2 video-specific header extension contained in that packet if the T bit is set to 1, or the picture header for the current picture may be available from previous packets belonging to the same picture. The transmitter's strategy for inclusion of the MPEG-2 video-specific header extension may depend on a number of factors. This header may not be needed when (a) the information has been transmitted sufficiently often in previous packets to assure reception with the desired probability, (b) the information is transmitted over a separate reliable channel, (c) expected loss rates are so low that missed frames are not a concern, or (d) conserving bandwidth is more important than error resilience,and so on.

If T=1 and E=0, there may be extensions present in the original video bitstream that are not included in the current packet. The transmitter may choose not to include extensions in a packet when they are not necessary for decoding or if one of the cases listed above for not including the MPEG-2 video specific header extension in a packet applies only to the extension data.

If N=0, the picture header from a previous picture of the same type (I, P, or

B) may be used as long as at least one packet has been received for every intervening picture of the same type and the N bit was 0 for each of those pictures. Compliance may involve the following measures:

1. Saving the relevant picture header information that can be obtained from the MPEG-2 video-specific header extension or directly from the video bitstream for each picture type
2. Keeping validity indicators for this saved information based on the received N bits and lost packets
3. Updating the data whenever a packet with N=1 is received

If the necessary information is not available from any of these sources, data deletion until a new picture start code is advised.

Whenever an RTP packet is lost (which can be detected by a gap in the RTP sequence number), the receiver may discard all packets until it receives one with the Beginning-of-slice bit set. At this point, the stream contains sufficient state information to allow processing by an MPEG decoder starting at the next slice boundary (possibly after reconstruction of the GOP_header and/or Picture_Header, as described above).

Packet losses can be detected from a combination of the sequence number and the timestamp fields of the RTP fixed header. The extent of the loss can be determined from the timestamp, the slice number, and the horizontal location of the first slice in the packet. The slice number and the horizontal location can be determined from the slice header and the first macroblock address increment, which are located at fixed bit positions.

If lost data consists of slices all from the same picture, new data following the loss may simply be given to the video decoder, which will normally repeat missing pixels from a previous picture. The next audio frame must be played at the appropriate time determined by the timestamp and the audio offset contained in the received packet. Appropriate audio frames (e.g., representing background noise) may need to be fed to the audio decoder in place of the lost audio frames to keep the lip-synch and/or to conceal the effects of the losses.

If the received new data after a loss is from the next picture (i.e., no complete picture loss) and the N bit is not set, previously received headers for the particular picture type (determined from the P bits) can be given to the video decoder followed by the new data. If N is set, data deletion until a new picture start code is advisable unless headers are made available to the receiver through some other channel.

If data for more than one picture is lost and headers are not available, unless N is zero and at least one packet has been received for every intervening picture of the same type and the N bit was 0 for each of those pictures, resynchronization to a new video sequence header is advisable.

In all cases of heavy packet losses, if the correct headers for the missing pictures are available, they can be given to the video decoder and the received data can be used irrespective of the N-bit value or the number of lost pictures.

Use of frequent video sequence headers makes it possible to join in a program at arbitrary times. This measure also reduces the resynchronization time after severe losses.

11.4.4   H.263+

As a recently developed standard, H.263+ contains several coding options that are designed particularly for packetized delivery of video. The recommended uses of these options for the Internet delivery using RTP by RFC 2429 (37) are discussed next.

11.4.4.1   Slice Structured Mode.
Slice-structured mode, as described in the standard (38, Annex K) can be used to obtain natural breakpoints consistent with a given path MTU. In slice-structured mode, the motion vector predictors in a slice are restricted to slice boundaries. This is similar to a picture segment that begins with a group-of-blocks (GOB) header; however, slices provide much greater freedom in the selection of the size and shape of the area, which is represented as an independently decodable region. Slices can have a dynamically selected size to allow the data for each slice to fit into a packet consistent with the path MTU. For the Internet transport, slices should not be fragmented across packet boundaries. Optimally, each packet will contain only one slice.

11.4.4.2   Independent Segment Decoding (ISD).
The standard (38, Annex R) for ISD does not allow any data dependency across slice or GOB boundaries in the reference pictures. It can be utilized to further improve resiliency in high-loss conditions. If ISD is used in conjunction with the slice structure, the rectangular slice submode must be enabled and the dimensions and quantity of the slices present in a frame must remain the same between each two intra-coded frames (I frames), as required in H.263+. The individual ISD segments may also be entirely intra-coded from time to time to realize quick error recovery without adding the latency time associated with sending complete intra pictures.

11.4.4.3   Reference Picture Selection Mode.
The standard (38, Annex N) for reference picture selection mode allows the use of any older reference picture rather than the one immediately preceding the current picture. Usually, the last transmitted frame is implicitly used as the reference picture for interframe prediction. If the reference picture selection mode is used, the data stream carries information enabling dertermination of the reference frame that should be used.

This mode can be used with or without a back channel, which provides information to the encoder about the internal status of the decoder.

11.4.4.4 Bitstream Scalability Mode. Three kinds of scalability are included in the standard: temporal, signal-to-noise ratio (SNR), and spatial scalability. Temporal scalability is achieved via the disposable nature of bidirectionally predicted frames, or B frames. A low-delay form of temporal scalability known as P-picture temporal scalability can also be achieved by using the reference picture selection mode described in Section 11.4.4.3.

11.4.4.5 Payload Format. For each RTP packet, the RTP header is followed by a variable size H.263+ payload header. The payload format includes provisions for proper byte alignment of the start codes and removal of start code preambles when they are implied by the packet structure.

The H.263+ payload-specific header is structured in Figure 11.7, with individual headers as follows:

P: indicates the picture start or a picture segment (GOB/slice) start or a video sequence end (EOS or EOSBS). This bit allows the omission of the two first bytes of the start codes, thus improving the compression ratio.

V: indicates the presence of an 8-bit field containing information for video redundancy coding (VRC), which follows immediately after the initial 16 bits of the payload header.

PLEN: length in bytes of the extra picture header. If PLEN is nonzero, the extra picture header is attached immediately following the rest of the payload header.

PEBIT: indicates the number of bits that shall be ignored in the last byte of the picture header.

11.4.4.6 Video Redundancy Coding Header Extension. VRC header extension (39) is an optional mechanism intended to improve error resilience over packet networks. Implementing it in H.263+ requires the Reference Picture Selection mode. Since there are multiple "threads" of independently inter-frame-

0	1	2	3	4	5	6	7	8	9	1 0	1 1	1 2	1 3	1 4	1 5
MBZ						P	V	PLEN			PEBIT				

Figure 11.7 H.263+ payload-specific header.

predicted pictures, damage on an individual frame will cause distortions only within its own thread, leaving the other threads unaffected. From time to time, all threads converge to a so-called sync frame (an intra picture or a non-intra picture, which is redundantly represented within multiple threads); from this sync frame, the independent threads are started again.

P-picture temporal scalability is another use of the reference picture selection mode and can be considered to be a special case of VRC in which only one copy of each sync frame may be sent. It offers a thread-based method of temporal scalability without the increased delay caused by the use of B pictures. In this use, sync frames sent in the first thread of pictures are also used for the prediction of a second thread of pictures, which fall temporally between the sync frames to increase the resulting frame rate. In this use, the pictures in the second thread can be discarded to obtain a reduction of bit rate or decoding complexity without harming the ability to decode later pictures. More threads can be added as well, but each thread is predicted only from the sync frames (which are sent at least in thread 0) or from frames within the same thread. While a VRC data stream, like all H.263+ data is totally self-contained, it may be useful for the transport hierarchy implementation to have knowledge about the current damage status of each thread. On the Internet, this status can easily be determined by observing the marker bit, the sequence number of the RTP header, and the thread ID and a circling "packet per thread" number. The latter two numbers are coded in the VRC header extension.

The format of the VRC header extension is illustrated in Figure 11.8, with the following individual headers.

> *TID*: thread ID. Up to 7 threads are allowed. Each frame of H.263+ VRC data will use as reference information only sync frames or frames within the same thread. By convention, thread 0 is expected to be the "canonical" thread, which is the thread from which the sync frame should ideally be used. In the case of corruption or loss of the thread 0 representation, the decoder can use a representation of the sync frame with a higher thread number. Lower thread numbers are expected to contain equal or better representations of the sync frames than higher thread numbers in the absence of data corruption or loss.
>
> *TRUN*: monotonically increasing (modulo 16) 4-bit number counting the packet number within each thread.

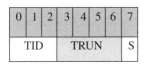

Figure 11.8 VRC header extension.

S: A bit that indicates that the packet content is for a sync frame. An encoder using VRC may send several representations of the same "sync" picture, to ensure that regardless of which thread of pictures is corrupted by errors or packet losses, the reception of at least one representation of a particular picture is ensured (within at least one thread). The sync picture can then be used for the prediction of any thread. If packet losses have not occurred, the sync frame contents of thread 0 can be used and those of other threads can be discarded (and similarly for other threads). Thread 0 is considered the "canonical" thread, the use of which is preferable to all others. The contents of packets having lower thread numbers are considered to have a higher processing and delivery priority than those with higher thread numbers. Thus packets having lower thread numbers for a given sync frame are delivered first to the decoder under loss-free and low-time-jitter conditions. This results in the discarding of the sync contents of the higher numbered threads as specified in Annex N of the standard (38).

11.5 DISCUSSIONS

The Internet protocols, some standardized and some in draft form, collectively provide a complete set of tools for implementing real-time multimedia stream delivery over the Internet. A fundamental principle of Internet architecture is to divide a complicated application into well-defined pieces that are common to many other applications, and solve each of them synergistically. Following this principle, several aspects of video transmission over the Internet are handled by various protocols as discussed in Chapter 3 and elsewhere (40).

A thorough understanding of all these protocols is beneficial for multimedia application designers. Familiarity with the transport protocol is particularly essential for video codec designers targeting Internet delivery because effective use of the transport layer requires in-depth knowledge of the underlying video coding methods as well. As demonstrated in the preceding sections, the transport protocol, being at the intermediate level of the real-time data transmission architecture, is very closely related to the way the multimedia payload types are organized and used.

At the current time, RTP seems to be the transport protocol of choice for many vendors for multimedia transport over the Internet. Moreover, it is a part of the ITU's H.323 recommendation (41) and thus is being employed by all H.323-compatible products used for multimedia communications. Although some real-time multimedia applications of today use transport protocols that are proprietary or not intended for multimedia transport (e.g., HTTP), almost all these applications are expected to support RTP in the near future. This is mainly because of RTP's flexibility in accommodating the needs of different media payloads through its payload format definition mechanism, while offering the basic functions needed by all real-time transport applications.

Unless the codec and the network properties are jointly considered, it is very difficult, if not impossible, to design a cost-effective video delivery system. The lower layer protocols have a fundamental impact on the performance and usability of video coding techniques in a networked application. For example, if the network offers some service guarantees, such as delay bounds or guaranteed packet deliveries (no loss), it may be preferable to use video coding techniques that sacrifice error resilience for better compression efficiency. If appropriate data flow control is done at the lower layers, application designers need not worry about network buffer overflows due to short-term high output data rates as in the case for I frames in MPEG video.

In many cases, the additional services offered by the lower protocol layers or the network infrastructure are not free, and a price–performance compromise may be obtained by using layered coding techniques. This way specialized services are needed for transmitting only a portion (layer) of the encoded video. Although a large number of publications on layered video can be found in the literature, currently, no commercial products exist. Presently unclear are the type of layering to be used and the division of the video data among the layers. One reason for this may be the nonexistence of a QoS infrastructure and an associated price structure. However, these are expected to materialize in the near future, making the selection of a layered codec a pressing issue.

This chapter outlines the common techniques used for effective video delivery over the Internet. The payload format design techniques are presented through a detailed analysis of selected payload formats. As in learning many other architecture-related works, studying earlier designs is beneficial for new designs. The reader is encouraged to study other payload formats also.

APPENDIX A
IETF COPYRIGHT NOTICE

The following copyright notice applies to References 24, 31, 34–36, and 38.

of developing Internet standards in which case the procedures for copyrights defined in the Internet Standards process must be followed, or as required to translate it into languages other than English.

REFERENCES

1. S Shenker, J Wroclawski. Network element service specification template. Internet Engineering Task Force Request for Comment 2216, September 1997.
2. H Schulzrinne, S Casner, R Frederick, V Jacobson, RTP: A transport protocol for real-time applications. Internet Engineering Task Force Request for Comment 1889, January 1996.
3. D E Comer Internetworking with TCP/IP. Englewood Cliffs, NJ, Prentice-Hall, 1991.
4. V Paxson. End-to-end Internet packet dynamics. Proceedings of ACM SIGCOMM '97, pp 139–152.
5. C Perkins, O Hodson. Options for repair of streaming media. Internet Engineering Task Force Request for Comment 2354, June 1998.
6. J M Boyce, R D Gaglianello. Packet loss effects on MPEG video sent over the public Internet. Proceedings of ACM Multimedia '98, pp 181–190.
7. D Clark and D Tennenhouse. Architecture considerations for a new generation of protocols. Proceedings of ACM SIGCOMM '90, September 1990, pp 201–208.
8. H Schulzrinne, S Casner, R Frederick, V Jacobson. RTP: A transport protocol for real-time applications. Internet Engineering Task Force AVT Work-in-progress, draft-ietf-avt-rtp-new-04.txt, Section 2.4, June 1999.
9. M Civanlar, G Cash, B Haskell. AT&T's error resilient video transmission technique. Internet Engineering Task Force Request for Comment 2448, November 1998.
10. Reliable Multicast Transport Working Group, Internet Engineering Task Force, http://www.ietf.org/html.charters/rmt-charter.html
11. J Rosenberg, H Schulzrinne. An RTP payload format for generic forward error correction. Internet Engineering Task Force AVT Work-in-progress, draft-ietf-avt-fec-08.txt.
12. S Blake, D Black, M Carlson, E Davies, Z Wang, W Weiss. An architecture for differentiated services," Internet Engineering Task Force Request for Comment 2475, December 1998.
13. D L Mills. Network Time Protocol (Version 3) Specification, implementation and analysis. Internet Engineering Task Force Request for Comment 1305, March 1992.
14. J-C Bolot, T. Turletti. A rate control mechanism for packet video in the Internet. Proceedings of IEEE Infocom '94, June 1994.
15. J-C Bolot, T Turletti, I Wakeman. Scalable feedback control for multicast video distribution in the Internet. Proceedings of ACM SIGCOMM '94, August, 1994, pp. 58–67.
16. I Busse, B Deffner, H Schulzrinne. Dynamic QoS control of multimedia applications based on RTP. Comput Commun, 19:49–68, January 1996.

17. S McCanne, V Jacobson, M Vetterli. Receiver-driven layered multicast. Proceedings of ACM SIGCOMM '94, August 1996, pp. 117–130.

18. B Braden, D Clark, J Crowcroft, B Davie, S Deering, D Estrin, S Floyd, V Jacobson, G Minshall, C Partridge, L Peterson, K Ramakrishnan, S Shenker, J Wroclawski, L Zhang. Recommendations on queue management and congestion avoidance in the Internet. Internet Engineering Task Force Request for Comment 2309, April 1998.

19. S Cen, C Pu, J Walpole. Flow and congestion control for Internet media streaming applications. Proceedings of Multimedia Computing and Networking 1998.

20. R Rejaie, D Estrin, M Handley. Quality adaptation for congestion controlled video playback over the Internet. Proceedings of ACM SIGCOMM '99, February 1999.

21. J Mogul, S Deering. Path MTU Discovery. Internet Engineering Task Force Request for Comment 1191, November 1990.

22. P Nee, K Jeffay, G Danneels. The performance of two-dimensional media scaling for Internet videoconferencing. Proceedings of the Seventh NOSSDAV, May 1997, pp. 237–248.

23. S Casner, V Jacobson. Compressing IP/UDP/RTP headers for low-speed serial links. Internet Engineering Task Force Request for Comment 2508, February 1999.

24. T Turletti, T Huitema,C Huitema. RTP payload format for H.261 video streams. Internet Engineering Task Force Request for Comment 2032, October 1996.

25. S MacCanne, V Jacobson. vic: a flexible framework for packet video. Proceedings of ACM Multimedia '95, Nov. 1995 pp 511–522.

26. IPTV, Cisco.

27. Real Player G2, Real Networks.

28. T Turletti. INRIA Videoconferencing tool (IVS). Available by anonymous ftp from zenon.inria.fr in the "rodeo/ivs/last_version" directory. See also http://www.inria.fr/rodeo/ivs.html

29. S Pingali, D Towsley, J F Kurose. A comparison of sender-initiated and receiver-initiated reliable multicast protocols. Proceedings of IEEE GLOBECOM '94.

30. M R Civanlar, G L Cash. Networked viewgraphs—NetVG. Proceedings of the International Workshop on Packet Video' 99, New York, April 1999. http://www.research.att.com/~mrc/PacketVideo99.html

31. L Berc, W Fenner, R Frederick, S McCanne, P Stewart. RTP payload format for JPEG-compressed video. Internet Engineering Task Force Request for Comment 2435, October 1998.

32. ISO DIS 10918-1. Digital compression and coding of continuous-tone still images (JPEG). CCITT Recommendation T.81.

33. C Kent, J Mogul. Fragmentation considered harmful. Proceedings of the ACM SIGCOMM '87 Workshop on Frontiers in Computer Communications Technology, August 1987.

34. The JPEG File Interchange Format. Maintained by C-Cube Microsystems, Inc. Available in ftp://ftp.uu.net/graphics/jpeg/jfif.ps.gz.

35. D Hoffman, G Fernando, V Goyal, M R Civanlar. RTP payload format for MPEG1/MPEG2 video," Internet Engineering Task Force Request for Comment 2250, January 1998.

36. M R Civanlar, G L Cash, B G Haskell. RTP payload format for bundled MPEG. Internet Engineering Task Force Request for Comment 2343, May 1998.
37. C Bormann, L Cline, G Deisher, T Gardos, C Maciocco, D Newell, J Ott, G Sullivan, S Wenger, C Zhu. RTP payload format for the 1998 version of ITU-T Recommendation H.263 Video (H.263+). Internet Engineering Task Force Request for Comment 2429, October 1998.
38. ITU-T Recommendation H.263. Video coding for low bit rate communication. International Telecommunications Union, Geneva, January 1998.
39. S Wenger. Video redundancy coding in II.263+. Proceedings of Audio-Visual Services over Packet Networks. Aberdeen, September 1997.
40. M Reha Civanlar. Protocols for real-time multimedia data transmission over the Internet. Proceedings of IEEE ICASSP '98, Seattle, 1998.
41. ITU-T, Recommendation H.323. Multi-media conferences for packet-based network environments. International Telecommunications Union, Geneva.

12
Wireless Video

Bernd Girod
*Department of Electrical Engineering, Stanford University,
Stanford, California*

Nikolaus Färber
*Telecommunications Laboratory, University of Erlangen–Nuremberg,
Erlangen, Germany*

12.1 INTRODUCTION

In the last decade, both mobile communications and multimedia communications
have experienced unequaled rapid growth and commercial success. Naturally, the
great—albeit separate—successes in both areas fuel the old vision of ubiquitous
multimedia communication: being able to communicate from anywhere at any
time with any type of data. The convergence of mobile and multimedia is now under way. Building on advances in network infrastructure, low-power integrated
circuits, and powerful signal processing/compression algorithms, wireless multimedia services will likely find widespread acceptance in the next decade. The
goals of current second-generation cellular and cordless communications standards—supporting integrated voice and data—are being expanded in third-generation wireless networks to provide truly ubiquitous access and integrated
multimedia services. This vision is shared by many. For example, Ericsson's
GSM pioneer Jan Uddenfeldt writes, "The tremendous growth of Internet usage is
the main driver for third-generation wireless. Text, audio, and image (also moving) will be the natural content, i.e., multimedia, for the user" (1).

Video communication is an indispensable modality of multimedia, most
prominently exemplified by the Internet-based World Wide Web today. After the
web browser itself, audio/video streaming decoders have been the most frequently downloaded Internet application, and they will be part of the browser

software by the time this chapter appears in print. Real-time audiovisual communication will also be an integral part of third-generation wireless communication services. The current vision includes a small handheld device that allows the user to communicate from anywhere in the world with anyone in a variety of formats (voice, data, image, and full-motion video). This next generation of wireless multimedia communicators is expected to be equipped with a camera, a microphone, and a liquid crystal color display, serving both as a videophone and computer screen. The conventional laptop keyboard is likely to be replaced by a writing tablet, facilitating optical handwriting recognition and signature verification. With progressing miniaturization of components, wristwatch "Dick Tracy" communicators are expected to follow soon after.

Of all modalities desirable for future mobile multimedia systems, motion video is the most demanding in terms of bit rate, hence is likely to have the strongest impact on network architecture and protocols. Even with state-of-the-art compression, television quality requires a few Megabits per second, while for low-resolution, limited-motion video sequences, as typically encoded for picturephones, a few tens of kilobits per second will give satisfactory picture quality (2). Today's "second-generation" cellular telephony networks, such as Global System for Mobile Communications (GSM), typically provide 10–15 kbit/s, suitable for compressed speech, but too little for motion video. Fortunately, the standardization of higher bandwidth networks, such as Universal Mobile Telecommunications System (UMTS) (3,4), is well under way, and, together with continued progress in video compression technology, wireless multimedia communicators with picturephone functionality and Internet videoserver access will be possible.

Beyond the limited available bit rate, wireless multimedia transmission, an area reviewed recently (5), offers a number of interesting technical challenges. One of the more difficult issues stems from the inability of mobile networks to provide a guaranteed quality of service, because high bit error rates occur during fading periods. Transmission errors of a mobile wireless radio channel range from single bit errors to burst errors or even an intermittent loss of the connection. The classic technique to combat transmission errors is forward error correction (FEC), but its effectiveness is limited because of widely varying error conditions. A worst-case design would lead to a prohibitive amount of redundancy. Closed-loop error control techniques like automatic repeat request (ARQ) (6) have been shown to be more effective than FEC and have been successfully applied to wireless video transmission (7,8). Retransmission of corrupted data frames, however, introduces additional delay, which might be unacceptable for real-time conversational or interactive services. As a result, transmission errors cannot be avoided with a mobile radio channel, even when FEC and ARQ are combined. Therefore, the design of a wireless video system always involves a trade-off between channel coding redundancy that protects the bitstream and source coding redundancy deliberately introduced for greater error resilience of the video decoder.

Without special measures, compressed video signals are extremely vulnerable against transmission errors. Basically, every bit counts. Considering specifically low bit rate video, compression schemes rely on interframe coding for high coding efficiency; that is, they use the previous encoded and reconstructed video frame to predict the next frame. Therefore, the loss of information in one frame has considerable impact on the quality of the following frames. Since some residual transmission errors will inevitably corrupt the video bitstream, this vulnerability precludes the use of low bit rate video coding schemes designed for error-free channels without special measures. These measures must be built into the video coding and decoding algorithms themselves, and they form the "last line of defense" if techniques like FEC and ARQ fail.

A comprehensive review of the great variety of error control and concealment techniques that have been proposed during the last 10–15 years has been presented in an excellent paper by Wang and Zhu (9) and is also included in Chapter 6 of this book. For example, one can partition the bitstream into classes of different error sensitivity (often referred to as data partitioning) to enable the use of unequal error protection (10–12). Data partitioning has been included as an error resilience tool in the MPEG-4 standard (13). Unequal error protection can significantly increase the robustness of the transmission and provide graceful degradation of picture quality in the case of a deteriorating channel. Since unequal error protection does not incorporate information about the current state of the mobile channel, the design of such a scheme is a compromise that accommodates a range of operating conditions. Feedback-based techniques, on the other hand, can adjust to the varying transmission conditions rapidly and make more effective use of the channel. This leads us to the notion of *channel-adaptive source coding.*

ITU-T Study Group 16 has adopted feedback-based error control in their effort toward mobile extensions of the successful Recommendation H.263 (see Chapter 1) for low bit rate video coding. The first version of H.263 already included *error tracking,* a technique that allows the encoder to accurately estimate interframe error propagation and adapt its encoding strategy to mitigate the effects of past transmission errors (14,15). The second version, informally known as H.263+, was adopted by the ITU-T in February 1998. Among many other enhancements, it contains two new optional modes supporting reference picture selection (Annex N) and independent segment decoding (Annex R) as an error confinement technique (16,17). Additional enhancements—for example, data partitioning, unequal error protection, and reversible variable-length coding— are under consideration for future versions of the standard, informally known as H.263++ and H.26L.

Most of the error control schemes for wireless video do not generalize; rather, they are pragmatic engineering solutions to a problem at hand. The tradeoffs in designing the overall transmission chain are not well understood and need further study that ultimately should lead to a general theoretical framework for joint optimization of source coding, channel coding and transport protocols, coding schemes with superior robustness and adaptability to adverse transmission condition, and multimedia-aware transport protocols that make most efficient use of limited wireless network resources. In the meantime, we must be content with more modest goals.

In this chapter, we investigate the performance and trade-offs characteristic of the use of established error control techniques for wireless video. We set the stage by discussing the basic trade-off between source and channel coding redundancy in Section 12.2 and introduce the distortion–distortion function as a formal tool for comparing wireless video systems. In Section 12.3, we briefly discuss how to combat transmission errors by channel coding and illustrate the problems that are encountered with classic FEC applied to a fading channel. We also discuss error amplification that can occur with IP packetization over wireless channels. In Section 12.4, we discuss error resilience techniques for low bit rate video, with particular emphasis on techniques adopted by the ITU-T as part of the H.263 Recommendation. These techniques include feedback-based error control, yielding in effect a channel-adaptive H.263 encoder. The various approaches are compared by means of their operational distortion–distortion function under the same experimental conditions.

12.2 TRADING OFF SOURCE AND CHANNEL CODING

Naturally, the problem of transmitting video over noisy channels involves both source and channel coding. The classic goal of source coding is to achieve the lowest possible distortion for a given target bit rate. This goal has a fundamental limit in the rate distortion bound for given source statistics. The source-coded bitstream then needs to be transmitted reliably over a noisy channel. Similar to the rate distortion bound in source coding, the channel capacity quantifies the maximum rate at which information can be transmitted reliably over the given channel. Hence, the classic goal of channel coding is to deliver reliable information at a rate that is as close as possible to the channel capacity. According to Shannon's *separation principle,* it is possible to independently consider source and channel coding without loss in performance (18). However, this important information-theoretic result is based on several assumptions that might break down in practice. In particular, it is based on (a) the assumption of an infinite block length for both source and channel coding (hence infinite delay) and (b) an exact and complete knowledge of the statistics of the transmission channel. As a corollary of (b), the separation principle applies only to point-to-point communications and is not valid for multiuser or broadcast scenarios (18). Therefore, *joint source–channel coding* (JSC coding) can be advantageous in practice.

A joint optimization of source and channel coding can be achieved by exploiting the redundancy in the source signal for channel decoding (*source-controlled channel decoding:* see, e.g., Ref. 19) or by designing the source codec for a given channel characteristic (*channel-optimized source coding:* see, e.g., Ref. 20). In either case, source and channel coding can hardly be separated anymore and are truly optimized jointly. Unfortunately, joint source–channel coding schemes for video are in their infancy today. A pragmatic approach for today's state-of-the-art is to keep the source coder and the channel coder separate, but optimize their parameters jointly. This approach is followed in this chapter. A key problem of this optimization is the bit allocation between the source and channel coder, as discussed below. To illustrate the problem, we first consider the typical components of a wireless video system. For more information on separate, concatenated, and joint source–channel coding for wireless video see Reference 21.

12.2.1 Components of a Wireless Video System

Figure 12.1 shows the basic components of a wireless video system. The space–time discrete input video signal $i[x, y, t]$ is fed into a video encoder. The video encoder is characterized by its operational distortion–rate function $D_e(R_e)$, where $e[x, y, t]$ is the reconstructed video signal at the encoder, and R_e and D_e are the average rate and average distortion, respectively. After source coding, the compressed video bitstream is prepared for transmission over a network.

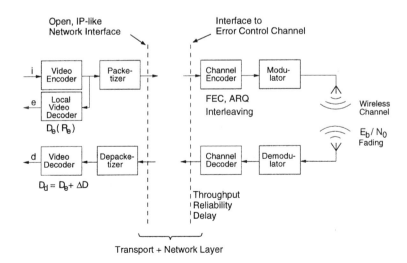

Figure 12.1   Basic components of a video transmission system.

Often, this involves packetization. This is particularly the case for transmission employing the Internet Protocol (IP). The correct delivery of packets requires a multitude of functionalities that need to be provided by the network, such as routing, handover, packet fragmentation and reassembly, and flow control. These functionalities are covered in Chapter 3, and, for now, we assume that the corresponding protocol layers are transparent and do not introduce losses. In practice, this assumption is not always justified, and thus we revisit this issue in Section 12.3.4.

In wireless video systems, the end-to-end transmission typically comprises one or two wireless radio extensions to a wired backbone, at the beginning and/or the end of a transmission chain. Therefore, the packetized bitstream is transmitted at least once over a wireless channel as illustrated in Figure 12.1. In contrast to the wired backbone, the capacity of the wireless channel is fundamentally limited by the available bandwidth of the radio spectrum and various types of noise and interference. Therefore, the wireless channel can be regarded as the "weakest link" of future multimedia networks; hence it requires special attention, especially if mobility gives rise to fading and error bursts. The resulting transmission errors require *error control* techniques. A classic technique is FEC, which can be combined with *interleaving* to reduce the effect of burst errors. On the other hand, closed-loop error control techniques like ARQ are particularly attractive if the error conditions vary in a wide range. These error control techniques are part of the channel codec and are discussed in more detail in Section 12.3.

The bitstream produced by the channel encoder is represented by an analog signal waveform suitable for the transmission channel by the modulator. The power of the channel noise that is superimposed to the transmitted signal must be evaluated with respect to the energy that is used for the transmission of each bit. Therefore, the ratio of bit energy to noise spectral density (E_b/N_o) is often used to characterize the noisiness of the channel. Other parameters that describe the correlation of errors are also of importance. After demodulation, the channel decoder tries to recover from transmission errors by exploiting the error correction capability of the FEC scheme or by requesting a retransmission of corrupted data frames.

The term *error control channel* refers to the combination of the channel codec, the modulator/demodulator (modem), and the physical channel (22). Ideally, the error control channel would provide an error-free binary link with a guaranteed bit rate and maximum delay to the video codec. However, as we will see in Section 12.3, the effectiveness of channel coding is limited in a mobile environment when data must be transmitted with low delay. Essentially, only a compromise between *reliability, throughput,* and *delay* can be achieved. This fundamental trade-off is typical for the communication over noisy channels and must be considered for the design of wireless video systems.

Because the error control channel must balance reliability, throughput, and delay, some residual transmission errors usually remain after channel decoding, especially for low-latency applications. In this case, the video decoder must be capable of processing an erroneous bitstream. The residual errors cause an additional distortion ΔD such that the decoded video signal $d[x, y, t]$ contains the total average distortion $D_d = D_e + \Delta D$.

12.2.2 Distortion Measures

For a quantitative analysis of wireless video systems, we require measures for the video signal distortion introduced by the source encoder (D_e) or the distortion at the output of the video decoder (D_d). Clearly, since the decoded video signal is ultimately played back to a human observer, a distortion measure should be consistent with the perceived subjective quality. In practice, the most common distortion measure for video coding is *mean-squared error* (MSE). Though notorious for its flaws as a measure of subjective picture quality, MSE provides consistent results as long as the video signals to be compared are affected by the same type of impairment (23). For example, the subjective quality produced by a particular video codec at two different bit rates for the same input signal can usually be compared by MSE measurements because both decoded signals contain similar quantization and blocking artifacts. Hence, we define the distortion at the encoder as follows:

$$D_e = \frac{1}{XYT}\sum_{x=1}^{X}\sum_{y=1}^{Y}\sum_{t=1}^{T}(i[x,y,t] - e[x,y,t])^2 \tag{1}$$

for a frame size of $X \times Y$ pixels and T encoded video frames. If the distortion is to be calculated for individual frames, we can obtain $D_e[t]$ by calculating the MSE for each frame separately.

The obvious approach to measuring the distortion at the decoder after transmission is to calculate the MSE between the received video signal $d[x, y, t]$ and the original video signal $i[x, y, t]$. In fact, this is frequently done in the literature to evaluate video transmission systems (24–26). The probabilistic nature of the channel forces one to consider the distortion averaged over many different realizations of the channel. For a particular constellation of the wireless video system (i.e., FEC rate, E_b/N_0, encoding parameters of video codec, . . .), we therefore obtain decoded signals for each realization l, denoted as $d_l[x, y, t]$. Assuming L realizations, the MSE at the decoder is then calculated as follows:

$$D_d = \frac{1}{XYTL}\sum_{x=1}^{X}\sum_{y=1}^{Y}\sum_{t=1}^{T}\sum_{l=1}^{L}(i[x,y,t] - d_l[x,y,t])^2 \tag{2}$$

Sometimes it is necessary to also calculate the distortion D_e at the encoder by averaging over many realizations of the channel, similar to Eq. (2). In particular, this is the case for channel-adaptive source coding, where the operation of the encoder depends on the behavior of the channel as discussed in Section 12.4.

Note that two types of distortion appear in the decoded video signal d: the distortion due to source coding and the distortion caused by transmission errors. While the former is adequately described by D_e, we define

$$\Delta D = D_d - D_e \tag{3}$$

to describe the latter. Typically, D_e is the result of small quantization errors that are evenly distributed over all encoded frames, while ΔD is dominated by strong errors that are concentrated in a small part of the picture and are (hopefully!) present only for a short time. Because such errors are perceived very differently, an average measure such as D_d alone can be misleading if not applied carefully. Instead, both D_e and ΔD should be considered for the evaluation of video quality simultaneously, as discussed in the next section.

Before concluding this section, we note that MSE is commonly converted to peak signal-to-noise ratio (PSNR) in the video coding community. PSNR is defined as $10 \log_{10}(255^2/\text{MSE})$, where 255 corresponds to the peak-to-peak range of the encoded and decoded video signal (each quantized to 256 levels). It is expressed in decibels (dB) and increases with increasing picture quality. Though the logarithmic scale provides a better correlation with subjective quality, the same limitations as for MSE apply. As a rule of thumb for low bit rate video coding (with clearly visible distortions), a difference of 1 dB generally corresponds to a noticeable difference, while acceptable picture quality requires values greater than 30 dB. Since PSNR is more commonly used than MSE, we will use Eqs. (4)–(6) instead of Eqs. (1)–(3) in our presentations of experimental results.

$$\text{PSNR}_e = 10 \log_{10} \frac{255^2}{D_e} \tag{4}$$

$$\text{PSNR}_d = 10 \log_{10} \frac{255^2}{D_d} \tag{5}$$

$$\Delta \text{PSNR} = \text{PSNR}_e - \text{PSNR}_d = 10 \log_{10} \frac{D_e}{D_d} = 10 \log_{10} \frac{D_e}{D_e + \Delta D} \tag{6}$$

Now, after having defined the necessary distortion measures, we return to the problem of bit allocation between source and channel coding by introducing the distortion–distortion function.

12.2.3 Distortion–Distortion Function

Consider again the wireless video transmission system illustrated in Figure 12.1. Assume that a modulation scheme is used that provides a constant "raw" bit rate R_c. By operating the video encoder at a bit rate $R_e \leq R_c$, the remaining bit rate $R_c - R_e$ can be utilized for error control information to increase the reliability of the transmission. Thus, the *residual word error rate* (RWER), which describes the probability of residual errors after channel decoding, is reduced. As noted above, there is a fundamental trade-off between throughput and reliability, corresponding to the bit allocation between source and channel coding characterized by the code rate $r = R_e/R_c$.

Altering the bit allocation between source and channel coding has two effects on the picture quality of the video signal d at the decoder output. First, a reduction of r reduces the bit rate available to the video encoder and thus degrades the picture quality at the encoder regardless of transmission errors. The actual $PSNR_e$ reduction is determined by the operational distortion rate function $D_e(R_e)$ of the video encoder. On the other hand, the residual error rate is reduced in connection with the reduction of r, determined by the properties of the error control channel, that is, the channel codec, the modulation scheme, and the characteristic of the channel. Finally, a reduction in RWER leads to a reduction in $\Delta PSNR$ depending on several implementation issues, such as resynchronization, packetization, and error concealment, all of which are associated with the video decoder. The interaction of the various characteristics are illustrated in Figure 12.2. The upper right-hand graph shows the resulting trade-off between $PSNR_e$ and $\Delta PSNR$ and provides a compact overview of the overall system behavior. Because the curve shows the dependency between two distortion measures, we refer to it as the operational *distortion–distortion function* (DDF). Note that the overall picture quality at the decoder, $PSNR_d$, increases from top left to bottom right as illustrated in Figure 12.2. Therefore, if desired, DDFs can also be used to evaluate the overall distortion.

The DDF is a useful tool to study the influence of parameters or algorithms in the video codec for a given error control channel. Instead of building a combined distortion measure, both distortion types are available to evaluate the resulting system performance without additional assumptions with respect to how they are to be combined, as long as subjective quality decreases with both increasing D_e and increasing ΔD.

As pointed out in Section 12.2.2, D_e is a useful distortion measure for source coding as long as the video signal is impaired by the same kind of distortion. More formally, let Q be the average subjective video quality as perceived by a representative group of test persons. For D_e to be useful for coder optimization, we require that $Q \approx f(D_e)$ for the set of impaired video sequences considered, where $f(.)$ is a monotonically decreasing function. The exact form of $f(.)$ is

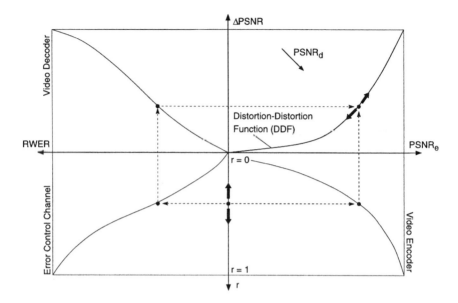

Figure 12.2 Interaction of system components when the bit allocation is varied be-tween source and channel coding, characterized by the channel code rate r. PRNR$_e$ is the picture quality after encoding and ΔPSNR is the loss of picture quality caused by residual errors. An important system parameter of the error control channel is the residual word er-ror rate (RWER). The upper right-hand curve is the distortion–distortion function (DDF) of the wireless video system and is a compact description of the overall performance.

irrelevant. With a similar argument, ΔD is useful to optimize the error control channel and the video decoder, if the subjective quality $Q \approx g(\Delta D)$, where $g(.)$ is monotonically decreasing.

For the joint optimization of source and channel coding, we require a sub-jective quality function $Q \approx h(D_e, \Delta D)$ that captures the superposition of the two different types of distortion. Unfortunately, measuring $h(., .)$ would require te-dious subjective tests, and no such tests have been carried out to the authors' best knowledge. Nevertheless, we can safely assume that $h(., .)$ would be monotoni-cally decreasing with D_e and ΔD, and, fortunately, this monotonicity condition is often all we need when using DDFs to evaluate and compare error resilience techniques. In many situations, DDFs to be compared do not intersect in a wide range of D_d and ΔD. In this case it is possible to pick the best scheme for any $Q \approx h(D_e, \Delta D)$ as long as the monotonicity condition holds. This greatly simplifies the evaluation of video transmission systems, since the difficult question of a combined subjective quality measure for source coding and transmission error distortion is circumvented.

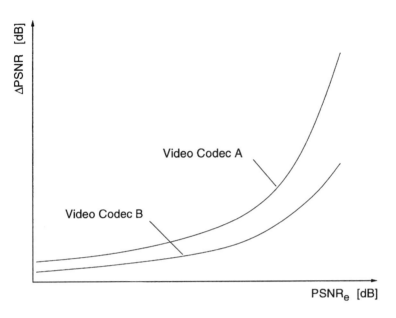

Figure 12.3 DDF of two video codecs. Because codec B consistently provides a smaller PSNR loss (ΔPSNR) for the same picture quality at the encoder (PSNR$_e$), it is the superior scheme.

Figure 12.3 illustrates two typical DDFs using PSNR$_e$ and ΔPSNR as a quality measure. Because video codec B consistently suffers a smaller PSNR loss as a result of transmission errors, it is the better choice. Note that DDFs do *not* solve the problem of optimum bit allocation between source and channel coding, since this requires the knowledge of $h(.,.)$. In practical system design, the best bit allocation can be determined in a final subjective test, where different systems are presented that sample the best obtained DDF.

12.3 COMBATING TRANSMISSION ERRORS

Before discussing error resilience techniques in the video encoder and decoder, we provide an introduction to error control techniques in the channel codec. Because the characteristics of the physical channel play an important role, we consider first the properties of the mobile radio channel and the issue of modulation. For error control, we focus on Reed–Solomon codes, interleaving, and automatic repeat request. Because of the increasing importance of open, Internet-style packet networks, we also consider the effect of packetization, which can cause error amplification.

The following discussion also includes a description of the simulation environment that is used throughout this chapter. For modulation and channel coding we use standard components rather than advanced coding and modulation techniques. This is justified by our focus on video coding and by the fact that the selected standard components are well suited to illustrate the basic problems and trade-offs. Most of the conclusions that are derived in later sections also apply to other scenarios because the underlying concepts are very general. For more information on coding and modulation techniques that are employed in the next generation mobile networks, we refer to Chapter 5 (Wireless Systems and Networking). These are not discussed in detail below because the interface to the error control channel will behave similarly, resulting in similar problems and solutions on the source coding level.

12.3.1 Characteristics of the Mobile Radio Channel

The mobile radio channel is a hostile medium. Besides absorption, the propagation of electromagnetic waves is influenced by three basic mechanisms: reflection, diffraction, and scattering. In conjunction with mobility of the transmitter and/or receiver, these mechanisms cause several phenomena, such as time-varying delay spread or spectral broadening, which can severely impair the transmission. These are briefly discussed in the following. More information can be found in Chapter 5 and in References 27–29. This section shows that the underlying physical mechanisms result in fundamental performance limits for wireless transmission. As a result, the use of error control techniques in the video codec is of increased importance.

When a mobile terminal moves within a larger area, the distance between the radio transmitter and receiver often varies significantly. Furthermore, the number and type of objects between transmitter and receiver usually changes and might cause *shadowing*. The resulting attenuation of radio frequency (RF) power is described by the *path loss*. In an outdoor environment, the path loss is affected by hills, forests, or buildings. In an indoor environment, the electromagnetic properties of blocking walls and ceilings are of importance. The effect of these objects and the distance to the transmitter can be described by empirical models (27,29). Usually, these models include a mean path loss as a function of distance (nth power law) and a random variation about that mean (log-normal distribution). For our experimental results in this chapter we assume that the path loss is constant for the duration of a simulation (approximately 10 seconds), hence assume constant (average) E_b/N_0.

Besides *large-scale fading* as described by path loss, small changes in position can result in dramatic variations of RF energy. This *small-scale fading* is a characteristic effect in mobile radio communication and is caused by *multipath propagation*. In a wireless communication system, a signal can travel from transmitter to receiver over multiple reflective paths. Each reflection arrives from a different direction with a different delay, hence, for a narrowband signal, undergoes a different attenuation and phase shift. The superposition of these individual signal components can cause constructive and destructive interference alternating at a small scale (as small as half a wavelength). For a moving receiver, this space-variant signal strength is perceived as a time-variant channel, where the velocity of the mobile terminal determines the speed of fluctuation. Small-scale fading is often associated with *Rayleigh fading* because, if the multiple reflective paths are large in number and equally significant, the envelope of the received signal is described by a Rayleigh probability density function (pdf).

An important problem caused by multipath propagation is *delay spread*. For a single transmitted impulse, the time T_m between the first and last received components of significant amplitude represents the *maximum excess delay*, which is an important parameter for the characterization of the channel. If T_m is bigger than the symbol duration T_s, neighboring symbols interfere with each other, causing *intersymbol interference* (ISI). This channel type requires special mitigation techniques such as equalization and is not considered further here. Instead, we focus on *flat fading* channels, with $T_m < T_s$. In this case, all the received multipath components of a symbol arrive within the symbol duration and no ISI is present. Here, the main degradation is the destructive superposition of phasor components, which can yield a substantial reduction in signal amplitude. Note, however, that the error resilience techniques described in Section 12.4 are also applicable to ISI channels given appropriate channel coding.

Similar to the delay spread in the time domain, the received signal can also be spread in the frequency domain. For a single transmitted sinusoid, the receiver may observe multiple signals at shifted frequency positions. This *spectral broadening* is caused by the Doppler shift of an electromagnetic wave observed from a moving object. The amount of shift for each reflective path depends on the incident direction relative to the velocity vector of the receiver. The maximum shift magnitude is called the Doppler frequency f_D, which is equal to the mobile velocity divided by the carrier wavelength. For the dense-scatterer model, which assumes a uniform distribution of reflections from all directions, the resulting *Doppler power spectrum* has a typical bowl-shaped characteristic with maximum frequency f_D [also known as the Jakes spectrum (28)]. This model is frequently used in the literature to simulate the mobile radio channel and is also used in this chapter. Note that the Doppler power spectrum has an important influence on the time-variant behavior of the channel because it is directly related to the temporal correlation of the received signal amplitude via the

Fourier transform. For a given carrier frequency, the correlation increases with decreasing mobile velocity, such that slowly moving terminals encounter longer fades (and error bursts). Therefore, f_D is often used to characterize how rapidly the fading amplitude changes.

In summary, mobile radio transmission must cope with time-varying channel conditions of both large and small scale. These variations are mainly caused by the motion of the transmitter or the receiver resulting in propagation path changes. As a result, errors are not limited to single bit errors but tend to occur in bursts. In severe fading situations the loss of synchronization may even cause an intermittent loss of the connection. As we will see, this property makes it difficult to design error control techniques that provide high reliability at high throughput and low delay.

12.3.2 Modulation

Since we cannot feed bits to the antenna directly, an appropriate digital modulation scheme is needed. Usually, a sinusoidal carrier wave of frequency f_c is modified in amplitude, phase, and/or frequency depending on the digital data that shall be transmitted. This results in three basic modulation techniques, known as amplitude shift keying (ASK), frequency shift keying (FSK), and phase shift keying (PSK). However, other schemes and hybrids are also popular. In general, the modem operates at a fixed symbol rate R_s, such that its output signal is cyclostationary with the symbol interval $T_s = 1/R_s$. In the most basic case, one symbol corresponds to one bit. For example, binary PSK (BPSK) uses two waveforms with identical amplitude and frequency but a phase shift of 180 degrees. Higher order modulation schemes can choose from a larger set of waveforms, hence can provide higher bit rates for the same symbol interval, but they are also less robust against noise for the same average transmission power.

The choice of a modulation scheme is a key issue in the design of a mobile communication system because each scheme possesses different performance characteristics. In most cases, however, the selection of a modulation scheme reduces to a consideration of the power and bandwidth availability in the intended application. For example, in cellular telephony the principal design goal is the minimization of spectral occupancy by a single user, such that the number of paying customers is maximized for the allocated radio spectrum. Thus, an issue of increasing importance for cellular systems is to select bandwidth-efficient modulation schemes. On the other hand, the lifetime of a portable battery also limits the energy that can be used for the transmission of each bit, E_b; hence power efficiency is also of importance. A detailed discussion of modulation techniques is beyond the scope of this chapter, and the reader is referred to References 30 and 31 for detailed information.

We conclude this section by describing the modulation scheme and para-meters that are used for simulations in this chapter. Some of the modem parameters are motivated by the radio communication system DECT (digital enhanced cordless telecommunications). Though DECT is a standard originally intended by the European Telecommunications Standards Institute (ETSI) for cordless telephony, it provides a wide range of services for cordless personal communications, which makes it very attractive for mobile multimedia applications (29,32). Similar to DECT, we use BPSK for modulation and a carrier frequency of f_c = 1900 MHz. For moderate speeds (35 km/h) a typical Doppler frequency is f_D = 62 Hz, which is used for the simulations in the remainder of this chapter. According to the double-slot format of DECT, we assume a total bit rate of R_c = 80 kbit/s, which is available for both source and channel coding. For simplicity we do not assume any TDMA structure and use a symbol interval of T_s = 1/80 ms. Note that the Doppler frequency f_D and T_s determine the correlation of bit errors at the demodulator. Example bit error sequences shown in Figure 12.4 exhibit severe burst errors.

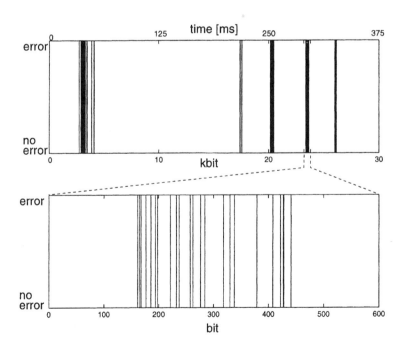

Figure 12.4 Illustration of burst errors encountered for Rayleigh fading channel (Doppler frequency f_D = 62 Hz, E_b/N_0 = 18 dB) and BPSK modulation (symbol interval T_s = 1/80 ms).

12.3.3   Channel Coding and Error Control

In this section, we discuss two main categories of channel coding and error control: FEC and ARQ. The latter requires a feedback channel to transmit retransmission requests, while FEC has no such requirement. We also address interleaving as a way to enhance FEC in the presence of burst errors. In the following we discuss the trade-off between *throughput, reliability,* and *delay* of the error control channel and present some simulation results for illustration.

12.3.3.1   Forward Error Correction.
FEC techniques fall in two broad categories: block coding and convolutional coding. Though they are very different in detail, they follow the same basic principle.

At the transmitter, parity check information is inserted into the bitstream such that the receiver can detect and possibly correct errors that occur during transmission. The amount of redundancy is usually expressed in terms of the *channel code rate r,* which takes on values between zero (no payload information) and one (no redundancy). Though convolutional codes are as important in practice as block codes, we will use block codes to explain and illustrate the performance of FEC.

For block coding, the bitstream is grouped into blocks of k bits. Then, redundancy is added by mapping k information bits to a *codeword* containing $n > k$ bits. Thus, the code rate of block codes is given by $r = k/n$. The set of 2^k codewords is called the *channel code C(n, k).* For a *systematic code,* the k information bits are not altered and $n - k$ check bits are simply appended to the payload bits. Decoding is achieved by determining the most likely transmitted codeword, given a received block of n bits.

The error correction capability of a $C(n, k)$ code is primarily influenced by the *minimum Hamming distance* d_{min}. The Hamming distance of two binary codewords is the number of bits in which they differ. For a code with minimum Hamming distance d_{min}, the number of bit errors that can be corrected is at least

$$t = \lfloor (d_{min} - 1)/2 \rfloor$$

Therefore, the design of codes (i.e., the selection of 2^k codewords from the set of 2^n possible codewords) is an important issue, since d_{min} should be as large as possible. For large n, this is not straightforward, especially when the problem of decoding is considered, as well. Furthermore, there are fundamental limits in the maximization of d_{min}, such as the *Singleton bound*

$$d_{min} \le n - k + 1$$

Fortunately, channel coding is a mature discipline that has come up with many elegant and clever methods for the nontrivial tasks of code design and decoding algorithms. In the following, we limit the discussion to *Reed–Solomon* (RS) codes as a particularly useful class of block codes that actually achieve the Singleton bound. Other block codes of practical importance include Bose–Chaudhuri–Hocquenghem (BCH), Reed–Muller, and Golay codes (22).

Reed–Solomon codes are used in many applications, ranging from the compact disc (CD) to mobile radio communications (e.g., DECT). Their popularity is due to their flexibility and excellent error correction capabilities. RS codes are nonbinary block codes that operate on multibit symbols rather than individual bits. If a symbol is composed of m bits, the RS encoder for an $RS(N, K)$ code groups the incoming data stream into blocks of K information symbols (Km bits) and appends $N - K$ parity symbols to each block. For RS codes operating on m-bit symbols, the maximum block length is $N_{max} = 2^m - 1$. By using *shortened* RS codes, any smaller value for N can be selected, which provides a great flexibility in system design. Additionally, K can be chosen flexibly, allowing a wide range of code rates. Later on, we will take advantage of this flexibility to investigate different bit allocations between source and channel coding.

Let us now consider the error correction capability of an $RS(N, K)$ code. Let E be the number of corrupted symbols in a block containing N symbols. Note that a symbol is corrupted when any of its m bits is in error. Though this seems to be a drawback for single bit errors, it can actually be advantageous for the correction of burst errors, as typically encountered in the mobile radio channel. As RS codes achieve the Singleton bound, the minimum number of correctable errors is given by

$$T = \lfloor (N - K)/2 \rfloor$$

and the RS decoder can correct any pattern of symbol errors as long as $E \le T$. In other words, for every two additional parity symbols, an additional symbol error can be corrected. If more than E symbol errors are contained in a block, the RS decoder can usually detect the error. For large blocks, undetected errors are very improbable, especially when the decoder backs off from the Singleton bound for error correction (*bounded distance decoding*). The probability that a block cannot be corrected is usually described by the *residual word error rate* (RWER). In general, the RWER decreases with increasing K and with increasing E_b/N_0.

The performance of RS codes for the mobile radio channel discussed previously is shown in Figure 12.5. On the left we show the RWER for a variation of r. For a given value of E_b/N_0, the RWER can be reduced by approximately one to two orders of magnitude by varying the code rate in the illustrated range. This gain in RWER is very moderate owing the bursty nature of the wireless channel. For channels without memory, such as the additive white Gaussian noise (AWGN) channel, the same reduction in r would provide a significantly higher reduction in RWER. In this case it is possible to achieve very high reliability (RWER < 10^{-6}) with only little parity-check information, and resilience tech-

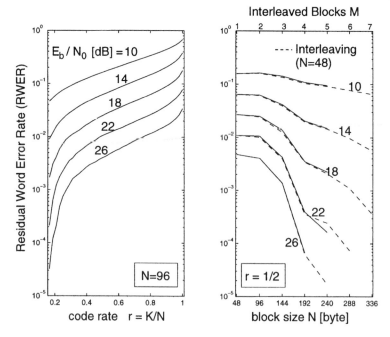

Figure 12.5 Residual word error rate (RWER) for the variation of channel code rate r (left) and block size N (right). Rayleigh fading with BPSK modulation and Reed–Solomon codes operating on 8-bit symbols are assumed.

niques in the video codec would hardly be necessary. For bursty channels, however, the effectiveness of FEC is limited because the error correction capability is often exceeded when a block is affected by a burst. Note that the left-hand side of Figure 12.5 illustrates the trade-off between throughput (r) and reliability (1-RWER) of the error control channel.

The right-hand side of Figure 12.5 shows the RWER for a variation of the block length N. The dashed lines are considered later. From the solid lines it can be seen that the increase in block length can be very effective for high E_b/N_0. Note that the throughput is not affected, since the code rate is kept constant at $r = 1/2$. However, the trade-off between *reliability* (1-RWER) and delay (N) must be considered in the choosing of N. On the one hand, the error correction capability of a block code increases with the block length. On the other hand, long blocks introduce additional delay (assuming constant code rate and source rate). Usually the acceptable delay is determined by the application. For file transfer, high delays in the order of several seconds are acceptable. For conversational services, such as voice or video telephony, a maximum round-trip delay of 250 ms should not be exceeded. For low-delay video applications, the frame interval usually sets the upper bound. For example, assuming 12.5 frames/s video and a total bit rate of $R_c = 80$ kbit/s, the resulting maximum block length is $n = 6400$ bits. However, shorter blocks are preferable because other effects also contribute to the overall delay.

Besides the limitations on N imposed by delay considerations, there are implementation and complexity constraints. In particular the *decoding* of block codes in case of errors is a task that becomes computationally demanding for large N. The number of bits that are combined to symbols in RS codes is usually less than and most commonly equal to 8, thus allowing a maximum block length of $N_{max} = 2^m - 1 = 255$ bytes.

Note that a limited block length can cause severe problems for FEC schemes when the transmission channel tends to burst errors. Either a block is affected by a burst, in which case the error correction capability is often exceeded, or the block is transmitted error-free and the additional redundancy is wasted. To overcome this limitation, FEC is often enhanced by the technique known as *interleaving*.

12.3.3.2 Interleaving.

The idea behind interleaving is to spread the error burst in time. In a simple block interleaver, encoded blocks of N symbols are loaded into a rectangular matrix row by row. After M rows have been collected, the symbols are read out column by column for transmission. At the receiver, this reordering of symbols is inverted and the blocks are passed to the FEC decoder. For burst errors, this effectively reduces the concentration of errors in single code words; that is, a burst of b consecutive symbol errors causes a maximum of b/M symbol errors in each code word. For large M, the interleaver–deinterleaver pair thus creates in effect a memoryless channel. Though interleaving can be implemented with low complexity, it suffers from increased delay, depending on the number of interleaved blocks M. The dashed lines on the right-hand side of Figure 12.5 illustrate the effectiveness of interleaving in the given error control channel. As the basic block length we use $N = 48$ symbols. For the same delay, essentially the same performance can be achieved as for increased block length, providing the same trade-off between reliability and delay. However, also larger blocks than $N_{max} = 255$ can be obtained at reduced complexity. Therefore interleaving is a frequently used technique for bursty channels if the additional delay is acceptable.

12.3.3.3 Automatic Repeat Request.

Another error control technique that can be used to exchange reliability for delay and throughput is *automatic repeat request* (ARQ). In contrast to FEC, ARQ requires a feedback channel from the receiver to the transmitter and therefore cannot be used in systems that do not have such a channel available (e.g., broadcasting).

For ARQ, the incoming bitstream is grouped into blocks, similar to FEC.

Each block is extended by a header including a *sequence number* (SN) and an error detection code at the end of each block—often a *cyclic redundancy check* (CRC). This information is used at the receiver for error detection and to request the retransmission of corrupted blocks using *positive acknowledgments* (ACKs) and/or *negative acknowledgments* (NACKs), which are sent back via the feedback channel. Usually, retransmissions are repeated until error-free data are received or a time-out is exceeded.

This basic operation can be implemented in various forms with different implications on throughput, complexity, and delay. There are three basic ARQ schemes in use: *stop and wait* (SW), *go back N* (GN), and *selective repeat* (SR) (6). Though SR-ARQ requires buffering and reordering of out-of-sequence blocks, it provides the highest throughput. Another possible means of enhancing ARQ schemes is the combination with FEC, which is known as *hybrid ARQ*. For a detailed analysis of throughput the reader is referred to References 22 and 33, both of which also consider the case of noisy feedback channels. Furthermore, the application of ARQ in fading channels is analyzed in Reference 34, while Reference 35 proposes an ARQ protocol that adapts to a variable error rate by switching between two modes.

One critical issue in ARQ is delay, because the duration between retransmission attempts is determined by the *round-trip delay* (RTD). Thus, if the number of necessary retransmission attempts is A, the total delay until reception is at least $D = A \cdot \text{RTD}$. Since A depends on the quality of the channel, the resulting delay and throughput are not predictable and vary over time. For applications in which delay is not critical, ARQ is an elegant and efficient error control technique, and it has been used extensively [e.g., in the *Transport Control Protocol* (TCP) of the Internet]. For real-time video transmission, however, the delay associated with classic ARQ techniques is often unacceptable.

The situation has improved slightly in the past few years through delay-constrained or *soft* ARQ protocols. One simple approach to limit delay with ARQ is to allow at most $A = D/\text{RTD}$ retransmissions, where D is the maximum acceptable delay. Because this may result in residual errors, the trade-off between *reliability* and *delay* must be considered. A given maximum delay constraint can also be met by adjusting the source rate of the video codec. If a close interaction between source and channel coding is possible, the rate of the video codec can be directly controlled by the currently available throughput (36,37). The effectiveness of this approach for wireless video transmission over DECT was demonstrated as long ago as 1992 (7). If such a close interaction is not possible, scalable video coding must be used (8,38,39). Other refinements of ARQ schemes proposed for video include the retransmission of more strongly compressed video (40) or the retransmission of multiple copies (9) in a packet network. Nevertheless, ARQ can be used only for applications with relatively large acceptable delay and/or very low RTDs—or limited reliability.

12.3.4   IP over Wireless

Future wireless video applications will have to work over an open, layered, Internet-style network with a wired backbone and wireless extensions. Therefore, common protocols will have to be used for the transmission across the wired and wireless portions of the network. These protocols will most likely be future refinements and extensions of today's protocols built around the Internet Protocol. One issue that arises when operating IP over a wireless radio link is that of *fragmentation and reassembly* of IP packets. Because wireless radio networks typically use frame sizes that are a lot smaller than the maximum IP packet size, big IP packets must be fragmented into several smaller blocks for transmission and reassembled again at the receiving network node. Unfortunately, if any one of the small blocks is corrupted, the original big packet will be dropped completely, thus increasing the effective packet loss rate. One way to avoid fragmentation is to use the minimum packet size along the path from the transmitter to the receiver. However, this information is usually not available at the terminal. Furthermore, the overhead of the IP packet headers (typically 48 bytes with IP/UDP/RTP) may become prohibitive.

The resulting error amplification is illustrated in Figure 12.6 for the investigated error control channel, where the fragments of the IP packet are mapped to FEC blocks. Clearly, the packet error rate increases with the number of blocks

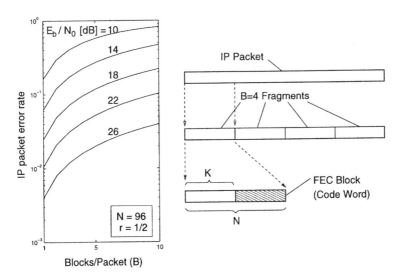

Figure 12.6   Packet error rate after fragmentation and reassembly of an IP packet into *B* blocks. Rayleigh fading with BPSK modulation and Reed–Solomon codes operating on 8-bit symbols are assumed.

that are necessary to convey the original packet. This problem must be considered for the design of future multimedia-aware protocols (e.g., by allowing corrupt fragments within the reassembled IP packet, which are indicated in the header). However, we will not further discuss problems that arise from intermediate network layers. Here, our intention is merely to point out that the avoidance of unnecessary performance degradation calls for consideration of certain important protocol enhancements.

12.4 ERROR RESILIENCE TECHNIQUES FOR LOW BIT RATE VIDEO

In this section we focus on error resilience techniques that can be used in the video codec to improve the overall performance. As an example, we use the important H.263 video compression standard. Most of the ideas discussed can also be applied to other video coding algorithms, and are also covered in Chapter 8 (Error Resilience Coding). We assume that the reader is familiar with the basic concepts and terms of the H.263 video compression standard. For a review, refer to the chapters of Part 1 of this book or to the literature (41,42).

Although we restrict our investigation to methods that are supported by the current H.263 syntax, it is still very difficult to provide a complete analysis. On the one hand, H.263 includes various optional coding modes that can be used for error resilience in many combinations. On the other hand, the operation of the encoder is not standardized, such that the present syntax can be used in a very flexible way. The clever combination of existing options that may not even be intended for error resilience can significantly increase the performance of a wireless video system. Furthermore, the operation of the decoder in the case of errors is not covered by the current version of the H.263 standard. Although ITU-T Study Group 16 intends to include error detection and error concealment in future versions of Recommendation H.263, this area is not covered at present, and the performance of the decoder therefore depends heavily on a particular implementation. Because of this flexibility in mode combinations and decoder operation, we can discuss only the most common and effective error resilience techniques.

12.4.1 Input Format and Rate Control

To achieve high compression, as required for transmission over mobile radio channels at low bit rates, both the spatial resolution and the frame rate must be reduced compared to standard television pictures. We use QCIF (Quarter Common Intermediate Format, 176 × 144 pixels) for our simulations, which is the most common input format at the range of bit rates considered. As a typical frame rate we use 12.5 frames/s. Though a variable frame rate in the range of

5–15 frames/s may be advantageous for subjective quality, we maintain a fixed rate of 12.5 to allow a fair comparison between different approaches based on PSNR values. Unless otherwise stated, we use sequences of 300 frames (i.e., 150 encoded frames covering a time period of 12 seconds). Because the transmission over an unreliable channel introduces random errors, several simulations are performed for different channel realizations to obtain averaged results according to Eq. (2). For each investigated error resilience technique and parameter setting (FEC, E_b/N_0, Intra percentage, . . .) we use $L = 30$ channel realizations.

We use a simple rate control in our simulations. Each frame is encoded with a fixed quantizer step size, which is adapted frame by frame to obtain a given target bit rate. The adaptation of the quantizer step size is performed as follows. First the mode decision is performed according to TMN5 (43) for the whole frame, and then the resulting prediction error is transformed and quantized with different quantizer step sizes. Finally, the value that minimizes the deviation from a desired buffer fullness is selected. This rate control reduces buffer variations to an acceptable amount, hence allows the transmission over a constant bit rate channel with limited delay. In practice, more sophisticated quantizer control algorithms could be used that can further reduce buffer fluctuations at improved rate distortion performance. For more information on rate control algorithms and their implications on performance and delay, see Chapter 9 (Variable Bit Rate Video Coding).

12.4.2 Error Detection and Resynchronization

Transmission errors can be detected in a variety of ways. With FEC, errors can often be detected with high reliability by the channel decoder, even if the correction capability of the code is exceeded. For example, H.261 and H.263 allow the use of an optional FEC framing to detect errors within a BCH(511,493) codeword. If a packet protocol stack such as IP is used, lower layers often provide error detection as a basic service. For example, this is the case for the packet video standard ITU-T Recommendation H.323 (see Chapter 13 on networked video systems standards, ITU-T and DAVIC). For our simulations, an RS code is used with a block size of 88 bytes. This block size corresponds to the average size of one GOB for the given input format (QCIF, 12.5 frames/s) and bit rate (80 kbit/s). The packetization delay in the order of a GOB can be neglected, even for low-latency applications.

In some transmission systems, reliability information can be obtained for each received bit when the receiver provides channel state information, or when the channel decoder provides reliability information (44,45). This information is then passed on to the video decoder. In addition, the video decoder itself can detect transmission errors. The video bitstream contains some residual redundancy, such that violations of syntactic or semantic constraints will usually occur quickly after a loss of synchronization (13,46–48). For example, the decoder might not find a matching variable-length code (VLC) word in the code table (a syntax violation), or detect that the decoded motion vectors, discrete cosine transform (DCT) coefficients, or quantizer step sizes exceed their permissible range (semantic violations). Additionally, the accumulated run that is used to place DCT coefficients into an 8×8 block might exceed 64, or the number of macroblocks in a GOB might be too small or too large. Especially for severe errors, the detection can further be supported by localizing visual artifacts that are unlikely to appear in natural video signals. However, these inherent error detection capabilities of a video decoder have a limited reliability and cannot exactly localize errors. Usually, several erroneous code words are processed by the video decoder before syntactic or semantic constraints are violated, and the distance between error location and error detection can vary significantly. Therefore, external error detection mechanisms, such as FEC framing, should be used if available.

A more difficult problem than error detection is resynchronization after a detected error. Because the multiplexed video bitstream consists of VLC words, a single bit error often causes a loss of synchronization and a series of erroneous codewords at the decoder. Residual redundancy in noncompact VLCs can be used to design self-synchronizing codes, such that valid symbols may be obtained again after some slippage (49). However, even if resynchronization is regained quickly, the appropriate location of the decoded information within the video frame is no longer known, since the number of missing symbols cannot be determined. Moreover, the subsequent codewords are useless if the information is encoded differentially, as it is often the case, for example, for motion vectors. The common solution to this problem is to insert unique synchronization codewords into the bitstream at regular intervals, usually followed by a block of "header" bits. Since any conditional encoding across the resynchronization point must be avoided, the header provides anchor values (e.g., for absolute location in the image or current quantizer step size). Although the length of a synchronization codeword can be minimized (50), relatively long synchronization codewords are used in practice to reduce the probability of accidental emulation in the bitstream.

Recently, more advanced techniques for resynchronization have been developed in the context of MPEG-4 and H.263++. Among several error resilience tools, *data partitioning* has been shown to be effective (13). Especially when combined with *reversible variable-length coding* (RVLC), which allows bitstreams to be decoded in either the forward or the reverse direction, the number of symbols that must be discarded can be reduced significantly. Because RVLCs can be matched well to the statistics of image and video data, only a small penalty in coding efficiency is incurred (51,52). A recently proposed technique can even approach the efficiency of Huffman codes by combining a prefix and suffix codeword stream by delayed XORing (53).

Another elegant technique that is not part of any current video coding standard has been proposed by Redmill and Kingsbury as *error-resilient entropy coding* (EREC) (54). Similar to data partitioning, EREC involves a reordering of the bitstream. Instead of clustering all symbols of the same type into one partition, EREC reorganizes VLC image blocks such that each block starts at a known position within the bitstream, and the most important information is closest to these synchronization points. More information on RVLCs and EREC can also be found in Chapter 8 (Error Resilience Coding).

Considering H.263, the most basic way of improving resynchronization is to use more GOB headers, which can be inserted optionally as resynchronization points at the beginning of each GOB. In QCIF format, 9 GOBs are encoded which consist of 11 macroblocks in one row. All GOBs may include a GOB header, although this is essential only for the first GOB, which always starts with the picture header. The unique synchronization word that is used in H.263 as a preamble for the GOB header consists of 16 consecutive 0-bits followed by a 1-bit ("0000000000000001"). The encoding of anchor values in the header that follows the sync word require 12 bits, such that the total number of bits for a GOB header is 29. In addition to this overhead, the rate distortion performance is further reduced by less effective prediction of motion vectors. However, this reduced coding efficiency is usually well compensated by improved error resilience, as shown below.

Because all information between two resynchronization points can be used independently from previous information in the same frame, the corresponding set of macroblocks is often used as the basic unit for decoding. In the following we use the term *slice* to refer to this set of macroblocks. In the baseline mode of H.263, a slice always corresponds to an integer number of GOBs because the placement of resynchronization points is restricted to the start of a GOB. However, in the *sliced-structure mode* of H.263 (Annex K), a resynchronization point can be placed after each macroblock providing increased flexibility. On the one hand, the number of resynchronization points per frame, which is restricted to 9 in QCIF baseline mode, can be further increased. On the other hand, it is possible to adapt the size of slices to the size of packets or FEC blocks. When Annex K is enabled, GOB headers are to be replaced by slice headers with very similar functionality but slightly increased overhead (34 bits including sync word).

Typically, if a transmission error is detected within a slice, it is discarded entirely and error concealment is invoked for all its macroblocks. This approach is also taken throughout this chapter for the experiments. Because we employ an FEC framing with fixed block size, several slices may overlap with a single FEC block. In this case, the decoder invokes error concealment for each slice that overlaps with the corrupted block. To reduce the number of discarded macroblocks, it is therefore particularly important to reduce the size of slices. In the *sliced-structure mode,* overlap of an FEC block with two adjacent slices can be

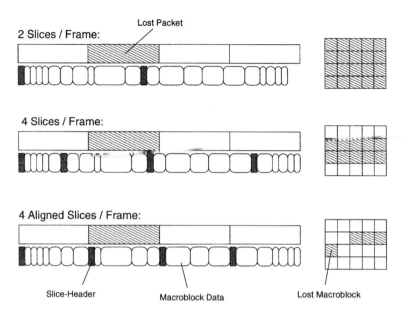

Figure 12.7   Resynchronization techniques that can be used in H.263. Left: the variable-length macroblocks in the bitstream are illustrated together with the fixed-size packets used for transmission. Right: the discarded macroblocks in the reconstructed frame. For clarity, a reduced frame size of 5 × 4 macroblocks is used instead of the 11 × 9 macroblocks in the QCIF format.

avoided by starting a new slice at the beginning of the next block. This results in fixed-length "video packets" that include a variable number of macroblocks. In MPEG-4, this technique has already proven to be effective. However, this ideal packetization requires a close interworking between source and channel coding, which may be difficult in some situations. For example, in a call through a gateway, the source coding is done in a terminal, while the packetization is done in the gateway. Figure 12.7 schematically illustrates the advantage of using an increased number of slices per frame and the additional advantage of alignment with packets. Finally, Figure 12.8 illustrates the performance of H.263 using different numbers of sync words per frame. The sliced-structure mode is not enabled, but the number of sync words is increased by inserting additional GOB headers. Discarded macroblocks are concealed by simply copying the corresponding image data from the reference frame (see Section 12.4.3). The left-hand side of Figure 12.8 indicates that the maximum number of headers (1 picture header and 8 GOB headers) is always advantageous for $E_b/N_0 = 26$ dB. Though the loss in picture quality ΔPSNR is only slightly improved by using

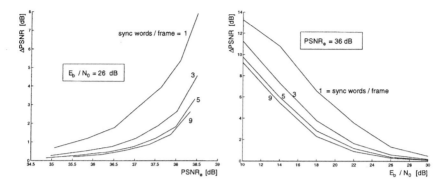

Figure 12.8 Evaluation of video quality with different numbers of sync words per frame. Left: operational DDF for fixed channel. Right: ΔPSNR for fixed PSNR$_e$. The test sequence is Mother and Daughter.

more than 5 sync words per frame, the increased overhead for 9 sync words is still justified. However, it can be expected thata significantly higher numbers, as would be possible with Annex K, would finally result in a reduced performance. Chapter 8 investigates the optimum amount and location of sync words for the sliced-structure mode. The right-hand side of Figure 12.8 shows the loss in picture quality when a PSNR of 36 dB is required at the encoder output. For the whole range of investigated E_b/N_0 values, 9 sync words/frame provides the optimum performance. For all other simulations in this chapter we therefore use GOB headers for each GOB.

12.4.3   Error Concealment

The severeness of residual errors can be reduced if error concealment techniques are employed to hide visible distortion as well as possible. Since typically an entire GOB (i.e., 16 successive luminance lines) is affected, spatial interpolation is less efficient than temporal extrapolation. Only in the case of very complex motion or scene cuts, it can be advantageous to rely on the spatial correlation in the image (55,56), or to switch between temporal and spatial concealment (48,57). In the simplest and most common approach, *previous frame concealment,* the corrupted image content is replaced by corresponding pixels from the previous frame. This simple approach yields good results for sequences with little motion (46). However, severe distortions are introduced for image regions containing heavy motion.

    If the combination of data partitioning and strong error protection for motion vectors is used, one might rely on the transmitted motion vectors for motion-compensated concealment. If motion vectors are lost, they can be reconstructed by appropriate techniques, for example, by spatial interpolation of the motion vector field (58), which can be enhanced by additionally considering the smoothness of the concealed macroblock along the block boundaries (59,60). The interested reader is referred to Chapter 6 on error concealment or to Reference 9 for a comprehensive overview of concealment techniques. All error resilience techniques discussed in the sequel benefit similarly from better concealment. Hence, it suffices to select one technique, and we present experimental results for the simple *previous frame concealment* in the following sections. In this section, however, we also investigate a second concealment technique, which we refer to as *encoded motion concealment*. In this approach, the motion vectors used at the encoder for prediction are also used at the decoder for motion-compensated concealment. Though this approach cannot be implemented in practice because it assumes error-free transmission of motion vectors, it provides an upper bound for the performance of motion-compensated concealment. Therefore it becomes possible to relate the gains obtained by error concealment to the gains obtained by other error resilience techniques. However, as pointed out above, error concealment is always an enhancement of, not a replacement for, other error resilience techniques.

The left-hand side of Figure 12.9 illustrates the possible gain of encoded motion concealment over previous frame concealment for $E_b/N_0 = 22$ dB. The improvement in ΔPSNR becomes most obvious for high residual error rates: that is, when fewer bits are assigned to the channel codec and the video encoder can obtain high values for $PSNR_e$. At $PSNR_e = 36$ dB the loss in picture quality is reduced from 1 dB to 0.5 dB. However, it should be noted that the test sequence used contains only moderate motion. For sequences with more complex motion,

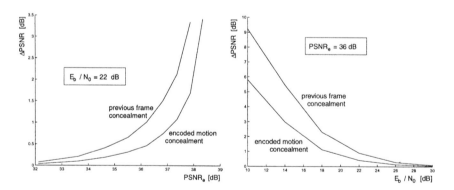

Figure 12.9 Evaluation of video quality with different error concealment techniques. Left: Operational DDF for fixed channel. Right: ΔPSNR for fixed $PSNR_e$. The test sequence is Mother and Daughter.

the difference is more severe. The right-hand side of Figure 12.9 indicates that the gain obtained by error concealment can be converted into improved power efficiency for the transmission. For a given loss in picture quality (e.g., ΔPSNR = 1 dB), the required value of E_b/N_0 can be reduced by approximately 4 dB. In practice, however, this reduction in transmission power may have to be paid for by increased computation for error concealment. Nevertheless, concealment is an important error resilience technique because it provides significant gains at no overhead in bit rate.

12.4.4   Mitigation of Interframe Error Propagation

Like error concealment, resynchronization reduces the amount of image distortion that is introduced for a given error event (e.g., a packet loss). However, such techniques do not prevent error propagation, which is the most dominant and annoying error effect in video coding. Error propagation is caused by the recursive structure of the decoder when operating in the interframe mode, that is, with the previously decoded frame used as a reference for the prediction of the current frame. Errors remaining after concealment therefore propagate to successive frames and remain visible for a long period of time. In addition, the accumulation of several errors can result in very poor image quality, even if the individual errors are small. Figure 12.10 illustrates the typical transmission error effects for the loss of one GOB in frame 4. Not only does the error propagate temporally, but it also spreads spatially as a result of motion-compensated prediction. In the remainder of this chapter, we focus on error resilience techniques that mitigate the effect of error propagation in various ways. In general, three basic approaches are possible to remove errors from the prediction loop, once they have been introduced:

> The prediction from previous frames is omitted by using the intra mode.
> The prediction from previous frames is restricted to error-free image regions.
> The prediction signal is attenuated by *leaky prediction.*

From a theoretical point of view, the first and last items are related, since intra coding can be considered to be an extreme form of leaky prediction, where the

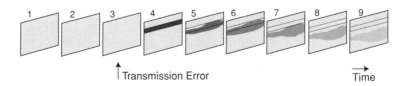

Figure 12.10   Illustration of spatiotemporal error propagation.

prediction signal is completely attenuated. By using the intra mode for a certain percentage of the coded sequence, it is also possible to adjust the average attenuation. However, leaky prediction is a more general scheme that provides additional flexibility. Furthermore, leaky prediction is not explicitly supported by existing standards for improved error resilience. We therefore discuss these items separately.

12.4.4.1 Leaky Prediction.

Leaky prediction is a well-known technique for increasing the robustness of differential pulse code modulation (DPCM) systems by attenuating the energy of the prediction signal (61). Because the attenuation is applied in each time step, the energy of superimposed errors decays over time and is finally reduced to a negligible amount. In contrast to speech and still image coding, this technique has not received a lot of attention in recent contributions to error-resilient video coding, even though the idea is not new (58,62). Nevertheless, the underlying effect plays an important role in interframe error propagation of current video codecs, because leakage is introduced as a side effect by spatial filtering in the motion-compensated predictor.

H.263 and all recent video compression standards employ bilinear interpolation for subpixel motion compensation, which acts as a low-pass filter. Spatial filtering in the motion-compensated predictor is a necessary ingredient for good compression performance of a hybrid coder (63,64). Even with integer-pixel accurate motion compensation, a "loop filter" should be employed. For example, in H.261, which uses integer-pixel motion compensation, the PSNR gain due to the loop filter is up to 2 dB (2,42). As low-pass filtering attenuates the high spatial frequency components of the prediction signal, leakage is introduced in the prediction loop. While error recovery is also improved at the same time, this is really a side effect, and the leakage in the DPCM loop of standardized video codecs by itself is not strong enough for error robustness. For this purpose, additional leakage, such as more severe low-pass filtering, could be introduced. Although this would reduce coding efficiency, the trade- off between coding efficiency and error resilience may be more advantageous than for intra coding because of increased flexibility in the design of the loop filter.

Considering the standardized H.263 syntax, the possible influence on the spatial loop filter and the leakage in the prediction loop is limited, especially for operations in the baseline mode. Though it is possible to prefer half-pel motion vectors over integer-pel motion vectors, the obtained gain is usually small. However, several coding modes of H.263 add additional spatial filtering to the motion-compensated predictor. For example, the *advanced prediction mode* (Annex F) uses overlapped block motion compensation (OBMC), and the *deblocking filter mode* (Annex J) introduces additional filtering at the borders of coarsely quantized blocks. Since these options also improve coding efficiency, they can have a twofold advantage for a wireless video transmission system.

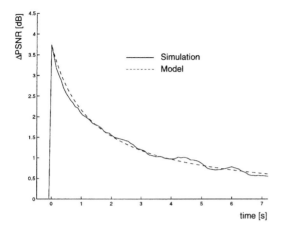

Figure 12.11 Recovery of picture quality after previous frame concealment of one GOB. Leakage introduced by spatial filtering is the cause of this recovery.

Also in the baseline mode, the influences of leakage on interframe error propagation in H.263 cannot be neglected. This is shown in Figure 12.11, which illustrates the recovery of ΔPSNR after the loss of one GOB under conditions of previous frame concealment. The QCIF sequence *Foreman* is coded in the baseline mode at 100 kbit/s and 12.5 frame/s, resulting in an average PSNR_e of about 34 dB in the error-free case. Using the reconstructed frames at the encoder as the baseline, the loss in picture quality is calculated for each reconstructed frame at the decoder output. Figure 12.11 shows the average degradation when each individual GOB in the fifth encoded frame is lost, one at a time. Though the error energy decays over time, a residual loss of 1 dB still remains in the sequence after 3 seconds. Note that no macroblocks are encoded in intra mode, and therefore the decay is entirely caused by spatial filtering. In contrast to leaky prediction in one-dimensional DPCM systems, where the error energy decays exponentially, it can be shown that the decay in MSE is roughly proportional to $1/t$ in hybrid video coding (65,66). More precisely, the MSE at the decoder, after a transmission error that introduces the additional error MSE_0, can be modeled by

$$\mathrm{MSE}_d[t] = \mathrm{MSE}_e + \frac{\mathrm{MSE}_0}{1 + \gamma t}$$

where γ is a parameter that describes the effectiveness of the loop filter to remove the introduced error, typically in the range $0 < \gamma < 1$, and MSE_e is the MSE at the encoder; t is the frame index, with the transmission error occurring at $t = 0$.

As Figure 12.11 shows, this model can describe experimental results quite accurately when the parameters are chosen appropriately.

Because the amount of leakage in H.263 is too small to be useful for error resilience, other techniques are needed to limit interframe error propagation. The most common approach, which can be implemented easily in H.263, is the regular intra update of image regions.

12.4.4.2 Intra Update.

A reliable method to stop interframe error propagation is the regular insertion of I frames (i.e., pictures that are encoded entirely in intra mode). Unfortunately, for the same picture quality I frames typically require several times more bits than frames encoded with reference to previous frames. Therefore, their use should be restricted as much as possible, especially for low bit rates. Because the regular insertion of I frames causes a significant variation in bit rate, which must be smoothed by buffering for constant bit rate transmission, additional delay in the order of several frame intervals is introduced. To avoid this, intra coding can be distributed over several frames, such that a certain percentage of each frame is updated.

The correct choice of the intra percentage is a nontrivial issue that is influenced by the error characteristic of the channel, the decoder implementation, and the encoded video sequence. Obviously there is a trade-off to be considered. On the one hand, an increased percentage helps to reduce interframe error propagation. On the other hand, the coding efficiency is reduced at the same time. Besides the appropriate choice of intra percentage, there is great flexibility in the update pattern. Because the intra mode can be selected by the coding control of the encoder for each macroblock, it is up to the implementer to decide on the most effective scheme. For example, a certain number of intra-coded macroblocks can be distributed randomly within a frame or clustered together in a small region.

In a very common scheme, which is also requested in H.263, each macroblock is assigned a counter that is incremented if the macroblock is encoded in interframe mode. If the counter reaches a threshold T, the macroblock is encoded in intra mode and the counter is reset to zero. If a different initial offset is assigned to each macroblock, the update time of macroblocks will be distributed uniformly within the intra update interval T. However, the main reason for intra updates in H.263 is the *inverse DCT (IDCT) mismatch* rather than improved error resilience. IDCT mismatch may cause an accumulation of errors in the prediction loop if encoder and decoder use slightly different implementations of the inverse DCT. Because this effect is usually small, a rather long update interval is sufficient. The H.263 standard requests a minimum value of $T = 132$. However, lower values are advantageous for error resilience. In our simulations we use a very similar update scheme and refer to it as *periodic intra update*. The only difference is that we also increment the counter for skipped macroblocks to guarantee a regular update of all image regions.

Other update schemes have been proposed in the literature to further improve the effectiveness of intra coding. Thus it has been shown (58,67) that it is advantageous to consider the image content when deciding on the frequency of intra coding. For example, image regions that cannot be concealed very well should be refreshed more often, whereas no intra coding is necessary for completely static background. This idea can also be included in a rate distortion optimized encoding framework as proposed elsewhere (25,68) and also discussed in more detail in Chapter 8. Finally, different intra coding patterns, such as nine randomly distributed macroblocks, 1×9, or 3×3 groups of macroblocks, have been compared by Zhu and Kerofsky (24). Though the shape of different patterns slightly influences the performance, the selection of the correct intra percentage has a significantly higher influence. We employ the *periodic intra update* scheme described above.

The results for the simulated transmission over a Rayleigh channel are presented in Figure 12.12. From the distortion–distortion function (DDF: left), it can seen that a choice of 6% intra macroblocks results in the optimum performance for the Rayleigh fading channel at E_b/N_0 = 18 dB. Note that lower as well as higher percentages reduce the performance at a given value of PSNR$_e$. In particular, the loss in ΔPSNR is as much as 4 dB for 6% intra versus 0% intra at PSNR$_e$ = 36 dB. The right-hand side of Figure 12.12 shows that 6% intra macroblocks is also the optimum choice for the whole range of channel conditions that are investigated. Therefore we use this number in all following simulations. In fact, the results we presented above also use the described intra update scheme and 6% intra macroblocks. Note, however, that the optimum intra percentage depends on the encoded sequence as well as the RWER and the

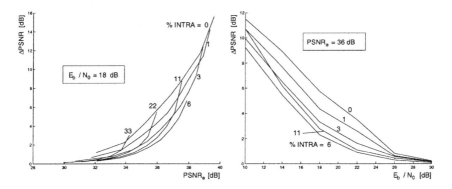

Figure 12.12 Evaluation of video quality by means of different amounts of intra-coded macroblocks. Left: Operational DDF for fixed channel. Right: ΔPSNR for fixed PSNR$_e$. The test sequence is Mother and Daughter.

concealment algorithm employed. In practice, it is therefore difficult to select the correct intra percentage.

12.4.4.3 Error Confinement.
Leaky prediction and intra coding mainly address the problem of temporal error propagation. However, interframe error propagation also results in a spatial error spreading, as illustrated in Figure 12.10. Motion-compensated prediction may cause errors to move from their original location to other parts of the frame and even to spread over the whole image. In some situations it is easier to combat the error by confining it to a well-defined subregion of the frame. This can be achieved by restricting the range of motion vectors, such that no information outside the subregion is used for prediction. In effect, the video sequence is partitioned into *subvideos* that can be decoded independently.

Though the restriction of motion vectors could be guaranteed by the coding control of the encoder without any additional changes to the syntax, H.263 offers an optional mode for such a subvideo technique to allow a clearer and easier implementation. The *independent segment decoding mode* (ISD mode) is described in Annex R of H.263. It can also be combined with the sliced structure mode, but we restrict the discussion to the case in which a segment is identical to a GOB (assuming GOB headers for each GOB). In the ISD mode, each GOB is encoded as an individual subvideo independently from other GOBs. All GOB boundaries are treated just like picture boundaries. This approach significantly reduces the efficiency of motion compensation, particularly for vertical motion, since image content outside the current GOB must not be used for prediction. To reduce the loss of coding efficiency, the ISD mode is therefore often combined with the *unrestricted motion vector mode* (UMV mode), which allows motion vectors pointing outside the coded picture area by extrapolating the image (or subvideo) borders. In spite of the UMV mode, typical losses in PSNR in the range of 0.2–2.0 dB often must be accepted.

In the case of transmission errors, the ISD mode assures that errors inside a GOB will not propagate to other GOBs, as illustrated in Figure 12.13. Of course, the ISD mode alone does not solve the problem of temporal error propagation. It

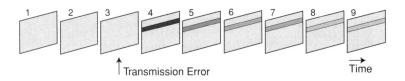

Figure 12.13 Illustration of the reduction of spatio temporal error propagation when the independent segment decoding mode is used.

only simplifies keeping track of the error effects. However, intra coding can also be used within each subvideo with very similar results. Because the ISD mode alone does not influence the overall performance significantly, we do not provide specific wireless video simulation results. Instead, we use this mode in combination with other modes described below.

12.4.5 Feedback-Based Error Control

As shown in Section 12.4.4, the remaining distortion after error concealment of corrupted image regions may be visible in the video sequence for several seconds. Although intra update schemes, as discussed above, help to limit the duration of error propagation, they also reduce coding efficiency. Furthermore, the optimum intra percentage is difficult to select in practice. In this section we discuss error resilience techniques that overcome these problems by utilizing a feedback channel from the receiver to the transmitter. Because this approach assumes a special system architecture, we treat it in a separate section. The reader is also referred to Chapter 10 (Feedback of Rate and Loss Information for Networked Video) for further techniques that utilize a feedback channel.

In our context, the feedback channel indicates which parts of the bitstream were received intact and/or which parts of the video signal could not be decoded and had to be concealed. Depending on the desired error behavior, negative acknowledgment (NACK) or positive acknowledgment (ACK) messages can be sent. Typically, an ACK or an NACK refers to a series of macroblocks or an entire GOB. NACKs require a lower bit rate than ACKs, since they are sent only when errors actually occur, while ACKs must be sent continuously. In either case, the required bit rate is very modest compared to the video bit rate of the forward channel. The feedback message is usually not part of the video syntax but is transmitted in a different layer of the protocol stack where control information is exchanged. For example, in conjunction with H.263, ITU-T Recommendation H.245 (69) allows reporting of the temporal and spatial location of macroblocks (MBs) that could not be decoded successfully and had to be concealed. Since the information is transmitted by means of a retransmission protocol, error-free reception is guaranteed. However, additional delay may be introduced in the case of errors. In the following we assume that ACKs/NACKs are received reliably after a relatively large round-trip delay of 300 ms.

12.4.5.1 Error Tracking. The error tracking approach uses the intra mode for selected MBs to stop interframe error propagation but limits its use to severely affected image regions. During error-free transmission, the more effective inter mode is used, and the system therefore adapts effectively to varying channel conditions. This is accomplished by processing the NACKs from a feedback channel in the coding control of the encoder. Based on the information of a NACK, the encoder can reconstruct the interframe error propagation at the decoder. The coding control of a forward-adaptive encoder can then effectively stop interframe error propagation by avoiding the reference to severely affected MBs (e.g., by selecting the intra mode). If error concealment is successful and the error of a certain MB is small, the encoder may decide that intra coding is not necessary. For severe errors, a large number of MBs is encoded in intra mode, and the encoder may have to use a coarser quantizer to maintain constant frame rate and bit rate. In this case, the overall picture quality at the source encoder decreases with a higher frequency of NACKs. Unlike retransmission techniques such as ARQ, error tracking does not increase the delay between encoder and decoder. It is therefore particularly suitable for applications that require a short latency.

Figure 12.14 illustrates error tracking for the example presented in Figure 12.10. As soon as the NACK is received with a system-dependent round-trip delay, the impaired MBs are determined and error propagation can be terminated by intra coding these MBs (frames 7–9). A longer round-trip delay just results in a later start of the error recovery. Note that it is necessary to track the shifting location of the errors to stop error propagation completely. To reconstruct the interframe error propagation that has occurred at the decoder, the encoder could store its own output bitstream and decode it again, taking into account the reported loss of GOBs. While this approach is not feasible for a real-time implementation, it illustrates that the encoder, in principle, possesses all the information necessary to reconstruct the spatiotemporal error propagation at the decoder, once the NACKs have been received. For a practical system, the interframe error propagation must be estimated with a low-complexity algorithm, as described elsewhere (14,15,70), for a macroblock-based coder, such as H.263. A worst-case estimate of error propagation that does not consider the severity of errors is proposed by Wada (71).

The basic idea of the low-complexity algorithm is to carry out error tracking with macroblock resolution rather than pixel resolution. This is sufficient because the intra/inter mode decision at the coder and the error concealment de-

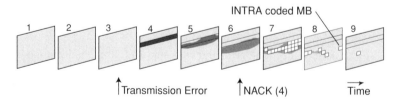

Figure 12.14   Illustration of spatiotemporal error propagation when *error tracking* is used.

cision at the decoder are carried out for entire MBs as well. A cyclical buffer for all MBs of the last several frames stores the spatial overlap of MBs in successive frames due to motion-compensated prediction, along with the error energy that would be introduced if concealment had to be used. If a NACK is received that indicates an error a few frames back, this error energy is "released" and "ripples" through the directed graph of frame-to-frame dependencies to the macroblocks of the current frame. Since all calculations are carried out on the MB level, the computational burden and memory requirements are small compared to the actual encoding of the video. For example, at QCIF resolution, there are only 99 MBs in each frame, as opposed to 38,016 luminance and chrominance samples.

Error tracking is particularly attractive because it does not require any modifications of the bitstream syntax of the motion-compensated hybrid coder. It is therefore fully compatible with standards such as H.261, H.263, or MPEG. The ITU-T recommends using previous frame concealment and error tracking with baseline H.263 and includes an informative appendix (Appendix 1) with Recommendation H.263. In addition, minor extensions of the H.245 control standard were adopted to include the appropriate NACK messages.

Figure 12.15 evaluates the error tracking approach by means of the described simulation environment. For comparison, the *periodic intra update* scheme using 1 and 6% intra macroblocks is included. Even when the optimum intra percentage is selected by the encoder (which is difficult in practice), channel-adaptive error tracking shows significant gains. Note that error tracking would provide additional gains for round-trip delays shorter than the 300 ms assumed here.

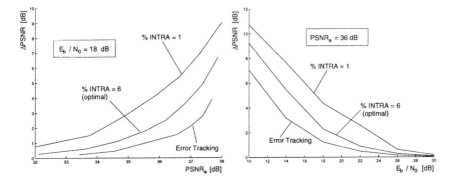

Figure 12.15 Evaluation of video quality using feedback information from the decoder and *error tracking*. Left: Operational DDF for fixed channel. Right: ΔPSNR for fixed PSNR$_e$. The test sequence is Mother and Daughter.

12.4.5.2 Reference Picture Selection. Rather than switching to intra mode at the encoder to stop interframe error propagation at the decoder, the encoder could predict the current frame with reference to a previous frame that has been successfully decoded. This *reference picture selection* (RPS) approach can lower the excess bit rate due to NACK-induced intra coding (17,72). It is also described in Chapter 8 on error resilience coding.

H.263+ has included RPS as an option, described in Annex N. As for the discussion of the ISD mode, we again consider the case in which GOBs are used and each GOB starts with a header. Then, in H.263, the reference picture is selected on a GOB basis; that is, the same reference picture is used for all MBs within one GOB. Future versions of H.263 are likely to contain an enhanced reference picture selection mode on the basis of MBs. To stop error propagation while maintaining the best coding efficiency, the last frame available without errors at the decoder should be selected. The RPS mode can be combined with the ISD mode for error confinement, or, for better coding efficiency, with an error tracking algorithm.

Reference picture selection can be operated in two different modes. When the encoder receives only *negative* acknowledgments, the operation of the encoder is not altered during error-free transmission, and the GOBs of the previous frame are used as a reference. After a transmission error, the decoder sends a NACK for an erroneous GOB and thereby requests that older, intact frames provide the reference GOB. Typical transmission error effects are illustrated in Figure 12.16, where the selection of reference GOBs is indicated by arrows. Note that the use of the ISD mode is assumed, and the indicated selection is valid only for the erroneous GOB. The encoder receives a NACK for frame 4 before the encoding of frame 7. The NACK includes the explicit request to use frame 3 for prediction, which is observed by the encoder. Similar to the error tracking approach, the quality degrades until the requested GOB arrives at the decoder, (i.e., for the period of one round-trip delay). Therefore, the sequence of loss of picture quality after a transmission error and recovery after receiving a NACK is very similar to that found in basic error tracking. The advantage of the RPS mode over simply switching to intra mode lies in the increased coding efficiency. Fewer bits are needed for encoding the motion-compensated prediction error than for the video signal itself, even if the time lag between the reference frame and the current frame is several frame intervals.

In the *positive* acknowledgment mode, all correctly received GOBs are acknowledged and the encoder uses only those GOBs as a reference. Since the encoder must use older reference pictures for motion-compensated prediction with increasing round-trip time, the coding performance decreases even if no transmission errors occur. On the other hand, error propagation is avoided entirely, since only error-free pictures are used for prediction.

Reference picture selection requires additional frame buffers at the encoder

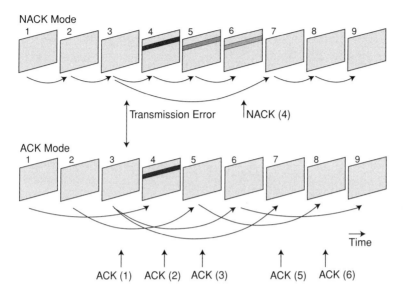

Figure 12.16 Illustration of spatiotemporal error propagation when the *reference picture selection* is used.

and decoder to store enough previous frames to cover the maximum round-trip delay of NACKs or ACKs. In the NACK mode, the storage requirements of the decoder can be reduced to two frame buffers. Furthermore, if only error-free GOBs are to be displayed, one frame buffer is sufficient. In the ACK mode no such storage reduction is possible unless a combination of both modes is allowed (72). Increased storage requirements may still pose a problem for inexpensive mobile terminals for some time. Beyond that, there are proposals for increased coding efficiency in low bit rate video codecs, which use several or even many previous frames for prediction (73–75). When RPS is used, the additional frames can also serve to simultaneously increase robustness with respect to errors (76).

For experimental evaluation of H.263 by means of reference picture selection, we use a combination of the RPS, ISD, and UMV modes. We assume that only NACKs are returned and use the same round-trip delay as in the preceding section (i.e., 300 ms). Even though the UMV mode helps to reduce the loss in coding efficiency that is caused in the ISD mode by restricted prediction, we observe that the overall loss in coding efficiency compared to the baseline mode is still considerable. Therefore, compared with error tracking, the overall gain by avoiding intra coding is diminished. For the test sequence shown we even observe that error tracking actually performs better, as can be seen from Figure 12.17. However, the difference is not significant, and the order might be reversed

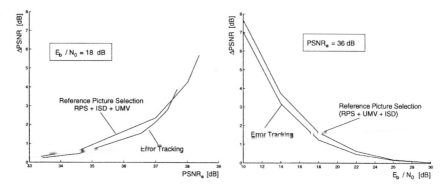

Figure 12.17   Evaluation of video quality by means of feedback information from the decoder and RPS. Left: Operational DDF for fixed channel. Right: ΔPSNR for fixed PSNR$_e$. The test sequence is Mother and Daughter.

for other test sequences. We therefore conclude that the two feedback-based approaches perform equally well and offer significant gains over error resilience schemes without feedback.

12.5 CONCLUSIONS AND OPEN PROBLEMS

In this chapter we have discussed the transmission of video over wireless channels with an emphasis on the interaction and trade-offs between system components. For evaluation, two types of distortion in the decoded video signal must be considered: distortions due to source coding and distortions caused by transmission errors. Altering the bit allocation between source and channel coding usually has opposite effects on the two distortion types: that is, one increases while the other is reduced. To represent this trade-off formally, we introduced the distortion–distortion function (DDF), which can be used as a tool for comparing wireless video systems.

For wireless video there are two major problems directly related to the transmission medium:

1. Only low bit rates are available, owing to the limited availability of the radio spectrum.
2. Path loss and multipath fading cause time-variant error rates.

In designing the digital transmission system, there is a fundamental trade-off among *throughput, reliability,* and *delay.* The actual amount by which, for example, reliability can be increased for a reduction in throughput depends on the components of the error control channel (i.e., the channel, the modem, and the channel codec). This trade-off has been illustrated for the mobile radio channel assuming Rayleigh fading, BPSK modulation, and RS block codes. Especially for the mobile radio channel, the underlying physical mechanisms result in fundamental performance limits that require special measures in the video codec as the "last line of defense."

In Section 12.4 we discussed such measures for low bit rate video, with particular emphasis on techniques with relevance to the H.263 Recommendation. These error resilience techniques fall into two major categories: techniques that reduce the amount of introduced errors for a given error event (*resynchronization, error concealment*) and techniques that limit interframe error propagation (*leaky prediction, intra update*). The influence of both categories on the overall performance can be significant, as has been demonstrated by means of operational DDFs. For example, for a given PSNR at the encoder, the loss in PSNR caused by transmission errors can be reduced from more than 10 dB to less than 2 dB when existing options are combined appropriately.

Additional gains can be obtained by using channel-adaptive source coding. The use of feedback information on the source coding level is an efficient and elegant technique for real-time multimedia communication over networks with heterogeneous quality of service. Feedback schemes, such as error tracking or reference picture selection, are suitable for interactive, individual communications, but they have inherent limitations outside this domain. They are particularly powerful if the round-trip delay is short. If the round-trip delay increases, they become less efficient and ultimately useless. Also, feedback schemes rapidly deteriorate with increasing number of users. Their strength is in point-to-point communications, and extensions to a few users are possible at a loss in performance.

There are several other approaches to error-resilient video transmission that could not be covered in this chapter. In particular, data partitioning and scalable video coding are of increased importance when feedback from the channel is not available. Instead, these approaches rely on priority mechanisms that are part of the network congestion management or are provided implicitly through unequal error protection. Such techniques scale well with the number of users and are suitable for multicasting and broadcasting. On the other hand, they are less efficient than feedback schemes for point-to-point communications. Hybrid techniques that combine the advantages of channel-adaptive source coding based on feedback and scalable coding are not known today. Data partitioning and scalable video coding are covered in more detail in Chapter 7 (Layered Coding). These techniques can be very effective in practice.

Also, so-called multiple-description coding (MDC) schemes, tailored toward graceful degradation for randomly selected subsets of the bitstream, are in their infancy today. The multiple-description coding problem in its simplest form attempts to transmit a signal to three receivers, where the first receiver receives a first bitstream, the second receiver receives a second bitstream, and a third receiver gets both bitstreams. Such scenarios are directly relevant to broadcasting systems and transmission over erasure channels or best-effort networks. Since Shannon's separation principle for source and channel coding does not hold, even the fundamental information-theoretic performance limits for such schemes are unknown, let alone efficient algorithms that perform close to these limits. The situation becomes even more complicated when the influence of a delay constraint for real-time transmission is considered. More information on MDC is also included in Chapter 8 (Error Resilience Coding).

Besides the investigation of new coding schemes, the joint consideration of network and application layers will play an important role in the future. The close interaction between these layers may seem to require a vertical system integration in a closed-network architecture. However, exactly the opposite architecture is becoming more and more important—horizontal integration with an IP-like spanning middle layer for seamless communication across network boundaries. Any efforts that require or assume closed-network architectures are likely to be irrelevant in the future. Instead, the same interface/protocol will have to work across both wired and wireless portions of the future multimedia network.

There are two ways for multimedia applications to evolve within an open system architecture. On the one hand, end-to-end transport and error control for video/multimedia can be implemented in the terminals. On the other hand, the IP protocol stack can be refined and extended to offer additional services and functionalities that are required for efficient real-time transmission. Such multimedia-aware transport protocols need to consider the implications of wireless channels as the weakest link in the transmission chain. Otherwise, unnecessary performance degradation cannot be avoided. Judging from current efforts, both possibilities—end-to-end error control and multimedia-aware extensions of current transport protocols—will continue to evolve and contribute to the ultimate success of wireless video.

REFERENCES

1. J Uddenfeldt. Digital cellular—Its roots and its future. Special issue on the Mobile Radio Centennial Proc IEEE. 86 (7):1319–1324, July 1998.
2. B Girod, N Färber, E Steinbach. Performance of the H.263 video compression standard. J VLSI Signal Process: Syst Signal, Image, Video Technol 17:101–111, November 1997.
3. E Berruto, M Gudmonson, R Menolascino, W Mohr, M Pizarroso. Research activities on UMTS radio interface, network architectures, and planning. IEEE Commun Mag 36(2):82–95, February 1998.

4. D. Grillo, ed. Special section on third-generation mobile systems in europe. IEEE Personal Commun Mag 5(2):5–38, April 1998.

5. P Bahl and B Girod, eds. Special section on wireless video. IEEE Commun Mag 36(6):92–151, June 1998.

6. S Lin, D J Costello, M J Miller. Automatic repeat error control schemes. IEEE Commun Mag 22:5–17, December 1984.

7. A Heron, N MacDonald. Video transmission over a radio link using H.261 and DECT. IEE Conference Publication. 354. Institution of Electrical Engineers, London, 1992, pp 621–624.

8. M Khansari, A Jalali, E Dubois, P Mermelstein. Low bit-rate video transmission over fading channels for wireless microcellular system. IEEE Trans Circuits Syst Video Technol 6(1):1–11, February 1996.

9. Y Wang, Q-F Zhu. Error control and concealment for video communication: A review. Proc IEEE 86(5):974–997, May 1998.

10. R Fischer, P Mangold, RM Pelz, G Nitsch. Combined Source and channel coding for very low bitrate mobile visual communication systems. Proceedings of the International Picture Coding Symposium (PCS), Melbourne, Australia, March 1996, pp 231–236.

11. K Illgner, D Lappe. Mobile multimedia communications in a universal telecommunications network. Proceedings of SPIE Visual Communications and Image Processing (VCIP), Taipei, Taiwan, May 1995, vol 2501, pp 1034–1043.

12. B Girod, U Horn, B Belzer. Scalable video coding with multiscale motion compensation and unequal error protection. In: Y Wang, S Panwar, S P Kim, H L Bertoni, eds. Multimedia Communications and Video Coding. New York: Plenum Press, 1996, pp 475–482.

13. R. Talluri. Error-resilient video coding in the MPEG-4 standard. IEEE Commun Mag 36(6):112–119, June 1998.

14. E Steinbach, N Färber, and B Girod. Standard compatible extension of H.263 for robust video transmission in mobile environments. IEEE Trans Circuits Syst Video Technol 7(6): 872–881, December 1997.

15. B Girod, N Färber, E Steinbach. Error-resilient coding for H.263. In: D Bull, N Canagarajah, A Nix, eds. Insights into Mobile Multimedia Communication. New York: Academic Press, 1999, pp 445–459.

16. S Wenger, G Knorr, L Ott, F Kossentini. Error resilience support in H.263+. IEEE Trans Circuits Syst Video Technol 8(7): 867–877, November 1998.

17. S Fukunaga, T Nakai, H Inoue. Error resilient video coding by dynamic replacing of reference pictures. Proceedings of IEEE Global Telecommunications Conference (GLOBECOM), London, November 1996, vol 3, pp 1503–1508.

18. T M Cover, J A Thomas. Elements of Information Theory. New York: Wiley, 1991.

19. G Buch, F Burkert, J Hagenauer, B Kukla. To compress or not to compress? Proceedings of Communication Theory Conference in conjunction with IEEE Global Telecommunications Conference (GLOBECOM), London, November 1996, pp 198–203.

20. H Jafarkhani, N Farvardin. Channel-matched hierarchical table-lookup vector quantization for transmission of video over wireless channels. Proceedings of

IEEE International Conference on Image Processing (ICIP), Lausanne, Switzerland, September 1996, vol 3, pp 755–758.

21. R E Van Dyck, D J Miller. Transport of wireless video using separate, concatenated, and joint source-channel coding. Proc IEEE 87(10): 1734–1750, October 1999.

22. S B Wicker. Error Control Systems. Englewood Cliffs, NJ: Prentice-Hall, 1995.

23. B Girod. Psychovisual aspects of image communication. Signal Process 28(3): 239–251, September 1992.

24. Q-F Zhu, L Kerofsky. Joint source coding, transport processing, and error concealment for II.323-based packet video. Proceedings of SPIE Visual Communication and Image Processing (VCIP), San Jose, CA, January 1999, vol 3653, pp 52–62.

25. S Wenger, G Côté. Using RFC2429 and H.263+ at low to medium bit-rates for low-latency applications. Proceedings of Packet Video Workshop (PVW), New York, April 1999.

26. A Ortega, K Ramchandran. Rate-distortion methods for image and video compression. IEEE Signal Process Mag 15(6): 23–50, November 1998.

27. B Sklar. Rayleigh fading channels in mobile digital communication systems. Part I. Characterization. IEEE Commun Mag 35(9): 136–146, September 1997.

28. W C Jakes. Microwave Mobile Radio Reception. New York: Wiley, 1974.

29. P Wong, D Britland. Mobile Data Communications Systems. Norwood MA: Artech House, 1995.

30. J G Proakis. Digital Communications. 2nd ed. New York: McGraw-Hill, 1989.

31. B Sklar. Digital Communications, Fundamentals and Applications. Englewood Cliffs, NJ: Prentice-Hall, 1988.

32. J E Padgett, C Günther, T. Hattori. Overview of wireless personal communications. IEEE Commun Mag 33(1): 28–41, January 1995.

33. R Cam, C Leung. Throughput analysis of some ARQ protocols in the presence of feedback errors. IEEE Trans Commun 45(1): 35–44, January 1997.

34. M Zorzi, R Rao, L B Milstein. Error statistics in data transmission over fading channels. IEEE Trans Commun 46(11): 1468–1477, November 1998.

35. Y Yao. An effective go-back-N ARQ scheme for variable-error-rate channels. IEEE Trans Commun 43(1): 20–23, January 1995.

36. C Hsu, A Ortega, M Khansari. Rate control for robust video tranmission over wireless channels. Proceedings of SPIE Visual Communication and Image Processing (VCIP), San Jose, CA, February 1997, vol 3024, pp 1200–1211.

37. C Hsu, A Ortega, M Khansari. Rate control for robust video tranmission over burst-error wireless channels. IEEE J Selected Areas Commun 17(5): 756–772, May 1999.

38. M Podolsky, S McCanne, M Vetterli. Soft ARQ for layered streaming media. Technical Report UCB/CSD-98-1024. Computer Science Division, University of California, Berkeley, November 1998.

39. N Färber, B Girod. Robust H.263 compatible video transmission for mobile access to video servers. Proceedings of IEEE International Conference on Image Processing (ICIP), Santa Barbara, CA, October 1997, vol 2, pp 73–76.

40. P Cherriman, L Hanzo. Programable H.263-based video transceivers for interfer-

ence-limited environments. *IEEE Trans Circuits Syst Video Technol* 8(3): 275–286, June 1998.

41. T Gardos. H.263+: The new ITU-T recommendation for video coding at low bit-rates. Proceedings of *IEEE International Conference on Acoustics, Speech, and Signal Processing (ICASSP)*, Seattle, May 1998, vol 6 pp 3793–3796.

42. G Côté, B Erol, M Gallant, F Kossentini. H.263+: Video coding at low bit-rates. *IEEE Trans Circuits Syst Video Technol* 8(7): 849–866, November 1998.

43. Telenor Research. Video codec test model, TMN5, 1995, PD software. http://www.nta.no/brukere/DVC

44. J Huber, A Rüppel. Zuverlässigkeitsschätzung für die Ausgangssymbole von Trellis-Decodern. *Arch Elektron Übertragungstech* 44(1): 8–21, January 1990.

45. J Hagenauer, P Höher. A Viterbi algorithm with soft-decision output and its applications. Proceedings of *IEEE Global Telecommunications Conference (GLOBE-COM)*, Dallas, TX, November 1989, pp 47.1.1–47.1.7.

46. C Chen. Error detection and concealment with an unsupervised MPEG2 video decoder. *J Visual Commun Image Represent* 6(3): 265–278, September 1995.

47. W-M Lam, AR Reibman. An error concealment algorithm for images subject to channel errors. *IEEE Trans Image Process* 4(5): 533–542, May 1995.

48. J W Park, J W Kim, SU Lee. DCT coefficients recovery-based error concealment technique and its application to the MPEG-2 bit stream. *IEEE Tran. Circuits Syst Video Technol* 7(6): 845–854, December 1997.

49. T J Ferguson, JH Rabinowitz. Self-synchronizing Huffman codes. *IEEE Trans. Inf Theory* IT-30(4): 687–693, July 1984.

50. W-M Lam, AR Reibman. Self-synchronizing variable length codes for image transmission. Proceedings of *IEEE International Conference on Acoustics, Speech, and Signal Processing (ICASSP)*, San Francisco, March 1992, vol 3, pp 477–480.

51. J Wen, J D Villasenor. A class of reversible variable length codes for robust image and video coding. Proceedings of *IEEE International Conference on Image Processing (ICIP)*, Santa Barbara, CA, October 1997, vol 2, pp 65–68.

52. J Wen, J D Villasenor. Reversible variable length codes for efficient and robust image and video coding. Proceedings of the *Data Compression Conference (DCC)*, Snowbird, UT, March 1998, pp 471–480.

53. B Girod. Bidirectionally decodable streams of prefix code words. *IEEE Commun Lett* 3(8): 245–247, August 1999.

54. DW Redmill, NG Kingsbury. The EREC: An error-resilient technique for coding variable length blocks of data. *IEEE Trans Image Process* 5:565–574, April 1996.

55. Y Wang, Q-F Zhu, L Shaw. Maximally smooth image recovery in transform coding. *IEEE Trans Commun* 41:1544–1551, October 1993.

56. H Sun, W Kwok. Concealment of damaged block transform coded images using projection onto convex sets. *IEEE trans Image Process* 4:470–477, April 1995.

57. H Sun, J Zedepski. Adaptive error concealment algorithm for MPEG compressed video. Proceedings of SPIE *Visual Communication and Image Processing (VCIP)*, Boston, November 1992, vol 1818, pp 814–824.

58. P Haskell, D Messerschmitt. Resynchronization of motion compensated video affected by ATM cell loss. Proceedings of *IEEE International Conference on Acoustics, Speech, and Signal Processing (ICASSP)*, San Francisco, March 1992, vol 3, pp 545–548.

59. W-M Lam, A R Reibman, B Lin. Recovery of lost or erroneously received motion vectors. Proceedings of *IEEE International Conference on Acoustics, Speech, and Signal Processing (ICASSP)*, Minneapolis, MN, April 1993, vol 5, pp 417–420.

60. P Salama, N Shroff, EJ Delp. A fast suboptimal approach to error concealment in encoded video streams. Proceedings of *IEEE International Conference on Image Processing (ICIP)*, Santa Barbara, CA, October 1997, vol 2, pp 101–104.

61. N S Jayant, P Noll. *Digital Coding of Waveforms*. Englewood Cliffs, NJ: Prentice-Hall, 1984.

62. DJ Connor. Techniques for reducing the visibility of transmission errors in digitally encoded video signals. *IEEE Trans Commun* COM-21(6): 695–706, June 1973.

63. B Girod. The efficiency of motion-compensating prediction for hybrid coding of video sequences. *IEEE J Selected Areas Commun* SAC-5(7): 1140–1154, August 1987.

64. B Girod. Motion-compensating prediction with fractional-pel accuracy. *IEEE Trans Commun* 41(4): 604–612, April 1993.

65. B Girod, N. Färber. Feedback-based error control for mobile video transmission. *Proc IEEE*. Special issue on video for mobile multimedia 97(10): 1707–1723, October 1999.

66. N Färber, K Stuhlmüller, B Girod. Analysis of error propagation in hybrid video coding with application to error resilience. *Proceedings of IEEE International Conference on Image Processing (ICIP)*, Kobe, Japan, October 1999, vol 2, pp 550–554.

67. J Liao, J Villasenor. Adaptive intra update for video coding over noisy channels. *Proceedings of IEEE International Conference on Image Processing (ICIP)*, Lausanne, Switzerland, September 1996, vol 3, pp 763–766.

68. T Wiegand. Personal communication, July 1998.

69. ITU-T Recommendation H.245. Control protocol for multimedia communication. International Telecommunications Union, Geneva, 1996.

70. N Färber, E Steinbach, B Girod. Robust H.263 compatible video transmission over wireless channels. *Picture Coding Symposium (PCS)*, Melbourne, Australia, March 1996, pp 575–578.

71. M Wada. Selective recovery of video packet loss using error concealment. *IEEE J Selected Areas Commun* 7(5): 807–814, June 1989.

72. Y Tomita, T Kimura, T Ichikawa. Error resilient modified inter-frame coding system for limited reference picture memories. *Proceedings of the International Picture Coding Symposium (PCS)*, Berlin, September 1997, pp 743–748.

73. T Wiegand, X Zhang, B Girod. Motion-compensating long-term memory prediction. *Proceedings of IEEE International Conference on Image Processing (ICIP)*, Santa Barbara, CA, October 1997, vol 2, pp 53–56.

74. T Wiegand, X Zhang, B Girod. Long-term memory motion-compensated prediction. *IEEE Trans Circuits Syst Video Technol* 9(1): 70–84, February 1999.

75. B Girod, T Wiegand, E Steinbach, M Flierl, X Zhang. High-order motion compensation for low bit-rate video. *Proceedings of the European Signal Processing Conference (EUSIPCO)*, Island of Rhodes, Greece, September 1998 vol 1, pp 253–256. Invited paper.

76. T Wiegand, N Färber, B Girod. Error-resilient video transmission using long-term memory motion-compensated prediction. *IEEE J Selected Areas Commun*, June 2000.

13
ITU-T and DAVIC Systems Standards

Sakae Okubo
Waseda Research Center, Telecommunications Advancement Organization of Japan, Tokyo, Japan

13.1 INTRODUCTION

The concept of networked video services, also called audiovisual multimedia services, is well known and has a checkered implementation history. Just after the invention of television technology in the early 1930s, experiments on its application to the videophones were conducted in New York (1). Since then a number of other trials have been conducted to investigate the use of video as part of the communications media. Commercial networked video service did not start until the mid 1980s, with the introduction of digital videoconferencing (2). Limited availability of wideband analog or high-speed digital networks and expensive audiovisual terminal equipment had been the two major obstacles. Progress in digital video compression technology, communication network digitalization, and microelectronics opened the way to a variety of audiovisual multimedia services.

Audiovisual multimedia services can be characterized in terms of the attributes and values in Table 13.1(3).

We can use combinations of these attributes to identify some typical commercial audiovisual multimedia services:

Multimedia conversational service; videophone and videoconferencing (point-to-point, multipoint)
Multimedia retrieval service
Multimedia distribution service
Multimedia message service
Multimedia collection service

Table 13.1 Attributes and Values of Audiovisual Multimedia Services

Attributes	Value
Communication configuration	Point-to-point
	Point-to-multipoint
	Multipoint-to-point
	Multipoint
Symmetry of information flow	Unidirectional
	Bidirectional–symmetric
	Bidirectional–asymmetric
Transmission control entity	Source
	Source and sink
	Third party
Time aspects	Real time
	Near–real time
	Non–real time
	Specified time
Media components	Audio
	Video
	Text
	Still picture
	Graphics, data
Media component interrelations	Synchronized
	Independent
Time continuity	Isochronous
	Nonisochronous (i.e., supported by local storage)

This chapter first addresses the standards developed by ITU-T for the multimedia conversational service. Then it covers the standards developed by DAVIC for the multimedia retrieval and distribution services. These three services are now widely deployed.

Videophone and videoconferencing differ somewhat from the customer perspective[*]; videophone is typically for one-to-one communication, while videoconferencing is for communication among several persons. The systems, however, are practically identical from the technical specification perspective, and interworking is possible. Hence the standards for videophone and videoconferencing systems are described together in this chapter.

Section 13.2 summarizes the activities of the standardization bodies, then

---

[*] ITU-T F.700(3) separates multimedia conference services from multimedia conversational services.

Sections 13.3 and 13.4 detail the standards for the two categories, and finally Section 13.5 touches on their future directions.

13.2 STANDARDIZATION OF AUDIOVISUAL MULTIMEDIA SYSTEMS

There are two types of standardization body; one is a formal international standardization organization (e.g., ITU, ISO, IEC); the other is an industry forum or consortium. The standards for videophone and videoconferencing systems have been produced by ITU-T (International Telecommunication Union—Telecommunication Standardization Sector, formerly CCITT until March 1993) (4), while those of multimedia information retrieval and distribution systems have been produced under the initiative of DAVIC (Digital Audio-Visual Council) (5), an industry consortium. This chapter covers both the ITU-T and DAVIC standards. Although they are not described in this chapter, other industry consortiums are active in closely related fields, including the following:

IETF (Internet Engineering Task Force) (6) formed for the evolution of the Internet architecture and the smooth operation of the Internet

IMTC (International Multimedia Teleconferencing Consortium) (7) formed for the development and implementation of interoperable multimedia teleconferencing solutions based on international standards

The ATM Forum (8) formed for accelerating the use of products and services in the asynchronous transfer mode through rapid convergence of interoperability specifications

Chapter 3 of this book addresses alternative architectures developed by IETF for the audiovisual multimedia services.

Standardization for the videophone system started with a new question during the CCITT study period of 1965–1968 to study the "seeing while talking" system. Actual study was carried out during the next study period, 1969–1972, and afterward. The study was motivated by the emergence of AT&T's Picturephone (9) and other systems in various countries around 1970.

The original videophone system concept was to enhance ordinary telephony with a visual capability. Therefore it focused on a head-and-shoulder picture of the user. The picture format was unique with about 250 lines, 2:1 interlaced. The analog transmission and exchange systems used a 1 MHz bandwidth. In spite of an enormous amount of effort, the videophone was not found to be commercially viable. One of the reasons was system cost, but the human factor was also involved as a more serious problem. People sometimes did not want to be seen while they made a telephone call.

New efforts were devoted to find effective business uses for the videophone technology. Videoconferencing was found to be one of the most promising applications for people wanting to increase the productivity of their business (10). A significant change in the technical approach that emerged during the study period 1973–1976 was to use standard broadcasting equipment rather than to develop videophone-specific equipment.

The first CCITT visual telephone system standard H.61 [later revised into H.100 (11)] was produced during the study period of 1977–1980. The visual telephone system was defined in a generic way as "two-way telecommunication service which uses a switched network of broadband analog and/or digital circuits to establish connections among subscriber terminals, primarily for the purpose of transmitting live or static pictures." H.61 specified the picture format as conforming to the local television standard. It also specified a videoconferencing scene representation method, termed "split-screen," where central parts of the two images are shown at the same time. For example, three participants in each part are stacked at the transmitting side and they can be separated at the receiving side for side-by-side displays of the six participants in a row (see Figure 13.1). For the transmission technology, it was at this point that the shift from analog to digital occurred, as digital video compression technology became practical.

Standardization of the digital video compression scheme and the videoconferencing system capitalizing on it took place during the CCITT study period of 1981–1984. In 1984 three H.100 series recommendations (12–14) were introduced for coding video as well as multiplexing audio, video, and other data into a digital primary rate circuit of 2 or 1.5 Mbit/s (the current revisions are listed in the references). These standards, however, are based on the regional digital hierarchy as well as the regional television standard; hence they contain substantially two incompatible videoconferencing systems.

At the end of the 1981–1984 study period, a new CCITT experts' group was formed to develop a worldwide single video coding standard more efficient than H.120, and thus able to utilize the narrowband ISDN (N-ISDN) rates; 384

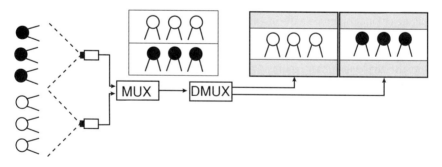

Figure 13.1.   Split-screen technique.

kbit/s, 64 kbit/s or their multiples (15). This activity successfully resulted in Recommendation H.261. The videophone and videoconferencing system using this video coding standard, together with H.200 series of multimedia multiplex and other component standards, was first established in 1990 as Recommendation H.320 (16).

After the standardization of the first-generation H.320 system, CCITT/ITU-T continued to adapt the videophone and videoconferencing systems to various network environments such as broadband ISDN (B-ISDN), GSTN*, LAN, and other packet-based networks (17–19). The outcome is several second-generation H.300 series recommendations as detailed in the sections that follow. It should be noted that these system standards are supported by the development of new tools such as audio coding, video coding, multimedia multiplexing, and communication procedure component standards.

Standardization of the multimedia retrieval systems by DAVIC started in 1994 just after the audio, video, and systems specifications of MPEG-2 had been finalized. One of the most attractive applications of the high-quality MPEG-2 audiovisual coding standards, in addition to digital broadcasting, was thought to be video on demand (VoD) or movie on demand (MoD). DAVIC was established in August 1994 to define tools and dynamic behavior of the audiovisual interactive system for end-to-end interoperability across countries, industries, and applications. DAVIC specifications cover the spectrum horizontally from the consumer system to the content provider system through the network and service provider systems as well as the delivery systems. They also cover vertically the whole protocol stack, including physical, network, transport, presentation, and application layers.

The first set of specifications, called DAVIC 1.0, was published in January 1996 and subsequently enhanced as the series of 1.1 (September 1996), 1.2 (December 1996), 1.3 (September 1997), and 1.4 (June 1998) (20). Furthermore, the DAVIC 1.3.1 specification was adopted in 1999 for the ISO/IEC International Standard 16500 and Technical Report 16501 through the PAS (publicly available specifications) procedure(21). Amendments will be made to cover DAVIC 1.4 or later specifications.

13.3   VIDEOPHONE AND VIDEOCONFERENCING SYSTEM

13.3.1   Generic System Configuration

A generic configuration of audiovisual communication systems including some representative standards is shown in Figure 13.2. It consists of terminals, a net-

---

*General switched telephone network. A generic name for ordinary telephone networks.

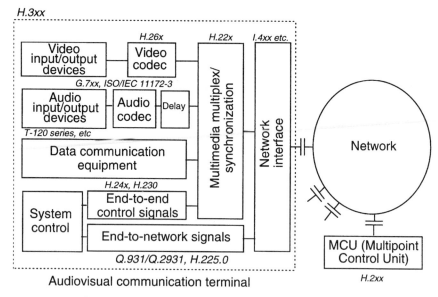

Figure 13.2   Generic configuration of the audiovisual communication system.

work, and one or more multipoint control units (MCU). An MCU is connected to three or more terminals and allows multipoint communication among them. Figure 13.2 also shows the following constituent functional elements of a terminal:

Audio input and output devices
Audio coding
Video input and output devices
Video coding
Delay compensation between audio and video processing
Data device and coding to provide visual aids such as whiteboard, still pictures, computer applications
Multimedia multiplex and synchronization
Communication control (end-to-end system control, end-to-network call control)
Network interface

Several types of digital network can be used for audiovisual communication, as shown in Figure 13.3. It indicates the range of available bit rates and the characteristic of each network type. The GSTN provides analog channels having a

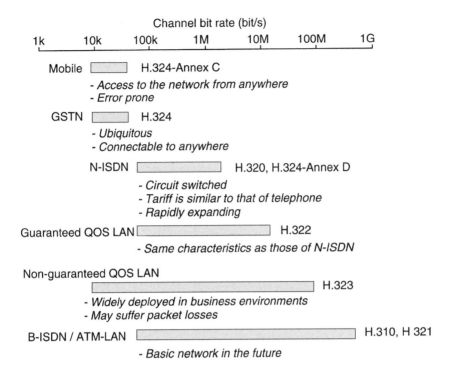

Figure 13.3 Networks and H.300-series audiovisual communication systems.

bandwidth of 3.1 kHz, but by use of modems, it also functions as a digital network providing up to 33.6 kbit/s (56 kbit/s if asymmetrical in channel configuration) digital channels.

ITU-T is standardizing the audiovisual communication system for each type of network as an H.300 series Recommendation. Figure 13.4 shows the history of development of such H.300 series system standards by indicating the respective work periods terminating at the point of establishment of each recommendation. Although not noted in the diagram, revision of each standard is continuing to enhance the system capabilities and to utilize new technologies.

The guiding principle for these system standard developments is to allow as much interworking as possible among different types of terminal. The use of common audio, video, and data coding methods has been sought with individual adaptation layers to different types of network. In the case of the bidirectional communication system, a communication control protocol is utilized by which two entities, such as terminal or MCU, can negotiate the capabilities they have and reach the best mode of operation. The system standard defines a minimum

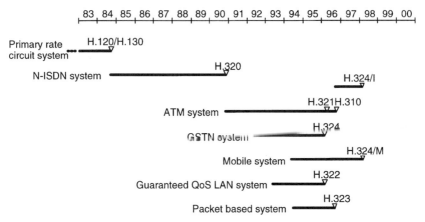

▽ *indicates the date when the Recommendation is first established.*

Figure 13.4 Development of H.300-series recommendations for audiovisual communication systems.

set of mandatory requirements for basic interoperability, but also allows the choice of optional operation modes for enhanced functionality.

Tables 13.2 and 13.3 show the ITU-T or ISO/IEC audio and video coding standards, respectively, for use in the H.300 series terminals. The applications over the data channel opened by the H.300 series systems are commonly defined in the T.120 series recommendations (22) for audiographic and audiovisual teleconference applications.

13.3.2 H.320 N-ISDN Systems

13.3.2.1 Overview. The narrowband integrated services digital network (N-ISDN) is a public circuit-switched network that provides one or more digital channels of 64 kbit/s (called B channel) or 384 kbit/s (H0 channel). These rates are common around the world. N-ISDN also provides a channel of 1536 kbit/s (H11 channel) or 1920 kbit/s (H12 channel) depending on the region. There are two network access methods for N-ISDN: basic access of 2B+D channels, where the D channel is for signaling at 16 kbit/s and primary rate access of mainly 23B+D, and 30B+D channels, where the D channel is for signaling at 64 kbit/s. Since basic access is provided over a normal telephone line and the charge of communication over one B channel is generally equivalent to that for ordinary telephony, N-ISDN is widely deployed in many countries for audiovisual communications. Channel aggregation, defined in H.221, allows the use of any number of B channels as a single channel (e.g., 2B channels as a 128 kbit/s channel).

Table 13.2 Audio Coding for Audiovisual Communication Systems

Audio bandwidth	Bit rate (kbit/s)					
	5, 6	8	16	24	48, 56, 64	> 128
Telephone: 4 kHz	G.723.1 G.729-Annex D	G.729	G.728		G.711	
Wideband audio: 7 kHz:				[a]	[a]	G.722
Sound: 15 kHz						MPEG-1[b] MPEG-2[c]

[a] Under development in ITU-T
[b] ISO/IEC 11172-3 (Ref. 54).
[c] ISO/IEC 13818-3 (Ref. 55), 13818-7.

Table 13.3 Video Coding for Audiovisual Communication Systems

Picture format		Bit rate	
Size	Scanning	10 kbit/s– 2 Mbit/s	> ~2 Mbit/s
288 lines × 352 pels × 30 Hz 144 lines × 176 pels × 30 Hz	Progressive	H.261	
1152 lines × 1408 pels × 30 Hz 576 lines × 704 pels × 30 Hz 288 lines × 352 pels × 30 Hz 144 lines × 176 pels × 30 Hz 96 lines × 128 pels × 30 Hz	Progressive	H.263	
576 lines × 704 pels × 25 Hz 480 lines × 704 pels × 30 Hz	Interlace		H.262|ISO/IEC 13818-2[a] (MPEG-2)
Many other formats	Progressive or interlace		

[a] Common text standard between ITU-T and ISO/IEC JTC1 (per Ref. 53).

ITU-T Recommendation H.320 defines the system on N-ISDN or other digital networks based on 64 kbit/s service (23).

Figure 13.5 shows the protocol stack of the H.320 system. The terminal must support G.711 audio coding (24) and H.261 video coding (25). It may support any other audiovisual and data coding as options that can be used if both ends agree. Call control for the network access, such as call setup and teardown, is specified by Q.931 (26).

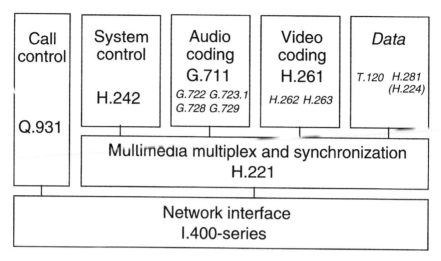

Figure 13.5 H.320 protocol stack.

13.3.2.2 H.221 Multimedia Multiplex. The audiovisual communication system utilizes audio, video, data, and system control, which are combined into a single bitstream at the transmitter and presented to the end user with synchronism at the receiver. Audio and video are synchronized to achieve "lip sync," by which users perceive the voice coming from the mouth of talker on the screen. These functions are called multimedia multiplexing and synchronization, respectively.

There are two types of multimedia multiplex method: bit multiplex and packet multiplex. The bit multiplex relies on synchronization words (one or more bits) regularly spaced in the bitstream for identifying the media type. At the receiver, once the position of a synchronization word has been found, the media type each bit represents is determined by its position relative to the synchronization word. The multiplexing pattern is given by outside means such as a predetermined bit order. The bit multiplex is rooted in telephone network technology. On the other hand, the packet multiplex relies on the packet header content to identify the type of media each packet carries. At the receiver, the starting point of each packet is first found by the delineating word; then the packet header is read, and finally the packet payload is passed to the appropriate media decoder. The multiplexing pattern can be dynamically changed. Packet-based multiplexing is rooted in computer network technology.

The H.320 system adopts the bit multiplex method defined in H.221 for its multimedia multiplex and synchronization (27). This is largely because video-phone and videoconferencing services have developed as an extension of the telephone service. Figure 13.6 shows the structure of the H.221 multiplex for a 64 kbit/s channel. Each 10 ms length of the stream constitutes a frame containing 80 octets. FAS (frame alignment signal) is the 8-bit synchronization word, while BAS (bit-rate allocation signal) is the 8-bit control command or indication word. For example, if G.728 16 kbit/s audio is used in a 64 kbit/s videophone session, audio is carried in subchannels 1 and 2 while video occupies the remaining avail-able bits that are not assigned to data or FAS/BAS. The H.221 frame has a struc-ture of 20 ms submultiframes and 160 ms multiframes, as shown in Figure 13.6. The multimedia multiplex pattern is controlled by the BAS command, which can change once every submultiframe. The transmitter and the receiver synchro-nously change the multiplex pattern at the start of the submultiframe following the one containing the changed BAS command. H.221 does not have a particular mechanism for media synchronization. Implicit synchronization, where the re-ceived media stream is presented as soon as decoded, works because different media are interleaved in a very small unit.

H.221 also provides a mechanism to synchronize two or more B (or H0) channels to use them as a single bundled channel. Different B or H0 channels

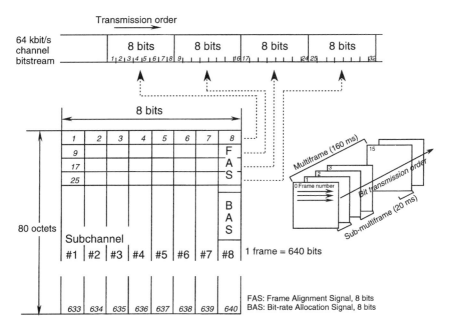

Figure 13.6 H.221 frame structure.

may traverse different network paths in N-ISDN even if they originate from the same terminal. A 4-bit multichannel numbering word inserted in the FAS provides 16 different phases of multiframe, giving a 2560 ms cycle. This allows detection of differential delay up to 1280 ms.

13.3.2.3   H.242 Communication Control.   Since N-ISDN is a versatile network, it may accommodate terminals of many different types. Any two terminals should be connected only when they can intercommunicate. Q.931 has information elements such as BC (bearer capability), LLC (low-layer compatibility) and HLC (high-layer compatibility) to indicate the characteristics of the requested communication. This is called out-band signaling. After a connection has been established, there remains the need to negotiate the features of the two terminals to reach an appropriate mode of operation. This is carried out by in-band signaling. H.242 defines several communication control procedures for this purpose (28). Its control codes are defined as BAS codes and are transmitted through the H.221 BAS channel having 400 bit/s throughput. Each 8-bit BAS code in an H.221 frame is protected by an 8-bit error correcting code in the subsequent frame.

The principle of H.242 communication control is illustrated in Figure 13.7. The receiving side indicates its audio, video, data, transfer rate, and other receiv-

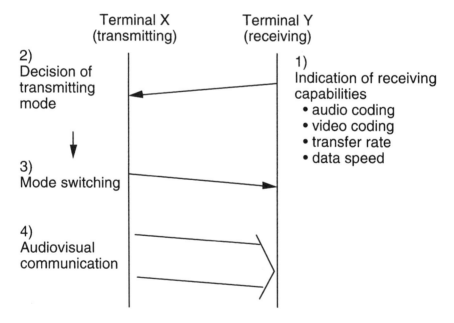

Figure 13.7   H.242 communication control procedures.

ing capabilities to the transmitting side, which then compares them with its transmitting capabilities to determine the best common mode. The transmitter sends the control commands indicating the operational mode with corresponding media information. Since the two directions are controlled independently, an asymmetrical mode of operation may be invoked.

In addition to the capability exchange and mode switching, H.242 defines several other communication procedures, such as the following:

Mode initialization to recover from error conditions
Use of multiple channels
Activation and deactivation of data channels
Operation in the restricted networks in North America (e.g., providing 56 kbit/s instead of 64 kbit/s)
Use of nonstandard modes of operation

13.3.2.4 Multipoint System. In a multipoint videoconferencing system configuration (see, e.g., Figure 13.8), more than two terminals in different locations join a conference via a multipoint control unit (MCU). An MCU accommodates multiple terminals with star-shaped connections, and multiple MCUs can be connected in cascade. ITU-T Recommendation H.231 (29) describes the general principles of such multipoint communication and the characteristics of MCU, while H.243 (30) specifies the control procedures such as establishment of connections between terminals and an MCU, audiovisual processing, chair control, data broadcasting, and MCU-to-MCU interconnection.

There are two types of video presentation in multipoint videoconferencing systems; one has video switching (i.e., the terminal displays a single location at a time), and the other contains video mixing (i.e., the terminal displays an image an MCU has composed from images from multiple locations). The latter is also called a "continuous presence" system.

In the video switching system, the MCU selects the video signal of a particular terminal out of all the incoming video signals and sends it to each terminal. In one basic algorithm, the image of the current speaker's location is sent to all others and the image of the previous speaker's location is sent to the current speaker. If the optional chair control is supported by both the MCU and the terminals, the chair can control who sees what. Similarly, the terminal can also optionally select an image of a particular location regardless of the current speaker. In the video mixing system, the MCU may implement a composition method—for example, quadrature composition, where four quarter-sized pictures from different locations are composed into a full-size picture. The video mixing process can be carried out in the coded bitstream domain or in the original pulse code modulation (PCM) video domain.

Audio signals from all locations are collected at the MCU and decoded to PCM signals; then all signals except that from the terminal to which they

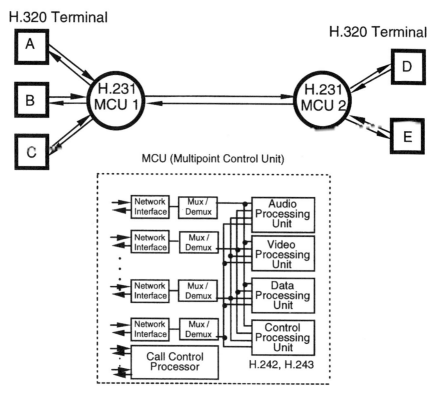

H.320 Terminal

H.320 Terminal

MCU (Multipoint Control Unit)

Figure 13.8 Multipoint videoconferencing system.

will be transmitted are mixed. Thus each terminal participating in a multipoint videoconference can hear all the sounds from all the other locations. Some sounds may be suppressed at the MCU to avoid excessive background noise.

Since the multipoint communication system was standardized after the basic point-to-point communication system, any terminal can join the multipoint communication without any change. An MCU behaves like another H.320 terminal with respect to the communication procedures; thus the H.242 protocol is applicable. If a terminal supports the multipoint procedures defined in H.243, it can enjoy enhanced services. For example, it can act as chair in a chair-controlled videoconference, whereas a terminal supporting only H.242 cannot.

13.3.3 H.324 GSTN Systems

13.3.3.1 Overview. The term, general switched telephone network (GSTN) describes an ordinary telephone network that provides analog telephone channels of 300—3400 Hz bandwidth. Since the infrastructure of GSTN is largely digitalized as a circuit-switched 64 kbit/s network, and high-speed modem technologies have rapidly progressed, GSTN can appear as a digital circuit-switched network providing digital channels of up to 33.6 kbit/s. Thanks to the progress of audiovisual coding technology and also digital signal processing technology, which allows cheap implementation of videophone equipment operating at low bit rates, the videophone-over-GSTN option received much interest after the H.320 system over N-ISDN had been standardized. Seeing the emergence of incompatible implementations in the marketplace, CCITT started the system standardization in 1992. This effort resulted in the H.324 suite of ITU-T recommendations in March 1996: H.324 for system definition (31), G.723.1 for audio coding at 5.3 or 6.3 kbit/s, H.263 for video coding at low bit rates such as 10–20 kbit/s, H.223 for multimedia multiplex, and H.245 for system control. A typical application of the H.324 system is visual telephony, in which speech communication is enhanced by the associated video. H.324 was later extended to cover mobile networks by adding more error resilience to H.223, and also the N-ISDN environments.

The H.324 protocol stack is shown in Figure 13.9. Mandatory audio coding is described in G.723.1 (32) specifically developed for the H.324 system. It operates at 5.3 or 6.3 kbit/s and uses linear predictive analysis-by-synthesis coding, with the excitation signal of algebraic-code-excited linear prediction (ACELP) for the low-rate coder and multipulse maximum likelihood quantization (MP-MLQ) for the high-rate coder. The mandatory video coding mode is described in H.263 (33), also specifically developed for the H.324 system. In addition to H.263, H.261 is mandated to facilitate the H.324 system interworking with the H.320 system. It should be noted that G.723.1 and H.263 are common tools for use in other H.300 series systems, though they were first developed to achieve the low bit rate operation of the H.324 systems. The call connection control protocol is in accordance with national standards for ordinary telephone services. Although not indicated in Figure 13.9, H.324 has a provision for multilink operation according to H.226, where multiple independent physical connections are aggregated together to provide a higher total bit rate (34).

13.3.3.2 H.223 Multimedia Multiplex. On top of the telephone network interface and modem, there sits a packet-based multimedia multiplex, H.223 (35). The packet multiplex has flexibility to cope with dynamically changing modem and payload data rates and is easier to implement in software. The H.223 scheme consists of a MUX layer for multiplexing and an AL layer for adaptation of the

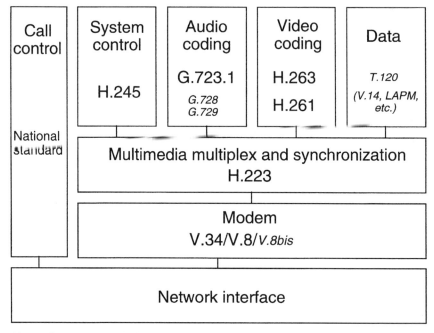

Note - Components in italics are optional; others may be included.

Figure 13.9   H.324 protocol stack.

different media streams to the modem channel characteristics. Each media stream has its own requirements regarding sensitivity to delay and channel errors. There are three types of AL layer, as shown in Table 13.4, to accommodate the different requirements of the various media.

One of the most outstanding features of H.223 is the achievement of the low delay necessary for conversational services. The packet multiplex method suffers from packetization delay, particularly at low bit rates. H.223 solves this problem by carrying multiple media information in a packet. This method provides both low delay and high transmission efficiency. The combination of different media information in a MUX packet is defined by one of the 16 tables, all except one of which are sent from the transmitter to the receiver at the start of communication. The exception is the fixed table #0, for H.245 system control information, which occupies the entire payload. Each MUX packet header has a field to indicate the table in use. The MUX packet is delineated by one or more high-level datalink control (HDLC) flags ("01111110") whose code is kept unique by inserting "0" after all occurrences of five consecutive "1"s in the multiplexed stream.

Figure 13.10 illustrates the H.223 multiplex mechanism. A MUX packet

Table 13.4   H.223 AL layer

Type	Functions	Media
AL1	No error detection or correction	Higher layer provides necessary error control
		System control, data
AL2	8-bit CRC	Delay-critical but error-tolerant information
	Optional sequence number	Audio
AL3	Provision for retransmission	Delay and error requirements between AL1 and AL3
		Video

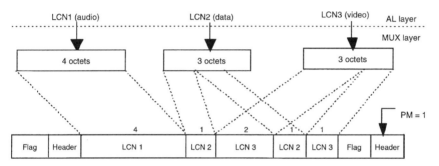

AL: Adaptation Layer
LCN: Logical Channel Number
MUX: Multiplex
PM: Packet Marker

Figure 13.10   H.223 multimedia multiplex.

consists of a header (1 octet) and, subsequently, a payload. The MUX-SDU (multiplex service data unit) consists of 4 octets from LCN1 (audio), 3 octets from LCN2 (data), and 3 octets from LCN3 (video). Audio is nonsegmentable, while data and video are segmentable. The multiplex pattern in use is as follows:

{audio 4 octets, (data 1 octet, video 2 octets), (data 1 octet, video 2 octets), (data 1 octet, video 2 octets), . . . }

Since all the segmentable video octets in the MUX-SDU are sent in the MUX packet, the MUX packet is terminated and PM (packet marker) in the next header is set to "1" to indicate the boundary of MUX-SDU to the receiver.

Figure 13.11 shows the mobile extension of the H.223 multiplex, where three layers of error resilience in the MUX layer are hierarchically defined for

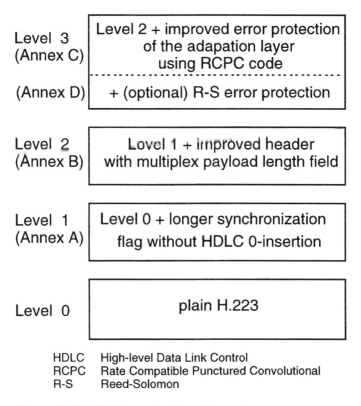

Level 3 (Annex C)	Level 2 + improved error protection of the adapation layer using RCPC code
(Annex D)	+ (optional) R-S error protection

| Level 2
(Annex B) | Level 1 + improved header
with multiplex payload length field |

| Level 1
(Annex A) | Level 0 + longer synchronization
flag without HDLC 0-insertion |

| Level 0 | plain H.223 |

HDLC   High-level Data Link Control
RCPC   Rate Compatible Punctured Convolutional
R-S   Reed-Solomon

Figure 13.11   H.223 extension for mobile environments.

error-prone mobile channels (36)–(39). Note that since layer 0 is identical to the basic H.223 specification, an H.324 mobile terminal can interwork with an existing H.324 terminal, at least at this layer.

13.3.3.3 H.245 Communication Control. H.324 systems use the H.245 communication control protocol (40). This was developed as a common protocol for all the second-generation audiovisual and other communication systems, such as H.310, H.323, H.324, and V.70 (digital simultaneous voice and data), which use packet-based multimedia multiplexes. H.245 adopts the acknowledged procedures using confirmation (ACK, NACK) every time a message is sent. This may require complex processing at the terminal, but it ensures communication by defining the state changes of both sending and receiving terminals.

The H.245 control protocol was developed to reflect the experience of H.242, which uses unacknowledged procedures, has a tight relationship with the H.221 multiplex, and has insufficient separation between different control functions. A basic assumption of H.245 is that the channel for carrying H.245 messages is error-free; thus the control procedures need not consider transmission errors. The error-free stack of an H.324 system for the H.245 channel is shown in Figure 13.12 as an example. Simple Retransmission Protocol (SRP) or optional LAPM/V.42 provides a reliable link layer to H.245 messages. The H.245 control protocol is described in terms of ASN.1 syntax (41), its semantics and message exchange procedures being represented by specification and description language (SDL) diagrams. The functions of H.245 are as follows:

Master–slave determination: for resolving conflicts such as the simultaneous invocation of similar events when only one such event is allowed (e.g., two terminals attempting to open a bidirectional channel).

Capability exchange: for ensuring that the only multimedia signals to be transmitted are those that can be received and treated appropriately by the receive terminal. It includes not only fixed capabilities but also combinations of simultaneous capabilities such as sharing the processing power between audio and video coding.

Logical channel signaling: for opening and closing logical channels that carry the audiovisual and data information. It includes both unidirectional and bidirectional logical channels.

Receive terminal-close logical channel request: for allowing a receive terminal to request the closure of an incoming logical channel.

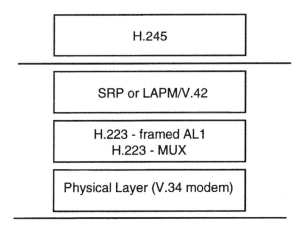

SRP: Simple Retransmission Protocol
LAPM: Link Access Procedures for Modems

Figure 13.12   Reliable H.245 control channel for the H.324 system.

H.223 multiplex table entry modification: for allowing a transmitting terminal to specify and inform the receiver of new H.223 multiplex table entries. Also allows a receiving terminal to request the retransmission of a multiplex table entry.

Audiovisual and data mode request: for allowing a terminal that receives transmission capabilities from the remote terminal to request a particular mode to be transmitted to it.

Round trip delay determination: for measuring the round-trip delay between a transmit terminal and a receive terminal.

Maintenance loops: for establishing various loops for maintenance and checking the remote terminal availability.

Commands and indications: for forcing the remote terminal to take a particular action or indicating audiovisual or other states.

As an example of H.245 procedures, Figure 13.13 shows the primitives and messages in the capability exchange signaling. The set of procedures for capability exchange signalling is referred to as the capability exchange signaling entity (CESE). For each communication direction there is an outgoing CESE at one terminal and a corresponding incoming CESE at another terminal. There are three consequences for sending out a capability message: acceptance, rejection, and timer expiration. Figure 13.14 shows the dynamic flow of the capability exchange primitive and the message as well as the CESE state. The outgoing CESE starts the timer (T101) and sends Terminal Capability Set, a message containing multiplex, audio, video, data, and other capabilities to the peer incoming CESE. The incoming CESE returns the message Terminal Capability Set Ack if it accepts the capability message; otherwise it returns Terminal Capability Set Reject, indicating the cause of rejection. When the timer expires before the outgoing

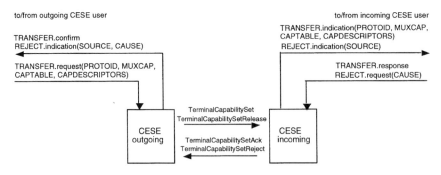

Figure 13.13 H.245 primitives and messages in the capability exchange signalling entity.

state - 0: IDLE, 1: AWAITING RESPONSE

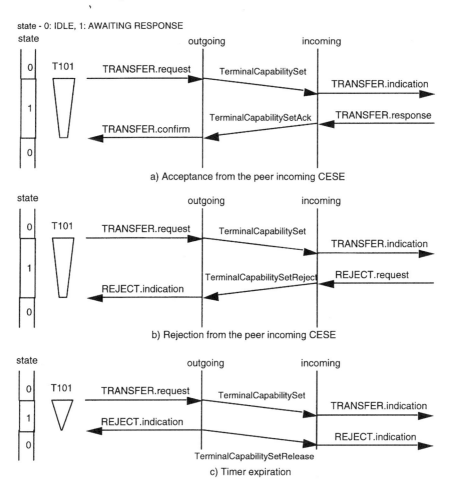

Figure 13.14   H.245 capability exchange message flow.

CESE has received Terminal Capability Set Ack, it sends Terminal Capability Set Release to indicate failure of the capability exchange.

13.3.3.4   H.324 Communication.   H.324 communication starts with the establishment of a call on the analog telephone network. Then modem-to-modem communication procedures are invoked according to V.8 (or optionally V.8bis) for starting sessions of data transmission over GSTN (42, 43). In the case of V.8, initialization of the V.34 modem for digital communication starts immediately, while V.8bis first allows analog telephone conversation and subsequently initializes the V.34 modem for digital data exchange only in response to user input or command from the remote terminal (44). In the digital communication phase, H.245 capability exchange and other communication control messages are first exchanged; then an appropriate mode of operation is established by opening logical channels, and finally audiovisual communication starts between the two terminals.

13.3.4   H.323 Packet-Based Network Systems

13.3.4.1   Overview.   The first-generation H.320 terminal for videoconferencing in office environments has evolved from the room type, where equipment is designed to be a part of dedicated conferencing room, to the roll-about type, where a compact set of equipment can be moved from one room to another, and then to the desktop type, which is mostly implemented as an enhancement to a personal computer. PCs are usually connected to local-area networks; hence the need was identified around mid-1993 to use LANs for connecting desktop videoconferencing and videophone terminals on corporate networks. Also contributing to this need were the low penetration of ISDN PBXs and the emergence of data applications for the desktop computer, such as the T.120 series. At that time ITU-T started standardization of audiovisual communication systems over LANs in response to this need. The first work was oriented to the Quality of Service (QoS) guaranteed LAN, such as ISLAN16-T (45), which provides N-ISDN equivalent services with respect to ensured bandwidth, stable network clock, and address resolution. This resulted in Recommendation H.322 (46), which was approved in March 1996.

The second work addressed more ubiquitous LAN types, such as Ethernet [IEEE 802.3 (47)], which provide best-effort services (nonguaranteed QoS). Thus technologies over and above those of H.320 were required. This work resulted in H.323 (48), H.225.0 (49) and other associated recommendations, which were first approved in November 1996 and have been revised with enhancements. It should be noted that H.323 does not deal with the LAN itself nor the transport layer, but defines higher layers above the packet-based network. Though the IP network including the Internet is a typical packet-based network, the H.323 scope is not limited to it. The primary design considerations in the development of H.323 were as follows:

> Interoperability, especially with N-ISDN and H.320
> Controlling access to the LAN to avoid congestion
> Multipoint call models
> Scalability from small to medium size networks

Since the H.323 system has been widely used across the Internet, it is also accepted as a standard way of IP telephony.

13.3.4.2   System Configuration.   The H.323 system consists of several components, as shown in Figure 13.15: terminal (T), gatekeeper (GK), gateway

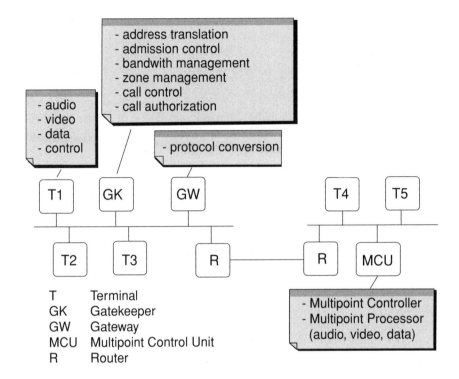

Figure 13.15   H.323 system configuration (zone).

(GW), router (R), and MCU. The gatekeeper is an H.323-specific component that carries out address translation for and network access control of H.323 terminals, gateways, and MCUs (collectively called "end points"). It may also provide other services to the end points such as bandwidth management and locating gateways. In contrast to other networks for H.320 and H.324 systems, typical packet-based networks do not have their own network access control entity; hence the H.323 system requires gatekeeper definition. In this sense H.323 is based on a communication model that differs from those of other recommendations in the H.300 series. The gateway provides real-time, two-way communications between H.323 terminals on the packet-based network and other H.300 series terminals on other networks. The MCU enables multipoint communication among three or more H.323 terminals and gateways. MCU functionally consists of multipoint controller (MC) that processes H.225.0 and H.245 control plane signals and multipoint processor (MP) that processes audiovisual and other user-plane signals.

A collection of those components in Figure 13.15 is called a zone. A zone has one and only one gatekeeper as its managing entity. It may be independent of network topology and may comprise multiple network segments connected through routers or other devices. Alias addresses [terminal identifier in the form of E.164 number (50), e-mail-like address, transport address, or other] must be unique with in a zone.

H.323 multipoint conferences are of two types: centralized and decentralized. The former is similar to the H.320 multipoint system described in Section 13.3.2. The latter utilizes the multicast function of the packet-based network whereby audiovisual signals from each transmitting terminal are delivered to all receiving terminals. In the decentralized conference, no MP is required for audio and video. Determining the ways of mixing audio and switching or mixing video at the receiving terminal is left to the terminal designer. This is the reason for decomposing the MCU into MC and MP in H.323.

13.3.4.3 Protocol Stack. The H.323 protocol stack is shown in Figure 13.16. Audio is mandatory, but video is optional. Mandatory audio coding is specified as G.711 for interworking with H.320. If the channel bit rate is lower

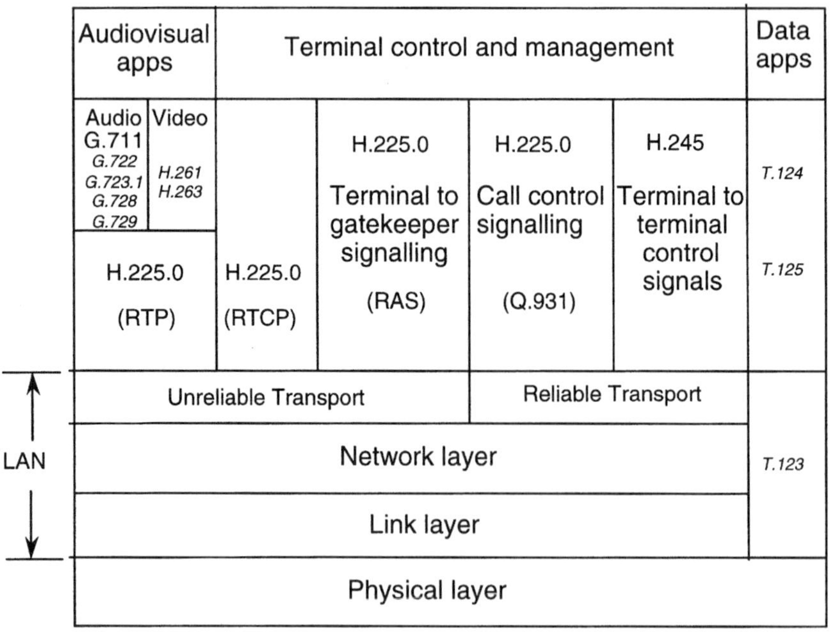

Audiovisual apps			Terminal control and management			Data apps
Audio G.711 *G.722* *G.723.1* *G.728* *G.729*	Video *H.261* *H.263*		H.225.0 Terminal to gatekeeper signalling (RAS)	H.225.0 Call control signalling (Q.931)	H.245 Terminal to terminal control signals	*T.124*
H.225.0 (RTP)	H.225.0 (RTCP)	H.225.0				*T.125*
Unreliable Transport				Reliable Transport		
Network layer						*T.123*
Link layer						
Physical layer						

Note - Components in italics are optional; others may be included.

Figure 13.16 H.323 protocol stack.

than 56 kbit/s, as typically occurs in Internet telephony, G.711 cannot be used. In such low bit rate cases, H.323 recommends G.723.1 for multimedia communications and G.729 for audio-only communications. If video is supported, H.261 is mandated for the same reason as G.711 audio coding. Any other optional audiovisual coding can be activated through the H.245 capability exchange. Each media stream is packetized into an RTP packet according to the Real-Time Transport Protocol and associated Real-Time Transport Control Protocol (RTCP) of the IETF standard (51). See Chapter 3 of this book for details of RTP and RTCP. This approach allows different error treatment for each media stream as appropriate, since a packet-based network is much more susceptible to burst errors in form of packet losses than the N-ISDN. Synchronization between media streams is accomplished by use of RTP timestamps.

The H.323 system control is divided into the following categories:

H.225.0 network access signaling between end point and gatekeeper
H.225.0 call signaling between end point and gatekeeper (or end point)
H.245 end-to-end signaling between two end points

The first category message is carried over the registration, admission, and status (RAS) channel. The second category is based on Q.931 messages that were originally developed for the N-ISDN call control. The third category is defined in the H.245 communication control protocol, which is common across the second-generation audiovisual communication systems.

The transport or lower layers are outside the scope of Recommendation H.323. The H.323 system utilizes the two types of transport provided by the packet-based network according to the error and delay requirements of each information channel:

Unreliable transport (such as UDP over IP): H.225.0 RTP/RTCP, H.225.0 RAS
Reliable transport (such as TCP over IP): H.225.0 call signaling, H.245

13.3.4.4 H.323 Communication.

H.323 includes a variety of system configurations depending on the allocation of terminal, gatekeeper, gateway, and MCU. An example of communication procedures is described here for the two terminals being managed by the same gatekeeper and the gatekeeper having chosen the direct call signaling between the two terminals. It is assumed that each terminal has discovered the gatekeeper and registered its transport and alias addresses to the gatekeeper by use of H.225.0 RAS signaling in advance of the actual audiovisual communication with the remote terminal.

The gatekeeper discovery may be manual or automatic. In the former case the terminal has a priori knowledge of the gatekeeper with which it is associated. In the latter case, the terminal first multicasts an H.225.0 Gatekeeper Request (GRQ) message "Who is my gatekeeper?" to the gatekeeper's well-known multicast address, and one or more gatekeepers may respond with an H.225.0 GatekeeperConfirmation (GCF) message "I can be your gatekeeper," including its transport address of the RAS channel. Now the terminal can register to the gatekeeper of its choice. An exchange of Registration Request (RRQ) and Registration Confirm (RCF) allows the gatekeeper to store the correspondence between the transport address and one or more aliases of the terminal for address resolutions.

13.3.4.4.1 Phase A: Call Setup (see Figure 13.17).

1. Calling end point 1 sends an Admission Request (ARQ) message, containing the alias address of end point 2 (the called end point), the bandwidth, and other parameters, to the gatekeeper through the RAS channel.
2. The gatekeeper returns Admission Confirm (ACF) with notification of the maximum bandwidth allowed, the H.225.0 call signaling channel

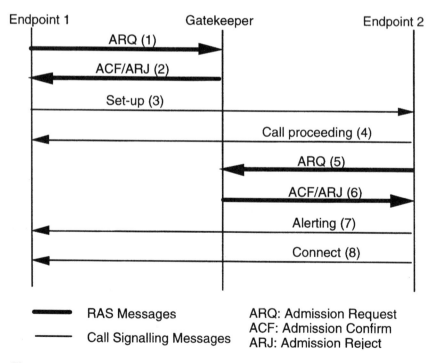

Figure 13.17   Direct call signaling with both terminals registered to the same gatekeeper.

transport address (such as IP address) of end point 2, and other parameters. Otherwise Admission Reject (ARJ) is returned.

3. Calling end point 1 sends a Setup message to destination end point 2 through the H.225.0 call signaling channel, using the transport address advised in step 2. The Setup message includes bearer capability, called party number, and other information necessary for call establishment.

4. The called end point acknowledges the receipt of Setup with a Call Proceeding message indicating that the received message is being processed.

5. If the called end point wishes to accept the call, it first requests admission (ARQ) from the gatekeeper as in step 1.

6. The gatekeeper returns acknowledgment (ACF) as in step 2.

7. After permission has been received from the gatekeeper, the called end point 2 returns an Alerting message indicating that the user is being notified of the incoming call.

8. If the called user responds, end point 2 returns a Connect message to calling end point 1 through the H.225.0 call signaling channel with the H.245 message channel transport address to be used in the next phase and other parameters.

13.3.4.4.2 Phase B: Initial Communication and Capability Exchange.
Through the H.245 message channel designated by phase A, capability exchange is carried out between the two end points to negotiate an appropriate mode of operation. The master–slave determination is also carried out at this phase.

13.3.4.4.3 Phase C: Establishment of Audiovisual Communication.
According to the H.245 logical channel signaling procedures, various media stream logical channels are established in this phase. Audio and video packets are transferred over the unreliable transport as shown in Figure 13.16. Each stream requires establishment of a pair of logical channels for RTP and its associated RTCP. Since RTCP packets are periodically sent to all the destinations of the RTP packets with the same delivery mechanism, they can be used for monitoring the network performance such as packet losses and eventually for controlling the number of packets sent from the terminal.

13.3.4.4.4 Phase D: Call Services. During a communication session, there may arise a need for change of bandwidth for some reason. An end point can change the bandwidth in use at any time through the H.245 logical channel signaling procedures if it is within the maximum value permitted by the gatekeeper. If a higher bandwidth is required, the end point must ask the gatekeeper through Bandwidth Request (BRQ) and wait for its response of Bandwidth Confirm (BCF) or Bandwidth Reject (BRJ).

H.323 defines optional procedures for the ad hoc multipoint conference that expands a point-to-point call involving MC to a multipoint conference. Various supplementary services, such as call transfer and call forwarding, are specified in separate H.450.× series recommendations.

13.3.4.4.5 Phase E: Call Termination. When a call is to be terminated, transmissions of media signals are first ceased; then relevant logical channels are closed according to the H.245 logical channel signaling procedures, and an H.245 command for ending the session (End Session Command) is sent. The connection is next closed with the H.225.0 signaling Release Complete. Finally the bandwidth is released to the gatekeeper, if involved, with the exchange of H.225.0 RAS Disengage Request (DRQ) and Disengage Confirm (DCF).

13.3.4.5 Communication Between Administrative Domains. The overall H.323 network consists of smaller subsets of H.323 entities, each of which is organized as an administrative domain. An administrative domain may contain one or more zones (i.e., one or more gatekeepers). The function of the administrative domain is supported by an entity called a border element, which serves as the public access point for the outside world of the domain to complete calls with the inside of the domain. Annex G to H.225.0 (52) defines a protocol for communication between administrative domains covering address resolution, access authorization, and usage reporting. Two border elements may exchange addressing and other database information at any time.

When an end point T1 in domain A places a call to another end point T2 in domain B, the communication progresses as shown in Figure 13.18. T1 issues an ARQ message to the associated gatekeeper GK$_A$, which then discovers the asso-

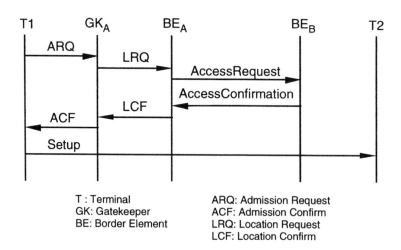

Figure 13.18 H.323 interdomain communication.

ciated border element BE_A by issuing a Location Request (LRQ) message in a similar way to the gatekeeper discovery with GRQ. BE_A talks with BE_B for resolution of the requested alias address by exchanging Access Request and Access Confirmation messages. The transport address of T2 is returned to T1, which then sets up a call to T2.

This protocol expands the H.323 capability from intrazone communications to interdomain communications, thus to global communications.

13.3.4.6   Interworking with Other H.300 Series Terminals.   An H.323 terminal may interwork with another H.300 series terminal through a gateway. The gateway terminates both sides. Thus it looks like an H.323 terminal to the packet-based network and like an H.320 terminal to N-ISDN, for example. Necessary conversions for audiovisual coding, multimedia multiplex, system control protocol, and call control protocol are carried out inside the gateway.

13.3.5   H.310/H.321 B-ISDN Systems

13.3.5.1   Overview.   In the late 1980s, the next-generation public network was envisaged as broadband ISDN (B-ISDN) based on asynchronous transfer mode (ATM). Customer premises networks were also moving to ATM, and so seamless network services were expected. ATM networks provide many opportunities for new and improved services, but also pose new problems that must be solved before these services can be offered, as summarized in Table 13.5. Standardization of the audiovisual communication systems in ATM environments started in mid-1990.

Table 13.5   ATM Network Characteristics

Opportunities
    Availability of high bandwidths
    Flexibility in bandwidth usage
    Variable bit rate capability
    Service integration
    Use of cell loss priority (CLP)
    Multipoint distribution in the network
    Flexibility in multimedia multiplexing or
        multiple connections
    Cell loss
Limitations
    Cell delay variation (jitter)
    Packetization delay
    Usage parameter control (peak and/or average rates)

The objective of standardizing audiovisual communication systems in ATM environments is to allow interoperability among different systems and interoperability with terminals connected to other networks, while fully utilizing the opportunities and alleviating the limitations of ATM. In particular, it is an essential requirement that the new-generation systems interwork with the existing ones; that is, the ATM audiovisual communication systems should be able to interwork with H.320 systems situated in the N-ISDN.

One of the greatest opportunities of B ISDN is the high bandwidth available, which may be up to several hundred megabits per second compared to only 1.5 or 2 Mbit/s for N-ISDN. Generally, higher bandwidth brings higher quality. A video coding standard, ITU-T Recommendation H.262|ISO/IEC 13818-2 (53) known as MPEG-2 Video, gives pictures of broadcast television quality at around 5–10 Mbit/s. High-quality stereo sound with subjective quality equal or close to that of compact discs is obtained at 384 kbit/s or lower bit rates by using ISO/IEC 11172-3 (54), known as MPEG-1 Audio. Its extension to multi channel and lower sampling frequencies is also available as ISO/IEC 13818-3 (55), MPEG-2 Audio. H.222.0|ISO/IEC 13818-1 (56), a packet multiplex known as MPEG-2 Systems, meets the requirements for multimedia multiplex and synchronization. When these tools are used, ATM audiovisual systems can realize high quality.

Another outstanding feature of the ATM network is its capability to achieve service integration. Cells and virtual channels can transport information media of any type once they have been digitized and packetized. Different types of service can share the same network. This is seen by the user as an opportunity to access a number of different services through a single terminal. Hence ATM audiovisual communication systems should be able to cover as many applications as required in a harmonized way. Possible applications include conversational services, distributive services, retrieval services, messaging services, video transmission, and video surveillance.

The high bandwidth of the ATM network also provides a possibility of low delay for conversational services. N-ISDN audiovisual systems use H.261 video coding, which incurs a buffering delay of at least four times the frame period (133 ms in total) plus any display delay due to picture skipping. ATM audiovisual systems should significantly improve the end-to-end delay, and therefore a target of less than about 150 ms has been set. This value corresponds to the "acceptable for most user applications" level of specification in ITU-T Recommendation G.114 (57) for one-way transmission time in speech systems.

To meet the above-mentioned requirements, ITU-T developed two recommendations for audiovisual communication systems in ATM environments, H.321 (58) and H.310 (59). They were first approved in March 1996 and November 1996, respectively, and have since been revised with enhancements. Recommendation H.321 specifies the adaptation of H.320 visual tele-phone terminals to B-ISDN environments, so satisfying the requirement that ATM terminals interwork with those connected to N-ISDN. Recommendation H.310 includes the H.320/H.321 interoperation mode but also defines a native mode, which takes advantage of the opportunities provided by ATM to pro-vide higher quality audiovisual communication. The H.310 terminal is man-dated to interwork with the H.320 terminal, and constitutes a superset of H.321.

Though the ATM technology and the standards for audiovisual communi-cation systems in ATM environments are ready now, it has to be noted that the use of ATM is mostly in the backbone part of the network at the moment. It re-mains to be seen when the ATM will come to the user–network interface and the H.310 native ATM system will be widely deployed.

13.3.5.2 Protocol stack. Figure 13.19 shows the H.310 protocol configura-tion, which includes the H.310 native mode and the H.320/H.321 interoperation mode. The latter part is the same as the protocol configuration of H.321. The whole protocol stack consists of the following:

Out-of-band network access signaling stack for DSS2 [digital subscriber signaling no. 2; Q.2931 (60) and others] signals

In-band communication control stack for H.245 or H.242 messages

H.320/H.321 interoperation mode stack using H.221 multimedia multiplex for audiovisual signals

H.310 native mode stack using H.222.1/H.222.0 multimedia multiplex for audiovisual signals

Optional data stack such as T.120

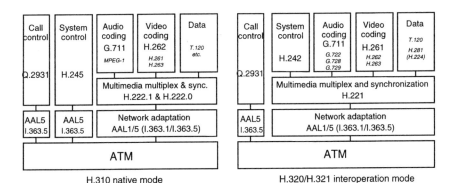

Note - Components in italics are optional; others may be included.

Figure 13.19 H.310 protocol stack.

The first two stacks are used for the call management, while the other three are used for the audiovisual content of the call. Elementary streams such as audio, video, data, video frame synchronous control, and indications signals, each of which may be standardized or private, are multiplexed into a serial packet stream according to H.222.0. H.222.1/H.222.0 functions include multiplexing, timebase recovery, media synchronization, jitter removal, buffer management, security and access control, subchannel signaling, and trick modes, which are mechanisms to support video-recorder-like control functionalities, (e.g., fast forward, rewind). Recommendation H.222.1 (61) specifies elements and procedures from the generic H.222.0, for their use in ATM environments, and also specifies code points and procedures for ITU-T-defined elementary streams. H.222.1 allows use of both the H.222.0 program stream and the H.222.0 transport stream. Only single-program transport streams are allowed. A particular call may consist of multiple program streams or transport streams, each carried in separate ATM virtual channels, and all referring to a common system time clock.

Subchannel signaling is the process by which a subchannel for audio, video, or other elementary stream is established and released between peer send and receive H.222.1 entities. Although H.222.1 specifies an unacknowledged signaling procedure by means of the program stream map for H.222.0 program streams and program-specific information for H.222.0 transport streams, as well as an acknowledged signaling procedure, H.310 specifies that the acknowledged signaling procedure to be used because it offers improved call phase synchronization and reliability. This signaling is defined in Recommendation H.245, where it is known as logical channel signaling, and is transported through the reliable H.245 message channel. AAL1 provides convergence sublayer (CS) functions such as clock recovery, jitter removal, bit error correction, cell loss recovery, and data structure preservation, while AAL5 CS functions include bit error detection, cell loss detection, and data structure preservation.

The H.320/H.321 interoperation mode stack is the same as that of H.320 except for the network interface and the call control. In ATM environments, the AAL1 layer or the AAL5 layer plus the network adaptation layer on top of ATM provides a constant bit rate service to the higher layer, which is equivalent to that of a N-ISDN B, H0 or H11/H12-channel. The call control is according to DSS2 instead of DSS1 for N-ISDN terminals. Communication between an H.321 terminal on B-ISDN and an H.320 terminal on N-ISDN is supported by the interworking function at the boundary of the two networks according to Recommendation I.580 (62).

13.3.5.3 Network Adaptation.

From the H.310 terminal design perspective, the audiovisual and other data elementary stream coding as well as their multiplexing had already been specified, as had the ATM layer specifications. Consequently, a prime area of the standardization work involved specification of the intermediate network adaptation. The network adaptation specifications are covered by Recommendations I.363.1 (63), I.363.5 (64) and H.222.1. The network adaptation for H.310 required consideration of the choice of AAL, the need for error resilience, and the means for jitter removal.

ITU-T considered the use of AAL1 and AAL5. AAL1 offered the benefit of being defined for transport of constant bit rate (CBR) traffic with provision of a constant bit or byte stream at the AAL service access point, and would be present in the terminal in any case for the H.320/H.321 interoperation mode. AAL5 offered an apparently ready availability of AAL5 chips in the marketplace and wide deployment in computing equipment (65), and was present for user–network signaling, as shown in Figure 13.19. Considering that the requirements of network adaptation are application dependent, and that the network performance may differ in different environments, ITU-T decided to define two terminal profiles based on AAL1 and AAL5 and their interworking arrangement through a conversion gateway.

The network performance with respect to bit errors and cell losses was one of the factors considered during the specification of the network adaptation. A practical criterion for evaluating the error effects was that perceived corruption should be less than once per session of about one hour. Experimental results showed that performance was enhanced if errors could be detected, and corrupted data not passed to the elementary stream decoders. The CRC32 error detection capability of AAL5 provides for this, and forward error correction (FEC) without interleaving was added to AAL1 to provide it with the same level of error resilience capability.

For the AAL1 profile, taking into account harmonization with J.82 for television signal transmission (66), which adopts the Reed–Solomon (128,124) long interleaver to enable cell loss correction, H.310 specifies the use of one of the following options: no FEC, RS(128,124) without interleaving, and RS(128,124) with interleaving. The actual choice of an option is carried out as part of the H.245 capability exchange. It is expected that as field experience increases, the most appropriate option will be established and its implementation will prevail.

For the AAL5 profile, there is no cell loss or bit error correction capability, since error detection and concealment were considered to be sufficient. The damaged part of the picture may be replaced by, for example, the corresponding part of the previous frame.

Another important function of the ATM network adaptation is to reduce the effect of cell delay variation, or jitter, caused by ATM cell multiplexing. The most significant effect of cell delay variation is on the reproduction of clocks in the decoder. Clock transmission and reproduction are defined in Recommendation H.222.0|ISO/IEC 13818-1, by means of timestamps called clock references. Jittered clock references may cause residual jitter in the reproduced clocks, which then affects the reproduced audiovisual and other data (e.g., as variation of reproduced

Table 13.6 Definition of H.310 Terminal Types

Audiovisual transport		AAL		
		AAL1	AAL5	AAL1 and 5
Unidirectional	ROT	ROT-1	ROT-5	ROT-1 and 5
Unidirectional	SOT	SOT-1	SOT-5	SOT-1 and 5
Bidirectional	RAST	RAST-1	RAST-5	RAST-1 and 5

color due to jittered color subcarrier), or it may require a long time for lock-in of the reproduced clock. The jitter can, however, be reduced to an acceptable level at various parts of the decoder system (network adaptation, source decoder, etc.). Hence Recommendation H.222.1 describes its functionality, but the means to achieve it is left to the implementers. Different methods of jitter reduction at the decoder do not affect interoperability between the encoder and the decoder.

13.3.5.4 Terminal profile. The definition of H.310 terminal types had to be flexible enough to provide for a wide range of audiovisual applications, over networks whose characteristics were not fully known, while minimizing the cost of interoperability among different types. H.310 defines the nine terminal types as shown in Table 13.6, taking consideration into the following aspects:

> *Audiovisual transport*: receive-only terminal (ROT), send-only terminal (SOT), receive-and-send terminal (RAST)
> *AAL*: AAL1, AAL5, both AAL1 and AAL5

13.3.5.6 H.310 Communication. While N-ISDN allows only a small number of transfer rates (i.e., 64, 384, 1536, and 1920 kbit/s), B-ISDN allows a wide range of transfer rates in almost an infinite number of steps. This provides an obvious benefit of flexibility, but also causes a potential interoperability problem: it may happen that one terminal supports a group of transfer rates and another supports a different group of transfer rates with no value in common. Recommendation H.310 solves this problem by first defining the transfer rate to be a multiple of 64 kbit/s, then mandating the two rates: $96 \times 64 = 6144$ kbit/s and $144 \times 64 = 9216$ kbit/s. Other optional transfer rates can be negotiated through the H.245 capability exchange procedures. The two mandatory rates correspond to the MPEG-2 main profile at main level (MP@ML) medium-quality services and high-quality services, respectively.

Audiovisual communication requires the following phases to be completed before audiovisual communication can take place (see Figure 13.20):

> Initial virtual channel (VC) setup for the H.245 signaling
> Capability exchange, through the initial VC, to identify the available common modes of operation

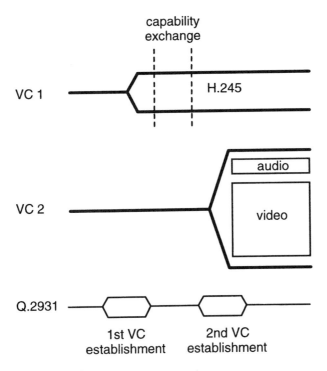

Figure 13.20   H.310 start-up procedures.

>   Additional VC setup
>   Logical channel establishment for audiovisual and data communication
>   through the additional VC

This set of procedures ensures the establishment of a VC with the necessary minimum bandwidth for the audiovisual and data communication because the capability negotiation through the initial VC gives the information for this purpose. The initial VC is symmetrical, with 64 kbit/s bandwidth and AAL5, while the additional VC may be symmetrical or asymmetrical depending on the application.

All H.310 terminals, when operating in the native ATM mode, use the H.245 control protocol. Not all audiovisual devices using ATM transport support H.245; for example, the device defined by DAVIC uses the DSM-CC protocol for system control flows, as described in Section 13.4 Since H.310 and the DAVIC specifications have many elements in common, it is possible that a composite terminal will be able to support both protocols, particularly in a personal computer or workstation implementation. At the start of the call, compatibility checking by means of user–network signaling (Q.2931) should take place to establish the call only if the two terminals are interoperable. H.310 allows the calling terminal to indicate a set of terminal protocol identifications, and the called terminal to select one of them, through the Q.2931 signaling.

13.3.5.7 Broadband multipoint communication. Multipoint communication procedures for the H.310 terminal are defined in Recommendation H.247 (67). In addition to the n-point tightly coupled connection (e.g., multipoint videoconference), which is very similar to the multipoint conference described in Section13.3.2, H.247 also defines point-to-multipoint connection without return channels (e.g., broadcast conference) utilizing the ATM multicast capability and a combination of the two (e.g., broadcast panel conference).

13.4 INFORMATION DISTRIBUTION AND RETRIEVAL SYSTEMS

This section describes another major category of networked video systems; digital audiovisual systems standardized by DAVIC (20) for distributing and retrieving high-quality multimedia information. DAVIC specifications define the minimum tools and the dynamic behavior at defined reference points for end-to-end interoperability across countries, applications, and services. To achieve this interoperability, DAVIC specifications describe the requirements and the framework of the overall system, provide architectural guides, and define the technologies and information flows to be used within and between the major components of generic digital audiovisual systems.

The DAVIC specifications include the descriptions of a specific set of requirements, functions, and technologies (called "contour") for some marketable application systems: enhanced digital broadcast (EDB), interactive digital broadcast (IDB), and institutional multimedia retrieval (IMR).

13.4.1 DAVIC System Reference Model

The system reference model with reference point definition is used as a guide for the design of open systems to achieve interoperability in multivendor environments. Figure 13.21 shows a DAVIC system reference model consisting of the following subsystems:

> *Service Consumer System (SCS)*: provides the user interface, accepts incoming information for presentation to the user or for control of the system, and passes addressed information to the delivery system.
> *Delivery System (DS)*: accepts and delivers information from/to the SPS or SCS, with an agreed quality level, to an appropriate destination.
> *Service Provider System (SPS)*: consists of a collection of system blocks

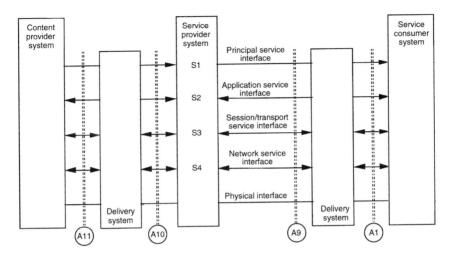

Figure 13.21 DAVIC system reference model.

that accept, process, and present addressed information for delivery to a service consumer system.

Content Provider System (CPS): uses the services of the CPS-SPS delivery system to load content into the service provider system.

Intersubsystem interfaces are defined at the reference points A1, A9, A10, and A11. Further reference points A2–A8 are defined inside the delivery system as shown in Figure 13.22. The service consumer system has internal reference points A0 (between the network interface unit and other internal set-top box elements) and A20 (set-top unit dataport interface or home local-area network interface) to indicate the interfaces for the set-top box decomposition*. It has another type of reference point, CA1 (between STU and security device) and CA0 (between security device and Smartcard) for conditional access interfaces.

Figures 13.21 and 13.22 are structured to indicate the service layers according to the properties that are important for peer-to-peer interactions. They are, from top to bottom, principal service layer, application service layer, session and transport service layer, and network service layer. Some service layer information is terminated at a particular subsystem, but some other service layer information is transparent at the subsystem.

---

*A set-top box (STB) is a module that comprises both STU and network–interface unit (NIU) functional elements; a set-top unit (STU) is a module that contains the network-independent functionalities of an STB.

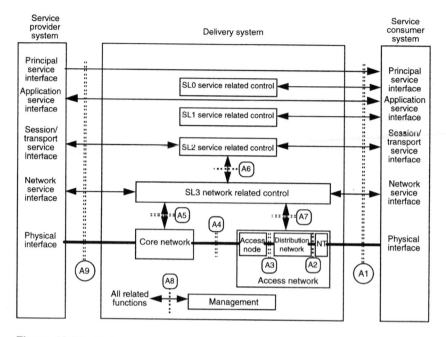

Figure 13.22   Delivery system architecture.

13.4.2   Information Flow at Reference Points

The DAVIC system is specified in terms of the following types of information
flow through the reference points:

S1 *flow*: Flow of content (e.g., audio, video, or data) information on the
user plane of the principal service layer (SL0).

S2 *flow*: Flow of control information on the user plane of the application
service layer (SL1). Presentation includes end-to-end controls (e.g.,
play, stop, fast forward of a movie).

S3 *flow*: Flow of control information on the control plane of the session
(e.g., messages to establish, modify, or terminate a session; negotiate resource requirements; or report exceptions) and transport service layer
(SL2).

S4 *flow*: Flow of control information on the control plane of the network
service layer (SL3). Messages to establish or release connections, and to
communicate addresses, port information, and other routing data are examples of connection information.

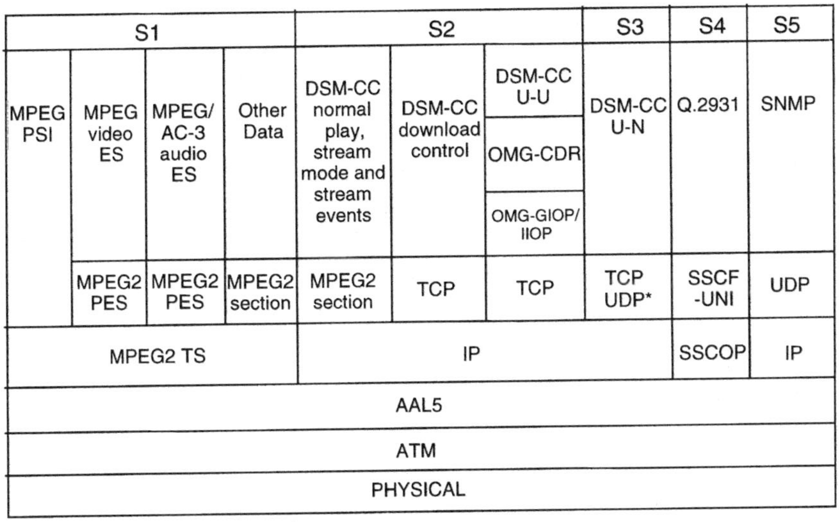

S1				S2			S3	S4	S5
MPEG PSI	MPEG video ES	MPEG/AC-3 audio ES	Other Data	DSM-CC normal play, stream mode and stream events	DSM-CC download control	DSM-CC U-U / OMG-CDR / OMG-GIOP/ IIOP	DSM-CC U-N	Q.2931	SNMP
MPEG2 PES	MPEG2 PES	MPEG2 section	MPEG2 section	TCP	TCP		TCP UDP*	SSCF -UNI	UDP
MPEG2 TS				IP				SSCOP	IP
AAL5									
ATM									
PHYSICAL									

* TCP at the server side, UDP at the STU side.

DSM-CC	Digital Storage Media - Command and Control	PSI	Program Specific Information
DSM-CC U-N	DSM-CC User-to-Network	SNMP	Simple Network Management Protocol
DSM-CC U-U	DSM-CC User-to-User	SSCF-UNI	Service Specific Coordination Function for Support of
ES	Elementary Stream		Signaling at the User Network Interface (Q.2130)
IP	Internet Protocol	SSCOP	Service Specific Connection Oriented Protocol (Q.2110)
OMG-CDR	Object Management Group - Common Data	TCP	Transmission Control Protocol
	Representation	TS	Transport Stream
OMG-GIOP	OMG - Generic Inter-ORB Protocol	UDP	User Datagram Protocol
PES	Packetized Elementary Stream		

Figure 13.23   DAVIC protocol stacks.

S5 flow: Flow of management information (e.g., pinging) on the management plane of any service layer.

13.4.3   DAVIC Protocol Stacks

Figure 13.23 gives an overview of a DAVIC system protocol suite. It indicates the specified stacks for each of the S1–S5 flows in the system reference model. The lower layer is ATM in Figure 13.22, where the MPEG transport stream contains one and only one program (single-program TS) but can also be non-ATM if the access network is of the hybrid fiber coaxial (HFC) type, where multiprogram TS is used instead of AAL5/ATM. Video coding is in accordance with MPEG-2 Video (H.262|ISO/IEC 13818-2) up to and including the HDTV resolution (1080 lines $\times$ 1920 pels), while audio coding is in accordance with MPEG-1 Audio (ISO/IEC 11172-3) for single channel, dual channel, joint stereo, or stereo; advanced television systems committee (ATSC) A/52 (68) Audio for multichannel surround sound; or MPEG-2 Audio (ISO/IEC 13818-3) for scalable audio. For system control flows S2 and S3, DSM-CC (ISO/IEC 13818-6) is specified.

13.4.4 Communication Procedures

DAVIC specifications include system dynamic behavior and physical scenarios. They detail the locations of the control functional entities along with the normative protocols needed to support the systems behavior in the form of protocol walk-throughs that use the specified protocols to rehearse both the steady state and dynamic operation of the system at relevant reference points.

As an example, we describe a session and call/connection setup scenario for a video-on-demand system in the environment of the simple ATM access network switched virtual circuit (SVC). Figure 13.24 shows the key dynamic functional entities for a DAVIC VoD system for each service layer: audiovisual, end-to-end control, session control, and call/connection control. The basic session and call/connection setup goes through the following procedures:

1. The STU sends a session setup request indication to the network session entity (ses_u to ses_n, S3 flow).
2. The network sends a session setup request indication to the server (ses_n to ses_p, S3 flow).
3. The server session entity instructs the server call/connection entity to

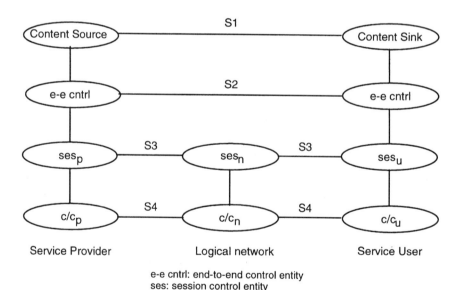

Figure 13.24 Functional entities and relationships of a DAVIC video-on-demand system.

setup S1 and S2 connections from the server to the STU (ses_p to c/c_p, primitive).

4. Network connection control signaling is used to establish S2 and optionally S1 (c/c_p to c/c_n to c/c_u, S4 flow).
5. The server call/connection entity informs the server session entity of completion of connection establishment (c/c_p to ses_p, primitive).
6. The server confirms session setup to the network (ses_p to ses_n, S3 flow).
7. The network informs STU of the added connection and confirms session setup (ses_n to ses_u, S3 flow).
8. User-plane communication begins between STU and server via S1 and S2 (S1 flow and S2 flow).

13.5 FUTURE DIRECTIONS

ISDN (N-ISDN and B-ISDN) has been a concept to provide integrated services through a unified user–network interface. Now, however, we see the use of networks of various different types. This is the background for the development of a series of second-generation H.300 series system standards. It now becomes important to realize interworking among different types of audiovisual communication system because for the end user only the terminal is visible, not the network, and all the H.300-series-compatible terminals look very similar.

There are several approaches to achieve interworking between different standard systems:

Switchable terminal: A terminal has multiple protocol stacks and network interfaces.

H.246 gateway between two different networks: A gateway carries out protocol conversion (69).

Use of minimum common capability: Audio-only communication, for example.

Use of layered coding: The base layer supports backward compatibility (interworking with the existing systems).

Interworking is one of the areas requiring further standardization work and efforts by industrial groups.

The new century will see the third-generation audiovisual communication system. It will use emerging advanced audiovisual coding and adapt to the network evolution. An interesting question is whether the current diversified communication networks will continue as a mixture of circuit-based and packet-based services, or the network services will converge to a single user–network interface like that of the IP packet-switched network. In any event, the performance of the new-generation system should be much better than that of the current systems in audiovisual quality, delay, and error resilience. The third-generation systems should also interwork with the second- and first-generation systems in one of the above-mentioned way, or in a new way yet to be figured out.

In the information distribution and retrieval area, the change of broadcasting systems from analog to digital will begin in many more countries. Digital television programs are much easier to deliver, exchange, store, and reuse than analog ones. DAVIC has defined the following systems:

> *TV anytime* By use of in-home storage, users can access various TV programs and other audiovisual contents at any time. Materials may be loaded onto a home storage device from broadcast content in real time, and also in non-real-time, when the broadcast content is intended solely for recording. Materials may also be loaded onto the home storage device from a remote storage system, in the manner of a "virtual video shop," by means of a video file transfer.

> *TV anywhere* The capability of IP-based systems to carry audiovisual materials in digital form creates the opportunity to deliver audiovisual materials to any location that has a connection of sufficient capacity and quality. This enables users to access services and content from remote locations. Services considered here encompass television and audio-only services, from high-quality music to low bit rate speech.

Based on these system types, further development of the application systems to utilize digital television programs and digital video materials will take place.

Standards for networked video systems in the new century will be largely affected by the computer and its network technologies. The direction of future networked video system standards will be determined by the manner of the eventual convergence or divergence of the technologies of communication, broadcasting, and computers.

REFERENCES

1. JA Baird. The Picturephone system. Foreword. Bell Syst Tech 50(2): 219–220, February 1971.
2. JE Thompson. Objectives and results of Project COST 211. IEEE GLOBECOM'82, D4.1, 1982, pp 802–804.
3. ITU-T. Framework recommendation for audiovisual/multimedia services. Recommendation F.700, 1996.
4. ITU. http://www.itu.ch/
5. DAVIC. http://www.davic.org/
6. IETF. http://www.ietf.org/
7. IMTC. http://www.imtc.org/

8. The ATM Forum. http://www.atmforum.com/

9. I Dorros. Picturephone. Bell Lab Record 47(5):136–141, May/June 1969.

10. JE Haworth. Confravision. Post Off Elect Eng 64(4): 220–225, 1972.

11. ITU-T. Visual telephone systems. Recommendation H.100, 1988.

12. ITU-T. Hypothetical reference connections for videoconferencing using primary digital group transmission. Recommendation H.110, 1988.

13. ITU-T. Codecs for videoconferencing using primary digital group transmission. Recommendation H.120, 1993.

14. ITU-T. Frame structures for use in the international interconnection of digital codecs for videoconferencing or visual telephony. Recommendation H.130, 1988.

15. S Okubo. Reference model methodology—A tool for the collaborative creation of video coding standards. Proc IEEE 83(2):139–150, February 1995.

16. M Yamashita, ND Kenyon, S Okubo. Standardization of audiovisual systems in CCITT. IMAGE'COM 90, Bordeaux, November 1990, pp 42–47.

17. D Lindbergh. The H.324 multimedia communication standard. IEEE Commun 34(12):46–51, December 1996.

18. GA Thom. H.323: The multimedia communications standard for local area networks. IEEE Commun 34(12): 52–56, December 1996.

19. S Okubo, S Dunstan, G Morrison, M Nilsson, H Radha, DL Skran, G Thom. ITU-T standardization of audiovisual communication systems in ATM and LAN environments. IEEE J Selected Areas Commun 15(6): 965–982, August 1997.

20. DAVIC. DAVIC 1.4 Specifications. June 1998.

21. H Yasuda, H Ryan. DAVIC and interactive multimedia services. IEEE Commun 36(9): 137–143, September 1998.

22. ITU-T. Data protocols for multimedia conferencing. Recommendation T.120, 1996.

23. ITU-T. Narrow-band visual telephone systems and terminal equipment. Recommendation H.320, 1999.

24. ITU-T. Pulse code modulation (PCM) of voice frequencies. Recommendation G.711, 1988.

25. ITU-T. Video codec for audiovisual services at $p \times 64$ kbit/s. Recommendation H.261, 1993.

26. ITU-T. Digital subscriber signalling system no. 1 (DSS 1)—ISDN user–network interface layer 3 specification basic call control. Recommendation Q.931, 1998.

27. ITU-T. Frame structure for a 64 to 1920 kbit/s channel in audiovisual teleservices. Recommendation H.221, 1999.

28. ITU-T. System for establishing communication between audiovisual terminals using digital channels up to 2 Mbit/s. Recommendation H.242, 1999.

29. ITU-T. Multipoint control units for audiovisual systems using digital channels up to 1920 kbit/s. Recommendation H.231, 1997.

30. ITU-T. Procedures for establishing communication between three or more audiovisual terminals using digital channels up to 1920 kbit/s. Recommendation H.243, 1997.

31. ITU-T. Terminal for low bit rate multimedia communication. Recommendation H.324, 1998.

32. ITU-T. Dual rate speech coder for multimedia communications transmitting at 5.3 and 6.3 kbit/s. Recommendation G.723.1, 1996.

33. ITU-T. Video coding for low bit rate communication. Recommendation H.263, 1998.
34. ITU-T. Channel aggregation protocol for multilink operation on circuit-switched networks. Recommendation H.226, 1998.
35. ITU-T. Multiplexing protocol for low bit rate multimedia communication. Recommendation H.223, 1996.
36. ITU-T. Multiplexing protocol for low bit rate multimedia mobile communication over low error-prone channels. Recommendation H.223, Annex A, 1998.
37. ITU-T. Multiplexing protocol for low bit rate multimedia mobile communication over moderate error-prone channels. Recommendation H.223, Annex B, 1998.
38. ITU-T. Multiplexing protocol for low bit rate multimedia communication over highly error-phone channels. Recommendation H.223, Annex C, 1998.
39. ITU-T. Optional multiplexing protocol for low bit rate multimedia communication over highly error prone channels. Recommendation H.223, Annex D, 1999.
40. ITU-T. Control protocol for multimedia communication. Recommendation H.245, 1999.
41. ITU-T. Information technology—Abstract Syntax Notation One (ASN.1)—Specification of basic notation. Recommendation X.680, 1994.
42. ITU-T. Procedures for starting sessions of data transmission over the public switched telephone network. Recommendation V.8, 1998.
43. ITU-T. Procedures for the identification and selection of common modes of operation between data circuit terminating equipment (DCEs) and between data terminal equipment (DTEs) over the general switched telephone network and on leased point-to-point telephone-type circuits. Recommendation V.8bis, 1996.
44. ITU-T. A modem operating at data signalling rates of up to 33,600 bit/s for use on the general switched telephone network and on leased point-to-point 2-wire telephone-type circuits. Recommendation V.34, 1998.
45. IEEE. IEEE Standard for Local and Metropolitan Area Networks—Supplement to Integrated Services (IS) LAN Interface at the Medium Access Control (MAC) and Physical (PHY) Layers: Specification of ISLAN16-T. Standard 802.9a-1995, 1995.
46. ITU-T. Visual telephone systems and terminal equipment for local area networks which provide a guaranteed quality of service. Recommendation H.322, 1996.
47. ISO/IEC. Information technology—Local and metropolitan area networks, Part 3. Carrier sense multiple access with collision detection (CSMA/CD) access method and physical layer specifications. ISO/IEC 8802-3 [ANSI/IEEE Standard 802.3, 1993 ed], 1993.
48. ITU-T. Packet-based multimedia communications systems. Recommendation H.323, 1999.
49. ITU-T. Call signalling protocols and media stream packetization for packet-based multimedia communication systems. Recommendation H.225.0, 1999.
50. ITU-T. The international public telecommunication numbering plan. Recommendation E.164, 1997.
51. H Schulzrinne, S Casner, R Frederick, V Jacobson. RTP: A transport protocol for real-time applications. IETF Request for Comments 1889, January 1996.
52. ITU-T. Communication between administrative domains. Annex G to Recommendation H.225.0, Annex G,1999.

53. ITU-T, ISO/IEC. Information technology—Generic coding of moving pictures and associated audio information: Video. Recommendation H.262|ISO/IEC 13818-2, 1995.

54. ISO/IEC. Information technology—Coding of moving pictures and associated audio for digital storage media at up to about 1.5 Mbit/s. Part 3. Audio. ISO/IEC 11172-3, 1993.

55. ISO/IEC. Information technology—Generic coding of moving pictures and associated audio. Part 3. Audio. ISO/IEC 13818-3, 1995.

56. ITU-T, ISO/IEC. Information technology—Generic coding of moving pictures and associated audio information. Systems. Recommendation H.222.0|ISO/IEC 13818-1, 1995.

57. ITU-T. One-way transmission time. Recommendation G.114, 1996.

58. ITU-T. Adaptation of H.320 visual telephone terminals to B-ISDN environments. Recommendation H.321, 1998.

59. ITU-T. Broadband audiovisual communication systems and terminals. Recommendation H.310, 1998.

60. ITU-T. Digital Subscriber Signalling System No. 2–User-network interface (UNI) layer 3 specification for basic call/connection control. Recommendation Q.2931, 1995.

61. ITU-T. Multimedia multiplex and synchronization for audiovisual communication in ATM environments. Recommendation H.222.1, 1996.

62. ITU-T. General arrangements for interworking between B-ISDN and 64 kbit/s based ISDN. Recommendation I.580, 1995.

63. ITU-T. B-ISDN ATM adaptation: Type 1 AAL. Recommendation I.363.1, 1996.

64. ITU-T. B-ISDN ATM Adaptation: Type 5 AAL. Recommendation I.363.5, 1996.

65. The ATM Forum. Audiovisual multimedia services: Video on demand specification 1.1. AF-SAA-0049.001, 1997.

66. ITU-T. Transport of MPEG-2 constant bit rate television signals in B-ISDN. Recommendation J.82, 1996.

67. ITU-T. Multipoint extension for broadband audiovisual communication systems and terminals. Recommendation H.247, 1998.

68. ATSC. Digital Audio Compression (AC-3) Standard. ATSC A/52, 1995. (see http://www.atsc.org/   for ATSC).

69. ITU-T. Interworking of H-series multimedia terminals with H-series multimedia terminals and voice/voiceband terminals on GSTN and ISDN. Recommendation H.246, 1998.

Index